# NURSE'S MANUAL OF
# Laboratory Tests and Diagnostic Procedures

# LOUISE M. MALARKEY, EdD, RN

*Professor, Department of Nursing, College of Staten Island, City University of New York, Staten Island, New York*

# MARY ELLEN McMORROW, EdD, RN, CCRN

*Professor, Department of Nursing, College of Staten Island, City University of New York, Staten Island, New York*

# Nurse's Manual of
# Laboratory Tests
# and Diagnostic Procedures

SECOND EDITION

**W.B. SAUNDERS COMPANY**
*A Division of Harcourt Brace & Company*

Philadelphia   London   Toronto   Sydney   Montreal   Tokyo

**W.B. SAUNDERS COMPANY**
*A Division of Harcourt Brace & Company*

The Curtis Center
Independence Square West
Philadelphia, Pennsylvania 19106

**Library of Congress Cataloging-in-Publication Data**

Malarkey, Louise M.
Nurse's manual of laboratory tests and diagnostic procedures /
Louise M. Malarkey, Mary Ellen McMorrow.—2nd ed.

p.    cm.

Includes bibliographical references and index.

ISBN 0–7216–7812–2

1. Diagnosis, Laboratory—Handbooks, manuals, etc.  2. Diagnosis—
   Handbooks, manuals, etc.  3. Nursing—Handbooks, manuals, etc.
   I. McMorrow, Mary Ellen.  II. Title.
   [DNLM:  1. Laboratory Techniques and Procedures—nurses'
   instruction.    QY 4 M237n 2000]

RB38.2.M34 2000     616.07′54—dc21

DNLM/DLC                                          99–11885

NURSE'S MANUAL OF LABORATORY TESTS AND DIAGNOSTIC PROCEDURES          0–7216–7812–2

Printed in the United States of America

Last digit is the print number:     9    8    7    6    5    4    3    2    1

*This book is dedicated to our families,*
*with love*


*To my grandchildren, Christopher, Travis, Madison,*
*Mary Claire, and Sarah*

L.M.M.


*To my sisters, Lydia, Peggy, and Ruth*
*and my daughter, Mary*

M.E.M.

# REVIEWERS

Patricia Cryer, RN, MS, MSN, CFNP
Tyler Junior College
Tyler, Texas

Marlene Dey, MSN, CNS-C, NP-C, RN
Essex County College
Newark, New Jersey
Somerset Medical Center
Somerville, New Jersey

Ann Putnam Johnson, EdD, MSN, RN, CS
Western Carolina University
Cullowhee, North Carolina

Cynthia Glawe Mailloux, RN, MSN
Penn State University, Worthington Scranton
Scranton, Pennsylvania

Bruce Austin Scott, MSN, RN, CS
San Joaquin Delta College
Saint Joseph's Medical Center
Stockton, California

Anita Thorne, RN, BSNEd, MA
Arizona State University
Tempe, Arizona

Phyllis Waits, RN, MSN, EdD
Alabama Southern Community College
Monroeville, Alabama

Written for nurses and nursing students, the second edition of this book presents current and comprehensive knowledge of tests and diagnostic procedures. The nursing content provides the focus on patient care for a safe and accurate outcome.

The first part of the book addresses the nursing role and responsibilities in laboratory and diagnostic testing, including the procedures used for all specimen collections. Parts II and III provide in-depth content for those laboratory tests and diagnostic procedures that can be used for the assessment of many systems and areas of the body. Part IV is organized by body systems and consists of the specific tests and procedures that assess the functions of those systems.

The organizational framework of the body systems chapters presents the information in such a way that it can be incorporated readily into nursing care in the clinical setting. Generally, the patient must undergo multiple tests that assess a particular area and function of the body. This book also serves the nurse or nursing student who uses a laboratory book as a reference source. Each test is written with total information, and any specific test can be located easily by using the index.

This book is compatible with the major textbooks that are used in the education of the nursing student. The content supplements and complements the knowledge provided by nursing faculty in the classroom and clinical settings. This book can be used throughout the nursing curriculum and in all patient care settings because of its comprehensive focus.

The scope of the book includes nursing considerations across the life span and normal test values for all age groups. The array of tests includes those that assess health as well as illness. Information includes testing in ambulatory and hospital settings. The approach includes the nursing process for generalized aspects of care. In the specific clinical tests, the nursing approach concerns the implementation of physical care, psychosocial support, and patient education.

Each test or procedure is presented with a consistent organizational format. The **Background Information** incorporates knowledge of anatomy, physiology, and pathophysiology to explain the test and to help make the results more meaningful. The **Purpose of the Test** and **Procedure** sections provide brief explanations of why and how the test is done. The **Implications of the Findings** section lists the actual and possible diagnoses that may cause an abnormal test result. The **Interfering Factors** are the elements that will invalidate the test or its findings. The **Nursing Implementation** section focuses on nursing care of the patient before, during, and after the test.

Many special features are included in this book, as follows:

**Critical Thinking Questions.** A popular feature from the first edition is the critical thinking situations that appear in the book margins. Each question pertains to a specific laboratory test or procedure. It is designed to stimulate the reader to solve a problem, search for alternatives, or consider the issues associated with the test. These questions may present a problem, a challenging situation, or an ethical dilemma. There is no single answer to this type of question, but some aspects of the thinking are presented in discussions at the end of the book. These discussions are new to the second edition.

**Complications.** Complications can occur, particularly when an invasive diagnostic procedure is performed. When a risk of complications exists, this material is presented at the end of the test discussion. A table of complications and nursing assessments is included. The nurse can use each table to identify abnormal assessment findings and notify the physician at an early stage of the problem.

**Quality Control.** This feature identifies the nursing actions that are needed to insure a valid procedure and an accurate test result.

**Critical Values.** This new feature identifies an extremely abnormal laboratory test result, sometimes called a "panic value." The abnormal value may be a very decreased or a very elevated result. In either case, the critical value indicates that the patient's problem is extreme and that his or her life is at risk. When the nurse receives a laboratory report with such a value, he or she must notify the physician immediately. The nurse should also obtain an up-to-date assessment of the patient's health status and prepare for nursing intervention, as appropriate to the situation. In the future, critical values will continue to be defined and revised as research increases the knowledge base.

**Home Testing.** A trend in our society is to provide specific types of laboratory tests to be purchased over the counter and used at home by individuals. More than a dozen different tests are available, with more in development. The concept of home testing is somewhat controversial, as discussed in Chapter 1. Specific home test procedures are presented in the clinical chapters of the book.

The authors found the home test kits to be expensive and some of the instructions to be complicated, lengthy, and difficult to understand. In addition, published research indicates that patients find it difficult to use the kits accurately. For the nurse and nursing student, this book includes information about specific home tests. The nurse can assist the person who chooses to do home testing so that the procedure is performed accurately. When abnormal results occur, the nurse can encourage the person to go for retesting and examination by a qualified health care professional.

**Genetic Testing.** The field of genetics and the development of genetic tests have increased considerably and continue to evolve at a rapid pace. This edition of the book includes a new chapter on genetic testing. Specific genetic tests are presented in Chapter 13, with additional information included in the pertinent clinical chapters of the book.

**Illustrations.** This edition of the book has many additional figures and illustrations to support the written discussion. Images of computed tomographic scans, x-rays, nuclear scans, ultrasound images, and graph recordings provide visualization of normal or abnormal results. The original line drawings help clarify concepts, illustrate techniques, and visualize abnormal findings.

The amount of information on laboratory and diagnostic testing has increased rapidly in the past few years. Sophisticated equipment, changes in technology, and advances in research all have combined to increase the information and the number of tests and procedures. In addition, the measurement of test results and the quality of imaging are more detailed and specific, thereby improving the diagnostic results.

As authors, we have worked to consolidate and organize the information into a usable textbook and resource book. The wide range of tests is designed to meet the needs of the learner, from the beginning nursing student to the advanced practice nursing professional. We also hope that the book is interesting, appealing, and helpful to our readers.

LOUISE M. MALARKEY
MARY ELLEN McMORROW

# ACKNOWLEDGMENTS

No book is ever written without the help and support of many people. The authors wish to acknowledge and thank all of those who shared in our endeavor.

The nursing students who question, challenge, and seek knowledge are a constant source of stimulation and renewal for us as teachers and writers. The nursing faculty and professionals have our admiration because of their dedication to the learning of new knowledge, to communicating with and teaching others, and, above all, to maintaining commitment to high standards of nursing excellence.

Special recognition and appreciation are extended to Thomas B. Eoyang, Vice President and Editor in Chief, Nursing Books, at W.B. Saunders Company. His creativity, vision, and wisdom have been a major influence on our work. He provided the support and confidence that remained an ongoing strength for us throughout the project. Special thanks are also extended to Terri Wood, Senior Nursing Editor, and Kevin Law, former Senior Developmental Editor at W.B. Saunders Company. Their abilities and efforts changed a plain manuscript into an effective and informative book.

The writing of a textbook requires extensive library work and supporting documentation. We received the help of librarians in universities and medical centers all across the country, as they sent us the requested journal articles from so many different sources. Special thanks go to the librarians and library staff of the College of Staten Island. Particular recognition and appreciation are extended to Wilma Jones, Raja Jayatilleke, and Angela DeMartinis for their assistance, expertise, and patience.

Most important, each of us offers our thanks to our close friends and our families. As this project progressed, they accepted our delays and absences with understanding. They maintained ongoing interest, corrected our computer mistakes, and listened to our talk (or silence). Their support and caring are very meaningful.

# CONTENTS

PART **IV**

Laboratory and Diagnostic Tests of Specific Body Systems

CHAPTER **20**

Endocrine Function   550

CHAPTER **24**

## Musculoskeletal Function    766

CHAPTER **25**

## Sensory Function    800

APPENDIX **A**

## Therapeutic Drug Monitoring    837

APPENDIX **B**

## Toxic Substances    840

APPENDIX **C**

## Abbreviations Associated with Laboratory and Diagnostic Testing    842

APPENDIX **D**

## Symbols and Units of Measurement    848

APPENDIX **E**

## Normal Values: Whole Blood, Serum, and Plasma Tests    849

APPENDIX **F**

## Normal Values: Urine Tests    865

APPENDIX **G**

## Normal Values: Body Fluids    869

# PART I

# Nursing Responsibilities in Laboratory Tests and Diagnostic Procedures

# CHAPTER 1

# The Nursing Role

Laboratory tests and diagnostic procedures involve two broad areas of nursing performance. The first area pertains to the procedure itself and to the nursing measures that ensure completion of the testing in an accurate and timely manner. The second area concerns the nursing interactions with the patient who must undergo the diagnostic test or procedure. The nursing process is used to organize patient care and meet the patient's needs.

The nursing role in patient care for individuals undergoing diagnostic tests and procedures may be direct or indirect. Often, it involves an interdisciplinary approach to the planning and implementation of care.

Direct care is provided by the nurse when the patient is hospitalized or enters an outpatient setting for performance of the laboratory or diagnostic test. The nurse may perform some aspects of the care or supervise paraprofessional workers in the delivery of care, particularly during the pretest and posttest periods. For some of the more complex or invasive tests, a nurse is present during the procedure to provide care to the patient and assist the physician who performs the test.

Indirect care often occurs when the patient is at home for the pretest and posttest phases of the diagnostic testing. The nurse may be responsible for guiding or instructing the patient in preparing for the test or in recovery after the test. The patient performs self-care, or a family member assists the patient according to the instructions that are given.

In many instances, diagnostic work is an interdisciplinary function that involves coordination and communication among the nurse, several physicians, and technicians of the laboratory, radiology department, or diagnostic specialty units. The nurse's role is often pivotal in the transmission of information to and from the testing center. The nurse must explain specific laboratory or diagnostic pretest requirements to the patient or must perform specific pretest procedures on the patient. Additionally, the specific needs or problems of the patient are explained to the testing center personnel. The goal is to accomplish the diagnostic work accurately, safely, and in a timely manner.

The process of laboratory or diagnostic testing can be conceptualized as a cycle that has four phases of operation: (1) the pretest phase, (2) the test phase, (3) the posttest phase, and (4) analysis of the results (Fig. 1–1). Appropriate nursing roles and responsibilities for the test or procedure, as well as appropriate aspects of nursing care for the patient, are pertinent to each phase.

## Procedural Role and Nursing Responsibilities

### Pretest Phase

**Scheduling of a Diagnostic Test.** This involves communication among the individual who prescribes the test, the patient, and the individual who performs the test. The nurse or unit coordinator is often responsible for accurate transcription of the orders, completion of the requisition form, and scheduling of the test.

When multiple tests are prescribed, it is sometimes necessary to prioritize the test schedule, because the method of conducting one test can interfere with the results of another test. For example, x-ray studies that use iodinated contrast medium are performed before x-ray studies that use barium contrast material. This timing is necessary because residual barium remains in the intestine for several days, and its opacity obscures the view of the other tissues, such as the biliary tract and abdominal vasculature. Likewise, blood tests that

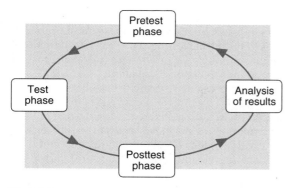

**Figure 1–1**

The cycle of laboratory or diagnostic testing. Both the nurse and the patient are involved in each phase of the cycle. After analysis of the test results, the cycle may be restarted for additional testing, as needed.

■

*Critical Thinking 1–1*

What are the potential risks when the laboratory specimen is obtained from the wrong patient or the specimen container is labeled incorrectly?

use a radioimmunoassay method of analysis must be performed before or 7 days after a nuclear scan, because the radioisotopes of the scan would interfere with the radioimmunoassay method of analysis of the blood and alter the test results.

When these interfering factors involve tests performed by a single department, such as the laboratory, the priorities are routinely sorted out by the laboratory personnel. When the interfering factors involve two departments, such as the laboratory and the radiology department, the nurse consults with the departments to clarify the priorities and to plan appropriately.

Some priorities in scheduling are determined by the acuity of the patient. Particular test results are needed rapidly for the assessment of the patient's status, for correct medical diagnosis and treatment, or for evaluation of the patient's response to treatment. Blood tests may be performed serially, for example, every hour for 4 hours; at frequent intervals such as daily; or immediately (stat). The request may specify the urgency and the desired times for the tests.

The nurse monitors each situation, ensuring that the tests are performed on time and that the test results are reported to the physician or posted in the patient's chart, or both, as quickly as they become available. When a test is ordered with an immediate or urgent priority, the laboratory or diagnostic unit is notified by telephone, the scheduling arrangements are confirmed, and the tests are completed as requested.

Some tests can be performed at the bedside with immediate results, such as the basic metabolic panel and coagulation tests. Other tests are specialized, and the final results may not be available for several days or more.

Nonroutine or special tests must be scheduled in advance. For example, positron emission tomography (PET), a nuclear scan, is performed in large medical centers on a particular day of the week, because the radioisotopes must be made in a special laboratory. Fertility tests and genetic tests are other examples of tests that must be scheduled. The analysis may involve one or more laboratories with specialized equipment and personnel.

Whenever questions exist about scheduling, priorities, the availability of the test, or even the type of specimen container to be used, the nurse can consult the printed hospital reference manual or communicate with the appropriate laboratory or diagnostic unit for assistance.

**Requisition Forms.** These forms must be completed accurately because they are often the only form of communication used to request a test, and they are part of the identification process that ensures that the correct test is performed on the correct patient. The requisition form is used to request the specific test, including the time and date that it should be performed. The form contains the patient information, including the patient's name, identification number, and hospital room number, and the name of the physician. Some agencies require additional information, such as the patient's birth date, to help ensure correct identification.

The requisition slip includes additional information that is appropriate to the test as determined by the physician or the individual who prescribes the test. Examples include the patient's age and gender, date of the last menstrual period, gestation of the pregnancy in a pregnant woman, pertinent medical history, and suspected diagnosis. The information is used in the analysis of the specimen and in the interpretation of the results.

## Test Phase

The procedural responsibilities of the nurse vary considerably with different tests, and they vary somewhat among different institutions or units within an institution. When the specimen collection is performed by the physician or technician, the nurse may have only indirect responsibility for ensuring that the test is performed, that the specimen is labeled properly, and that it is sent to the laboratory.

If the hospitalized patient must go to the radiology department or to a special diagnostic unit, the nurse ensures that patient care is completed and that the patient is prepared for transport to the unit. Equipment, such as an intravenous line or a drainage system, must be functional and secured properly. The patient's chart goes with the patient.

In some cases, the nurse is directly involved in the collection of specimens. This may include the collection of blood, urine, stool, and culture specimens, as well as assistance with the collection of a sample of tissue or other body fluids. In these processes, the nurse shares in the responsibility for maintenance of quality controls, proper performance of the equipment, and accurate identification of the patient.

**Identification Procedures.**    It is essential to perform a correct identification before collecting the specimen and before starting a diagnostic procedure by labeling the specimen container before it is transported to the laboratory. To identify the patient, the person who performs the test compares the data on the patient's identification band (name, room number, bed number, and other data) with the data on the requisition slip. Also, the patient is asked to state his or her full name. If the patient cannot respond, the staff nurse or a relative is asked to verify the identity (Jacobs et al., 1996).

Once the specimen is obtained, the label is compared with the requisition slip and the patient's identification band. All three must be identical. Before leaving the patient's bedside or the examining room, the nurse applies the label to the specimen container. For specimens of tissue or body fluid, the labels and requisition slips must identify the source of the specimen.

**Quality Control.**    This often refers to the calibration or testing of instruments and the analysis of control specimens that ensure accurate measurement. Today, the concept has expanded in scope, and quality control is part of a more inclusive quality assurance program (Handorf, 1994).

Quality control and quality assurance activities are used to assess for human and mechanical problems in diagnostic testing. The goal is to prevent or eliminate problems that interfere with the accuracy and reliability of test results.

The nursing department is usually involved in some quality control efforts. Activities include preparation of the patient before the test, testing or calibration of the diagnostic equipment, and ensuring that specimen collection requirements and special requirements for the storage or transport of the specimens are met. In other quality control efforts, the nurse minimizes or eliminates many of the interfering factors that would affect the accuracy and validity of the test and its results.

Throughout this text, quality controls that pertain to nursing are identified. They include special requirements for the collection, storage, and transport of specimens. They also include restrictions and requirements the patient must follow before the test, optimal times for particular specimen collections, and special conditions, such as sterility, use of preservatives, and temperature controls that protect the specimen from contamination or deterioration.

**Alternative-Site Testing.**    This is a new and rapidly evolving aspect of laboratory testing. In the past, a central laboratory and its subsections were housed in a single location, often in a hospital or a single community location. Today, a growing move toward decentralization has resulted in an increase in the sites of laboratory services inside the hospital and outside the institution. The reasons for decentralization are politically and economically driven in part, but technologic developments also constitute a strong factor. Miniature, computerized, desktop analyzers and handheld analyzers have brought laboratory testing and analysis nearer to the patient. Home test kits place the laboratory testing completely in the hands of the patient.

Alternative-site laboratory testing refers to choices about where laboratory testing is performed (Fig. 1–2). Point-of-care testing includes alternative testing sites outside the central laboratory, but it specifically refers to methods of testing and analysis that bring the laboratory services nearer to the patient. Point-of-care testing and its subconcepts are pertinent to nursing because they involve changes in the nursing role, nursing procedures, and nursing practices (Lamb, Parrish, Goran, & Biel, 1995).

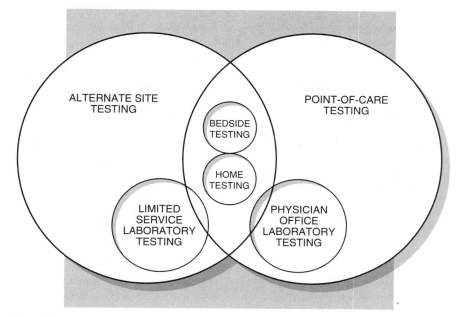

**Figure 1–2**

Alternative-site laboratory testing. The diagram represents the interrelationships of laboratory testing outside the traditional central location of the laboratory. (Modified with permission from Handorf, C. A. [1994]. Background—Setting the stage for alternate-site laboratory testing. *Clinics in Laboratory Medicine, 14,* 455.)

■

*Critical Thinking 1–2*

On your nursing unit, several recent laboratory specimens were rejected as "unsatisfactory." What steps can you take to prevent future problems?

**Point-of-Care Testing.**   This type of testing, also known as near-patient testing, brings laboratory testing and analysis to the patient or to the bedside. In many cases, satellite laboratories are established near or next to operating rooms, intensive care units, and emergency rooms. Sometimes a desktop analyzer is used in a clinic, an ambulatory care setting, a physician's office, or even the patient's home. With this new technology, automated analyzers are used to perform certain laboratory tests rapidly and with increased efficiency. Patient benefits include rapid turnaround time (the results are known within minutes), more prompt treatment, a smaller amount of blood loss with a decreased specimen volume requirement, and possibly lower costs and a shorter

hospital stay (Dirks, 1996; Kiechle & Ingram-Main, 1993; Lamb et al., 1995; Zalonga, 1993).

In critical care units and other hospital settings in which patients are acutely ill, the common tests that are performed and analyzed at the bedside include determination of blood gases, electrolytes, acid-base balance, osmolarity, and glucose levels; coagulation studies; and determination of hemoglobin and hematocrit values (Dirks, 1996; Woo & Henry, 1994). The results are available in a few minutes. When the patient is critically ill, many tests are performed at frequent intervals.

In addition to other laboratory test responsibilities, the nurse must ensure that all the results are charted in the correct order and time sequence. When computerized charting is used, the laboratory results must be transferred electronically to central computer systems (Horton, Utz, & Gibson, 1995).

With point-of-care methodology, some reference values are different from the values of the same tests analyzed in the central laboratory. Different reagents, test equipment, and procedures can create the differences in values. The nurse refers to the reference values provided by the laboratory or the manufacturer of the point-of-care equipment for correct analysis of the data. Sometimes, the manufacturer provides a printed conversion table to translate the data to a common reference value.

**Bedside Testing.**   This is one category of point-of-care testing and refers to the testing that is performed with small handheld instruments that analyze the patient's blood in a few minutes. The phrase *bedside testing* is inadequate, because the specimen is obtained and the blood analyzed wherever the patient is located, including the home or the workplace. The patient may be the one who performs the test as part of self-care responsibilities.

**Expanded Nursing Role.**   Point-of-care testing involves an expanded role for nurses that overlaps with that of laboratory technicians. The nurse may collect the blood sample, perform the analysis, and produce the test results. When the diabetic patient uses the glucometer, the nurse may have to teach the patient these same functions or evaluate the patient's performance and accuracy in using the equipment. In addition, nurses are involved in the selection and maintenance of the equipment located in the patient care units (Bickford, 1994).

To maintain accuracy, laboratory instruments are calibrated daily. In addition, the function of the equipment is evaluated, and a quality control check is performed to measure the accuracy of test results every day. This may be carried out by the laboratory technician or by the nurse. The biomedical department of the hospital usually is responsible for periodic maintenance of the equipment so that ongoing function is ensured.

Quality control measures are taken to ensure accurate performance by personnel (Handorf, 1994). A written protocol for equipment use is developed. Personnel are trained and evaluated on a routine basis. These requirements are now incorporated into the regulations of the Joint Commission on Accreditation of Healthcare Organizations (JCAHO) and other professional accrediting organizations (Travers, Wolke, & Stitak, 1994).

In some institutions, laboratory technicians are responsible for point-of-care testing; in other places, nurses, as the providers of direct patient care, use the automated analyzers. As part of the cross-training approach that is being used in hospitals, the nurse who uses this equipment must have formal training, certification that the training has been completed satisfactorily, and periodic reevaluation of performance. Without the training of nonlaboratory personnel, a high incidence of inconsistency of performance and inaccurate test results exists. Because of the turnover or rotation of nursing staff, the nurse manager of the unit must monitor the ongoing staff needs for continuing education.

**Home Testing.**   This type of point-of-care testing places the test entirely in the hands of the patient by use of home test kits. A proliferation of these kits or monitors can be purchased over the counter in the supermarket, medical supply store, and pharmacy. Depending on the test, the kits range from simple dipsticks to complex handheld analyzers that require periodic recalibration. Tests for human immunodeficiency virus (HIV) detection and drug tests for substance abuse detection require the specimens to be mailed to a designated laboratory for analysis. For these tests, the results are reported when the sender phones the laboratory. Only the laboratories with HIV and drugs-of-abuse test kits provide a tape recording or counseling services to explain a positive result and give advice about how to proceed with follow-up health care. The remainder of the test kits provide the results with printed instructions to seek medical advice for abnormal or positive results.

Health care professionals have expressed concern or caution regarding the use of these tests by laypeople. The concerns include reliance on one type of testing, when several tests are needed for a complete assessment; the inability of some patients to perform the test accurately; the patient's confusion about how to read the test results; his or her potential failure to seek medical assistance for an abnormal result; the lack of professional assistance or intervention for the patient; the consequences of a false-positive or false-negative result; and the high cost of home testing kits and materials (Anderson, Eccles, & Irvine, 1996; Burgess & MacGillis, 1995; Daviaud et al., 1993; Hicks, 1993; Tonnessen, 1995).

The benefits of home testing include convenience for the user, privacy regarding the results, improved methods of monitoring one's own health status, and increased self-care opportunities or empowerment regarding one's health.

An increasing number and variety of home tests are available. When the patient plans to use home testing, the nurse can best help by reviewing the instructions for use and explaining how to read the results. If there are abnormal results, the patient should be encouraged to return to the health care professional for repeat testing and follow-up care. Discussions of specific home tests are included in this text in the appropriate chapters.

**Infection Control: Standard Precautions.**   Standard precautions must be used when obtaining or handling a specimen of blood or body fluid. Gloves must be worn during the collection procedure. If splashing or contact with a mucous membrane is anticipated, the nurse wears a mask, protective eyewear, and a gown or protective clothing in addition to the gloves.

All specimens of blood or body fluids are placed in the correct containers with tightly fitted lids to prevent leakage during transport of the specimen to the laboratory. After the completion of the procedure, the gloves and disposable clothing are removed and discarded. Hands are washed with soap and water.

Precautions are taken to prevent the puncture or cutting of one's own skin with a contaminated needle, scalpel blade, or sharp instrument. To prevent needlestick injury, the needle-and-syringe unit is disposed of in a puncture-resistant container. The needle is not recapped, broken, bent, or removed from the syringe because of the risk of accidentally puncturing the hand.

Special reusable needles, such as those for a spinal tap or aspiration of a joint, are placed in puncture-resistant containers for transport to an area where they are cleansed and sterilized. After use, reusable instruments and diagnostic equipment are also cleansed and sterilized or disinfected according to established procedures.

The use of standard precautions is based on the premise that all patients are potentially infectious and that there is a risk of transmission of infection after exposure to blood or other body fluids. The precautions are used to protect all health care workers against bloodborne pathogens, including HIV.

## Posttest Phase

**Transport of the Specimen.**   The specimen is generally transported to the laboratory as soon as possible; however, some laboratory or pathology specimens become unstable within a short interval after they are collected. Specific factors, such as exposure to sunlight, warming, refrigeration, and exposure to air, can cause alteration or deterioration of particular specimens (Brunzel, 1994). As soon as the specimen is collected, quality control measures are used to protect it. The specific requirements and quality control measures are presented in the discussions of individualized tests located in Part IV of this volume.

For many blood tests, the untreated specimen begins to deteriorate within a few hours. To prevent this problem, the blood must be centrifuged and the serum extracted. With proper temperature control, serum has a longer period of stability than that of blood and can be stored for a specified period. The nurse ensures that all specimens are delivered promptly to the laboratory for immediate processing, storage, and analysis.

When a fresh tissue sample must be analyzed for cytologic features, the specimen cannot be placed in fixative or preservative. Because the specimen will dry out after some exposure to the air, it may be delivered directly into the hands of the pathologist or technician as soon as it is obtained. This coordination of activity provides immediate transport and tissue preparation so that the quality of the specimen is maintained.

Some specimens are obtained in the home and then transported to the laboratory. Other specimens must be mailed or transported to a reference laboratory in another city or another part of the country. These situations create an automatic delay before the specimen can be analyzed. General measures to protect the specimen from damage or deterioration include careful packaging, keeping blood cool and away from sunlight, extracting the serum from the cells by centrifuge, and adding a preservative tablet to urine samples. Specific directions are also provided by the laboratory, or they are included in the test kit and its mailing envelope.

**Rejection Criteria.**  When an unsatisfactory specimen is delivered to the laboratory, rejection criteria are applied. The causes of rejection are presented in Table 1–1. The nurse or staff member who is responsible can help ensure acceptance of the specimen by collecting a sufficient quantity, by complying with the written protocol of the test, and by carefully labeling the specimen container.

## Analysis of the Results

**Reference Values.**  Normal values, or reference values, are often presented in a range from the lower to the upper limits of normal. The reference values are used to interpret the results of the test, assist in making an accurate diagnosis, and evaluate the patient's response to treatment.

The reference values for a test vary with the different methods of analysis and different quantitative measurements that are used. For example, the test that measures the 5′-nucleotidase enzyme may be reported with different numeric reference values. The results can have different measurements, and the values are reported as units per liter (U/L), units per milliliter (U/mL), units (U), or Bodansky units. The nurse can use the reference values in this text as a general guide, but the reference values provided by the laboratory that performed the test are the most appropriate values for interpreting the findings in the clinical setting.

For some tests, there is no normal value because the particular substance should not be present at all. When it is not present, the result is described as negative. When it is found, the result is abnormal. The finding may be described as "present" or "positive," or it may be measured with a numeric value that quantifies the amount.

The phrase *critical value* refers to a test result that is extremely abnormal and indicates that the patient's life or health is in imminent danger. Identification of these extreme abnormalities helps the nurse and physician differentiate between abnormal results and the extremes that indicate a crisis.

**Variables.**  The normal reference values are determined by research studies that use human subjects with varying characteristics. These include the variables of demographics, age, gender, and race. Some of the tests, however, have additional reference values for particular groups of individuals because their normal values are influenced by differences in physiology.

Age differences create distinct sets of reference values for some tests. At one end of the life cycle, some reference values are different for the fetus, newborn, and child. In children, the reference values for some tests are different at particular ages. At the other end of the spectrum, age differences result in some variation of reference values in the older adult (Jacobs et al., 1996). For example, hormonal values in the postmenopausal woman are measurably different from those in the younger adult woman.

Gender is another variable that produces some differences in reference values. When differences between men and women occur, the variations are probably due to increased muscle mass in men and differences in hormones and hormone secretion between men and women (Henry, 1996).

Additional variations in the reference values for some tests are the result of differences in body weight, position (whether the patient is lying down

---

## Table 1–1   Criteria for Rejection of an Unsatisfactory Laboratory Specimen

Improper labeling of the specimen
Lack of a label on the specimen
Improper collection of the specimen
Lack of a preservative
Delay in delivery of the specimen to the laboratory
Improper preservation of the specimen
Improperly completed requisition form
Insufficient volume or quantity of the specimen
Inadequate pretesting preparation of the patient

or seated at the time of specimen collection), and pregnancy.

**SI Units.**    The International System of Units (Système International d'Unités, or SI) is a system that reports laboratory data in terms of standardized international measurements. This system of measurement is currently used in a number of countries, with the goal of worldwide use in the near future. Throughout this text, whenever possible, the reference values are presented in conventional units and also in SI equivalents.

## Patient-Nurse Interactions

### Dimensions of Nursing Care

The range of interactions between the patient and the nurse varies considerably with the complexity of the test or procedure. Blood tests that use specimens of blood, urine, or feces require some nursing intervention to ensure adequate patient preparation and quality control standards in the collection, storage, or transport of the specimens. Diagnostic procedures, however, require increased interaction with the patient, particularly when the procedure is invasive. Nursing responsibilities involve physical and psychosocial dimensions of patient care, with particular concern for the patient's safety.

Patient-nurse interactions involve direct or indirect care in the pretest, test, and posttest phases of the diagnostic procedure. The nursing process is applicable as a guide to the identification of the patient's needs and the development of the appropriate nursing interventions that lead to a positive outcome (Fig. 1–3).

**Changes in Health Care Delivery.**    These changes have resulted in shorter hospital stays for patients. Shorter periods of hospitalization limit the time for direct care during the acute phase of illness. For the acutely ill hospitalized patient, numerous diagnostic tests or procedures are often scheduled during a concentrated period. In addition to the routine pretest and posttest assessments of the patient, the nurse assesses the actual or potential complications that are related to the invasive diagnostic procedures.

The changes in health care delivery have also resulted in many diagnostic tests being performed on an outpatient basis while the patient continues to live at home. The patient has been

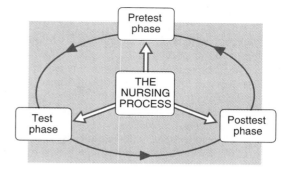

**Figure 1–3**
Application of the nursing process. In each phase of diagnostic testing, the nursing process is applied to provide safe, accurate, complete, and effective nursing care.

given greater self-care responsibility for pretest preparation and posttest recovery. The direct nursing interactions with the patient are often of short duration and may be limited to a brief pretest phase, the test phase, and the immediate posttest phase.

When a diagnostic procedure is performed in the outpatient setting, the patient receives pretest planning information and instructions regarding any special requirements that are necessary before or after the procedure. The clearly stated instructions are given to the patient or the family member who assists with the patient's care. If the instructions are complex, they should be given in writing so that the patient can refer to them as needed. Additionally, the patient needs the address and location of the laboratory or diagnostic unit as well as the time and date for which the test is scheduled.

In procedures requiring sedation or light anesthesia, the patient is instructed in advance that a responsible individual will be required to provide transportation home at the end of the test. When there is a possibility for a delayed complication in the posttest period, the patient receives instruction so that he or she will recognize abnormal symptoms and will notify the physician if they occur. All these measures are designed to provide continuity of care, even when the patient is some distance from the health care provider.

**Pediatric Patients.**    Modifications in communication and safety measures are required for pediatric patients. These measures should be compatible with the age and behavior of the child. When explanations can be understood, time should be taken to prepare the young child for the test or procedure. Honest, friendly explanations help the child cope with and endure the test. The child may fear pain, injections, or the large equipment of the radiology department or may fear the strangers who perform the test. Explanations are given simply and briefly. In some cases, the parents help prepare the child and provide calming reassurance (Torres, 1993).

Infants or active small children usually require restraints to protect them from harm and to maintain immobility during the test or procedure. The choice of restraint is based on the particular need; these restraints are used for tests of short duration. The choices include a sheet restraint, a mummy-style restraint, or a special commercial restraint that holds the patient in a particular position.

When the procedure requires a prolonged period of immobility, sedation is often used for infants and small children. Because of their young age, children cannot be expected to remain still for a long time. The procedures that use sedation in children include nuclear medicine scans, computed tomography, magnetic resonance imaging, electroencephalography, echocardiography, and some ultrasonography procedures.

**Geriatric Patients.**   These individuals may have specific needs that are age related or caused by a specific disease process. For the confused or depressed patient, instructions may need to be given slowly or repeated several times. The patient may have a hearing deficit or difficulty understanding speech or language. Alternative communication measures may include written pretest and posttest instructions, inclusion of a family member in the communications, or providing an interpreter to help the patient.

The elderly patient may take a considerable number of different medications, and some of them can interfere with particular laboratory tests. The physician is consulted regarding any alteration in the medication schedule, such as withholding the medication for a specified period.

Frail, elderly patients are at risk for injury from a fall. The common underlying problems include visual impairment, stiffness, weakness, mental confusion, dizziness, and the effects of medication. Care is taken to prevent accidental injury or a fall by assisting the patient out of the wheelchair and onto or off a gurney, examining table, radiography table, or toilet.

The elderly individual is often uncomfortable when lying on an x-ray table for a long time. The table is hard and the patient's joints are often stiff with arthritis. The room is usually cool, and some older patients complain about the temperature. It may not be possible to change the patient's position during x-ray studies or other diagnostic procedures because of the requirements of the test; however, warm blankets are usually provided so that at least the discomfort of chilling is removed.

## Pretest Phase

**Nursing Assessment.**   This assessment consists of the appraisal of the patient's physical and psychosocial status in relation to the requirements of the test. Pertinent findings in the psychosocial and physical history include any problems with the patient's vision, hearing, mobility, and comprehension of instructions. Current medications are listed. When iodinated contrast medium is used in the radiologic study, the nurse looks for any history of allergy to shellfish or iodine or of a previous reaction during a radiology test. Allergies to other foods and medications are also documented. If a female of childbearing age needs an x-ray study, she is questioned to determine whether there is any possibility of pregnancy.

Vital signs are taken to establish baseline values, particularly for invasive procedures or for when contrast medium, sedation, or anesthesia is used. The infant's or child's weight is recorded when the dose of medication or contrast medium must be calculated according to body weight.

For the purposes of consent, the patient is assessed for knowledge about the procedure, the pretest preparation, and other information that has been explained by the physician.

The nurse assesses the patient for signs of anxiety or fear. The cause can be apprehension about the test or procedure, or it may be fear of abnormal test results that indicate serious illness. If signs of distress are noted, the nurse asks about the cause or source of the anxiety.

The nurse also reviews the laboratory and other diagnostic test results and ensures that they are placed on the patient's chart. Some tests, such as prothrombin time, complete blood cell count, chest radiograph, and electrocardiogram, must verify a health clearance before some of the more invasive diagnostic tests are undertaken.

**Nursing Diagnoses.** Once the nursing assessment is completed, the nurse formulates nursing diagnoses that are appropriate to the patient who will undergo a procedure (NANDA, 1999). The pretest-phase nursing diagnoses are presented in Table 1–2.

**Expected Outcomes.** During the pretest period, the expected outcomes include the following:

1. When conscious sedation or anesthesia is anticipated, the patient arranges for a family member or friend to provide transportation home from the ambulatory test center.
2. The patient is free from all signs and symptoms of infection.
3. The patient communicates any history of allergic reaction to iodine, other allergens, and medications.
4. The patient's vital signs, coagulation studies, and other blood profiles remain within normal limits.
5. The patient requests information or clarification regarding the test and any special measures required in preparation for the test.

6. The patient, a family member, or a significant other demonstrates comprehension of the test and its preparation requirements.

## Nursing Implementation

Notify the physician of abnormal pretest results that indicate infection, clotting abnormality, fever, or irregularity in the vital signs. The diagnostic procedure may be postponed until the abnormality is corrected.

If the patient has allergies to food, medication, or contrast medium, post an allergy warning sticker on the outside of the patient's chart.

Provide the pretest instructions in a way that is understood by the patient. Pretest instructions often include the discontinuation of food and fluids for a specific period. They may also involve modification of activity or the temporary discontinuation of one or more medications for a specified period. Some abdominal or intestinal tests require a cleansing of the bowel by enema or cathartic, or both.

### Table 1–2    Pretest-Phase Nursing Diagnoses

| Nursing Diagnosis | Defining Characteristics | Related Factors |
|---|---|---|
| Risk for injury | Presence of risk factors such as developmental age, psychologic factors, or physical factors such as sensory or motor deficit | |
| Risk for infection or allergic reaction | Presence of risk factors such as altered immune function, history of chronic illness, impaired oxygenation of tissues, external factors such as allergens, or infectious agents | |
| Altered protection | Presence of risk factors such as altered clotting factors, immunosuppression, myelosuppression, or altered cardiovascular status | |
| Impaired verbal communication | Unable to speak dominant language, speaks with difficulty, disorientation, difficulty in comprehending | Cultural, developmental, or age-related factors; psychologic barriers, physiologic conditions |
| Anxiety | Presence of increased tension, uncertainty, fear of unspecific consequences, cardiovascular excitation, facial tension, quivering voice, insomnia, confusion | Threat to or change in health patterns |

When indicated, obtain the patient's signature of consent for the test or procedure. The patient should have received the physician's explanation of the procedure, the method of performing the test, and the potential risks involved. If the patient cannot give consent because of age or physical or mental impairment, obtain the signature of the person who is legally responsible for the patient's health care decisions. Once the consent form is signed and witnessed, enter it into the patient's chart.

Provide reassurance or information, as needed, to help reduce the patient's anxiety. Communicate with and assist the patient in an attentive and caring manner.

**Nursing Evaluation.** The pretest phase is completed successfully when the following have been accomplished:

1. The patient has followed all the pretest instructions accurately.
2. The patient's blood values, vital signs, and temperature measurement are within normal limits.
3. The patient appears calm and accepting about the test.

## Test Phase

**Nursing Assessment.** The nursing assessment during the test phase begins with the correct identification of the patient and the verification of the

procedure and the particular area to be tested (such as right or left leg, arm, breast, lung).

Monitoring of the physiologic status of the patient is carried out by a variety of measurements, depending on the complexity of the procedure and the use of conscious sedation or light anesthesia. Ongoing assessment of the patient may be performed through observation of the level of consciousness, repeated monitoring of vital signs, pulse oximetry, cardiac monitoring, or, in pregnant patients, fetal monitoring.

The skin is assessed for signs of infection or trauma, particularly at the site of intended venipuncture. The chart is also reviewed for the most recent laboratory findings and the pretest vital signs.

The nurse observes the patient for signs of discomfort, including shivering, trembling, pain, and tension. The patient is asked how he or she feels to encourage communication of any problems or concerns.

**Nursing Diagnoses.** Once the nursing assessment is completed, the nurse formulates nursing diagnoses that are appropriate to the patient who undergoes the procedure (NANDA, 1999). The test-phase nursing diagnoses are presented in Table 1–3.

**Expected Outcomes.** During the test period, the outcomes include the following:

1. The patient maintains adequate skin circulation and tissue perfusion.

### Table 1–3  Test-Phase Nursing Diagnoses

| Nursing Diagnosis | Defining Characteristics |
|---|---|
| Risk for impaired skin integrity | Disruption of the skin surface<br>Presence of internal or external risk factors, including skin compression, immobility, or altered circulation |
| Decreased cardiac output | Variations in blood pressure readings, arrhythmias, color changes of the skin, decreased peripheral pulses, dyspnea, increased heart rate |
| Impaired gas exchange | Cyanosis, restlessness, dyspnea, hypoxemia<br>Risk factors: administration of sedative analgesic medications, contrast medium, and potential allergic reaction |
| Risk for infection | Presence of risk factors such as inadequate primary defenses and performance of invasive procedures |
| Pain | Verbal report or expressive behavior, such as moaning, crying<br>Observed evidence, such as guarding behavior or grimacing |
| Anxiety | Verbalization of feelings about the test or its potential findings, changes in cardiovascular and respiratory rates |

2. Cardiopulmonary stability is maintained, with vital signs and results of monitoring devices in a normal range.
3. The puncture wound or incision remains clean and free from infection.
4. The patient expresses any pain or discomfort, including the location and characteristics of the sensation.
5. The patient describes any feelings of anxiety and helps identify the cause of those feelings.

## Nursing Implementation

Position the patient correctly for the procedure. Use padding, supportive devices, or restraints to promote safety and protect the patient's tissue against injury.

Continuously monitor the patient's cardiopulmonary status, including assessment of skin color and integrity, vital signs, breathing status, and level of consciousness.

Keep the emergency cart in a nearby location.

Ensure that all invasive equipment is sterile or has been properly cleaned and disinfected. Before the skin is punctured or opened, ensure that the skin is appropriately cleansed. Draping the area with sterile towels may also be indicated.

Offer reassurance through verbalization or physical support, particularly when the patient appears distressed by the procedure.

Administer prescribed pain medication as indicated.

**Nursing Evaluation.**   The test phase is completed when the following has been accomplished:

1. The patient demonstrates normal cardiopulmonary function as measured by normal vital signs and normal readings on all monitoring devices.
2. The patient maintains normal skin color and tone, with palpable peripheral pulses.
3. The patient experiences a lessening of pain, anxiety, or discomfort.
4. The patient has a clean, dry dressing with no signs of renewed bleeding, hematoma, swelling, or redness.

## Posttest Phase

**Nursing Assessment.**   The assessment is focused on the patient's physiologic, emotional, and mental status after the test is completed. Physiologic assessment is essential after an invasive procedure, conscious sedation, or anesthesia. The nurse assesses the expected alterations that occur because of the procedure or medications and also the potential complications.

When cardiac monitoring, fetal monitoring, and pulse oximetry are used during procedures, they are usually continued into the posttest period until the results remain stable in a normal range. Vital signs are taken to ensure that the hemodynamic status remains stable.

A risk of complications from an allergic response to the contrast medium and a risk of an embolus to a more distal location exist when an invasive neurologic, cerebrovascular, or peripheral arterial study is performed. Neurovascular assessments are performed to assess the integrity of the distal arterial blood flow and the responses of the neurologic tissues that are supplied by that blood flow. Vital signs also are monitored frequently to identify any untoward changes in cardiorespiratory status.

The nurse also uses observation to perform many assessments. When the diagnostic procedure is invasive, the nurse examines the site of the incision, penetration of the needle, or insertion of the instrument. The tissue is examined for signs of swelling, discharge, bleeding, or discoloration. Some pain or soreness may be present because of the incision or the manipulation of internal tissue. The nurse asks the patient to describe and locate the pain or tenderness. Sometimes the patient does not have immediate pain because of the lingering effects of the anesthetic or narcotic-analgesic medications. The nurse also examines the dressings. They are normally clean, dry, and intact.

The nurse can usually perform an emotional assessment by asking general questions about how the patient feels and observing the patient's responses. Most patients are relieved to have completed the test and are ready to return to their hospital rooms or to their residences. If there has been a period of fasting, they often express the desire to eat.

The assessment of mental status is appropriate when the patient has received conscious sedation or anesthesia or after a cerebrovascular invasive test. The nurse assesses the level of consciousness as well as clarity of thinking and speech. During the initial recovery from conscious sedation or anesthesia, the patient may be somewhat confused or drowsy, with diminished affect. As the medications are metabolized and excreted, increasing responsiveness and clarity of thinking are noted.

Before discharge, the patient who has had an invasive procedure is assessed for knowledge about continued requirements for care at home until healing is complete. The patient may be able to perform self-care, or there may be a need for family assistance for the remainder of the day. Assessment for infection or inflammation continues for several days, because the symptoms take time to develop. The patient or family member is taught to continue this assessment at home.

**Nursing Diagnoses.** Once the nursing assessment has been completed, the nurse formulates nursing diagnoses (NANDA, 1999) that are appropriate to the patient during the posttest phase of care. The posttest-phase nursing diagnoses are presented in Table 1–4.

**Expected Outcomes.** During the posttest period, the outcomes include the following:

1. The patient is conscious and alert.
2. Oxygenation and tissue perfusion are sustained, including circulation to the extremities.
3. Adequate cardiac output is maintained.
4. The skin remains warm, with normal color and no evidence of swelling or bleeding.
5. The patient does not fall or experience trauma.
6. After medication is administered, the patient expresses relief from pain.
7. The site of puncture or incision remains infection free.
8. The patient, family member, or significant other verbalizes understanding of posttest instructions regarding patient care.

## Nursing Implementation

After the completion of a diagnostic procedure in which conscious sedation or a light anesthesia was used, position the patient on his or her side to maintain a patent airway.

Oxygen may be administered, and the intravenous fluid replacement continues until the patient is able to drink fluids orally.

Administer the prescribed pain medication as needed. To help relieve discomfort, encourage the patient to change positions. Provide support with pillows.

Maintain sterile technique in the assessment of the wound or in changing the dressing.

To prevent a fall or an injury, assist the patient off the x-ray or examining table; also help the patient to the bathroom or with dressing in street clothes, as necessary. The patient may experience stiffness, pain, or drowsiness or may have diminished mental acuity as the result of the medication or procedure.

Inform the patient that the physician will discuss the diagnostic results with him or her as soon as this information is available. The patient with sutures is instructed to make an appointment

| **Table 1–4   Posttest-Phase Nursing Diagnoses** | |
| --- | --- |
| **Nursing Diagnosis** | **Defining Characteristics** |
| Altered tissue perfusion: cerebral, cardiopulmonary, peripheral | Changes in skin temperature, blood pressure changes, arrhythmias, dyspnea, decreased peripheral pulses, altered mental status |
| Pain | Verbal report about pain or discomfort |
| | Alteration in muscle tone, movement, or facial expression |
| | Expressive behavior, such as moaning, grimacing, and crying |
| Risk for injury | Presence of risk factors such as immobility, developmental age, or sensory-motor deficit |
| Risk for infection | Presence of risk factors such as exposure to pathogens, immunosuppression, or broken skin |
| Knowledge deficit regarding care after procedure | Verbalization of the problem, inaccurate follow-through of instructions |

with the physician for the evaluation of the incision and removal of the sutures.

Before discharge, instruct the patient about any additional restrictions that are recommended, such as instructions regarding activity, bathing, resumption of medication, the intake of fluids, or the care of the incision.

**Nursing Evaluation.**   The posttest phase is completed when the following have been accomplished.

1. The patient demonstrates normal vital signs, responsiveness to questions, and normal skin color and temperature.
2. The patient experiences a lessening of pain, anxiety, or discomfort.
3. The patient has a clean, dry dressing with no signs of renewed bleeding, hematoma, swelling, or redness.
4. The patient verbalizes his or her understanding of the postdischarge instructions.

## References

Anderson, R. A., Eccles, S. M., & Irvine, D. S. (1996). Home ovulation testing in a donor insemination service. *European Society for Human Reproduction and Embroyology, 11,* 1674–1677.

Baer, D. M. (1995). Hematology testing at the bedside. *Laboratory Medicine, 26*(1), 48–53.

Baer, D. M. (1996). POCT quality . . . . point of care testing. *Medical Laboratory Observer, 28*(6), 14.

Baer, D. M., & Belsey, R. E. (1993). Limitations of quality control in physicians offices and other decentralized situations: The challenge to develop new methods of test validation. *Clinical Chemistry, 39*(1), 9–12.

Bickford, G. R. (1994). Decentralized testing in the 1990's: A survey of United States hospitals. *Clinics in Laboratory Medicine, 14,* 623–650.

Brunzel, N. A. (1994). *Fundamentals of urine and body fluid analysis.* Philadelphia: W. B. Saunders.

Burgess, J., & MacGillis, A. (1995). HIV antibody testing in home test kits. *Connecticut Nursing News, 68*(5), 2A.

Daviaud, J., Fournet, D., Ballongue, C., Guillem, G. P., Leblanc, A., Casellas, C., & Pau, B. (1993). Reliability and feasibility of pregnancy home-use tests: Laboratory validation and diagnostic validation by 638 volunteers. *Clinical Chemistry, 39*(1), 53–59.

Dirks, J. L. (1996). Diagnostic blood analysis using point-of-care technology. *AACN Clinical Issues: Advanced Practice in Acute and Critical Care, 7,* 249–259.

Frizzell, J. (1998). Avoiding lab test pitfalls. *American Journal of Nursing, 98*(2), 34–38.

Goyzueta, F. G., Bailey, C. J., & Billett, H. H. (1996). Automated differential white blood cell counts in the young pediatric population. *Laboratory Medicine, 27*(1), 48–52.

Handorf, C. R. (1994). Background—Setting the stage for alternate site laboratory testing. *Clinics in Laboratory Medicine, 14,* 539–558.

Harris, H. R. (1994). Home testing for HIV. *Surgical Technologist, 26*(6), 14.

Henry, J. B. (1996). *Clinical diagnosis and management by laboratory methods* (19th ed.). Philadelphia: W. B. Saunders.

Hicks, J. M. (1993). Home testing: To do or not to do? *Clinical Chemistry, 39*(1), 7–8.

Horton, G. L., Utz, C., & Gibson, C. (1995). Managing information from bedside testing. *Medical Laboratory Observer, 27*(1), 28–32.

Jacobs, D. S., Demott, W. R., Grady, H. J., Horvat, R. T., Huestis, D. W., & Kasten, B. L. (Eds.). (1996). *Laboratory test handbook* (4th ed.). Baltimore: Williams & Wilkins.

Kiechle, F. L., & Ingram-Main, R. (1993). Bedside testing: Beyond glucose. *Medical Laboratory Observer, 25*(5), 65–66, 68.

Krenzischek, D. A., & Tanesco, F. V. (1996). Comparative study of bedside and laboratory measurements of hemoglobin. *American Journal of Critical Care, 5,* 427–432.

Lamb, L. S., Jr., Parrish, R. S., Goran, S. F., & Biel, M. H. (1995). Current nursing practice of point-of-care laboratory diagnostic testing in critical care units. *American Journal of Critical Care, 4,* 429–434.

Lowell, M. (1995). Consumer trends in self diagnosis, home testing, and over the counter medication: Implications for the registered nurse. *Kansas Nurse, 70*(5), 1–2.

NANDA (1999). *Nursing diagnoses: Definitions & classification 1999–2000.* Philadelphia: North American Nursing Diagnosis Association.

Schallom, L. (1999). Point of care testing in critical care. *Critical Care Nursing Clinics of North America, 11*(1), 99–106.

Tonnessen, D. (1995). How helpful are home cholesterol tests? *Women's Health Digest, 1*(1), 70–72.

Torres, L. S. (1993). *Basic techniques and patient care for radiologic technologists* (4th ed.). Philadelphia: J. B. Lippincott.

Travers, E. M., Wolke, J. C., & Stitak, M. M. (1994). Consolidating ancillary testing in multihospital systems. *Clinics in Laboratory Medicine, 14,* 493–524.

Woo, J., & Henry, J. B. (1994). The advance of technology as a prelude to the laboratory of the twenty-first century. *Clinics in Laboratory Medicine, 14,* 459–472.

Zalonga, G. P. (1993). Part 1. Rapid, accurate urine testing at the bedside. *Consultant, 33*(6), 90–92, 95–98.

# CHAPTER 2

# Specimen Collection Procedures

Three of the major sources of specimen samples are blood, stool, and urine, with the greatest number of tests performed on blood. The laboratory performs biochemical and microscopic analysis of these body substances to provide objective data about the patient's health and to identify disease processes.

In collection procedures, accurate technique is essential to obtaining a valid specimen and to preventing injury to the patient. In addition, quality control measures are used in maintaining accuracy in the identification of the patient and the specimen, in the method of obtaining the specimen, and in the transportation of the specimen to the laboratory.

## Laboratory Procedures

## Blood Collection: Arterial Puncture

**(Blood)**                    Synonyms: None

### Background Information

Arterial blood specimens are obtained for blood gas studies, including the measurement of oxygen, carbon dioxide, and pH. The assessment of arterial blood is usually performed on the patient who has an actual or potential problem with oxygenation. The nursing diagnoses may include ineffective airway clearance, ineffective breathing pattern, altered tissue perfusion: cardiopulmonary, and impaired gas exchange.

The procedure of arterial puncture is technically more difficult than that of venipuncture, but arterial blood is far more accurate for the measurement of oxygenation throughout the body. The usual site of the arterial puncture is either the radial or the brachial artery; the radial artery is preferred. Although the femoral artery can be used, the risk of hemorrhage at that site is greater.

Before an arterial puncture of the radial artery is carried out, the *Allen test* is performed to verify the presence of collateral circulation to the hand (Table 2–1). If arterial occlusion of the radial artery occurs after arterial puncture, the presence of collateral circulation protects the hand from ischemic damage. An alternative method of performing the Allen test is presented in Chapter 14.

Some institutions and settings permit the nurse with specialized training to draw blood via an arterial puncture. Refer to the institutional or laboratory protocol to determine who may do this procedure.

## Table 2–1   The Allen Test

**Purpose**

In preparation for a radial artery puncture, the Allen test assesses the adequacy of collateral circulation to the hand.

**Procedure**

Elevate the hand to diminish the arterial blood flow.

Use one or two fingers to compress the radial artery at its pulse point on the wrist.

Observe for a color change in the hand. The hand should become blanched because of diminished blood flow.

Maintain the arterial compression, lower the hand, and observe for a color change. There should be a brisk return of pinkness to the hand, indicating effective collateral circulation from the ulnar artery.

**Interpretation**

When collateral circulation is adequate, the radial artery can be used for arterial puncture.

When there is a poor response to the Allen test, the other arm should be tested to search for a better site.

Abnormal results can be caused by a thrombus or arterial spasm that affects the radial artery or ulnar artery, or both.

Poor collateral circulation bilaterally may be caused by a systemic problem, such as shock or poor cardiac output.

| | |
|---|---|
| **Purpose of the Test** | Arterial puncture is used to obtain a sample of arterial blood for analysis of blood gases and acid-base balance. |
| **Procedure** | A heparinized syringe and needle is used to collect 3 mL of arterial blood. For radial artery puncture, a 23- to 25-G needle is used. For brachial artery puncture, an 18- to 20-G needle is used. In many institutions, a prepackaged kit provides the equipment for blood gas studies. |
| **Interfering Factors** | • Poor collateral circulation to the extremities<br>• Inability to puncture the artery or withdraw blood<br>• Air mixed in with the blood specimen |
| **Nursing Implementation** | **Pretest** |

■

*Critical Thinking 2–1*
Why should the arterial site with the stronger pulse and stronger collateral circulation be selected?

Identify the patient by asking his or her name, checking the identification bracelet, and comparing the identification bracelet with the name on the requisition form.

When the radial artery is to be used, palpate the pulse of each wrist to select the site with the stronger circulation.

Perform the Allen test to assess the collateral circulation to the hand.

Position the hand so that the wrist is in slight dorsiflexion.

Explain to the patient that a sharp pain will be felt as the needle punctures the blood vessel. In some cases, a local anesthetic may be administered beforehand.

### During the Test

The interior of the syringe and needle must be coated with heparin. The syringe in the blood gas kit may be heparinized already. If heparin must be added, 1 mL (1,000 or 5,000 U/mL) is drawn into a 10-mL syringe. After the syringe is rotated to coat the entire interior surface, the heparin is expelled. A small amount of heparin remains in the dead space and within the shaft of the needle.

Clean the skin over the pulse point with povidone-iodine, using sterile gauze. Remove this solution by wiping the skin with 70% alcohol. Allow the skin to dry.

With the bevel of the needle up and the syringe placed at a 45- to 60-degree angle, slowly insert the needle into the artery (Fig. 2–1). Blood will pulse into the syringe without your having to draw back on the plunger.

Once the required amount of blood is in the syringe, remove the needle. The amount is usually 3 mL, but the volume can vary according to the type of syringe and the test protocol (Henry, 1996).

### Posttest

Use a sterile gauze to apply immediate pressure to the puncture site for 5 minutes.

Remove the needle from the syringe. If there is air in the syringe, expel it.

### Quality Control

> Any air in the syringe would be absorbed into the blood and alter the patient's blood gas values.

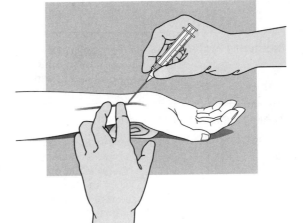

**Figure 2–1**

Technique for arterial puncture. Puncture of the radial artery can be performed only when both the radial and the ulnar arteries provide adequate circulation to the hand.

Place the airtight cap on the tip of the syringe.

Place the syringe on ice and arrange for immediate transport of the specimen to the laboratory.

Once the bleeding from the puncture site has stopped, apply a small sterile bandage.

Continue to assess the wrist and hand for signs of complications. It is common for the patient to complain of some temporary discomfort, such as aching, throbbing, or tenderness at the puncture site.

## Complications

The three complications of arterial puncture are hemorrhage, infection, and thrombus formation, but the incidence is low. A summary of the complications of arterial puncture is presented in Table 14–2.

## Blood Collection: Capillary Puncture

**(Blood)**    Synonyms: Microcapillary puncture, skin puncture

### Background Information

Capillary puncture is a technique whose use is likely to increase because of the changes in health care delivery. The trends of early patient discharge from the hospital and treatment in outpatient settings often require additional monitoring of the blood as part of the follow-up evaluation. Additionally, a growing trend is to perform point-of-care testing, meaning that laboratory analysis of the blood is performed at the patient's bedside. This method is used particularly in high-volume areas when rapid results are required. The laboratory analyzer performs multiple tests on a small blood sample from a fingerstick or heelstick source.

The traditional use of the capillary puncture is for patients with small or inaccessible veins. This method is useful in burn patients, in those who are extremely obese, and in patients in whom there is a tendency toward thrombus formation. It is the method of choice for obtaining blood samples from premature infants, neonates, and young babies. It may be used to preserve the total blood volume of the infant or small child, particularly when there is a need for multiple blood tests.

Because capillary blood is similar in composition to venous blood, capillary blood collection may be performed for a complete blood cell count, hematocrit determination, blood smear, coagulation studies, and most blood chemistry tests. The specimen source is always identified on the requisition slip, because there may be differences between venous and capillary blood concentrations of calcium, glucose, potassium, and total protein.

### Site of Collection

The available sites for collection of capillary blood include the finger, heel, and earlobe. The finger is often used for adults or older children. The locations most often used are the distal tips of the third and fourth fingers, slightly to the side (Fig. 2–2). Few calluses are located on the sides of the fingers, and the lancet can puncture the skin more easily. The frontal tips or pads of the fingers are not used because many nerve endings are located there, and the puncture would be more painful.

The heel is used for premature infants, neonates, infants, and small children and for special cases such as patients with thermal injury. With the heelstick technique, the medial or lateral plantar surface of the foot is used (Fig. 2–3). The heel and big toe are preferred. The central area of the plantar

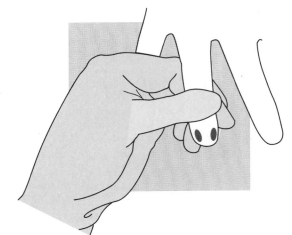

**Figure 2–2**
Capillary puncture sites in the finger. In adults, the middle or ring finger is the preferred site for a capillary blood sample. The sterile lancet punctures the skin in the distal tip slightly to the side of the finger pad.

surface of the foot is never used. There is a risk of damage to the calcaneus bone, Achilles tendon, or other tendons, nerves, and cartilage that are located in the central area of the foot.

The earlobe may be used as the alternative puncture site of last resort in adults and older children, but it cannot be used for infants and neonates. It is a preferred site for obtaining arterialized blood for measurement of pH and partial pressure of carbon dioxide ($P_{CO_2}$), because it is highly vascular tissue with few metabolic requirements. However, the blood values obtained from an earlobe site are unreliable in cases of low cardiac output and vasoconstriction. If the earlobe is used, the soft fleshy part is punctured, and the area of cartilaginous tissue is avoided.

In the selection of the skin puncture site, the tissue should not be edematous, inflamed, or recently punctured. These factors cause increased interstitial fluid to mix with the blood, and they also increase the risk of an infection.

The heelstick method is preferred for sampling blood in the premature

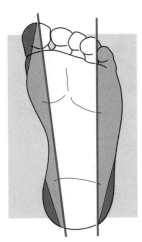

**Figure 2–3**
Heelstick sites for capillary puncture. The shaded areas are appropriate sites for neonates and infants, but the best sites are those of the heel and big toe, as indicated by areas of darker shading.

baby and infant. It is technically easier to perform and avoids the significant complications that can occur with arterial or venous puncture. Some special considerations must be made, however, because of the number of heel-stick punctures performed and the small size of the patients.

Increasingly, infants are discharged from the nursery after a short stay. This means that additional blood tests for bilirubinemia, phenylalanine, hemoglobinopathy, and galactosemia, as well as other screening tests, are performed on an outpatient basis. Some of these tests are performed serially, meaning that multiple blood samples are taken over time. The nurse in the outpatient setting assesses the heels of the infant for signs of complications that can occur from repeated punctures.

The premature infant also needs special consideration when multiple blood samples are obtained by the heelstick technique. The premature infant may weigh as little as 500 g. The heels are small, and there is little depth to the tissue for the many punctures and tests that are needed. Additionally, blood flow is often inadequate, and two or three punctures may be needed to obtain the required amount.

To help prevent injury to the calcaneus, the depth of the lancet must be controlled, and careful selection of the tissue site must be carried out. To help prevent infection and hematoma, aseptic technique and gentle handling of the tissue are needed whenever blood is drawn. Because of repeated trauma to the heels of the premature infant, the nurse assesses this tissue for signs of localized complications. These complications can occur during the stay in the neonatal unit, or they can develop years later.

| | |
|---|---|
| **Purpose of the Test** | Capillary blood collection is used when a small amount of blood is sufficient or the venipuncture method is not feasible. |
| **Procedure** | A sterile lancet is used to collect capillary blood from a skin puncture site. The blood is blotted onto special filter paper (Fig. 2–4) or collected in a narrow-diameter glass tube. The tube is called a micropipette, microtube, or capillary tube. |
| **Interfering Factors** | • Reduced cardiac output<br>• Vasoconstriction |

**Nursing Implementation**

**Pretest**

Identify the patient and check the requisition form with the patient's identification bracelet. Inform the patient that blood needs to be drawn from the designated site.

Particularly with small children, provide reassurance to help limit anxiety.

If pretest fasting or dietary restriction is required, verify that the instructions were followed for the correct period of time.

Assemble the equipment and put on a pair of gloves.

The patient may be seated or in the supine position.

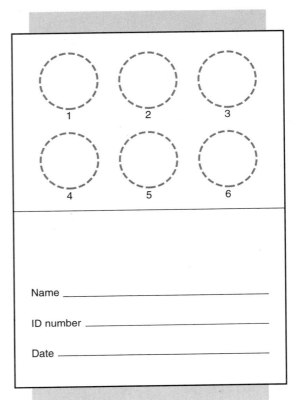

**Figure 2–4**
Capillary blood filter paper.
Droplets of blood are
blotted onto the filter paper at
each circle. The nurse must
saturate each circle before
moving on to fill the next one.
The nurse must not *partially*
fill some circles and then
return to complete them later.
To promote blood flow, the
hand is kept lower than
the heart, and the finger is
stroked in a distal direction.

## During the Test

Assess the skin site for color and temperature and the absence of infection and
   edema. If the skin is cool or pale, the circulation may be diminished. Put the
   hand in warm water or apply a warm, moist compress to the site for a few
   minutes. This helps increase circulation to the skin.
Use a gauze and 70% alcohol to cleanse the skin site and allow the skin to dry.
Holding the tissue between the thumb and the forefinger, use a firm, quick
   stroke to puncture the skin with the sterile lancet.
Wipe away the first drop of blood, because it contains tissue fluids. Collect the
   subsequent drops of blood in capillary tubes or on the blotting paper.
To help obtain more blood, the finger may be massaged gently. The tissue near
   the puncture should not be squeezed because tissue fluids will mix with the
   blood, and the blood will clot quickly (Stepp & Woods, 1998).
The capillary tubes are held horizontally to prevent air bubbles. They should be
   filled two-thirds to three-quarters full and then sealed with clay.
The circles on the filter paper are filled one at a time, until they are fully saturated. Allow the blood on the paper to air-dry for 10 minutes before it is
   placed in a collection envelope.

### Posttest

Once the specimen collection is completed, wipe the puncture site with alcohol.

Instruct the patient to place a sterile gauze on the site and apply pressure until the bleeding stops.

If the infant or small child is crying, provide comfort.

Label all specimens and arrange for their prompt transport to the laboratory.

## Complications

The most serious complications of heelstick puncture in infants is infection; fortunately, the incidence of this complication is low (Henry, 1996). The infection is usually localized in the soft tissue, and the most common causative organism is *Staphylococcus aureus*. Weeks later, however, the infection can develop into osteomyelitis. The source of the infection is poor aseptic technique, a contaminated lancet, or injury to the bone during the skin puncture.

Bruising, pain, scarring, and hematoma formation are more frequent complications (Wilson & Gaedeke, 1996). They occur from frequent skin punctures or excessive squeezing of the tissues during the collection of the blood samples.

The complications of heelstick puncture are presented in Table 2–2.

# Blood Collection: Venipuncture

**(Whole Blood, Serum, Plasma)**

Synonyms: Phlebotomy, venous blood collection

## Background Information

Venipuncture is performed by drawing and collecting a specimen of blood from a superficial vein. It is a quick method of obtaining a larger sample of blood, and the specimen can be used to perform many different laboratory analyses. Depending on the test to be performed, the analysis is carried out on whole blood, serum, or plasma.

Whole blood contains all the blood components. A centrifuge is used to separate the blood components and obtain either serum or plasma. If the blood has been collected in a tube containing anticoagulant, the centrifuge process produces

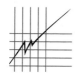

| Table 2–2 Complications of Heelstick Puncture | |
|---|---|
| **Complication** | **Nursing Assessment** |
| Infection | Localized redness and swelling |
| | Localized pain and tenderness |
| | Purulence or abscess formation |
| | Radiographic changes indicating osteomyelitis |
| Hematoma and bruising | Bruising and discoloration |
| | Firm swelling of the tissue |
| | Tenderness or pain |
| | Bleeding onto the skin |

plasma. If whole blood is collected in a tube without anticoagulant, the centrifuge process yields serum. Plasma is serum that contains fibrinogen.

---

**Site of Collection**

The most common site for venipuncture is the antecubital fossa, because several large superficial veins are available. The most commonly used veins are the median cubital, the basilic, and the cephalic veins (Fig. 2–5). Veins of the wrists, hands, or ankles may also be used.

---

**Intervening Variables**

When an intravenous line, shunt, or other intravenous device has been placed in one arm, the other arm or another venous site must be selected. The reason for avoiding these sites is that the administration of intravenous fluids alters the composition of the blood specimen. Additionally, venous shunts are established for specific treatments, and they can be damaged by excessive punctures.

For a variety of physiologic and age-related reasons, locating a suitable vein is sometimes difficult. When the patient is severely dehydrated or hypotensive, or both, the veins have less fluid volume. They are less visible and less palpable and may be partially collapsed. Reduced cardiac output also diminishes the volume of blood in the peripheral veins.

Severe obesity can be a problem, because the overlying layers of fat interfere with the location and palpation of a suitable vein. In the elderly, the superficial veins of the hands are highly visible and prominent, but it is difficult to use these sites. The veins are fragile, and venipuncture can cause a hematoma to form. Additionally, these veins move during the venipuncture process, making it difficult to enter the lumen of the vein. The excess movement is caused by the loss of supportive muscle and connective tissue associated with aging.

In the premature and newborn infant, the veins are small. Frequent venipuncture can cause severe complications, including damage to the veins and surrounding tissue.

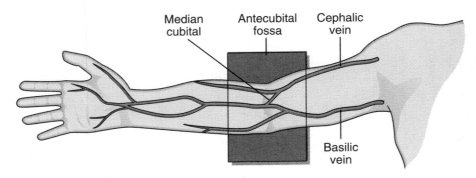

**Figure 2–5**

Preferred sites for venipuncture. The three primary veins in the antecubital fossa are preferred because they are usually visible and fixed in place by surrounding tissue. (Reproduced with permission from Lehmann, C. A. [1998]. *Saunders manual of clinical laboratory science* [p. 7]. Philadelphia: W. B. Saunders.)

If any of these interfering factors are present, causing difficulty with venipuncture, capillary puncture may be an acceptable alternative. If the hand veins are selected for venipuncture, a butterfly needle and a syringe are used to obtain the blood.

## Purpose of the Test

Venipuncture is used to obtain a venous blood sample for laboratory analysis. The serum component of the blood is used for most of the chemistry analyses.

## Procedure

Either a vacuum tube system or a needle, syringe, and test tube containers are used to collect the blood sample. The selection of the color-coded specimen tube is based on the requirements of the specific test. Each laboratory blood test discussed in this text lists the correct test tube to be used for that test.

## Interfering Factors

- Dehydration
- Hypotension
- Obesity
- Fragility of veins
- Prematurity and infancy

## Nursing Implementation

### Pretest

Identify the patient, and check the requisition form with the patient's identification bracelet.

Inform the patient that blood needs to be drawn from the designated site. Provide reassurance to help limit anxiety.

If pretest fasting or dietary restriction is required, verify that the instructions were followed for the correct period of time.

Assemble the equipment, and put on a pair of gloves.

The patient may be seated or in the supine position. The patient's arm is in extension, with easy access to the antecubital fossa.

■

*Critical Thinking 2–2*
What safety measures should be used in case the patient becomes faint or dizzy during the venipuncture procedure?

### During the Test

Inspect the antecubital fossae of both arms to select the best vein for the venipuncture. Ask the patient to open and close the hand a few times to help make the veins more visible.

Gently palpate the vein to determine its location, direction, width, and depth.

Cleanse the skin with 70% alcohol, and allow it to air-dry.

Apply the tourniquet about 2 to 3 in above the antecubital fossa.

Using your fingertips, anchor the vein above and below the puncture site.

With the bevel up, insert the needle at a 15-degree angle along the pathway of the vein (Fig. 2–6).

### Syringe Method

Once the needle is in the vein, gently aspirate blood into the syringe. Collect the volume of blood that is needed.

**Figure 2–6**
Needle placement during venipuncture. To obtain good blood flow, the needle is positioned correctly in the vein lumen. The needle should not rest against the upper wall of the vein or puncture through the vein wall on the opposite side.

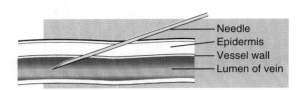

### Vacuum Tube System Method

Once the needle is in the vein, hold it firmly in place.

Push the blood collection tube fully into the holder so that the blood flows through the needle and into the vacuum tube (Fig. 2–7). When multiple specimens are needed, remove each full tube and insert the next tube firmly into the holder.

After all blood has been collected, release the tourniquet.

Place a sterile gauze over the puncture site. Remove the needle. Use the gauze and your finger to compress the puncture site.

### Quality Control

When you draw blood by syringe or the vacuum tube system method, the tourniquet should not remain tied for more than 1 minute. The prolonged compression of the vein and stasis of the blood flow caused by the tourniquet results in clumping or hemolysis of the erythrocytes, which interferes with the laboratory analysis and alters some test results.

### Posttest

Instruct the patient to continue compression of the puncture site for 2 to 5 minutes or until the bleeding stops.

If a syringe and needle were used, transfer the blood to the appropriate test tube containers.

Label every vial of blood with the patient's name and identification number, the time, and the date.

Perform any special measures that are needed to protect the specimen from deterioration. These measures are test specific and are described throughout this text.

Assess the patient's arm to ensure that the bleeding has ceased. Apply an adhesive bandage as needed.

Remove gloves and wash your hands.

Arrange for prompt transport of the specimen to the laboratory.

---

**Complications**

Hematoma formation occurs when the vein continues to leak blood under the skin. The result is a large bruised area. The problem can be prevented by continued compression of the puncture site until clotting occurs. The patient can also elevate the arm and rest it on top of the head. This reduces the blood volume and pressure on the walls of the vein.

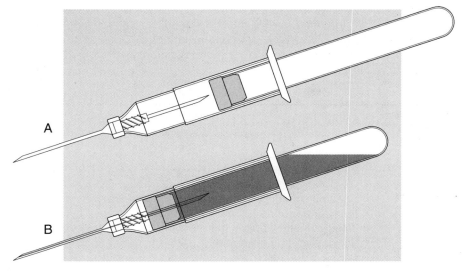

**Figure 2–7**

Function of the vacuum tube collection system. *A,* Before venipuncture, the vacuum tube is placed into the holder, resting on the tip of the sterile needle. *B,* Once the needle enters the vein, the tube is pushed to the front of the holder, and the needle penetrates the stopper of the tube. Because of the negative pressure in the tube, the blood is pulled from the vein, through the needle, and into the vacuum tube.

## Stool Collection

**(Feces)**    Synonym: Stool specimen

### Background Information

The laboratory testing of fecal matter may involve chemical analysis that identifies the abnormal composition of the feces or may involve microbiologic analysis that identifies infectious organisms. Once the abnormality has been identified, additional diagnostic tests or procedures are often needed to determine the cause and location of the problem.

One group of abnormal fecal test results is caused by diseases that damage the intestinal mucosa, alter the integrity of the intestinal tissue, or interfere with the functions of digestion, absorption, and elimination. The fecal changes may include the presence of blood or an alteration in the composition of the feces. Examples of these diseases include malignancy of the stomach or colon, peptic ulcer, regional ileitis, celiac disease, or scleroderma.

A second group of abnormal fecal test results is caused by abnormality in the organs and ducts that secrete into the intestinal tract. These organs include the liver, pancreas, and gallbladder. The fecal changes can include excess fat in the stool or a lack of fecal urobilinogen. Examples of these conditions include cystic fibrosis, pancreatic cancer, hepatitis, and bile duct obstruction.

A third category of abnormal fecal test results is caused by infectious organisms that infect the intestinal tract. The organisms are discovered by microscopic examination of the stool or stool culture. The infection may be of bacterial, viral, parasitic, or other origin, often infecting the small or large intestine. Sometimes the infection causes damage to the intestinal mucosa or underlying tissue, resulting in blood in the stool. In this example, more than one abnormality can be detected in the analysis of fecal matter.

| | |
|---|---|
| **Purpose of the Test** | Analysis of feces is used to screen for intestinal disease in an asymptomatic individual; to help identify abnormal intestinal function or abnormal function of the gallbladder, liver, or pancreas; and to help assess the patency of the biliary tree. |

**Procedure**

A half-pint waterproof container that is clean and dry and has a wide mouth with a tight-fitting lid is used to collect approximately 1 to 2 oz of fecal matter.

**Interfering Factors**

- Improper specimen collection
- Contamination of the specimen with water or urine
- Delay in transport of the specimen
- Failure to follow pretest dietary instructions
- Pretest ingestion of antibiotics, cathartics, or barium, or administration of an enema

**Nursing Implementation**

### Pretest

Ask the patient if he or she has had a recent barium x-ray study or recent treatment with oral antibiotics.

Schedule the test accordingly.

**Quality Control**

Barium sulfate interferes with the analysis of feces for approximately 2 weeks after ingestion. Stool culture is less likely to demonstrate the causative organism when antibiotics have been taken during the preceding 3 to 4 weeks.

Instruct the patient about any dietary restrictions that are part of specific test preparations. For some of the tests, such as those looking for fecal fat and fecal occult blood, pretest dietary modifications are required.

Instruct the patient not to ingest castor oil, mineral oil, antacids, or antidiarrheal medications or to administer an enema before the test.

**Quality Control**

These substances appear in the fecal matter and interfere with the chemical or microscopic analysis.

### During the Test

Instruct the patient to evacuate directly into the container or a clean, dry bedpan. Tongue blades can be used to transfer a small amount of feces from the bedpan into the collection container.

Urine, water, or toilet paper must not be mixed in with the fecal specimen.

Once the specimen is obtained, place the lid on the container and wash your hands.

### Posttest

Label the container with the patient's name and other appropriate data. Mark the time and date of the collection on the container and requisition slip.

Arrange for transport of the specimen within 30 minutes.

If there is a delay before transport, store the specimen in the refrigerator. The cool temperature preserves any microorganisms that may be present.

## Urine Collection

**(Urine)**                     Synonyms: None

### Background Information

Urine provides a major source of data about the status and function of the urinary tract. In addition, because urine is an ultrafiltrate of the plasma, it is used to assess various homeostatic and metabolic processes of the body. Urine is easily collected, but the procedure must be performed completely and accurately. If there is an error in procedure, false or invalid test results can occur.

The four basic urine collection procedures, which are based on the time or duration of the collection period, are as follows: the first morning specimen, the random specimen, the fractional specimen, and the timed specimen. Because the purposes and methods vary, each of these procedures is discussed separately in subsequent sections of this chapter.

In addition to spontaneous voiding, several other possible methods of collection are available. A description of the special collection methods is presented here. When urine cannot be collected by normal voiding, these special methods are used for any of the basic collection procedures.

### Special Collection Methods

**Catheterization.**   A catheterized specimen is used when the patient cannot void or when an indwelling catheter is already in place. For straight catheterization, a sterile catheter is inserted through the urethra and into the bladder. The urine flows from the bladder, through the catheter, and into the specimen container. Once the bladder has been emptied, the catheter is removed.

With an indwelling catheter, fresh urine is collected directly from the catheter in all types of tests except the timed specimen. For the single urine specimen collection, the catheter is clamped below the port temporarily. After a short interval, a sterile needle and syringe are used to remove the urine sample through a special port in the catheter. Then the clamp is removed, and the urine flow to the collection bag resumes. A timed specimen has a much longer collection period and requires a larger volume of urine. At the start of the test, a new, empty collection bag is attached to the indwelling catheter and its tubing. The urine is removed from the collection bag at intervals and is added to the specimen collection container until the time period is completed.

**Pediatric Specimens.**   If the child is toilet trained and can follow directions, the nurse can provide instructions to the parent or assist the child in the collection of the urine. For the infant or child who cannot control the release of urine voluntarily, a pediatric collection bag is used. The perineum is cleansed and dried, and then the bag is applied and fixed with an adhesive strip. For the male infant, the bag is placed over the penis. For the female infant, the bag is applied over the labia and perineum. In each gender, the rectum must be excluded to prevent the mixing of fecal matter with urine. Once the bag is in place, it is checked every 15 minutes until the urine is collected.

**Suprapubic Aspiration.** This method is used when an anaerobic culture is required or when there is a problem with external contamination of the urine culture, such as in infancy. With the use of sterile technique, the suprapubic aspiration is performed by the physician. A sterile needle is inserted through the abdominal wall above the symphysis pubis and then is advanced into the full bladder. A syringe is used to aspirate the urine specimen. The specimen is placed into a culture container, and the needle is removed. Complications with this procedure are rare (Henry, 1996).

## First Morning Specimen

(Urine)                    Synonyms: None

### Background Information

The first morning specimen is the first urine to be voided after the patient awakens from sleep. This urine has been retained in the bladder for about 6 to 8 hours. Because of the lack of fluid intake or exercise during the period of sleep, the urine is concentrated and somewhat acidic.

This type of specimen is preferred for routine screening. It is also preferred for the detection of specific substances, including nitrites, protein, and microorganisms. Concentrated urine or an incubation period is needed to readily detect these substances in the urine.

### Purpose of the Test

The first morning specimen is used for routine urinalysis that includes chemical and microscopic analysis. This specimen is also used to identify orthostatic proteinuria.

### Procedure

A clean, dry plastic or glass container with a lid is used to collect a midstream urine specimen.

### Interfering Factors

- Menstrual secretions
- Delay in the analysis of the urine
- Inadequate labeling of the specimen

### Nursing Implementation

**Pretest**

Provide a urine container with a lid.
Instruct the patient to collect a midstream voided specimen.
A midstream void means that the patient begins to urinate, and about halfway through the process the specimen is collected. With this method, the initial urine flow washes the bacteria out of the distal urethra before the specimen is collected.
In some protocols, a midstream clean-catch method is used. If this is the case, provide the patient with the materials and instructions, as presented in Table 2–3.

## Table 2–3    Midstream Clean-Catch Urine Procedure

### Purpose

This method of urine collection reduces the external sources of contamination before the urine is collected. The contaminants are the bacteria and secretions of the skin that surround the urethra and also reside in the distal portion of the urethra.

### Procedure

*Cleansing Process: Male*

The glans is exposed and cleansed with the use of three sterile cotton balls or gauze squares moistened with a mild antiseptic solution.

The first cotton ball cleanses the tissue from the urethral meatus to the ring of the glans in a single stroke. The cotton ball is then discarded. The process is repeated with the other two cotton balls, cleansing the remaining areas of the glans.

If the male is uncircumcised, the foreskin must be retracted and the tissue under the foreskin cleansed thoroughly before the preceding steps are taken.

*Cleansing Process: Female*

The labia minora are separated to expose the urinary meatus. They must then remain separated throughout the cleansing process and urine collection phase.

The exterior mucous membranes and the meatus are cleansed, with the use of three sterile cotton balls or gauze squares moistened with a mild antiseptic.

The first moist cotton ball cleanses the tissue on one side of the urinary meatus with a single stroke from front to back. The cotton ball is discarded. The second cotton ball cleanses the other side of the meatus with the same motion and direction. The third cotton ball cleanses the center of the meatus, wiping in a single motion, also from front to back.

### Midstream Collection

The patient begins to void into the toilet or bedpan. The urine washes residual bacteria and secretions from the distal urethra.

At about the midpoint of voiding, the urine stream is interrupted. On release of the urine, 1 to 3 oz of urine is collected in the specimen container.

The container must not touch the perineal tissues or hair either during or after collection. The patient's fingers must not touch the inside of the container or lid.

Once the amount of urine in the container is sufficient, the patient finishes voiding into the toilet or bedpan, and the remaining amount is discarded.

### Posttest

Seal the lid of the container completely to prevent leakage.

Label the container (not the lid) appropriately with the patient's name and other pertinent information, including the date and time of the collection.

Ensure that the specimen is delivered to the laboratory immediately. If a delay is anticipated, the specimen must be refrigerated or a preservative added to the urine container.

### Quality Control

With a delay of 2 hours or more before analysis is performed, the nonrefrigerated, unpreserved specimen can undergo a number of changes. The changes vary among the individual specimens, but almost every laboratory value can be altered.

## Random Specimen

(Urine)                           Synonyms: None

### Background Information

The random urine specimen is one that can be collected at any time. It is easy and convenient for the patient because there is no need to plan or schedule the test. Even though the daytime activities of fluid intake and exercise alter the composition of the urine, there is no need to control these variables. The specimen is usually satisfactory for the purposes of screening or routine urinalysis.

Cytologic studies are also performed on random urine samples. For this test, the patient must drink extra fluids before each of several urine sample collections. The goal is to flush out an increased number of cells so that the detection of abnormal cells is enhanced. Random samples are also used for urine cultures, with the goal of identifying microbial growth and the presence of infection.

### Purpose of the Test

The random specimen is used for routine urinalysis that includes chemical and microscopic examination. This method of collection is also used for bacterial culture and cytologic studies to help identify the cause of disease in the urinary tract.

### Procedure

For routine urinalysis or a random urine screen, a clean plastic or glass container with a lid is used to collect a urine sample at any time. A midstream clean-catch method is used (see Table 2–3).

For bacterial, fungal, or viral culture, a sterile plastic or glass container with a lid is used to collect the random urine sample. The midstream clean-catch method is used. In special cases, a catheter or suprapubic aspiration is used to obtain the random specimen.

For cytologic studies, the midstream clean-catch method is used to collect each specimen in a clean plastic or glass container with a lid. Daily specimens are collected for 3 to 5 consecutive days.

### Interfering Factors

- Menstrual secretions
- Delay in the analysis of the urine
- Inadequate labeling of the specimen
- Contamination of the specimen

### Nursing Implementation

**Pretest**

Provide written and verbal instructions regarding how to cleanse the urethral meatus and surrounding tissue and how to collect the specimen.

Provide the appropriate collection container or containers.

For cytologic studies, instruct the patient to drink 24 to 32 oz of water each hour for 2 hours before voiding.

In some laboratory protocols, the patient is also instructed to exercise for 5 minutes by skipping or jumping rope before voiding. The activity and fluid volume should increase the yield of cells needed for the study. This process is repeated daily for 3 to 5 days to provide for the analysis of three to five consecutive urine specimens (Brunzel, 1994).

## Posttest

Seal the lid of the container completely to prevent leakage.

Label the container (not the lid) appropriately with the patient's name and other pertinent information, including the date and time of the collection.

Ensure that the specimen is delivered to the laboratory immediately. If there is an anticipated delay, the specimen must be refrigerated or a preservative added to the urine container.

### Quality Control

With a delay of 2 hours or more before analysis is performed, the nonrefrigerated, unpreserved specimen can undergo a number of changes. The changes vary among the individual specimens, but almost every laboratory value can be altered.

## Fractional Specimen

**(Urine)**                    Synonym: Double-voided specimen

### Background Information

A fractional collection of urine is a method used to compare a particular component of the urine with the serum level of that component. Blood samples and urine samples are collected at specific times, and the laboratory analysis measures the amount of the component found in each specimen.

The serum sample is measured for the blood level during controlled conditions such as in a fasting state or after administration of a dye or solute. The urine samples are measured for the baseline and renal threshold values. One example of fractional collection is the glucose tolerance test, presented in Chapter 20.

### Purpose of the Test

Fractional collection is used to compare blood and urine values in screening for diabetes mellitus and in the diagnosis of some liver and kidney disorders.

### Procedure

Generally, baseline blood and urine specimens are obtained first. The patient then receives a measured intravenous or oral substance such as food, dye, or glucose. Thereafter, timed blood and urine specimens are collected.

### Interfering Factors

- Failure to complete the pretest preparation
- Failure to collect all urine specimens
- Failure to obtain all urine specimens at the correct times
- Failure to label all specimens accurately

**Nursing Implementation**

### Pretest

Provide the patient with written and verbal instructions. Some of these tests require nothing-by-mouth (NPO) status for 6 to 8 hours before the test. Some have instructions to void and discard the first morning specimen.

### During the Test

Administer the prescribed glucose solution, injectable dye, or other measured substance used in the test.

Collect each urine specimen in a separate container at the specific time interval required by the protocol.

Label each container (not the lid) with the patient's name and other appropriate identifying information. The time of each voided specimen is also recorded on the container (e.g., ½-hour specimen, 1-hour specimen).

### Posttest

Send all specimens to the laboratory together without delay.

### Quality Control

If a delay of more than 2 hours occurs, the specimens must be preserved by refrigeration. Many components of urine are altered when the specimen remains warm and a delay occurs in performing the analysis. In particular, the level of urinary glucose becomes falsely decreased because of cellular and bacterial glycolysis.

## Timed Specimen

**(Urine)**     Synonyms: None

## Background Information

Timed collection is used for the quantitative analysis of a specific urinary component. Circadian rhythms, diurnal rhythms, metabolism, exercise, and hydration all affect the excretion rate of substances in the urine. At certain times during a 24-hour period, the excretion of substances such as electrolytes, hormones, proteins, and urobilinogen increases, and at other times excretion decreases. By collecting the quantity of urine over a specified period, accuracy of measurement is greater than that with a random specimen.

Sometimes, an abnormal substance is not present consistently in the urine. Thus, the urine is collected for a longer period, in the hope of identifying small amounts of the component that are occasionally present. Urine cytologic testing requires a 2-hour collection period repeated over several days. The parasites *Schistosoma* and *Onchocerca* are detected in urine that is collected over a 24-hour period.

**Time Intervals**

The designated time period for a urine collection depends on the specific component to be tested. Some tests are for a *predetermined length of time,* such as a 2-hour, 12-hour, or 24-hour urine collection. Other tests are for a *specific time of day,* such as 12 PM to 4 PM. In these instances, the time frame reflects when the substance is maximally excreted in the urine each day.

| | |
|---|---|
| **Purpose of the Test** | The timed collection is used to perform quantitative urine assays and clearance tests and to identify abnormal cytology, or ova and parasites in the urine. |

**Procedure**

A large (3,000-mL) clear or brown glass or plastic container with a lid is used to collect all urine within the designated period.

**Quality Control**

To prevent changes in the quality of the urine over time, all timed specimen containers are kept cool in a basin of ice or in the refrigerator. Some tests require that a preservative be added to the container before the collections begin. Information about the additive is found in the written laboratory protocol for the particular test.

**Interfering Factors**

- Failure to discard the first voided specimen before the procedure begins
- Failure to collect all the urine voided during the test period
- Failure to refrigerate or preserve the urine specimen
- Improper labeling

**Nursing Implementation**

**Pretest**

Provide both written and verbal instructions regarding the collection of the urine. These instructions must include the specific times for the collection period.

Advise the patient who works or is in school that it is easiest to collect the specimen on the weekend.

For a 24-hour urine collection, advise the patient to moderately limit fluid intake during the collection period. Alcohol intake should be avoided for 24 hours before and during any timed collection of urine.

Other restrictions are part of specific test protocols. Some tests have specific dietary restrictions, and some medications need to be withheld for a specific period. Any special restrictions or modifications are included in the patient's pretest instructions.

**During the Test**

For all timed collections, maintain the specimen and container on ice or in the refrigerator during the collection period. Such measures prevent deterioration of the specimen.

During the time period, all urine is added to the collection container. If any urine spills or if a specimen is discarded accidentally, the test is invalid. The stored specimen is discarded, and a new collection period is started on the following day.

For the 24-hour urine collection, the first void of the morning is discarded, and the urine collection period begins at 8 AM. Place all urine for 24 hours into the container. This includes the first voided specimen of the next morning.

*Critical Thinking 2–3*
A 4-year-old child completed the 24-hour urine collection, but the mother states that the child "wet the bed during the night." What instructions do you give to the mother?

### Posttest

Label the container (not the lid) with the patient's name and other appropriate identifying data. Include the time and date of the start and the completion of the urine collection period.

Arrange for prompt delivery of the specimen to the laboratory.

## References

Abel, L., & Fuellen, G. (1996). Reduction of contaminated urine specimens in pregnant women. *Nurse Practitioner: American Journal of Primary Health Care, 21*(7), 6, 8, 11.

Adult urinalysis screening. (1995). *Nurse Practitioner, 20*(9), 55–56.

Baer, D. M. (1995). Blood waste draws. *Medical Laboratory Observer, 27*(7), 12.

Brunzel, N. A. (1994). *Fundamentals of urine and body fluid analysis.* Philadelphia: W. B. Saunders.

Chernow, B., Jackson, E., Miller, J., & Wiese, J. (1996). Blood conservation in acute care and critical care. *AACN Clinical Issues: Advanced Practice in Critical Care, 7*, 191–197.

Dech, Z. F., & Szaflarski, N. L. (1996). Nursing strategies to minimize blood loss associated with phlebotomy. *AACN Clinical Issues: Advanced Practice in Critical Care, 7*, 277–287.

Ernst, D. J. (1995). Flawless phlebotomy. Becoming a great collector. *Nursing 95, 25*(10), 54.

Henry, J. B. (1996). *Clinical diagnosis and management* (19th ed.). Philadelphia: W. B. Saunders.

Jacobs, D. S., Demott, W. R., Grady, H. J., Horvat, R. T., Huestis, D. W., & Kasten, B. L. (1996). *Laboratory test handbook* (4th ed.). Baltimore: Williams & Wilkins.

McConnell, E. (1997). Performing Allen's test. *Nursing 97, 27*(11), 26.

Millam, D. A. (1993). How to teach good venipuncture technique. *American Journal of Nursing, 93*(7), 38–41.

Stepp, C. A., & Woods, M. A. (1998). *Laboratory procedures for medical office personnel.* Philadelphia: W. B. Saunders.

Tietz, N. W. (1995). *Clinical guide to laboratory tests* (3rd ed.). Philadelphia: W. B. Saunders.

Wilson, J. R., & Gaedeke, M. K. (1996). Blood conservation in neonatal and pediatric populations. *AACN Clinical Issues: Advanced Practice in Critical Care, 7*, 229–237.

# PART II

# Multisystem Laboratory Tests

# CHAPTER 3

# Urinalysis Screen

Urinalysis is one of the oldest and most common laboratory tests in existence. It produces a large amount of information about possible diseases of the kidneys and lower urinary tract as well as about systemic diseases that alter the composition of the urine. Urinalysis is also valuable because normal results are used to exclude a number of possible alternative diagnoses.

Urinalysis has several additional advantages over more sophisticated alternatives, particularly in the initial stage of diagnosis. Urinalysis is economical, and the analysis can be performed rapidly. Furthermore, the specimen can be obtained easily, noninvasively, and without risk to the patient.

## Laboratory Tests

Urinalysis  38
   Color, clarity  39
   Specific gravity  39
   pH  40
   Protein  40
   Bilirubin  41

Urobilinogen  41
Glucose  41
Ketones  41
Occult blood  41
Red blood cells  41
White blood cells  42

Bacteria  43
Leukocyte esterase  43
Casts  43
Crystals  43

## Urinalysis

**(Urine)**  Synonym: UA

**Normal Values**

| | | | |
|---|---|---|---|
| Color: | Yellow, clear | Occult blood: | Negative |
| Specific gravity: | 1.003–1.029 | RBCs (male): | 0–3 per HPF |
| pH: | 4.5–7.8 | RBCs (female): | 0–5 per HPF |
| Protein: | Negative | WBCs: | 0–5 per HPF |
| Bilirubin: | Negative | Bacteria: | Negative |
| Urobilinogen: | Normal | Leukocyte esterase: | Negative |
| Glucose: | Negative | Casts: | 0–4 hyaline |
| Ketones: | Negative | | casts per LPF |
| Home test, blood: | Negative; normal | Crystals: | Few |
| Home test, bacteria: | Negative; normal | | |
| Home test, glucose: | Negative | | |
| Home test, protein: | Negative | | |

## Background Information

Analysis of the urine consists of two parts: the chemical analysis and the microscopic analysis. The chemical analysis is usually performed by dipstick method (Fig. 3–1). Microscopic analysis may be done routinely but is more likely done in response to a specific request or as a follow-up to an abnormal result in the chemical analysis.

The dipstick method is also used routinely in point-of-care testing, such as at the patient's bedside, in physicians' offices, and in home testing. With the reagent strips, the process of analysis is rapid, accurate, and inexpensive. Treatment can begin more promptly (Zalonga, 1993).

When microscopic analysis is performed in the laboratory, the initial phase is a scanning of the specimen under a low-power field (LPF). The purpose is to search for cells, casts, and crystals. If these components are located, the microscopic high-power field (HPF) is used to obtain greater detail about the findings.

**Color and Clarity.**  Normal urine is yellow and clear. The yellow varies in tone from pale to stronger yellow, depending on the urine's concentration and specific gravity. There are many possible changes of color or clarity, some of which are presented in Table 3–1. In addition, some medications and chemicals are responsible for changes in urine color.

**Specific Gravity.**  The specific gravity is a measurement of the ability of the kidneys to con- centrate and excrete the urine. The measurement indicates the proportion of dissolved solid components to water. In the normal elderly population, the specific gravity decreases proportionately with advancing years.

Concentrated urine has a higher specific gravity because the proportion of components to water in its composition is greater. For example, a specific gravity greater than 1.020 indicates concentrated urine with a composition of more solute or less water, or both. If glucose or protein is present in the urine, the specific gravity value also rises. The presence of these additional abnormal components must be considered in the evaluation of the findings.

Diluted urine has a lower specific gravity because it contains fewer components in proportion to the amount of water. For example, a specific gravity less than 1.009 indicates diluted urine with a composition of less solute or more water, or both.

In the individual with healthy renal function and normal fluid intake, the specific gravity of the initial glomerular filtrate is 1.010. In normal physiology, as the filtrate passes through the tubule system, an ongoing exchange of solutes and water alters the specific gravity of the filtrate and ultimately the urine. When the specific gravity of urine remains *fixed* (unvarying over time) at 1.010, that value is an indication of severe renal

**Figure 3–1**

Urinalysis: Dipstick method. A commercial reagent strip for urine chemistry testing and its container with color comparison chart. The reagent-impregnated test pads are fixed to an inert plastic strip. Once the strip has been wetted in a urine sample, a chemical reaction causes the reagent pad to change color. Results are obtained by comparing the color of the reagent pad to the appropriate analyte on the color chart. (Reproduced with permission from Brunzel, N. A. [1994]. *Fundamentals of urine and body fluid analysis* [p. 149]. Philadelphia: W. B. Saunders.)

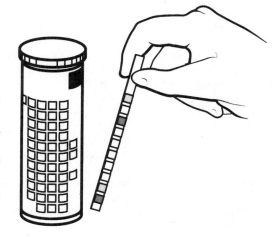

**Table 3–1 Causes of Change in Urine Color and Clarity**

| Characteristic | Cause |
| --- | --- |
| *Clarity* | |
| Cloudy, smoky, hazy | Pyuria |
| | Bacteriuria |
| | Phosphates in the urine |
| *Color* | |
| Colorless | Overhydration |
| | Diuretic therapy |
| | Diabetes mellitus |
| | Diabetes insipidus |
| Dark | Acute intermittent porphyria |
| Red or pink | Hematuria |
| | Ingestion of beets, berries, fava beans, red food coloring, rhubarb |
| Dark yellow or orange | Bile |
| Green | *Pseudomonas* bacteriuria |
| | Urinary bile pigments |

damage. When the specific gravity of the urine is the same as that of the glomerular filtrate, it indicates that the renal tubules cannot resorb water and effectively concentrate the urine.

**pH.** With an average dietary intake and normal metabolism, the body produces a continuous supply of hydrogen ions and acids. As part of the acid-base balance, the kidneys remove excess hydrogen ions from the blood and excrete them in the urine.

The urinary pH is affected by dietary intake. A large intake of acidic fruits or protein causes the urine to be more acidic, with a lower urinary pH value. A large intake of citrus fruits and vegetables causes the urine to be more alkaline, with a higher urinary pH value. A normal dietary intake produces slightly acidic urine, with an average pH value of 6.0.

In abnormal physiology, a urine pH greater than 6.5 indicates the presence of bicarbonate in the urine. Alkaline urine may occur because of systemic alkalosis (respiratory or metabolic). It also may occur because of a renal tubular disorder, with the decreased ability of the renal tubules to form ammonia and exchange hydrogen ions for cations such as sodium. Metabolic acidosis results from the tubular damage and the inability to regulate acid-base balance. In urine with a pH greater than 7.0, calcium carbonate, calcium phosphate, or magnesium ammonium phosphate stones can form.

A urinary pH less than 5.5 indicates the absence of bicarbonate ions in the urine. The cause of the problem may be systemic acidosis (respiratory or metabolic), with the excess hydrogen ions of the extracellular fluids spilling into the urine. Xanthine, cystine, or uric acid stones can form in highly acidic urine.

**Protein.** In normal physiology, minimal amounts of protein are excreted in the urine, mostly as albumin. The albumin is filtered out by glomeruli, with a greater amount released into the urine during the daytime or after strenuous exercise.

The presence of excess urinary albumin is an indicator of glomerular disease. The nephrotic syndrome produces a great loss of albumin in the urine. The renal loss may also be associated with systemic disease that causes glomerular damage (Gosling, 1995; Statland, 1993).

The dipstick method may be used to detect protein in the random urine sample. This rapid assessment method is useful in detecting albumin, but it is less sensitive to globulins and other plasma proteins that enter the urine (Zalonga, 1993). It cannot detect the small amounts of protein that appear in the urine during the early stage of renal damage, and the dipstick method is not sensitive enough to detect low-molecular-weight proteins in the urine. Because of decreased sensitivity to small amounts of protein and small protein molecules, the dipstick method may produce a false-negative result. (Additional discussion of urinary protein is presented in Chapter 21.)

**Bilirubin.** Bilirubinuria is an abnormal finding that results from an increase in the serum conjugated (direct) bilirubin. The level of urine bilirubin rises in some conditions of hepatocellular jaundice and liver disease. Bilirubinuria is frequently present in obstructive jaundice, with either intrahepatic or extrahepatic biliary obstruction. The test for bilirubin does not measure the unconjugated (indirect) bilirubin that is caused by hemolytic jaundice, because these bilirubin molecules cannot pass through the glomeruli easily. (Additional discussion of bilirubin is presented in Chapter 19).

**Urobilinogen.** This substance is normally excreted in the urine in small amounts. When the values are low or normal, the urobilinogen cannot be detected with the dipstick method and routine urinalysis. When urobilinogen levels are elevated, urinalysis indicates the need to follow up with a 2-hour urine urobilinogen test for specific measurement. The elevated level is an indicator of damage to the liver tissue, impaired liver function, or hemolytic anemia. (A discussion of the 2-hour urine urobilinogen test is presented in Chapter 19.)

**Glucose.** Glycosuria is usually an indicator of significant hyperglycemia and diabetes mellitus. When a fasting specimen is obtained, it is highly specific and accurate in the detection of glucose in the urine. The nonfasting random sample is much less specific.

The urine glucose test is best used as a screening test for the healthy population and in monitoring control of the type II diabetic patient. The dipstick method is not sensitive enough to be useful as a quantitative measure of glucose in the urine. Because of the poor sensitivity and inability to detect hypoglycemia, the urine glucose dipstick test also is not sufficient for monitoring of the type I diabetic patient.

**Ketones.** In starvation or abnormal carbohydrate metabolism, large quantities of ketone bodies appear in the urine before the serum levels of ketones are elevated. Urinalysis is useful in monitoring known diabetics, particularly when they are ill, hyperglycemic, or pregnant.

Ketonuria is not limited to diabetics. In children, ketonuria can occur during febrile illness or as the result of severe diarrhea and vomiting. It may also occur during a normal pregnancy. Additionally, elderly individuals can experience ketonuria as the result of fasting.

**Occult Blood.** A positive result from a dipstick test for occult blood in the urine occurs when intact erythrocytes, hemoglobin, or myoglobin is present. Like gross hematuria, microscopic hematuria is caused by diseases of the kidney or lower urinary tract or by a nonurinary problem of medical origin. When the occult blood test result is positive, a microscopic examination of the urine is performed to identify red blood cells (RBCs) and RBC casts. Additional laboratory or diagnostic tests are also indicated to diagnose and locate the cause of the bleeding.

Hematuria is a relatively common finding with many possible causes. It can be an indicator of serious disease. The bleeding can be intermittent and the blood loss minimal, but these patterns bear no relationship to the severity of the disease.

Myoglobin is released from injured skeletal or cardiac muscle into the blood. Myoglobin release has many possible causes related to muscle tissue damage, including damage of a toxic, traumatic, ischemic, or infectious origin. The myoglobin is then filtered from the blood by the glomeruli and excreted in the urine. Myoglobin is associated with renal failure, but the exact relationship is unknown.

**Red Blood Cells.** Normal urine may exhibit a few RBCs without any significant pathologic cause. The presence of a few cells is considered acceptable under HPF microscopic visualization. Significant hematuria is indicated by one episode of gross hematuria or one episode of high-grade microhematuria, with an RBC count greater than 100 cells per HPF. Significant hematuria is an indicator for further diagnostic evaluation.

When accompanied by proteinuria, red cell casts, or renal tubular cells, the hematuria is usually of renal or lower urinary tract origin. When there are RBCs but no casts and only minimal proteinuria, the disorder is likely to be of urologic origin. Glomerular diseases often cause the RBCs to be misshapen, fragmented, hypochromic, and small. The cause of these RBC changes is unknown, but they may be due to the passage of RBCs through damaged glomeruli or to osmotic changes in the renal tubules.

**White Blood Cells.** There are few to no white blood cells (WBCs) in normal urine. An elevated WBC count indicates pyuria. When WBCs are clumped, it indicates severe urinary tract infection. The microscopic urinalysis finding of 5 to 10 WBCs per HPF (5 to 10 WBCs/mm$^3$) is a significant elevation that indicates the presence of urinary tract infection (Regan & Pahira, 1995). The combination of an elevated WBC count and the presence of white cell casts is an indicator of infection of renal origin.

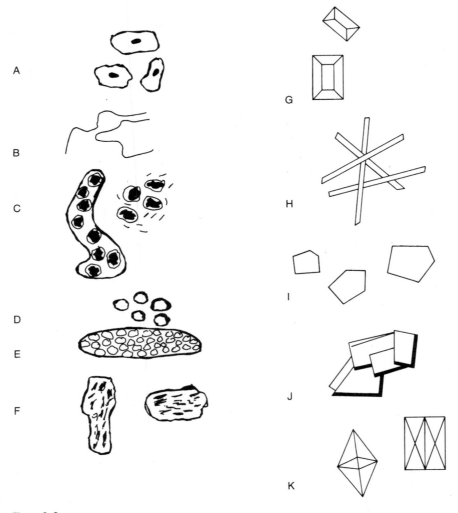

**Figure 3–2**

Elements of urinary sediment. *A*, Epithelial cells. *B*, Mucus-secreting cells. *C*, White blood cell cast, white blood cells, and bacteria. *D*, Red blood cells. *E*, Red blood cell cast. *F*, Waxy casts. *G*, Triple phosphate crystals. *H*, Calcium phosphate crystals. *I*, Cystine crystals. *J*, Uric acid crystals. *K*, Calcium oxalate crystals. (Reproduced with permission from Little, D. N., Thompson, M. E., & Thompson, D. E. [1989]. The diagnostic evaluation, urinalysis and imaging. *Primary Care, 16*, 864.)

**Bacteria.**  Most urinary tract infections are characterized by a significant number of bacteria in the urine. The bacteria are visualized during high-power microscopic examination of the centrifuged specimen. The bacteria can be characterized with a Gram's stain. The finding of a bacteria count greater than $10^5$ bacteria per milliliter is considered diagnostic of urinary tract infection.

Bacteria can also be detected with the nitrite dipstick method. In the presence of most urinary bacteria, the dipstick turns pink (positive result) within 60 seconds. This method does not measure the severity of infection or identify the type of bacteria, but it is an effective method to screen for asymptomatic bacteriuria.

**Leukocyte Esterase.**  The leukocyte esterase test is an indirect method used to detect bacteria in the urine. The dipstick method identifies lysed or intact WBCs (neutrophils). When these cells are present, the bacteria must also be present.

When leukocyte esterase is used as a screening test, it should be combined with the nitrite dipstick test to avoid false-negative results. This screening is recommended for older adults (older than 60 to 65 years), for patients with diabetes mellitus, and as part of preventive prenatal care for pregnant women (U. S. Department of Health and Human Services [USDHHS], 1995a).

When leukocytes or neutrophils are present in the urine, the leukocyte esterase dipstick turns blue in 1 minute. For greatest accuracy, the dipstick result is read in 5 minutes.

**Casts.**  Casts are globulin protein structures that are precipitated in the renal tubules. They are found in the urine sediment, and the different types are identified during microscopic examination (Fig. 3–2). The presence of a great number of casts is an indicator of renal parenchymal disease. Granular casts are associated with glomerulonephritis and renal pathologic conditions. Fatty casts are produced in the nephrotic syndrome. Cellular casts can have RBCs, WBCs, renal tubular cells, or a mix of these different cells. They are indicators of inflammation or infection of glomeruli, renal tubules, or renal interstitial tissue.

Hyaline casts are the most common type of cast, but their presence may or may not be significant. Hyaline casts can appear after strenuous exercise, with fever, or in congestive heart failure. Persistent large numbers of hyaline casts are an indication of renal disease.

**Crystals.**  Crystals are the end products of food metabolism and, when present, are found in urinary sediment. A variety of crystals can be identified by microscopic examination, based on their characteristic shapes (see Fig. 3–2). Crystals can be found in healthy urine, although most individuals have few or none present in urine.

Crystals are seen commonly in patients with urolithiasis, toxic damage to the kidneys, or chronic renal failure. Uric acid, xanthine, and cystine crystals or their calculi are often present in acidic urine. Calcium carbonate, calcium phosphate, and magnesium ammonium phosphate crystals or their calculi are often present in alkaline urine. The presence of cellular elements or crystals, or both, causes the urine to become cloudy.

**Home Testing**

Kits are available for the patient to perform some urine tests at home. Individual kits include tests for occult blood, bacteria, glucose, and protein. With home testing, the patient with a known urinary tract disorder can participate in the care. The home testing of urine can alert the patient to an early change in the condition and the need to return to the physician.

■
*Critical Thinking 3–1*
The result of the urinalysis shows an abnormally elevated count of RBCs and red cell casts. The patient does not believe that the test result is important, and he does not want to have further diagnostic tests. How should you respond?

**Purpose of the Test**

Urinalysis is performed to screen for urinary tract disorders, kidney disorders, urinary neoplasms, and other medical conditions that produce changes in the urine. This test is also used to monitor the effects of treatment of known renal or urinary conditions.

**Procedure**

A clean container with a lid is used to collect 15 mL or more of urine. A random sample may be used, but the first-voided specimen of the morning is preferred.

**Home Testing**

Collect enough urine in a container so that the reagent strip can be dipped into the specimen. The strip is dipped into the urine for about 1 second, ensuring that all chemical pads on the strip are moistened. After waiting the correct time interval (usually 1 minute), the color of the test reagent pad is compared to the corresponding color chart (Stepp & Woods, 1998). A random sample of urine may be used, but the first-voided specimen of the morning is preferred.

**Findings**

**Elevated Values**

SPECIFIC GRAVITY

Dehydration
Fever
Profuse sweating
Vomiting, diarrhea, or
  both

Glycosuria
Proteinuria
Congestive heart
  failure
Adrenal insufficiency

Altered secretion of
antidiuretic
hormone

pH

Metabolic alkalosis
Respiratory alkalosis
Bacteriuria (*Proteus*
  spp., *Pseudomonas*)

Vegetarian diet
Nasogastric
  suctioning
Prolonged vomiting

Fanconi's syndrome
Milkman's syndrome
Alkali therapy

PROTEIN

Nephrotic syndrome
Renal disorders
  associated with hy-
  pertension,
  diabetes mellitus,
  systemic lupus
  erythematosus,
  amyloidosis

UROBILINOGEN

Hemolytic anemia
Hepatitis

Cirrhosis

Congestive heart
  failure

KETONURIA

| | | |
|---|---|---|
| Acidosis | Diabetic ketoacidosis | Increased protein |
| Alcholic ketoacidosis | Fasting or starvation | intake |

CASTS

| | | |
|---|---|---|
| Glomerulonephritis | Nephrotic syndrome | Renal failure |
| Chronic renal disease | Bacterial pyelonephritis | |

OCCULT BLOOD

| | | |
|---|---|---|
| Glomerulonephritis | Goodpasture's | Poison (snake or |
| Urolithiasis | syndrome | spider bite) |
| Urinary tract infec- | Benign prostatic | Parasitic disease |
| tion | hypertrophy | Thermal or crush |
| Tumor, benign or | Blood dyscrasia, | injury |
| malignant | hemolysis of RBCs | Trauma |
| Polycystic kidney | Endocarditis | Severe exercise, |
| Renal infarct | Leukemia | jogging |
| Lupus nephritis | | |

BILIRUBIN

Hepatitis
Biliary obstruction

GLUCOSE

Hyperglycemia
Diabetes mellitus

CRYSTALS

| *Uric Acid Crystals* | *Calcium Oxalate* | *Triple Phosphate* |
|---|---|---|
| Gout | *Crystals* | *Crystals* |
| Rapid nucleic acid | Chronic renal failure | Obstructive uropathy |
| turnover | Ethylene glycol | Urinary tract infec- |
| Urolithiasis | ingestion | tion |
| | Urolithiasis | Urolithiasis |

RED BLOOD CELLS

| | | |
|---|---|---|
| Benign tumor | IgA neuropathy | Urinary tract infec- |
| Carcinoma | Lupus nephritis | tion |
| Urinary calculi | Sclerosis | Trauma from exercise |
| Glomerulonephritis | | |

WHITE BLOOD CELLS

Urinary tract infec-
tion (cystitis,
prostatitis, urethri-
tis, pyelonephritis)

BACTERIA

| Chronic urinary tract infection | Pyelonephritis | Cystitis, acute or chronic |

**Decreased Values**

SPECIFIC GRAVITY

| Overhydration | Pyelonephritis | Severe renal damage |
| Diuresis | Glomerulonephritis | Diabetes insipidus |
| Hypotension | Renal tubular dysfunction | |

pH

| Metabolic acidosis | Diarrhea | Emphysema |
| Respiratory acidosis | Starvation | Renal failure |
| Diabetes mellitus | | |

*Critical Thinking 3–2*
As a child recovers from acute glomerulonephritis, how do partic-ular urinalysis findings help evaluate the patient's response to treatment?

**Interfering Factors**

- Insufficient quantity of urine
- Contamination of the specimen
- Prolonged delay before analysis is performed
- Warming of the specimen

**Nursing Implementation**

**Pretest**

Instruct the patient to collect a sample of urine, preferably on arising in the morning. The specimen must not be contaminated by toilet paper, toilet water, feces, or secretions. Women should not collect urine during menstruation, to prevent contamination with bloody discharge.

**Posttest**

Label the container with the patient's name, the time, and the date of the voiding.
Arrange for transport of the specimen to the laboratory as soon as possible, because the most accurate results are obtained from warm, fresh specimens.

**Quality Control**

Refrigeration preserves the elements of the urine, but the delay can cause crystals to precipitate. If the specimen stands at room temperature for too long, the warmth causes decomposition of the bacteria and WBCs.

### Table 3–2  Accuracy in the Performance of Urinary Dipstick Testing

Keep the container of test strips tightly closed when it is not in use. To prevent deterioration of the chemicals, protect the strips from exposure to light, heat, and moisture.

Perform the test on a fresh sample of urine without delay.

As the reagent strip is removed from the urine, tap the strip gently on the specimen container to remove excess urine.

For each test, wait the required time before reading the results.

Read the test results in a setting that has good lighting. Hold the strip in a horizontal position to prevent the mixing of chemicals from one pad to another.

In comparing the test pad to the manufacturer's color chart, align the squares and tests accurately. Do not allow the moist strip to touch the chart and discolor the squares.

### Home Testing

Teach the patient to follow the manufacturer's instructions exactly (Table 3–2). The collection container must be free of any residual detergent, cleanser, and fabric softener. These contaminants can cause a false-positive result for albumin (Tietz, 1995).

Demonstrate how to perform the color comparison of the pads on the moistened test strip with the color chart, including recognition of normal and abnormal results.

Advise the patient to notify the physician of abnormal changes.

### Critical Value

**The presence of a massive amount of oxalate crystals in fresh urine**

This finding is an indication of intoxication with ethylene glycol (antifreeze). The physician must be notified of this result immediately because of the toxicity of the substance and the potential for central nervous system depression, cardiopulmonary symptoms, and renal damage.

## References

Brunzel, N. A. (1994). *Fundamentals of urine and body fluid analysis.* Philadelphia: W. B. Saunders.

Burtis, C. A., & Ashwood, E. R. (Eds.). (1999). *Tietz textbook of clinical chemistry* (3rd ed.). Philadelphia: W. B. Saunders.

Geyer, S. J. (1993). Urinalysis and urinary sediment in patients with renal disease. *Laboratory Clinics of North America, 13,* 13–20.

Gosling, P. (1995). Microalbuminuria: A marker of systemic disease. *British Journal of Hospital Medicine, 54,* 285–290.

Henry, J. B. (Ed.). (1996). *Clinical diagnosis and management by laboratory methods* (19th ed.). Philadelphia: W. B. Saunders.

Jacobs, D. S., Dermott, W. R., Grady, H. J., Horvat, R. T., Huestis, D. W., & Kasten, B. L. (Eds.). (1996). *Laboratory test handbook* (4th ed.). Baltimore: Williams & Wilkins.

Lehmann, C. A. (1998). *Saunders manual of clinical laboratory sciences.* Philadelphia: W. B. Saunders.

Monane, M., Gurwitz, J. H., Lipsitz, L. A., Glynn, R. J., Choodnovskiy, I., & Avorn, J. (1995). Epidemiologic and diagnostic aspects of bacteriuria: A longitudinal study in older women. *Journal of the American Geriatrics Society, 43,* 618–622.

Monferdini, D., Joinville, M., & Grove, W. (1995). Improving urine sediment analysis. *Laboratory Medicine, 26,* 660–664.

Regan, T. C., & Pahira, J. J. (1995). UTI in men: How to recognize, how to treat. *Consultant, 35,* 1162–1166.

Seidman, E. J. (1997). Office diagnosis of microscopic hematuria: Methodology and clinical significance. *Hospital Medicine, 33*(1), 22–26.

Statland, B. E. (1993). Urine albumin. *Medical Laboratory Observer, 25*(1), 14.

Stepp, C. A., & Woods, M. A. (1998). *Laboratory procedures for medical office personnel.* Philadelphia: W. B. Saunders.

Tietz, N. W. (Ed.). (1995). *Clinical guide to laboratory tests* (3rd ed.). Philadelphia: W. B. Saunders.

U. S. Department of Health and Human Services. (1995a). Clinical guidelines. Adult urinalysis screening. *Nurse Practitioner, 20*(9), 55–56.

U. S. Department of Health and Human Services. (1995b).

Put prevention into practice. Urinalysis. *Journal of the American Academy of Nurse Practitioners, 7*(3), 125–128.

Zalonga, G. P. (1993). Reagent testing: Rapid, accurate urine testing at the bedside . . . Part 1. *Consultant, 33*(6), 90–92, 95–98.

# CHAPTER 4

# Hematology Screen

The *cells* of the blood consist of erythrocytes (red blood cells), leukocytes (white blood cells), platelets, and lymphocytes. The bone marrow is responsible for hematopoiesis and some lymphocytopoiesis (Table 4–1). The marrow responds to stimuli from the microenvironment for the initiation and continuation of hematopoiesis. The blood cells originate from hematopoietic stem cells, with formation, differentiation along specific lines, proliferation, and maturation occurring during hematopoiesis. When the cells are mature enough, they are released into the blood.

The process of hematopoiesis is supported by colony-stimulating factors (Rodak, 1995). These hormonelike glycoproteins stimulate and regulate hematopoiesis so that sufficient numbers of specific cells are available in the blood. Under normal conditions, the number of circulating blood cells of each type remains constant, with a balance between the rate of cell loss and the rate of cell production.

The process of lymphocytopoiesis originates in the lymphoid stem cells. The lymphoid stem cells form lymphocytes along two different lines. In the bone marrow, B lymphocytes are formed and released into the blood and lymphatic fluids. With stimulation from antigens, the B lymphocytes become plasma cells and release antibodies. After the initial differentiation of the lymphoid stem cell in the marrow, the thymus gland and secondary lymphoid organs form the second line of lymphocytes—the T lymphocytes—which are released into lymphatic fluid and, ultimately, into the blood.

This chapter focuses on the basic tests of red blood cells, white blood cells, and platelets. The tests include those that determine the number, concentration, and structure of the cells. (Chapter 6 focuses on coagulation tests, and Chapter 17 addresses the diverse hematologic tests and procedures related to the blood cells and bone marrow.)

## Laboratory Tests

| | | |
|---|---|---|
| Complete Blood Cell Count 49 | Platelet Count 61 | Reticulocyte Count 70 |
| Hematocrit 53 | Platelet Indices 65 | White Blood Cell Count 71 |
| Hemoglobin 55 | Red Blood Cell Count 66 | White Blood Cell Differential |
| Peripheral Blood Smear 57 | Red Cell Indices 68 | Count 75 |

## Complete Blood Cell Count

**(Blood)**  Synonyms: None

**Normal Values**

**White Blood Cell Count (WBC)**
$4.5–11 \times 10^3/\mu L$ *or* SI $4.5–11 \times 10^9/L$
**Red Blood Cell Count (RBC)**
Male: $4.5–5.9 \times 10^6/\mu L$ *or* SI $4.5–5.9 \times 10^{12}/L$
Female: $4.5–5.1 \times 10^6/\mu L$ *or* SI $4.5–5.1 \times 10^{12}/L$

*Continued on following page*

*Continued*

**Hemoglobin**
Male: 14.0–17.5 g/dL *or* SI 140–175 g/L
Female: 12.3–15.3 g/dL *or* SI 123–153 g/L
**Hematocrit**
Male: 41.5%–50.4% *or* SI 0.415–0.504 (volume fraction)
Female: 35.9%–44.6% *or* SI 0.38–0.47 (volume fraction)
**Red Cell Indices**
Mean corpuscular volume (MCV): 80–96 ($\mu m^3$ *or* SI 80–96 fL
Mean corpuscular hemoglobin (MCH): 27.5–33.2 pg *or* SI 27.5–33.2 pg
**Mean Corpuscular Hemoglobin Concentration (MCHC)**
33.4%–35.5% *or* SI 0.334–0.355 (concentration fraction)
**Red Cell Distribution Width (RDW-CV)**
13.1% (range: 11.6%–14.6%) (Henry, 1996)
**Platelet Count**
Adult: 150,000–450,000 cells/$\mu$L *or* SI 150–450 × 10$^9$/L
Newborn (1–3 days): 150,000–400,000 cells/$\mu$L *or* SI 150–400 × 10$^9$/L (Lehmann, 1998)

---

**Table 4–1   Hematopoiesis and Lymphocytopoiesis**

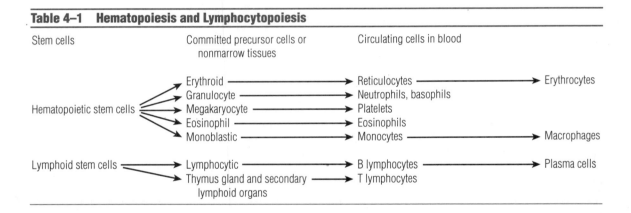

| Stem cells | Committed precursor cells or nonmarrow tissues | Circulating cells in blood |
|---|---|---|
| Hematopoietic stem cells | Erythroid → | Reticulocytes → Erythrocytes |
| | Granulocyte → | Neutrophils, basophils |
| | Megakaryocyte → | Platelets |
| | Eosinophil → | Eosinophils |
| | Monoblastic → | Monocytes → Macrophages |
| Lymphoid stem cells → | Lymphocytic → | B lymphocytes → Plasma cells |
| | Thymus gland and secondary lymphoid organs → | T lymphocytes |

---

## Background Information

The basic hematology screen consists of a complete blood cell count (CBC) and a peripheral blood smear. The CBC provides the count of each type of blood cell in the circulation, measurements of the hemoglobin and hematocrit, and measurements of the parameters of the erythrocyte by red cell indices. The WBC differential provides the counts of each type of leukocyte. The peripheral blood smear provides a microscopic view of the blood cells to verify the count and to identify abnormalities of cellular shapes and structures.

**Automated Analyzers.**   Today, the CBC is carried out by automated hematology analyzers. The defi-nition of the *complete* blood count has changed with the increasing sophistication of automation. The CBC is often an "abbreviated" blood count based on the technical capability of the particular analyzer used (Koepke, 1993). Generally, automated analyzers include analyses of the hemoglobin, hematocrit, red cell count, red cell indices, white cell count, and platelet count. Some CBC findings include some or all parts of the white blood cell (WBC) differential. Some of the CBC reports include platelet indices, although the interpretation and clinical use of this component is still undergoing scientific examination. In some institutions, the platelet count, the differential cell count, the reticulocyte count, and the peripheral smear are not part of the basic CBC and must be ordered separately.

**Technology of the Analyzers.**  The different types of analyzers are based on the principles of either *electric impedance* or *light scattering*. Based on the characteristics of the cells, the analyzers are able to identify the different cells and count them (Ward, Lehman, & Leiken, 1994).

In electric impedance methodology, the analyzer measures the difference in electric conductivity as each cell passes through a tiny opening in the electric field. The analyzer differentiates among the cells based on cell size. For the differential cell count, reagents are used to alter the cell's nucleus and cytoplasm. The analyzer can then differentiate among some or all of the types of leukocytes and count them.

In light scatter methodology, each cell passes through a quartz flow cell in the analyzer. As the cells pass through in single file, they cross a beam of laser light. As the cell interrupts the beam, it results in a scattering of light in all directions. The patterns of light scattering are detected, and the computer recognizes the distinct pattern that is characteristic of each cell type. The computer analysis provides the count and cell sizing for the different types of cells. The structures inside each blood cell are also identified by the scattering pattern of laser light so that hemoglobin, cell nuclei, and the characteristics of cytoplasm are identified and classified.

**Reference Values.**  The common reference values of the CBC are those obtained by manual analysis procedures. The manual methods produce values that are usually higher, because small amounts of plasma adhere to the walls of the collection tube as the fluid and cells are removed. This is particularly true when capillary tubes are used to collect the specimens.

The values of the automated analyzers are accurate and precise for most cell counts. Because there are many different types of analyzers and several methods of analysis, the interpretation of the values should be based on the reference values of the specific laboratory that performed the test.

This discussion of the CBC provides an overview of different parts of the test as performed for screening purposes. Each component is also presented later as an individual test, with more depth of discussion. The patient may be monitored by repeated CBC testing or by the specific component tests that are pertinent to the health problem and its treatment.

---

## Purpose of the Test

■

*Critical Thinking 4–1*
An infant has severe diarrhea, and you suspect that one of the nursing diagnoses is fluid volume deficit. Which components of the CBC are pertinent in this case? Why would the results be elevated?

The CBC is used to assess the patient for anemia, infection, inflammation, polycythemia, hemolytic disease, the effects of ABO incompatibility, leukemia, and dehydration status. It is also used to identify the cellular characteristics of the peripheral blood.

---

## Procedure

A purple-topped tube with ethylenediaminetetraacetic acid (EDTA) anticoagulant is used to collect 10 mL of venous blood. As an alternative, two purple-tipped capillary tubes can be used to collect blood from a heelstick, earlobe, or finger puncture.

For the peripheral blood smear, two slides are prepared immediately using drops of venous or capillary blood.

**Quality Control**

With venipuncture, the tourniquet should be tied lightly for a brief time to prevent pooling of cells in the vein at the site of blood collection. The venipuncture technique must be smooth, with a blood flow that fills the vacuum tube readily. If the blood demonstrates excessive turbulence because of a flawed venipuncture technique, the hemolysis of the erythrocytes will alter the test results. After the blood is collected, the tube is gently inverted 5 to 10 times to mix the anticoagulant and prevent clotting.

---

**Findings**

**Elevated Values**

WHITE BLOOD CELL COUNT

| Infection | Inflammation | Leukemia |

RED BLOOD CELL COUNT

| Polycythemia | Renal tumor | Hemoconcentration |

HEMOGLOBIN

| Polycythemia | Hemoconcentration |

HEMATOCRIT

| Polycythemia | Hemoconcentration |

RED BLOOD CELL INDICES

| MCV: Pernicious anemia, vitamin $B_{12}$ or folate deficiency | MCHC: Hereditary spherocytosis | RDW: Microcytic anemias |
| MCH: Hereditary spherocytosis | | |

PLATELETS

| Myeloproliferative diseases | Postsplenectomy response | Renal disease |
| Multiple myeloma | Hodgkin's disease | Infection or inflammation |
| Iron deficiency anemia | Lymphomas | |

**Decreased Values**

WHITE BLOOD CELLS

| Aplastic anemia | Pernicious anemia |
| Bone marrow depression | Some infectious or parasitic diseases |

RED BLOOD CELLS

| Hemorrhage | Aplastic anemia | Hemolysis of erythrocytes |
| Hemodilution | Bone marrow depression | |
| Anemia | | |

HEMOGLOBIN

| Hemorrhage | Hemolysis of | Hemodilution |
| Anemia | erythrocytes | |

HEMATOCRIT

| Hemorrhage | Hemolysis of | Hemodilution |
| Anemia | erythrocytes | |

RED BLOOD CELL INDICES

| MCV: Iron deficiency anemia, chronic inflammation | MCH: Iron deficiency anemia | MCHC: Iron deficiency anemia |

PLATELETS

| Idiopathic thrombo- cytopenic purpura | Disseminated intravascular coagulation | Systemic lupus erythematosus |
| Aplastic anemia | Bone marrow depression | Uremia |
| Anemias | | Liver disease |
| Malignancy of the spleen | | |

---

**Interfering Factors**

- Hemolysis
- Coagulation of the specimen
- Hemodilution

---

**Nursing Implementation**

Nursing care includes care of the venipuncture or capillary puncture site in addition to other implementation measures.

### During the Test

Ensure that the blood is not taken from the hand or arm that has an intravenous line. Hemodilution with intravenous fluids causes a false decrease in the values of some tests.

### Posttest

Arrange for prompt transport of the specimen. If there is an anticipated delay, refrigerate the specimen.

---

## Hematocrit

**(Blood)**   Synonyms: Hct, microhematocrit

---

**Normal Values**

Male: 41.5%–50.4% *or* SI 0.415–0.504 (volume fraction)
Female: 35.9%–44.6% *or* SI 0.359–0.446 (volume fraction)

## Background Information

The hematocrit is a measurement of the proportion of whole blood volume occupied by erythrocytes. The value is expressed as a percentage or fraction of cells to whole blood. For example, a hematocrit value of 40% means that there are 40 mL of erythrocytes in 1 dL of blood.

**Variations of Normal Values.**   In laboratory analysis performed by the manual method, the normal value is slightly higher than in that performed by the automated method. Additionally, regardless of the test methodology, the normal value for males is slightly higher than that for females. The pregnant female has a slightly lower normal value than that of the nonpregnant female because of the greater blood volume during pregnancy. In men older than 65 years, the normal value is slightly lower than that for younger males. For all individuals, the normal value can be 5% to 6% lower when blood is drawn with the patient in a recumbent position as opposed to an upright position (Jacobs et al., 1996).

**Elevated Values.**   The hematocrit rises when the number of erythrocytes increases or when the plasma fluid volume is reduced. When the fluid volume is decreased, the blood becomes concentrated, with increased viscosity.

**Decreased Values.**   The hematocrit falls to less than normal when an excessive loss of erythrocytes occurs, as in anemia or after excessive bleeding. It can also decrease because of excessive intravenous fluids that exert a dilution effect.

In bleeding or hemorrhage, the hematocrit drops several hours after the bleeding episode. The severity of the drop in value correlates directly with the amount of blood lost.

---

**Purpose of the Test**    The hematocrit is useful in the evaluation of blood loss, anemia, hemolytic anemia, polycythemia, and dehydration.

---

**Procedure**    A purple-topped tube with EDTA is used to collect 7 mL of venous blood. As an alternative, two purple-tipped capillary tubes can be used to collect blood from a heelstick, earlobe, or finger puncture.

### Quality Control

With venipuncture, the tourniquet should be tied lightly for a brief time to prevent pooling of cells in the vein at the site of blood collection. Venipuncture technique must be smooth, with a blood flow that fills the vacuum tube readily. If the blood shows excessive turbulence because of flawed venipuncture technique, the hemolysis of the erythrocytes will alter the test results. After the blood is collected, the tube is inverted gently 5 to 10 times to mix the anticoagulant and prevent clotting.

---

**Findings**

### Elevated Values

| | | |
|---|---|---|
| Polycythemia vera | Acute thermal injury | Dehydration |
| Secondary poly- cythemia | Extreme physical exertion | Chronic obstructive lung disease |
| Addison's disease | Hemoconcentration | |

### Decreased Values

| | | |
|---|---|---|
| Recent hemorrhage | Fluid retention | Hemodilution |
| Anemia | Cirrhosis | Leukemia |
| Fluid overload | Hemolytic anemia | Lymphoma |

| | |
|---|---|
| **Interfering Factors** | • Hemolysis<br>• Coagulation of the specimen<br>• Hemodilution |

**Nursing Implementation**

Nursing care includes care of the venipuncture or capillary puncture site in addition to other implementation measures.

**Pretest**

When the patient is hemorrhaging or has just had a severe bleeding episode, both hemoglobin and hematocrit values are monitored at regular intervals. The decreased results indicate the severity of the blood loss.

Likewise, after transfusion replacement of packed cells or whole blood, the same tests are used to monitor for rising values that indicate effectiveness of treatment. Ensure that the tests are performed at the indicated times.

**During the Test**

Ensure that the blood sample is not taken from a vein in the hand or arm with an intravenous line. Hemodilution with intravenous fluids or plasma will lower the hematocrit value falsely.

**Posttest**

Arrange for the prompt transport of the specimen to the laboratory. If there is an anticipated delay, refrigerate the specimen to prevent the deterioration of cells.

**Critical Values**

**>54% (SI >0.54 [volume fraction]) *or* <18% (SI <0.18 [volume fraction])**

The nurse should assess the patient, including vital signs. The physician must be notified immediately of a severely increased value and the assessment findings. A critical value usually occurs because of too few red blood cells (as after a hemorrhage) or too much intravascular fluid (as in fluid overload).

## Hemoglobin

**(Blood)**

Synonyms: Hgb, Hb

**Normal Values**

Male: 14.0–17.5 g/dL *or* SI 140–175 g/L
Female: 12.3–15.3 g/dL *or* SI 123–153 g/L
Child (5 years): 11.7–13.7 g/dL *or* SI 117–137 g/L
Infant (5–7 months): 10.8–12.2 g/dL *or* SI 108–122 g/L
Newborn (1 day): 17.3–21.5 g/dL *or* SI 173–215 g/L

## Background Information

Hemoglobin is the oxygen-carrying compound contained in each erythrocyte. The large amount of hemoglobin and the broad surface area of each erythrocyte enable the red blood cells to have a large oxygen-carrying capacity and to function with great efficiency.

Each hemoglobin molecule consists of the protein *globin* and the iron-containing pigment *heme*. At the lungs, the heme molecules combine with oxygen for transport to the cells. At the cell level, oxygen is released and the globin molecule combines with a molecule of carbon dioxide for the return trip to the lungs.

**Variation in Normal Values.**   The normal value of hemoglobin varies among individuals of different ages, genders, races, and geographic locations. The normal hemoglobin value is higher in males than in females. After age 10 years, the hemoglobin value is slightly lower in African Americans than in whites. Men older than 65 years have a slightly lower value than do younger men. The normal value is slightly higher in individuals who live in high-altitude areas. The value is 5% to 6% lower in patients who have their blood drawn when in a recumbent position as opposed to an upright position (Jacobs et al., 1996).

**Elevated Values.**   An elevated hemoglobin value may be a result of excess production of erythrocytes or a result of dehydration.

**Decreased Values.**   An individual generally is considered anemic when the hemoglobin value for the male is less than 13 g/dL (SI <130 g/L) and for the female is less than 11 g/dL (SI <110 g/L). The low value can be caused by a low red blood cell count, by a lack of hemoglobin in each erythrocyte, or by fluid retention. In fluid retention, red blood cell counts and hemoglobin values are relatively low because of the disproportionate amount of water in the blood.

## Purpose of the Test

The hemoglobin is used to measure the severity of anemia or polycythemia, and it monitors the response to treatment of anemia. It is also used to calculate the MCH and MCHC values.

## Procedure

A purple-topped tube with EDTA is used to collect 7 mL of venous blood. As an alternative, two purple-tipped capillary tubes can be used to collect blood from a heelstick, earlobe, or finger puncture.

### Quality Control

With venipuncture, the tourniquet should be tied lightly for a brief time to prevent pooling of cells in the vein at the site of blood collection. A smooth venipuncture technique will produce a blood flow that fills the vacuum tube readily. If the blood has excessive turbulence because of flawed venipuncture technique, the hemolysis of the erythrocytes will alter the test results. After the blood is collected, the tube is inverted gently 5 to 10 times to mix the anticoagulant and prevent clotting.

## Findings

### Elevated Values

| | | |
|---|---|---|
| Polycythemia vera | Acute thermal injury | Chronic obstructive |
| Secondary poly- | Dehydration | pulmonary disease |
| cythemia | Hemoconcentration | |

**Decreased Values**

| | | |
|---|---|---|
| Recent bleeding | Pregnancy | Cirrhosis of the liver |
| Fluid retention | Hemorrhage | Hyperthyroidism |
| Hemolysis of red blood cells | Anemia | |

## Interfering Factors

- Hemolysis
- Coagulation of the specimen
- Lipemia
- White blood cell count greater than $50 \times 10^3/\mu L$ (SI >$50 \times 10^9/L$)

## Nursing Implementation

Nursing care includes care of the venipuncture or capillary puncture site.

### Pretest

When the patient is hemorrhaging or has just had a severe bleeding episode, both hemoglobin and hematocrit measurements are taken at regular intervals. The results indicate the severity of the blood loss. Likewise, after transfusion replacement of packed cells or whole blood, the same tests are used to evaluate the effectiveness of treatment. Ensure that the tests are performed at the indicated times.

### During the Test

Ensure that the blood sample is not taken from the hand or arm that has an intravenous line in the vein because of the dilution effect on red blood cell concentration.

### Posttest

Arrange for prompt transport of the specimen to the laboratory. If a delay is anticipated, refrigerate the specimen to prevent deterioration of the cells.

■

*Critical Thinking 4–2*
At the nursing health center, a routine CBC for a 3-year-old child reveals a hemoglobin value of 10.6 g/dL (SI 106 g/L). To help validate the suspected nursing diagnosis of altered nutrition: less than body requirements, what additional assessment data are needed?

## Critical Values

**<6.0 g/dL (SI <60 g/L) *or* >18 g/dL (SI >180/L)**

The physician should be notified immediately of either of these extreme values. When the rate of change occurs slowly, the patient may not experience symptoms, particularly when resting. Further laboratory investigation is indicated to determine the cause of the abnormal finding.

## Peripheral Blood Smear

**(Blood)**    Synonym: Blood smear morphology

## Normal Values

Normal cell morphology

## Background Information

The peripheral blood smear is a visual microscopic examination of stained blood cells. In most hematologic diseases, characteristic changes can be seen in the blood cells. Changes in the size, structure, and shape of the cells or changes in the number and distribution of the cells may occur, or a combination of these changes may be seen. The microscopic visualization of these changes helps diagnose or confirm the hematologic diagnosis. The three hematologic lines of leukocytes, erythrocytes, and platelets can be examined in the peripheral blood smear.

For quality assurance or total quality management, a microscopic examination of slides is performed manually to check the accuracy of the cell counts performed by automated technology. The manual examination is also performed to visually identify abnormal cells that are flagged during the automated cell count. Lastly, the slides provide additional information when the patient's condition indicates unexplained or suspicious findings.

Digital image processing may also be used to perform some automated aspects of the examination. Slides are prepared, and the equipment performs the microscopic examination. The characteristics of the cells are compared with those of the cells in the computer memory. The normal cells match the computer software categories. They are identified, differentiated, and counted. Abnormal cells or unknown cells do not have a match in the computer data. The computer marks these cells and indicates their location on the slide. The technician or pathologist investigates the abnormalities in a second review.

### Morphologic Features of Red Blood Cells.
Normal erythrocytes are circular, nonnucleated discs of uniform size, color, shape, and cytoplasmic appearance. The cells are paler in the center than in the periphery. They are described as *normocytic* (normal in size) and *normochromic* (normal in color). The patient can be anemic despite these normal characteristics. A normocytic, normochromic anemia is one that is caused by hemolysis of erythrocytes or blood loss. The cells are normal, but too few of them exist.

Abnormal erythrocytes vary in size, color, hemoglobin content, shape, staining properties, and structure. The altered size is due to a defect in erythropoiesis. The bone marrow can be adversely affected by genetics, poor nutrition, changes in bone marrow cells, or changes in bone marrow function.

Abnormal color is due to an alteration in hemoglobin content. Too little hemoglobin causes a pale color. The problem may be due to iron deficiency or abnormal hemoglobin synthesis.

Poikilocytosis refers to abnormally shaped red cells. Abnormal erythrocyte structure includes the presence of a nucleus that identifies these cells as normoblasts, basophilic stippling, Howell-Jolly bodies, or Heinz bodies. The variations of some of the characteristics of erythrocytes, and their relationships to hematologic disease, are presented in Table 4–2.

### Morphologic Features of White Blood Cells.
The microscopic evaluation of leukocytes is the same as the differential count. There are five types of leukocytes: neutrophils, eosinophils, basophils, monocytes, and lymphocytes. These cells should be within a normal range in number, concentration, and stage of maturity. A complete discussion of these cells is presented later (see White Blood Cell Differential Count).

### Morphologic Features of Platelets.
The microscopic evaluation of platelets provides an estimate of the platelet count, with an evaluation of the size and structure of the cytoplasm of the cell. The increased concentration of large cells occurs in myeloproliferative diseases and immune thrombocytopenia.

---

**Purpose of the Test**   The cells of the blood are examined microscopically to help identify causes of anemia and to evaluate the function of the bone marrow. Abnormal cell counts, concentrations, or morphologic features are investigated, and the accuracy of cell counts performed by automated technology is also assessed.

**Table 4–2  Characteristics of Erythrocytes—Relationships to Hematologic Diseases**

| Characteristics | Interpretation | Pathophysiology | Associated Disorders |
| --- | --- | --- | --- |
| *Size* | | | |
| Normocytic | Normal cell size | Adequate response by the bone marrow | None |
| | | Shortened life span of the erythrocytes–increased hemolysis | Acute blood loss<br>Hemolytic anemia |
| | | Impaired release of iron from the reticuloendothelial system | Anemia of chronic disease |
| Macrocytic or megalocytic | Larger than normal cell size | Marrow disorder with defective DNA that affects cell development during erythropoiesis | Deficiency of vitamin $B_{12}$ or folic acid<br>Megaloblastic anemias |
| | | Uptake of cholesterol and bile salts by the erythrocyte membranes | Liver disease and obstructive jaundice |
| Microcytic | Smaller than normal cell size | Deficiency of heme, a lack of iron, or impaired hemoglobin synthesis | Iron deficiency anemia, thalassemia, sideroblastic anemia, lead poisoning, vitamin $B_6$ deficiency |
| *Color* | | | |
| Normochromic | Normal hemoglobin content | Normal iron stores, normal hemoglobin synthesis | Anemia due to hemorrhage, with loss of erythrocytes |
| Hyperchromic | Erythrocyte saturated with hemoglobin | A relative increase of hemoglobin within the erythrocyte that has a small diameter and small cell membrane; the cell is spherical | Spherocytosis |
| Hypochromic | Erythrocyte with diminished hemoglobin | Iron deficiency in proportion to erythropoiesis | Iron deficiency anemia |
| | | Defective hemoglobin synthesis | Thalassemia, lead poisoning, sideroblastic anemia |
| *Shape* | | | |
| Elliptocyte | Elliptical or oval shape | Cytoplasm and cholesterol in the cell membrane are polarized in areas of convexity; increased hemolysis can occur | Hereditary elliptocytosis, thalassema, iron deficiency anemia, sickle cell disease, other hemolytic diseases |
| Spherocyte | Sphere-shaped cell | Genetic disease of the bone marrow; the abnormal cells have a shorter life span | Hereditary spherocytosis, immune disease, and other hemolytic anemias |
| Target cell | Hemoglobin is distributed on the perimeter and in the center, giving a "target" appearance | Deficient hemoglobin for the normal cell size | Hemoglobin C, D, S diseases, thalassemia, iron deficiency anemia |
| | | Too large a cell membrane and cell size for a normal amount of hemoglobin | Obstructive jaundice, liver disease |

*(continued on the following page)*

**Table 4–2   Characteristics of Erythrocytes—Relationships to Hematologic Diseases** *(continued)*

| Characteristics | Interpretation | Pathophysiology | Associated Disorders |
|---|---|---|---|
| *Shape (continued)* | | | |
| Sickle cell | Crescent-shaped cells | In conditions of deoxygenation, the hemoglobin S becomes elongated and rigid; cell membranes also become sickle shaped | Sickle cell trait, sickle cell disease, other sickling hemoglobinopathies |
| Poikilocytosis | Varied, irregular shapes of cells (teardrop, tennis racket, horned, and helmet shapes) | Irreversible alteration of cell membrane from rapid erythropoiesis or extramedullary erythropoiesis | Megaloblastic anemia, hemolytic anemia, uremia, liver disease, metastatic cancer, toxicity, idiopathic myelofibrosis |
| Schistocyte | Red cell fragments | Partial splitting or phagocytosis of the cell, without loss of hemoglobin | Hemolytic anemia, disseminated intravascular coagulation, malignant hypertension, cancer, cardiac valve prosthesis, burns, uremia |
| *Structure* | | | |
| Nucleated | Normoblasts are immature red cells with nuclei | Normal in fetus or infant, but not in adults; extreme demand on bone marrow to produce cells rapidly | Erythroblastosis fetalis, thalassemia major |
| | | Extramedullary erythropoiesis | Idiopathic myelofibrosis |
| | | With neutrophilia, the bone marrow cells are altered | Leukemia, metastatic cancer of the bone marrow, multiple myeloma, Gaucher's disease |
| Basophilic stippling | Basophilic granules in cells | Abnormal hemoglobin synthesis and increased erythropoiesis | Lead poisoning, megaloblastic anemia |
| Howell-Jolly bodies | Remnants of nuclear material in cells | Abnormal erythropoiesis | Postsplenectomy, megaloblastic anemia, hemolytic anemia |
| Heinz bodies | Irregular patches of hemoglobin in cells | Genetic abnormality of hemoglobin formation; hemoglobin is oxidized and nonfunctional | Cell injury, hemoglobinopathy, hemolytic anemia |

**Procedure**   A purple-topped tube with EDTA is used to collect 7 mL of venous blood. As an alternative, two purple-tipped capillary tubes can be used to collect blood from a heelstick, earlobe, or finger puncture.

For the peripheral blood smear, two slides are prepared immediately using drops of venous or capillary blood.

### Quality Control

> With venipuncture, the tourniquet should be tied lightly for a brief time to prevent pooling of cells in the vein at the site of blood collection. A smooth venipuncture technique will allow the blood to flow into the vacuum tube readily. Flawed venipuncture technique will produce excessive turbulence, causing hemolysis of the erythrocytes and altering the test results. The tube is gently inverted 5 to 10 times after the blood is collected to mix the anticoagulant and prevent clotting.

**Findings**    See Table 4–2 for abnormal values.

**Interfering Factors**
- Hemolysis
- Coagulation
- Inadequate slide preparation technique

**Nursing Implementation**    Nursing care includes care of the venipuncture or capillary puncture site.

### During the Test

When collecting venous blood, the tube must be filled. This prevents degenerative changes in the cells because of too much EDTA.

When heelstick, finger, or earlobe puncture is used, do not use the first drop of blood or squeeze the tissue. This helps limit the presence of endothelial cells and damaged blood cells.

### Posttest

Arrange for prompt transport of the specimen to the laboratory.

### Quality Control

> Degenerative changes in neutrophils occur within 30 minutes. Enlargement of platelets occurs after 3 hours. If there is a delay before the blood is analyzed, the specimen must be refrigerated.

## Platelet Count
**(Blood)**    Synonym: Thrombocyte count

**Normal Values**    150,000–400,000 cells/µL *or* SI 150–400 × $10^9$/L

### Background Information

Platelets are the product of erythropoiesis of the bone marrow. After activity by the pluripotential and hematopoietic stem cells in the marrow, the line develops further through megakaryocyte cell division and the formation of the promegakaryocyte cell. During the next 7 to 10 days, a megakaryocyte matures, and fragments of its cytoplasm break off and enter the circulation as platelets. About

2,000 to 7,000 platelets are formed from one megakaryocyte. Two thirds of the total platelets are present in the circulation, and the remainder are stored in the spleen. The life span of the platelet in the circulation is 8 to 11 days (Dixon, 1997; Henry, 1996).

Platelets function to initiate the process of coagulation. When there is a nick or opening in a blood vessel, platelets quickly aggregate, adhere to the endothelial surface of the blood vessel, and plug the opening. As additional platelets and clotting factors arrive, the clot becomes firm and seals off the opening effectively (Fig. 4–1).

**Variation in Normal Values.** In laboratory testing, considerable variation exists in the normal platelet count reference range. Newborns have a wider range of normal values than do adults. The normal value is slightly decreased during menstruation and pregnancy. The platelet count is also reduced relative to the excess fluid in the blood. This dilution effect occurs with the administration of nonplatelet fluids, including intravenous fluids and packed red cell transfusions (Drew, 1996). When the platelets are counted, variation exists between the reference range performed by manual counting and that carried out by an automated counter. Analysis of the test results is based on the reference value provided by the laboratory that performs the cell count.

**Elevated Values.** *Thrombocytosis* is an excess number of platelets (>400,000 cells/μL *or* SI

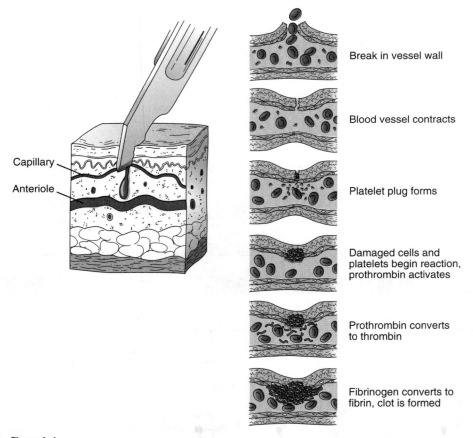

Capillary

Anteriole

Break in vessel wall

Blood vessel contracts

Platelet plug forms

Damaged cells and platelets begin reaction, prothrombin activates

Prothrombin converts to thrombin

Fibrinogen converts to fibrin, clot is formed

**Figure 4–1**
Process of clot formation. The platelets create a plug at the break in the blood vessel, followed by the process of clot formation. (Reproduced with permission from Stepp, C. A., & Woods, M. A. [1998]. *Laboratory procedures for medical office personnel* [p. 111]. Philadelphia: W. B. Saunders.)

>400 × 10⁹/L) in the blood. The condition may be reactive, in response to acute inflammatory disease, blood loss, or trauma. The platelets are produced at a faster rate in response to platelet loss. This condition rarely causes symptoms and is self-limiting. The level of platelets returns to a normal value as the underlying condition is corrected. Thrombocytosis may also be a symptom of myeloproliferative disease, such as chronic myelocytic leukemia. The platelet count rises severely, and potential exists for hemorrhage or thrombosis. Bleeding probably results from defects in the platelets and the inability to form a clot. Thrombosis in either veins or arteries can occur as platelets aggregate and trap erythrocytes in the microcirculation. Common sites of vascular occlusion include the splenic, hepatic, and pulmonary veins; the mesenteric and axillary arteries; and the fingers and toes (Rodak, 1995).

**Decreased Values.**    Thrombocytopenia is a decreased number of platelets (<100,000 cells/μL *or* SI <100 × 10⁹/L) in the blood. This condition causes a prolonged bleeding time because the the patient's clotting ability is seriously compromised. The decrease in platelets is caused by three possible categories of pathophysiologic change: (1) deficient platelet production, (2) rapid platelet destruction, and (3) abnormal pooling of the platelets (Table 4–3). The most common cause is the accelerated destruction of platelets. The bone marrow responds with accelerated production of new cells, but when the platelet destruction is rapid and extensive, the response of the marrow is inadequate. With inadequate numbers of platelets, the patient is vulnerable to bleeding, particularly into the skin.

---

## Purpose of the Test

The platelet count is used to assess the ability of the bone marrow to produce platelets and to identify the destruction or loss of platelets in the circulation. It is also used to evaluate the untoward effects of chemotherapy or radiation treatment.

---

## Procedure

A purple-topped tube with EDTA is used to collect 7 mL of venous blood. As an alternative, two purple-tipped capillary tubes are used to collect blood from a heelstick, earlobe, or finger puncture.

### Quality Control

When venipuncture is performed, the tourniquet should be tied lightly for a brief time to prevent pooling of cells in the vein at the site of blood collection. Venipuncture technique must be smooth, with a blood flow that fills the vacuum tube readily. If excessive turbulence of the blood results from flawed venipuncture technique, the erythrocytes will undergo hemolysis, altering test results. After the blood is collected, the tube is gently inverted 5 to 10 times to mix the anticoagulant and prevent clotting.

---

## Findings

■

*Critical Thinking 4–3*
Your patient's platelet count is 47,000 cells/μL (SI 47 × 10⁹ cells/L). What nursing actions should be implemented immediately?

### Elevated Values

Myeloproliferative
 diseases
Polycythemia vera
Myelofibrosis
Chronic myelocytic
 leukemia
Thrombocythemia
Posthemorrhage
 regeneration

Iron deficiency
 anemia
Multiple myeloma
Postsplenectomy
 response
Acute or chronic
 infection

Inflammatory
 diseases
Hodgkin's disease
Lymphoma
Chronic renal disease
Renal cysts

**Table 4–3 Pathophysiologic Causes of Thrombocytopenia**

| Category | Pathophysiology | Cause |
|---|---|---|
| Deficient platelet production | Impairment of bone marrow with reduced numbers of stem cells or megakaryocytes | Drugs, aplastic anemia, radiation chemotherapy, malignancy of the bone marrow |
| | Ineffective thrombopoiesis | Deficiency of iron, vitamin $B_{12}$, folic acid |
| | Defective production or regulation of thrombopoietin | Inherited genetic disorder |
| Platelet destruction | *Intracorpuscular destruction* | Inherited genetic disorder |
| | Defects in platelet structure with short platelet life span | |
| | *Extracorpuscular destruction* | Autoimmune processes |
| | Immunologic destruction of platelets by IgG antibodies | Infection |
| | Excess clotting or mechanical damage to platelets | Disseminated intravascular coagulation |
| | | Infection |
| | | Cardiac valve replacement |
| | | Microvascular clotting disorder |
| Abnormal distribution or pooling | Splenic disorder with hypersplenism | Malignancy, infection infiltrates, congestion |

**Decreased Values**

Idiopathic thrombocytopenic purpura
Megaloblastic anemia
Liver disease
Infection
Massive blood transfusion
Malignancy of the spleen
Radiation-chemotherapy

Fanconi's syndrome
Wiskott-Aldrich syndrome
Uremia
Systemic lupus erythematosus
Aplastic anemia
Severe iron deficiency anemia

Parasitic diseases (malaria, toxoplasmosis, histoplasmosis)
Disseminated intravascular coagulation
Thyroid disease
Eclampsia

**Interfering Factors**

- Platelet clumping
- Multiple transfusions

**Nursing Implementation**

**Pretest**

Instruct the patient to avoid strenuous exercise before the test, because exertion and stress elevate the test results temporarily.

**Posttest**

Assess the venipuncture site for signs of bleeding or ecchymosis.

To promote clotting, use sterile gauze to apply pressure to the site, or raise the arm above the head while maintaining pressure on the site.

When the platelet count is decreased, institute measures to protect the patient from trauma, bruising, or cuts. Do not advocate the use of aspirin for any reason, because this medication interferes with the platelets' ability to adhere in the clotting process.

| Critical Values | **<50,000 cells/µL (SI <50 × 10⁹/L) or >1,000,000 cells/µL** |
|---|---|

**<50,000 cells/µL (SI <50 × 10⁹/L) or >1,000,000 cells/µL**

The physician should be notified of the abnormal result immediately. When the platelet count is at or beyond either extreme value, the risk of spontaneous hemorrhage or thrombosis is increased. Superficial bleeding in the skin is evidenced by petechiae, purpura, or ecchymosis. Epistaxis (a nosebleed) or bleeding from the gingiva in the mouth may occur. Of more serious consequence is a hemorrhage into the brain, causing a stroke. Thrombosis can occur anywhere throughout the body, including the brain, abdominal organs, and heart (Rodak, 1995).

## Platelet Indices

**(Blood)**                    Synonyms: Platelet sizing, mean platelet volume (MPV), platelet distribution width (PDW)

| Normal Values | Mean platelet volume: 7.4–10.4 fL<br>Platelet distribution width: 2–4 µm in diameter |
|---|---|

### Background Information

Platelet indices evaluate the quality of the platelets by measurements of the volume and size of these cells. The automated cell counter can report the platelet cell size and mean platelet volume. This new test is similar in concept to the red cell indices that provide the measurements of erythrocytes. At this time, platelet indices have few clinical applications, and the significance of the data is not fully understood.

The mean platelet volume increases when the platelet count decreases. In patients with a low platelet count, the high mean platelet value correlates directly with a decreased tendency to bleed, and the patient has less risk of hemorrhage. Large-size platelets are usually newly released, young platelets. The larger platelets are thought to be more effective in hemostasis than those of smaller size and older age (Jacobs et al., 1996).

### Purpose of the Test

The platelet indices may be used in the diagnosis of hematologic disease, in assessment of platelet function, and in guiding the need for platelet transfusion in patients with thrombocytopenia.

### Procedure

A lavender-topped tube with EDTA is used to collect 7 mL of venous blood.

### Findings

**Elevated Values**

| MPV: Idiopathic thrombocytopenic purpura (ITP) | PDW: Idiopathic thrombocytopenic purpura (ITP) | Preeclampsia<br>Bernard-Soulier syndrome |
|---|---|---|

**Decreased Values**

| | | |
|---|---|---|
| PDW: Wiskott-Aldrich syndrome | Autoimmune thrombocytopenia Leukemia | Enlargement of the spleen |

---

**Interfering Factors**

- Platelet count of <10,000 cells/μL (SI <10 × 10⁹/L)

---

**Nursing Implementation**

**Posttest**

Assess the puncture site for signs of bleeding or ecchymosis.
To promote clotting, use sterile gauze to apply pressure to the site or raise the arm above the head while maintaining pressure on the site.

---

## Red Blood Cell Count

**(Blood)**        Synonyms: RBC, red cell count, erythrocyte count

---

**Normal Values**

> Male: $4.5–5.9 \times 10^6$ μL *or* SI $4.5–5.9 \times 10^{12}$/L
> Female: $4.5–5.1 \times 10^6$/μL *or* SI $4.5–5.1 \times 10^{12}$/L

---

### Background Information

Erythropoiesis, the formation of erythrocytes, occurs in the bone marrow. The red blood cell production begins with the division and maturation of the pluripotential and hematopoietic stem cells. In response to decreased oxygen tension and the stimulus of erythropoietin, the ongoing cell division, differentiation, and maturation proceed along the erythrocyte line until reticulocytes are produced. After remaining in the marrow for 1 to 2 days, the reticulocytes are released into the blood. The reticulocytes reach the final stage of maturity in 1 to 2 additional days in the blood. The erythrocytes function to transport oxygen from the lungs to the cells and to transport carbon dioxide from the cells to the lungs.

The maintenance of a normal number of erythrocytes in the blood is dependent on the ability of the bone marrow to continuously replace the erythrocytes that are lost or destroyed. Because of the fragility of the cell membrane, the life span of the RBC is approximately 120 days. The bone marrow must produce approximately 1 million new erythrocytes per second to maintain adequate replacement.

The stimulus for additional production of erythrocytes is cellular oxygen deficiency that triggers the flow of erythropoietin by the kidneys. Erythropoietin is a colony-stimulating factor that promotes erythropoiesis at various stages of differentiation in the bone marrow.

Numerous factors can create an imbalance between erythrocyte production and destruction. With excess production and a normal rate of destruction, the red blood cell count is elevated. With either diminished production or excess destruction of red cells in the blood, their number is decreased.

**Variation in Normal Values.** The normal red cell count is higher in men than in women, and it is higher in individuals who live at high altitudes (Jacobs, 1996). The normal value is lower in men older than 65 years than in younger men. The red cell count is 5% to 6% lower when the blood is drawn from a recumbent patient than from one in an upright position.

**Elevated Values.** Increases in the red cell count may be a result of hyperactivity of the bone marrow cells or a result of an increase in erythropoietin from renal disease. Relative polycythemia may also produce an increased red cell count. When this problem is caused by dehydration, there is a normal number of erythrocytes, but they are concentrated in the diminished fluid volume of the plasma.

Decreased Values.   Decreases in the red blood cell count can occur from an excessive loss of cells,

as in hemorrhage. It can also occur because of rapid or accelerated hemolysis of the red blood cells. When the bone marrow tissue is damaged by excess radiation or chemotherapy, or when a lack of erythropoietin from renal disease exists, too few red cells are produced, and the blood count is low.

## Purpose of the Test

The red cell count is used to evaluate anemia and polycythemia.

## Procedure

A purple-topped tube with EDTA is used to collect 7 mL of venous blood. As an alternative, two purple-tipped capillary tubes can be used to collect blood from a heelstick, earlobe, or finger puncture.

### Quality Control

With venipuncture, the tourniquet should be tied lightly for a brief time to prevent pooling of cells at the site of blood collection. A smooth venipuncture technique produces a blood flow that fills the vacuum tube readily. If the blood demonstrates excessive turbulence because of flawed venipuncture technique, the hemolysis of the erythrocytes will alter the test results. After the blood is collected, the tube is gently inverted 5 to 10 times to mix the anticoagulant and prevent clotting.

## Findings

### Elevated Values

| | | |
|---|---|---|
| Polycythemia vera | Renal carcinoma | Renal cyst |
| Secondary poly-<br>cythemia | Cerebral hemangio-<br>blastoma | |
| Hemoconcentration | | |

### Decreased Values

| | | |
|---|---|---|
| Anemia | Aplastic anemia | Glucose-6-phosphate |
| Immune response<br>with hemolysis | Recent hemorrhage<br>or blood loss | dehydrogenase<br>deficiency |
| Hemodilution or<br>excess intravenous<br>fluids | Bone marrow failure | |

## Interfering Factors

- Hemolysis
- Coagulation of the specimen
- Hemodilution

## Nursing Implementation

Nursing care includes care of the venipuncture or capillary puncture site.

### Pretest

Plan to obtain the specimen when the patient is calm and rested. Exercise, exertion, and fear all increase the red blood cell count.

### During the Test

Ensure that the arm or hand that has an intravenous line is not used to obtain the specimen. Intravenous fluid dilutes the blood and falsely decreases the cell count.

## Red Cell Indices

**(Blood)**   Synonyms: Erythrocyte indices, blood indices

| Normal Values | MCV: 80–96 µm³ *or* SI 80–96 fL <br> MCH: 27.5–33.2 pg *or* SI 27.5–33.2 pg <br> MCHC: 33.4%–35.5% *or* SI 0.334–0.355 (concentration fraction) <br> RDW-CV: 13.1% (range 11.6%–14.6%) (Henry, 1996) |
|---|---|

### Background Information

The red cell indices are a measure of the quality and characteristics of the erythrocyte and hemoglobin concentration. The abnormalities of the erythrocyte are used in the classification and evaluation of the different anemias. The indices consist of the MCV, MCH, and MCHC.

The values may be arithmetically calculated by using the values of the red cell count, the hemoglobin concentration, and the hematocrit. Today, however, most laboratories use automated blood analyzers, and the indices are automatically included in the CBC. In the automated count, a fourth category—the RDW—is also included. The reference values vary somewhat, depending on the method of analysis and the equipment used. To avoid misinterpretation, the evaluation of the test results should be based on the reference values of the laboratory that performs the procedure.

**Mean Corpuscular Volume.**   The MCV calculates the average erythrocyte size. The unit value may be expressed in femtoliters (fL) or cubic micrometers (µm³). The measurements are equivalent (1 fL = 1 µm³). If the MCV value is elevated, the erythrocytes are large, or *macrocytic*. If the MCV value is decreased, the erythrocytes are small, or microcytic.

**Mean Corpuscular Hemoglobin.**   The MCH calculates the weight of the hemoglobin in the average erythrocyte. The hemoglobin weight is expressed in picograms (pg). One picogram is equivalent to 1 micromicrogram (1 pg = 1 µµg). The MCH value is elevated when the erythrocyte is macrocytic and decreased when the erythrocyte is microcytic.

**Mean Corpuscular Hemoglobin Concentration.** The MCHC value measures the average concentration or percentage of hemoglobin in the average erythrocyte. When the MCHC value is elevated, a high concentration of hemoglobin exists in the erythrocyte, and the cell is hyperchromic. When the value is in a normal range, the red cell is normochromic. When the MCHC value is decreased, a lower concentration of hemoglobin exists, and the erythrocyte is hypochromic.

**Red Cell Distribution Width.**   The RDW is a numeric calculation of the range of sizes or widths of the erythrocytes. When the RDW value is elevated, the laboratory personnel review the blood film for *anisocytosis*, a variation in the size of erythrocytes. The presence and amount of anisocytosis is used to estimate the severity of anemia and to differentiate among the microcytic anemias. Some of the microcytic anemias cause an RDW elevation, and others cause minimal or no change in this laboratory value. Research is ongoing as to the significance and application of the RDW measurement (Jacobs et al., 1996; Koepke, 1995b).

**Purpose of the Test**

The red cell indices are used to help diagnose and classify anemias by measurement of size, hemoglobin weight, and hemoglobin concentration of the average erythrocyte.

**Procedure**

A purple-topped tube with EDTA is used to collect 7 mL of venous blood. As an alternative, two purple-tipped capillary tubes can be used to collect blood from a heelstick, earlobe, or finger puncture.

### Quality Control

With venipuncture, the tourniquet should be tied lightly for a brief time to prevent pooling of cells at the site of blood collection. The tube must be nearly filled. Venipuncture technique must be smooth so that the blood flow fills the vacuum tube readily. If the blood is excessively turbulent because of flawed venipuncture technique, erythrocyte hemolysis will alter the test results. After the blood is collected, the tube is inverted gently 5 to 10 times to mix the anticoagulant and prevent clotting.

**Findings**

### Elevated Values

MCV: Pernicious anemia, vitamin $B_{12}$ or folate deficiency

MCH: Hereditary spherocytosis

MCHC: Hereditary spherocytosis

RDW: Iron deficiency anemia, vitamin $B_{12}$ or folate deficiency

Diabetic ketoacidosis
Macrocytic anemia
Pernicious anemia

### Decreased Values

MCV: Iron deficiency anemia, lead poisoning, thalassemia minor, anemia of chronic disease, microcytic anemia

MCH: Iron deficiency anemia

MCHC: Iron deficiency anemia

RDW: None

**Interfering Factors**

- Hemolysis
- Coagulation of the specimen

**Nursing Implementation**

Nursing care includes care of the venipuncture or capillary puncture site.

### Pretest

Folic acid, pyridoxine, and vitamin $B_{12}$ alter the test results. If the patient takes these vitamins, the information should be recorded on the requisition slip.

### Posttest

Arrange for prompt transport of the specimen to the laboratory.

## Reticulocyte Count

(Blood)                                        Synonym: Retic count

**Normal Values**

> Adult: Percentage of cells: 0.5%–1.5% *or* SI 0.005–0.015 (number fraction)
> Cell count: 25,000–75,000/µL *or* SI 25–75 × 10$^9$/L
> Newborn: Percentage of cells: 3.0%–7.0% *or* SI 0.03–0.07 (number fraction)

## Background Information

Reticulocytes are immature erythrocytes. They are derived from pronormoblasts and their precursors in the bone marrow. Once they are formed, they remain in the marrow for 1 to 2 days to gain additional maturity. As the reticulocytes enter the blood, they still contain a bit of RNA and less than the full complement of hemoglobin. In the next 1 to 2 days in circulation, the reticulocytes complete their maturation and synthesis of hemoglobin.

Generally, few reticulocytes exist in the circulation in proportion to the number of erythrocytes. The normal reticulocyte count is expressed as a percentage of the erythrocyte count. Newborns have higher reticulocyte counts, but the count steadily decreases in the first 2 weeks of life (Jacobs et al., 1996). Thereafter, the normal value for the infant is the same as that for the adult.

The measurement of reticulocytes can be performed by manual counting of the cells, microscopic examination of stained slides, automated differential counts, or flow cytometry. The flow cytometry method can estimate the amount of RNA in the reticulocyte and thereby distinguish between immature and older reticulocytes. The term *left shift* means that more immature cells that contain greater amounts of RNA have been released from the bone marrow. This is an indicator of bone marrow "stress" and is an early response to anemia.

**Elevated Values.** An increase in reticulocytes indicates the ability of the bone marrow to produce erythrocytes. The elevated value is considered a healthy response after a loss of erythrocytes from hemorrhage or hemolysis occurs. It is also a healthy response to anemia or to a reduced amount of hemoglobin in the red blood cells. The reticulocyte count may also rise after treatment for anemia. When the demand for erythrocytes is high, the marrow releases very immature reticulocytes into the blood rather than allow these blood cells to mature for the full time in the marrow.

**Decreased Values.** The reduced number of reticulocytes indicates that erythropoiesis is diminished by the bone marrow. The cause may be a lack of stimulation by erythropoietin, a disease that affects the bone marrow cells, or a faulty maturation process in the bone marrow.

**Purpose of the Test**

The reticulocyte count is used to evaluate erythropoiesis, distinguish among different types of anemia, assess the severity of blood loss, and evaluate the bone marrow response to treatment of anemia (Dixon, 1997).

**Procedure**

A purple-topped tube with EDTA or a green-topped tube with heparin is used to collect 7 mL of venous blood. As an alternative, two purple-tipped capillary tubes can be used to collect blood from a heelstick, earlobe, or finger puncture.

**Quality Control**

With venipuncture, the tourniquet should be tied lightly for a brief time to prevent pooling of cells in the vein at the site of blood collection. Venipuncture technique must be smooth, with a blood flow that fills the vacuum tube readily. If excessive turbulence occurs in the blood because of flawed venipuncture technique, the hemolysis of the erythrocytes will alter the test results. After the blood is collected, the tube is inverted 5 to 10 times to mix the anticoagulant and prevent clotting.

**Findings**

**Elevated Values**

Iron deficiency
anemia treatment
Pernicious anemia
treatment

Hemolytic anemia
Hemorrhage

Chronic blood loss

**Decreased Values**

Aplastic anemia
Iron deficiency
anemia
Anemia of chronic
disease

Sideroblastic anemia
Red cell aplasia
Renal disease

Endocrine disease
Pernicious anemia

**Interfering Factors**

• Multiple blood transfusions
• Coagulation of the specimen
• Hemolysis

**Nursing Implementation**

Nursing care includes care of the venipuncture or capillary puncture site.

**Pretest**

If possible, schedule this test before a blood transfusion is started. Once blood is administered, dilution of the cells occurs, and the reticulocyte count decreases in proportion to the fluid volume. If multiple transfusions were already given, the results of this test are invalid. The reticulocytes are from the transfused blood and do not indicate the current status of the patient's bone marrow function.

**During the Test**

Do not permit the blood sample to be taken from the arm in which there is intravenous tubing. The fluid administration dilutes the blood and causes a low cell count.

## White Blood Cell Count

**(Blood)**                    Synonyms: WBC, leukocyte count, white count

| Normal Values | Adult: 4.5–11 × 10³/µL *or* SI 4.5–11 × 10⁹/L<br>Child (1 year): 6,000–17,500/µL *or* SI 6–17.5 × 10⁹/L<br>Newborn: 18,000–22,000 cells/µL *or* SI 18–22 × 10⁹/L |
| --- | --- |

## Background Information

Leukocytes maintain the general function of combating infection and inflammation. The five types of leukocytes are classified into two major groups: granular and nongranular. The granular leukocytes, consisting of neutrophils, eosinophils, and basophils, are formed by their precursor cells in the bone marrow. The nongranular lymphocytes, including some lymphocytes and all monocytes, are also formed by their precursor cells in the bone marrow. Some of the lymphocytes are formed by the thymus gland and lymph glands (Fig. 4–2).

Many of the leukocytes are phagocytic in their action. They are capable of rapid mobility to an area of infection or tissue damage, where they ingest many types of foreign cells, dead cells, or microorganisms. Each leukocyte capable of phagocytosis can ingest only some of this matter before its own metabolism is interfered with and it self-destructs. Other leukocytes function in allergy, hypersensitivity, or antigen-antibody responses. Each type of cell functions in specific ways, including vasodilation or the release of toxins or secretions that assist in the protective responses against foreign matter within the body.

The normal life span of these cells varies according to the type of leukocyte and the condition of the body at the time. In normal health, the life span is a bit longer than when infection or inflammation is present. Most neutrophils have a life span of only days or hours in the presence of infection. Nongranular leukocytes appear to have a much longer life span. The bone marrow must continuously replace destroyed leukocytes to maintain the normal complement of each type of cell. In the presence of infection or inflammation, the bone marrow activity increases greatly, and many leukocytes are produced to counteract the invasion by foreign cells or substances.

**White Blood Cell Count.** The leukocyte count is the total number of the five types of leukocytes present in 1 mm³ of blood. The leukocyte count is a general indicator of infection, tissue necrosis, inflammation, or bone marrow activity. More specific diagnostic information is obtained by the differential count that identifies the numbers of each type of white blood cell.

**Variation in Normal Values.** The leukocyte count can become falsely elevated with stress or exercise or after eating a heavy meal. The normal value is higher in children younger than 5 years. The normal leukocyte count is lower in African Americans than in whites.

**Elevated Values.** Leukocytosis, an elevated number of white blood cells, occurs in response to infection and is usually directly proportionate to the degree of bacterial invasion. The elevated value may also be caused by necrosis of tissue or malignancy of the bone marrow. A white blood cell count of 11,000 to 17,000 cells (11–17 × 10³/µL *or* SI 11–17 × 10⁹/L) is considered to be a mild to moderate leukocytosis.

**Decreased Values.** When the white blood cell count falls to less than normal limits, it is called leukopenia. Mild leukopenia is indicated by a white blood cell count of 3,000 to 5,000 cells (3–5 × 10³/µL *or* SI 3–5 × 10⁹/L). Any marked decrease is usually in neutrophils, although all five forms of leukocytes may be decreased. Decreases in the leukocyte count are usually a result of bone marrow depression or particular infection that has exhausted the supply of neutrophils and bone marrow reserves.

| Purpose of the Test | The white blood cell count indicates the possible presence and severity of infection or inflammatory response. When the results are abnormal, it may indicate |
| --- | --- |

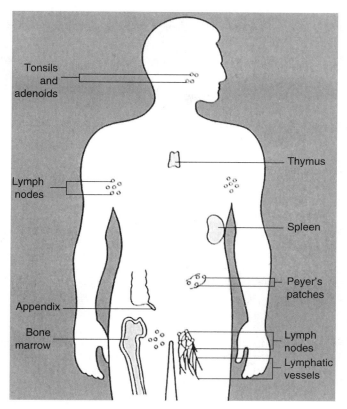

**Figure 4–2**

Organs of the immune system. The lymphocytes are produced in the bone marrow, thymus, and secondary lymphoid tissues. Some lymphocytes circulate in the blood, and others remain stored or are active in various parts of the immune system throughout the body. (Reproduced with permission from Schindler, L. W. [1988]. *Understanding the immune system* [NIH Publication No. 88-529, p. 3]. Washington, DC: U.S. Department of Health and Human Services, Public Health Service, National Institutes of Health.)

■

*Critical Thinking 4–4*
When the white blood cell count shows a result of $2.3 \times 10^3$ cells/µL (SI: $2.3 \times 10^9$ cells/L), how should the nursing plan be modified to protect the patient?

the need for additional tests such as a white blood cell differential or a bone marrow biopsy. The white blood cell count is used to monitor the bone marrow's response to chemotherapy, radiation treatment, toxic exposure to heavy metals, chemical poisons, or the untoward effects of some medications.

## Procedure

A purple-topped tube with EDTA is used to collect 7 mL of venous blood. As an alternative, two purple-tipped capillary tubes can be used to collect blood from a heelstick, earlobe, or finger puncture.

### Quality Control

> With venipuncture, the tourniquet should be tied lightly for a brief time to prevent pooling of cells at the site of blood collection. Venipuncture technique must be smooth, with a blood flow that fills the vacuum tube readily. If there is excessive turbulence in the blood because of flawed venipuncture technique, the hemolysis of the erythrocytes will alter the test results. After the blood is collected, the tube is inverted gently 5 to 10 times to mix the anticoagulant and prevent clotting.

## Findings

### Elevated Values

| | | |
|---|---|---|
| Bacterial infection | Tissue necrosis | Varicella |
| Lymphoma | (burns, gangrene, | Rubeola |
| Leukemia | myocardial | Leukemoid reaction |
| Chronic infection | infarction) | |
| Mumps | | |
| Cancer (liver, | | |
| intestine) | | |

### Decreased Values

| | | |
|---|---|---|
| Brucellosis | Malaria | Toxic ingestion of |
| Typhoid fever | Gaucher's disease | heavy metals or |
| Viral infections | Pernicious anemia | chemical poisons |
| (influenza, rubella, | Aplastic anemia | Systemic lupus |
| hepatitis) | Radiation | erythematosus |
| Typhus | Antineoplastic drugs | Felty's syndrome |
| Dengue fever | | |

## Interfering Factors

- Hemolysis
- Coagulation of the specimen
- Strenuous exercise
- Digestion of a heavy meal

## Nursing Implementation

Nursing care includes the care of the venipuncture or capillary puncture site.

### Pretest

Plan to obtain the specimen when the patient is calm and physically still.

When the test is planned in advance, instruct the patient to avoid strenuous exercise for 24 hours before the test.

Organize the care of the neonate so that minimal disturbance occurs before drawing the blood (Polinski, 1996).

Comfort the crying infant or child, because with stress or distress, the patient's adrenaline causes a rise in the white blood cell count for 15 to 30 minutes.

Instruct the patient to avoid a heavy meal before the test, because the digestion process causes a temporary rise in the white blood cell count.

### Posttest

In evaluating the white blood cell count of a newborn, plan for repeat testing several times. The same vascular source (vein, capillary) should be used.

This repetition helps provide accurate data and limits variations due to extraneous sources.

With a severe decrease in the white blood cell value, initiate measures to protect the patient from exposure to infection.

| Critical Values | |
|---|---|
| | **<2,500 cells/µL (SI <2.5 × 10⁹/L) *or* >30,000 cells/µL (SI >30 × 10⁹/L)** |

**Critical Values**

**<2,500 cells/µL (SI <2.5 $\times$ 10⁹/L) *or* >30,000 cells/µL (SI >30 $\times$ 10⁹/L)**

The physician should be notified immediately for either of these extreme or worse values. With severe leukopenia, the patient is at risk because there is little defense from infection. With severe leukocytosis, the patient may have an acute infection or inflammation, but the cell count may also be abnormal because of a bone marrow disorder, such as leukemia. *Hyperleukocytosis* is an extreme elevation of the white blood cell count and is a potential emergency. It is a value defined as >100,000 cells/µL (SI >100 $\times$ 10⁹/L). At this level, the patient may have a fatal hemorrhage in the lung or brain as the leukocytes clump or aggregate in the small blood vessels. Hyperleukocytosis is usually the result of a leukemia in crisis stage.

## White Blood Cell Differential Count

**(Blood)**    Synonyms: Differential leukocyte count, peripheral differential, white blood cell morphology, WBC differential

**Normal Values**

**NEUTROPHILS**
**Segmented Neutrophils**
Mean percent: 56% *or* SI 0.56 (mean number fraction)
Cell count (range): 1,800–7,800/µL *or* SI 1.8–7.8 $\times$ 10⁹/L
**Bands**
Mean percent: 3% *or* SI 0.03 (mean number fraction)
Cell count (range): 0–700/µL *or* SI 0–0.07 $\times$ 10⁹/L
**Eosinophils**
Mean percent: 2.7% *or* SI 0.027 (mean number fraction)
Cell count (range): 0–450/µL *or* SI 0–0.45 $\times$ 10⁹/L
**Basophils**
Mean percent: 0.3% *or* SI 0.003 (mean number fraction)
Cell count (range): 0–200/µL *or* SI 0–0.2 $\times$ 10⁹/L
**Lymphocytes**
Mean percent: 34% *or* SI 0.34 (mean number fraction)
Cell count (range): 1,000–4,800/µL *or* SI 1–4.8 $\times$ 10⁹/L
**Monocytes**
Mean percent: 4% *or* SI 0.04 (mean number fraction)
Cell count (range): 0–800/µL *or* SI 0–0.8 $\times$ 10⁹/L

## Background Information

The differential count identifies the five different types of leukocytes by microscopic visualization of the peripheral blood smear or by use of an automated analyzer that differentiates and counts the cells. The results indicate the percentage of each type of cell, and the cell counts indicate the number of each type of cell per measured volume of blood.

The leukocytes originate in the bone marrow, beginning with the division of the pluripotential stem cell. The subdivisions are the hematopoietic stem cell, the colony-forming units granulocyte, erythrocyte, macrophage, and megakaryocyte, and the lymphoid stem cell colony-forming unit lymphocyte.

Through increasing formation, maturation, and differentiation along specific cell lines, the hematopoietic stem cell ultimately produces monocytes and macrophages, neutrophils, eosinophils, and basophils. The lymphoid stem cell produces B cells from the bone marrow and T cells from the thymus and other lymphoid tissues (see Table 4–1).

**Neutrophils.**   The most active cells responding to tissue damage or infection are neutrophils. They are phagocytes that provide an early, rapid removal of cellular debris and a large number of bacteria. Of all the leukocytes, the neutrophils are the largest group. In normal health, only a small number circulate in the blood, with an additional supply in pools attached to the vascular endothelium. The largest supply is stored in the bone marrow and is released on demand. The circulating neutrophils have a life span of only 3 to 6 hours.

With increased demand, the body's first phase of response is to release the pools of neutrophils attached to the vascular endothelium. This is a rapid but brief response that occurs in minutes to hours. When the demand continues, the bone marrow releases greater numbers of neutrophils 4 to 24 hours following stimulation.

**Elevated Values.**   Neutrophilia occurs in response to bacterial infection, particularly that caused by staphylococci or streptococci. It also arises in response to inflammatory disease or conditions that cause tissue necrosis. Severe neutrophilia, particularly with a shift toward releasing immature neutrophils or even precursor marrow cells, may be caused by malignancy of the bone marrow, especially chronic myeloid leukemia.

**Decreased Values.**   Neutropenia may be caused by the depletion of the available pool of neutrophils during severe infection, damage to the circulating neutrophils, or damage to the bone marrow cells. Other conditions destroy not only neutrophils but also other types of blood cells and their precursor cells in the bone marrow. As a result, cytopenia or pancytopenia develops.

**Bands.**   Band neutrophils are the more immature form of a segmented neutrophil. An increase in bands is equivalent to a left shift, meaning that the marrow is releasing immature cells instead of neutrophils. It is believed that an increase in bands is an early indicator of sepsis. Although the bands are counted by an automated analyzer, the clinical usefulness of this part of the differential count is still being researched.

**Eosinophils.**   Eosinophils are granulocytes that contain toxic substances used to kill foreign cells in the blood. They also participate in the inflammatory response by phagocytosis, and they digest the antigen-antibody complexes and clean up the late stages of inflammation.

**Elevated Values.**   Eosinophilia occurs in response to allergic disorders, inflammation of the skin, parasitic infection in the tissues, some other infections and inflammations, metastatic malignancy, and tissue necrosis; it also occurs in some hematologic disorders that cause a change in the bone marrow (Statland, 1994).

**Decreased Values.**   Eosinopenia occurs with most infections that produce purulence.

**Basophils.**   Basophils are granulocytes involved in modifying or calming systemic allergic reactions and anaphylaxis. Mast cells are sometimes called tissue basophils. Mast cells and basophils are produced by the same precursor cells. The basophils release histamine, heparin, and serotonin into the circulation during an episode of inflammation.

**Elevated Values.**   Basophilia occurs during the healing phase of inflammation and in chronic inflammation. It occurs in the presence of hypersensitivity reactions to foods, pollens, and injected protein substances. It also occurs after radiation therapy and in myeloproliferative disorders, including myeloid leukemia.

**Decreased Values.**   Basopenia occurs during acute infection, hyperthyroidism, and stress.

**Lymphocytes.**   Lymphocytes are nongranulocytes produced in the bone marrow, thymus, and lymphoid organs. The two classes of lymphocytes are the B cells and the T cells: About 1 trillion lymphocytes exist in the body, and they are responsible for the activities of the immune system. All lymphocytes recognize foreign antigens in the circulation. Some of these antigens are attacked and destroyed by the lymphocytes in the blood. Other antigens are carried to the lymph glands via the lymphatic fluid. In the lymph nodes, the antigens become enmeshed with the immune cells, and the antigens are destroyed.

B cells are genetically programmed to make antibodies. Each cell is individualized for the manufacture of a specific antibody against a specific antigen. For example, one B cell makes antibodies against a respiratory bacillus, and another makes antibodies against an influenza virus. When the B cell encounters a specific antigen, it engulfs the antigen. With the help of a T cell and interleukins, the B cell complex gives rise to plasma cells that manufacture and release many antigen-specific antibodies (Fig. 4–3). The circulating antibodies are called immunoglobulins. Antibodies act in different ways to destroy antigens. Some release toxins on the antigens or coat them so that scavenger cells will engulf and destroy them. Other antibodies initiate the complement cascade to kill the antigen.

T cells of different kinds act to regulate the immune response. T helper cells activate the B cells and assist in the production of antibodies. Cytotoxic T cells are killer cells that destroy cells infected by virus, malignant cells, and foreign tissue cells, such as those of an organ graft. Suppressor T cells act to discontinue or reduce the manufacture of antibodies and suppress the immune response. In human immunodeficiency virus infection, T helper cells are destroyed by the virus. This activator of the immune response system is lost, and only suppressor T cells remain. The regulatory balance is gone, and the immune system remains suppressed.

**Elevated Values.** Lymphocytosis occurs in response to bacterial, viral, and other types of infection. It also occurs in some hematologic disorders, including lymphocytic leukemia (Brown, 1997).

**Decreased Values.** Lymphopenia occurs with impaired lymphatic drainage, some advanced cancers, bone marrow failure, and immunologic deficiency that decreases the T lymphocytes.

**Monocytes.** Monocytes are nongranulocytes that are released from the bone marrow while still in an immature form. Once in the circulation, the monocytes become macrophages capable of phagocytosis. Monocytes are long-lived cells unless they are destroyed by phagocytosis. In the tissues, the monocytes are the cells of the reticuloendothelial system. In the blood, they remove debris or foreign particles from the circulation. In phagocytosis, they perform the same work as neutrophils, but their numbers are greater, and they are capable of more work. They also participate in the immune response.

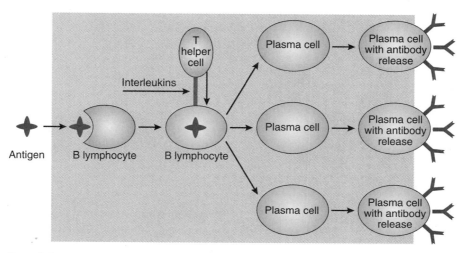

**Figure 4–3**

The process of antibody formation. The activation of B lymphocytes and T helper cells produces many plasma cells. The plasma cells produce and release many antigen-specific antibodies.

Elevated Values.   Monocytosis occurs in response to infection of all kinds as well as in granulomatosis, collagen disease, and some hematologic disorders.

Decreased Values.   Monopenia occurs because of bone marrow injury or failure and in some forms of leukemia.

## Purpose of the Test

The white blood cell differential assesses the ability of the body to respond to and eliminate infection. It also detects the severity of allergic reactions, parasitic infection, and other infection and identifies various stages of leukemia.

## Procedure

A purple-topped tube with EDTA is used to collect 7 mL of venous blood. As an alternative, two purple-tipped capillary tubes can be used to collect blood from a heelstick, earlobe, or finger puncture.

For the peripheral blood smear, two slides with coverslips are prepared immediately using drops of venous or capillary blood.

### Quality Control

With venipuncture, the tourniquet should be tied lightly for a brief time to prevent pooling of cells in the vein at the site of blood collection. Venipuncture technique must be smooth, with a blood flow that fills the vacuum tube readily. If the blood has excessive turbulence because of flawed venipuncture technique, the hemolysis of the erythrocytes will alter the test results. After the blood is collected, the tube is inverted gently 5 to 10 times to mix the anticoagulant and prevent clotting.

## Findings

### Elevated Values

NEUTROPHILS

Chronic myelogenous
  leukemia
Bacterial infection
Severe burns

Rheumatic fever
Ketoacidosis
Carcinoma or
  sarcoma

Myeloproliferative
  diseases
Down syndrome

EOSINOPHILS

Skin diseases (pemphigus, eczema,
  exfoliative
  dermatitis)
Trichinosis, *Echinococcus* disease
Scarlet fever

Chronic myelogenous
  leukemia
Myeloproliferative
  diseases
Hodgkin's disease
Malignancy

Rheumatoid arthritis
Sarcoidosis
Allergic reaction to
  drugs
Allergies (hay fever,
  hives, asthma)

BASOPHILS

Hypersensitivity
  reactions
Ulcerative colitis
Chronic hemolytic
  anemia

Hodgkin's disease
Myxedema
Chronic myelogenous
  leukemia

Polycythemia vera

LYMPHOCYTES

| | | |
|---|---|---|
| Infectious mononucleosis | Pertussis | Lymphocytic leukemia |
| Infectious hepatitis | Brucellosis | Lymphosarcoma cell leukemia |
| Cytomegalovirus infection | Tuberculosis | |
| | Syphilis | |

MONOCYTES

| | | |
|---|---|---|
| Acute infection (bacterial, viral, mycotic, rickettsial, protozoan) | Chronic myeloid leukemia | Acute monocytic leukemia |
| Tuberculosis | Myeloproliferative diseases | Myelomonocytic leukemia |
| Syphilis | Multiple myeloma | Lupus erythematosus |
| Brucellosis | Hodgkin's disease | Polyarteritis nodosa |
| Sarcoidosis | Non-Hodgkin's lymphoma | Rheumatoid arthritis |
| Ulcerative colitis | | |

**Decreased Values**

NEUTROPHILS

| | | |
|---|---|---|
| Infection | Aplastic anemia | Hypersplenism |
| Drug reaction | Radiation or chemotherapy | Cancer of the bone marrow |
| Autoimmune neutropenia | Megaloblastic anemia | |
| Maternal antibody production | | |

EOSINOPHILS

| | | |
|---|---|---|
| Allergies | Shock | Postsurgical response |
| Pyogenic infection | | |

BASOPHILS

| | | |
|---|---|---|
| Hyperthyroidism | Stress | Cushing's syndrome |
| Pregnancy | | |

LYMPHOCYTES

| | | |
|---|---|---|
| Thoracic duct drainage | Aplastic anemia | Renal failure |
| Right-sided heart failure | Human immunodeficiency virus infection | Terminal cancer |
| Hodgkin's disease | Miliary tuberculosis | |
| Systemic lupus erythematosus | | |

MONOCYTES

| | | |
|---|---|---|
| Hairy cell leukemia | Bone marrow failure | Aplastic anemia |

| **Interfering Factors** | • Temperature changes<br>• Exercise<br>• Pregnancy<br>• Pain<br>• Mental or physical stress<br>• Heightened emotion |
|---|---|

**Nursing Implementation**   Nursing care includes care of the venipuncture or capillary puncture site.

### Pretest

Because the differential count rises falsely in conditions of mental and physical stress, prepare the patient as follows:

Instruct the physically active patient to avoid strenuous activity for 24 hours before the test. The false rise is a result of the release of pooled neutrophils attached to vascular walls and an increase in circulating lymphocytes.

Calm the crying infant, and relieve the pain or distress experienced by the patient. Organize the care of the neonate so that he or she is calm at the time of the test (Polinski, 1996).

To minimize the patient's apprehension, provide reassurance about the simplicity of the procedure.

### Posttest

Arrange for prompt transport of the blood to the laboratory.

### Quality Control

If the blood remains standing in the tube, deterioration of the cells begins within 30 minutes. Different cells are affected at different rates, but the deterioration affects the nuclei and cytoplasm of the leukocytes.

## References

Borton, D. (1996). WBC count and differential. Reviewing the defensive roster. *Nursing 96, 26*(9), 26–32.

Brown, K. A. (1996). Hematology I: Erythrocyte metabolism and enzyme defects. *Laboratory Medicine, 27,* 329–333.

Brown, K. A. (1997). Nonmalignant disorders of lymphocytes. *Clinical Laboratory Science, 10,* 329–335.

Dixon, L. R. (1997). The complete blood count: Physiologic basis and clinical usage. *Journal of Perinatal and Neonatal Nursing, 11*(3), 1–18.

Drew, M. J. (1996). Blood banking. Pouring it in: Managing the massive transfusion. *Laboratory Medicine, 27,* 334–338.

Erikson, J. M. (1996). Anemia. *Seminars in Oncology Nursing, 12*(1), 2–14.

Fisher, M. (1996). The CBC—Part 1. WBC and differential. *Gynecologic Oncology Nursing, 6*(4), 40–41.

Goyzueta, F. G., Bailey, C. J., & Billett, H. H. (1996). Automated differential white blood cell counts in the young pediatric population. *Laboratory Medicine, 27*(1), 48–52.

Henry, J. B. (Ed.). (1996). *Clinical diagnosis and management by laboratory methods* (19th ed.). Philadelphia: W. B. Saunders.

Jacobs, D. S., Demott, W. R., Grady, H. J., Horvat, R. T., Huestis, D. W., & Klasten, B. L. (Eds.). (1996). *Laboratory test handbook* (4th ed.). Baltimore: Williams & Wilkins.

Koepke, J. A. (1993). Fitting the cell counter to the bed count. *Clinics in Laboratory Medicine, 13,* 817–829.

Koepke, J. A. (1995a). Estimating platelets on peripheral blood. *Medical Laboratory Observer, 27*(11), 20.

Koepke, J. A. (1995b). Anisocytosis. *Medical Laboratory Observer, 27*(7), 9.

Koepke, J. A. (1995c). Basophilia and its significance. *Medical Laboratory Observer, 27*(11), 17–18.

Lehmann, C. A. (1998). *Saunders manual of clinical laboratory science.* Philadelphia: W. B. Saunders.

Milne, J., Paes, B. A., Nanba, D., & Balmadres, D. (1996). Observer reliability of the manual immature to total neutrophil ratio in neonates. *Clinical Laboratory Science, 9,* 337–342.

Norris, M. K. G. (1994). Evaluating a WBC count with differential. *Nursing 94, 24*(8), 27.

Polinski, C. (1996). The value of the white blood count in the prediction of neonatal sepsis. *Neonatal Network: Journal of Neonatal Nursing, 15*(7), 13–23, 29–32.

Rodak, B. F. (1995). *Diagnostic Hematology.* Philadelphia: W. B. Saunders.

Savage, R. A. (1993). The red cell indices. *Clinics in Laboratory Medicine, 13,* 773–785.

Statland, B. E. (1994). Eosinophilia. *Medical Laboratory Observer, 26*(2), 12.

Steppe, C. A., & Woods, M. A. (1998). *Laboratory procedures for medical office personnel.* Philadelphia: W. B. Saunders.

Tietz, N. W. (Ed.). (1995). *Clinical guide to laboratory tests* (3rd ed.). Philadelphia: W. B. Saunders.

Ward, K. M., Lehman, C. A., & Leiken, A. M. (1994). *Clinical laboratory instrumentation and automation. Principles, application and selection.* Philadelphia: W. B. Saunders.

# CHAPTER 5

# Serum Electrolytes

Electrolytes are electrically charged particles that are dissolved in water. As ions, they exist in intracellular and extracellular body fluids and are capable of conducting electricity. Ions with a positive electrical charge are called cations, and those with a negative charge are called anions. The major cations in the body are sodium ($Na^+$), potassium ($K^+$), calcium ($Ca^{++}$), and magnesium ($Mg^+$), and the major anions are chloride ($Cl^-$), bicarbonate ($HCO_3^-$) and phosphate ($HPO_4^{--}$).

The concentration of the electrolytes is important in the maintenance of acid-base balance, hydration, and osmolarity. In addition, the concentration differences between intracellular and extracellular electrolytes regulate the functions of nervous system, cardiac, and muscle tissues (Henry, 1996).

In health, the concentration of electrolytes remains in a defined range, regulated by homeostasis. The intake of electrolytes in foods, the intake of water, the absorption of these elements by the intestines, the distribution of the electrolytes to the tissues, the influences of specific hormones, and the resorption or excretion abilities of the kidneys are all part of the homeostatic maintenance of fluid and electrolyte balance.

Imbalance in the electrolyte concentrations can occur for many reasons. The patient may not have sufficient intake of water or foods that contain specific electrolytes. Damage to the intestines or skin may cause excessive loss of fluid and electrolytes. Impaired renal function can alter the resorption or excretion of fluid and electrolytes.

An excessive amount of a particular substance, including electrolytes, in the blood is described with the prefix *hyper-* and the suffix *-emia,* as in hyperkalemia (excess potassium in the blood) or hypercalcemia (excess calcium in the blood). A decreased amount is described with the prefix *hypo-* and the suffix *-emia,* as in hypokalemia (decreased potassium in the blood) or hypomagnesemia (decreased magnesium in the blood). An electrolyte imbalance will affect many organs and the functions of cells. If uncorrected, the imbalance can reach a critical level, an extremely abnormal value. At this level, the patient exhibits symptoms of electrolyte imbalance, often affecting the functions of the brain, nervous system, respiratory system, and cardiovascular system. The uncorrected imbalance can become life-threatening, and death can occur.

Each of the electrolytes is presented individually in this chapter. The bicarbonate ion is estimated from the measurement of total carbon dioxide in the venous blood. The electrolyte imbalances and critical values are identified, with corresponding nursing assessments and interventions.

In laboratory protocols, serum sodium, serum potassium, serum chloride, and total carbon dioxide are often requested in an electrolyte panel or basic metabolic panel. These tests may be ordered as a routine screening of the patient's physiologic functions or as monitoring of the patient with an identified diagnosis or treatment that has a potential for electrolyte imbalance. These tests can also be ordered on a stat basis for specific and urgent health problems that have affected fluid or electrolyte balance. Serum magnesium, serum phosphorus, and serum and ionized calcium are requested as separate tests.

## Laboratory Tests

| | | |
|---|---|---|
| Carbon Dioxide, Total   83 | Chloride, Serum   89 | Potassium, Serum   96 |
| Calcium, Serum   84 | Magnesium, Serum   91 | Sodium, Serum   99 |
| Calcium, Ionized   87 | Phosphorus, Serum   94 | |

## Carbon Dioxide, Total

**(Whole Blood, Serum, Plasma)**    Synonyms: $CO_2$ content, $tCO_2$

**Normal Values**

2 years–adult (venous): 22–26 mEq/L *or* SI 22–26 mmol/L
2 years–adult (arterial): 23–29 mEq/L *or* SI 23–29 mmol/L
2 years–infant: 18–28 mEq/L *or* SI 18–28 mmol/L

## Background Information

Total carbon dioxide measures the combined forms of carbon dioxide in the blood. Some of the total carbon dioxide is dissolved in plasma; and some is combined with amino groups on hemoglobin molecules. The largest component is bicarbonate ion, composing 90% of the total carbon dioxide content in the blood. The total carbon dioxide content provides the principal extracellular buffer system, which is called the bicarbonate carbonic acid buffer. Buffer systems are needed in the regulation of acid-base balance. The concentration of carbon dioxide is controlled by the lungs, and the concentration of bicarbonate is controlled by the kidneys.

**Hypocapnia.**   A low serum level of carbon dioxide is called hypocapnia. It is caused by excess elimination of carbon dioxide, excess elimination of bicarbonate, excess accumulation of hydrogen ions in the blood, or a combination of these conditions. Hypocapnia is associated with respiratory alkalosis or metabolic acidosis.

**Hypercapnia.**   An elevated serum level of carbon dioxide is called hypercapnia. It often is caused by poor carbon dioxide excretion by the lungs or an inadequate respiratory drive. Hypercapnia is associated with respiratory acidosis, carbon dioxide retention, and metabolic alkalosis.

To fully evaluate acid-base disturbance, a total carbon dioxide determination is usually performed with pH and partial pressure of carbon dioxide ($P_{CO_2}$) monitoring. (Discussion of these additional tests and of acid-base balance is presented in Chapter 14.)

## Purpose of the Test

The total carbon dioxide determination is used to help evaluate acid-base balance and the bicarbonate buffer system.

## Procedure

For venous or arterial blood testing, a green-topped tube with heparin is used to obtain 5 mL of arterial blood.

### Quality Control

The rubber stopper must remain firmly in place so that the carbon dioxide cannot diffuse out and result in a falsely lowered value.

## Findings

### Elevated Values

| | | |
|---|---|---|
| Respiratory acidosis | Pulmonary edema | Severe, prolonged |
| Emphysema | Metabolic alkalosis | vomiting |
| Pneumonia | Hypokalemia | Cushing's syndrome |
| Cystic fibrosis | Excessive intake of | Primary aldoste- |
| Congestive heart | antacids | ronism |
| failure | | |

■
*Critical Thinking 5–1*
An adult male patient with emphysema has a venous carbon dioxide value of 40 mEq/L (SI 40 mmol/L). Identify the nursing measures that would help lower this laboratory test result.

### Decreased Values

| | | |
|---|---|---|
| Respiratory alkalosis | Diabetes mellitus | Renal failure |
| Hyperventilation | Severe diarrhea | Dehydration |
| Metabolic acidosis | Renal tubular acidosis | Hypovolemia |

## Interfering Factors

- Exposure of the specimen to air

## Nursing Implementation

Nursing measures include care of the artery or vein used to obtain the specimen. No other specific patient instruction or intervention is needed.

## Critical Values

**<15 mEq/L (SI <15 mmol/L) *or* >50 mEq/L (SI >50 mmol/L)**

If the total carbon dioxide reaches either critical value, the physician must be notified immediately. The blood pH and serum electrolytes are also likely to be in serious imbalance. The patient requires an immediate nursing assessment of all vital signs, with particular attention to abnormal changes in the rate and quality of respirations.

## Calcium, Serum

**(Serum)**

Synonyms: $Ca^{++}$, total serum calcium

## Normal Values

Adult: 8.6–10.0 mg/dL *or* SI 2.15–2.50 mmol/L
Child: 8.8–10.8 mg/dL *or* SI 2.20–2.70 mmol/L
Infant (0–10 days): 7.6–10.4 mg/dL *or* SI 1.90–2.60 mmol/L

## Background Information

Calcium is one of the essential mineral elements of the body. Almost all of it is concentrated in bone. The remainder is present in the cells or extracellular fluids, including the serum, in which about half the total calcium is in a free or ionized state and is physiologically active. A little less than half of the total calcium is bonded to albumin and other plasma proteins.

In the serum and other extracellular fluids, the normal level of calcium is maintained in homeostatic balance by the actions of the small intestine, bones, and kidneys. For the regulation of calcium, these target organs are governed by the interplay of parathyroid hormone, calcitonin hormone, and vitamin $D_1$, an active form of vitamin D.

Parathyroid hormone prevents hypocalcemia by increasing the amount of calcium in the extracellular fluids. It does this by (1) acting on bones to increase bone resorption, (2) acting on the kidneys to increase the resorption of calcium, and (3) acting on the kidneys to convert vitamin D to the active form vitamin $D_1$, which acts on the small intestine to absorb a greater amount of dietary calcium.

Calcitonin, a hormone manufactured by the thyroid gland, works in a manner opposite that of parathyroid hormone and vitamin $D_1$. Calcitonin prevents hypercalcemia by lowering the amount of calcium in the extracellular fluids. Its action is to decrease or limit the resorption of calcium by the bones and kidneys.

Calcium is needed for the process of bone formation and is an essential element in bone structure. It is also needed for many other physiologic functions, including coagulation of the blood, excitation of cardiac and skeletal muscle, maintenance of muscle tone, conduction of neuromuscular impulses, and synthesis and regulation of the endocrine and exocrine glands. On the cellular level, calcium preserves the integrity and permeability of the cell membrane, particularly for sodium and potassium exchange.

In normal physiology, calcium is obtained from dietary sources. About 20% of the daily intake is absorbed in the duodenum of the small intestine. As the absorbed calcium enters the blood, it is used in cells and bone formation, or it remains in the extracellular fluid. The glomeruli of the kidneys filter out the calcium from the blood. Most of it is then resorbed by the renal tubules and reenters the circulation and extracellular fluid. The excess dietary calcium is excreted in feces. The excess calcium in the extracellular fluid and serum is excreted by the kidneys, and a small amount is excreted in sweat (Fig. 5–1).

In the individual, the endocrine-regulating mechanisms maintain a steady serum calcium level with little variation. Daily, the normal level fluctuates in a diurnal rhythm, with a lower serum calcium level in the later afternoon. The reference values vary among laboratories because of dif-

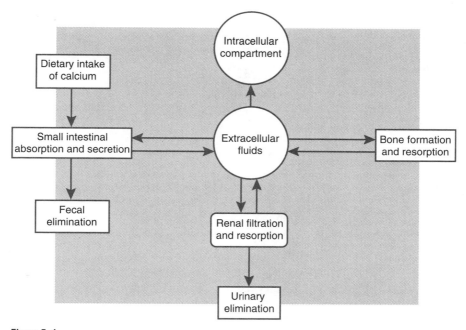

**Figure 5–1**

Calcium homeostasis in extracellular fluid. The normal serum calcium level is regulated by a complex interaction of intestinal, bone, and renal functions. Excess amounts of calcium are excreted from the body in feces and urine.

ferent methods of analysis. To ensure accuracy in laboratory testing, the specimen is always drawn in the early morning to minimize the diurnal variation. An abnormally elevated value is routinely validated by repeating the test two additional times.

**Hypercalcemia.**   An elevated level of calcium in the blood is called hypercalcemia. It alters the function of most body organs and can be a life-threatening complication. Hyperparathyroidism and malignancy are the most common causes of hypercalcemia. In hyperparathyroidism, an excess of parathyroid hormone increases the resorption of calcium from the bones and renal tubules. Ma-

lignancy and multiple myeloma increase the level of total serum proteins. The calcium level increases as the calcium bonds to the excess protein concentration.

**Hypocalcemia.**   A decreased level of calcium in the serum is called hypocalcemia. It causes neuromuscular hyperactivity, affecting many organs and functions. Very low calcium levels can be life-threatening. Total serum calcium is lowered in conditions that decrease plasma proteins, impair intestinal absorption, alter renal filtration and resorption functions, or decrease the amount of parathyroid hormone.

---

**Purpose of the Test**

The serum calcium level is measured to assist in the diagnosis of acid-base imbalance, coagulation disorders, pathologic bone disorders, endocrine disorders, cardiac arrhythmia, and muscle disorders.

---

**Procedure**

*Adult:* A red-topped tube is used to collect 10 mL of venous blood.
*Infant:* A capillary pipette is used to collect capillary blood via the heelstick method.

**Quality Control**

The tourniquet is applied briefly. Venipuncture technique must be smooth, with a flow of blood that fills the vacuum tube readily. If there is venous stasis and pooling or excessive hemolysis, the serum calcium level will be falsely elevated.

---

**Findings**

■

*Critical Thinking 5–2*
An older female patient has a serum calcium level of 7.6 mg/dL (SI 1.90 mmol/L). The hypocalcemia is due to inadequate nutrition. What approaches can you use to help her supplement her dietary intake of calcium?

**Elevated Values**

Hyperparathyroidism
Metastatic cancer
Multiple myeloma
Vitamin D intoxication
Milk-alkali syndrome

Overuse of calcium antacids
Paget's disease
Idiopathic hypercalcemia of infancy
Polycythemia vera

Pheochromocytoma
Sarcoidosis
Adrenal insufficiency
Thyrotoxicosis
Bacteremia
Dehydration

**Decreased Values**

Hypoparathyroidism
Vitamin D deficiency
Alcoholism
Chronic renal failure
Hypoalbuminemia
Massive blood transfusions

Prolonged intravenous fluid therapy
Acute pancreatitis
Anterior pituitary hypofunction

Renal tubular disease
Cirrhosis of the liver
Malnutrition
Neonatal prematurity

| **Interfering Factors** | • Upright position or prolonged activity before the test<br>• Venous stasis or hemolysis during the blood collection procedure<br>• Prolonged storage of the blood specimen |

**Nursing Implementation**

In addition to the care of the venipuncture site, review the following:

**Pretest**

Instruct the patient to fast from food and fluids for 8 hours. Arrange to have the blood drawn in the early morning (Jacobs et al., 1996).
Some medications (i.e., thiazides and other diuretics, lithium, and calcium salts) cause a rise in the serum value and also should be withheld during the period in which the patient fasts.

**Posttest**

Arrange for prompt transport of the specimen to the laboratory.

**Quality Control**

> The analysis must be performed on a fresh sample. Prolonged storage or a delay in performing the analysis results in a false elevation of the calcium value.

**Critical Values**

**<7.0 mg/dL (SI 1.75 mmol/L) *or* >12 mg/dL (SI > 2.99 mmol/L)**

If the serum calcium level lowers to the critical value of 7.0 mg/dL (1.75 mmol/L), the hypocalcemia can induce depression or psychosis, laryngeal stridor, tetany, convulsions, hypotension, and decreased myocardial contractility. A severe decrease to 6 mg/dL (SI 1.5 mmol/L) or less can be life-threatening.

If the serum calcium rises to the critical level of >12 mg/dL (SI >2.99 mmol/L), the hypercalcemia can induce polyuria, anorexia, nausea, and coma. A severe elevation of 14 mg/dL (SI 3.5 mmol/L) is more likely to induce coma and can cause death.

The nurse must notify the physician of any test result in these abnormal ranges. The nurse should also take the patient's vital signs and assess for specific symptoms that occur with calcium imbalance.

## Calcium, Ionized

**(Serum, Plasma, Whole Blood)**

Synonyms: Free calcium, $Ca_i$, $_iCa$

**Normal Values**

Adult (whole blood): 4.60–5.08 mg/dL *or* SI 1.15–1.27 mmol/L
Adult (plasma): 4.12–4.92 mg/dL *or* SI 1.03–1.23 mmol/L
Infant (24–48 hours, whole blood): 4.00–4.72 mg/dL *or* SI 1.00–1.18 mmol/L

## Background Information

Review the discussion of serum calcium in this chapter. Ionized calcium represents about half the total calcium value. Much of the remainder of the total serum calcium is in the form of calcium bound to protein. It is the ionized calcium that is physiologically active or free to be used by the body. Total calcium levels are influenced by serum albumin levels, but ionized calcium levels are not. Ionized calcium measurements are preferred for patients with altered serum proteins or disturbances in acid-base metabolism (Tietz, 1995).

| | |
|---|---|
| **Purpose of the Test** | This test is used to assess calcium abnormality and to avoid hypocalcemia, particularly in conditions of abnormal protein levels or in acid-base imbalance. |
| **Procedure** | Venipuncture is performed to fill a green- or red-topped tube. Exposure to air is prevented by using a vacuum tube. No tourniquet is used. |
| **Findings** | The level of ionized calcium in the blood is affected by any alteration of the blood pH. The following is, therefore, a partial listing. |

### Elevated Values

| | | |
|---|---|---|
| Primary hyperparathyroidism | Excess intake of vitamin D | Malignancy |
| Parathyroid hormone-producing tumors | | |

### Decreased Values

| | | |
|---|---|---|
| Primary hypoparathyroidism | Trauma | Major surgery |
| Pseudohypoparathyroidism | Pancreatitis | Sepsis |
| Post blood transfusion | Hemodialysis | Burns |
| | Vitamin D deficiency | Alkalemia |
| | Magnesium deficiency | |

| | |
|---|---|
| **Interfering Factors** | • Clotted specimen<br>• Exposure of the specimen to the air<br>• Warming of the specimen<br>• Diet high in calcium or deficient in vitamin D<br>• Multiple drugs, including antacids, anticonvulsants, aspirin, barbiturates, gentamicin, insulin, lithium, steroids, thiazide diuretics, and thyroid hormones |
| **Nursing Implementation** | The nurse provides actions similar to those of other venipuncture techniques. |

### Pretest

The patient maintains bedrest in a supine position for 30 minutes before the blood is drawn.

### Posttest

Refrigerate specimen or send it to the laboratory on ice immediately.

| Critical Values | **<3.02 mg/dL (SI <0.80 mmol/L)**<br><br>With a decrease in this critical level, the patient can develop neuromuscular irritability. The nurse notifies the physician of the laboratory value and assesses the patient for signs of depression or psychosis, laryngeal stridor, tetany, convulsions, hypotension, and decreased myocardial contractility. Generally, prescribed calcium replacement is initiated. A severe decrease to <2.08 mg/dL (SI <0.70 mmol/L) can be life-threatening (Jacobs et al., 1996). |
|---|---|

## Chloride, Serum

(Serum)                    Synonym: $Cl^-$

| Normal Values | Adult and child: 97–107 mEq/L *or* SI 97–107 mmol/L<br>Newborn: 96–106 mEq/L *or* SI 96–106 mmol/L<br>Premature infant: 95–110 mEq/L *or* SI 95–110 mmol/L |
|---|---|

## Background Information

Sodium ($Na^+$), potassium ($K^+$), bicarbonate ($HCO_3^-$), and chloride ($Cl^-$) are electrolytes with positive or negative charges. The positively charged electrolytes or ions are called cations, and the negatively charged electrolytes are called anions. In combination, the electrolytes determine the osmolarity, pH, and hydration status in intracellular and extracellular fluids. Chloride is a major extracellular anion.

Chloride generally increases or decreases in direct relationship to sodium. This means that as the concentration of sodium rises, chloride also rises, and as the concentration of sodium falls, chloride also falls. The concentration of chloride increases or decreases inversely with bicarbonate. This means that as the concentration of chloride increases, the bicarbonate level decreases, and as the concentration of chloride decreases, bicarbonate increases.

Chloride is ingested in food, and most of it is absorbed by the gastrointestinal tract. The glomeruli of the kidneys filter chloride out of the extracellular fluids, and the renal tubules resorb the amount of chloride needed to maintain homeostasis. The excess of this anion is excreted in urine. The normal serum level remains in a steady range, with a slight drop after meals. The postprandial decrease occurs as hydrochloric acid (HCl) is produced for digestion.

**Hyperchloridemia.**   An elevated level of chloride in the blood and extracellular fluid is called hyperchloridemia. It occurs during metabolic acidosis, resulting from excessive loss of bicarbonate fluids and electrolytes from the lower intestine, from renal tubular acidosis, and from mineralocorticoid deficiency. The chloride concentration may also rise with dehydration.

**Hypochloridemia.** A decreased level of chloride in the blood and extracellular fluid is called hypochloridemia. It occurs during a loss of hydrochloric acid from the upper gastrointestinal tract as well as from mineralocorticoid excess, salt-losing renal disease, or diabetic acidosis. The low level of chloride may also occur in conditions that cause a rise in bicarbonate or a decreased sodium concentration. Hypochloridemia may occur with overhydration.

## Purpose of the Test

Serum chloride measurements are obtained in the evaluation of electrolyte levels, water balance, and acid-base balance and in the measurement of the cation-anion balance (anion gap).

## Procedure

A red-topped tube is used to collect 10 mL of venous blood; or a green-topped tube is used to collect 5 mL of venous blood. In infants, a heelstick puncture and a capillary tube may be used to collect capillary blood.

### Quality Control

Venipuncture technique must be smooth, with a blood flow that fills the vacuum tube readily. If excessive turbulence occurs because of poor technique, the hemolysis of the erythrocytes will alter the test results.

## Findings

### Elevated Values

| | | |
|---|---|---|
| Dehydration | Acute renal failure | Hyperparathyroidism |
| Renal tubular acidosis | Diabetes insipidus | Adrenocortical |
| Prolonged diarrhea | Respiratory alkalosis | hyperfunction |

### Decreased Values

| | | |
|---|---|---|
| Prolonged vomiting | Metabolic alkalosis | Overhydration |
| Nasogastric drainage | Addison's disease | Syndrome of inappropriate antidiuretic hormone |
| Salt-losing nephritis | Congestive heart failure | |
| Chronic renal failure | Intestinal fistula | |
| Chronic respiratory acidosis | | Diuretic therapy |

## Interfering Factors

- Hemolysis
- Warming of the specimen

## Nursing Implementation

### Pretest

For a routine test, instruct the patient to discontinue all food and fluids for 8 hours before the test. This prevents the normal drop in value after eating. For tests performed on an urgent or emergency basis, the fasting status is omitted.

### Posttest

Arrange for prompt transport of the blood to the laboratory. The serum or plasma will require refrigeration until the analysis can be performed.

| Critical Values | >115 mEq/L (SI >115 mmol/L) *or* <80 mEq/L (SI <80 mmol/L) |
| --- | --- |
| | A severe elevation or loss of this electrolyte indicates serious fluid and electrolyte imbalance. The physician must be notified immediately. Specific medical treatment and nursing intervention depend on the cause of the problem, but immediate action must be taken to restore the electrolyte balance. |

## Magnesium, Serum

**(Serum)**                    Synonym: Mg⁺

| Normal Values | Adult: 1.6–2.6 mg/dL *or* SI 0.66–1.07 mmol/L |
| --- | --- |
| | Child (12–20 years): 1.7–2.2 mg/dL *or* SI 0.70–0.91 mmol/L |
| | (6–12 years): 1.7–2.1 mg/dL *or* SI 0.70–0.86 mmol/L |
| | (5 months–6 years): 1.7–2.3 mg/dL *or* SI 0.70–0.95 mmol/L |
| | Newborn: 1.5–2.2 mg/dL *or* SI 0.62–0.91 mmol/L |

## Background Information

Magnesium is one of the major intracellular cations of the body. Almost all magnesium is stored in soft tissue, muscle, and bone, with only 1% of the total magnesium present in the serum and extracellular fluid (Jacobs et al., 1996). Because so little of the magnesium is in the serum, total body magnesium is difficult to measure accurately.

Serum magnesium is maintained in homeostatic balance by the functions of gastrointestinal absorption and excretion and renal resorption and excretion. As seen in Figure 5–2, magnesium is obtained from food. The magnesium is absorbed in the small intestine and enters the blood and extracellular fluid. From there, the largest amount of magnesium is stored in bone. An equivalent amount is stored in the soft tissue and bones, and a small amount is stored in the erythrocytes. In the kidneys, the glomeruli filter the magnesium, and the renal tubules are responsible for resorption. Excess magnesium is removed from the body in feces and urine.

**Hypomagnesemia.**    A low level of magnesium in the blood is called hypomagnesemia. In a normal physiologic response to a low serum level of magnesium, the metabolites of vitamin D and the action of parathyroid hormone respond by increasing the amount of intestinal absorption of magnesium.

Additionally, parathyroid hormone causes the renal tubules to resorb a greater amount of magnesium, with less to be excreted in the urine. Renal tubular resorption exerts the most powerful effect on the conservation of magnesium and the restoration of the homeostatic balance. If these responses are inadequate, hypomagnesemia results. The deficiency of magnesium is usually associated with deficiencies of calcium and potassium.

Hypomagnesemia often occurs with inadequate food intake or impaired intestinal absorption or as a result of hemodialysis treatment. It may also occur during long-term hyperalimentation or intravenous fluid replacement. Hypomagnesemia together with hypokalemia is associated with a high rate of ventricular arrhythmias (Tsuji, Venditti, Evans, Larson, & Levy, 1994). Patients with a cardiac disorder or an acute myocardial infarction are particularly vulnerable to a depleted magnesium level (<2.0 mg/dL *or* SI <0.82 mmol/L), and ventricular arrhythmia or sudden death can occur. Hypomagnesemia is considered more serious than hypermagnesemia.

**Hypermagnesemia.**    An elevation of the serum value of magnesium in the blood is called hypermagnesemia. In a normal physiologic response to a rising level of magnesium in the blood, the intes-

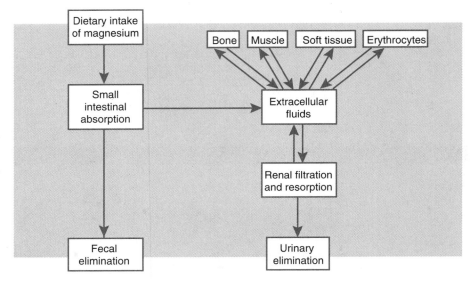

**Figure 5–2**
Homeostasis of magnesium in extracellular fluid. The normal serum magnesium level is regulated by intestinal and renal function. Most of the body's magnesium is stored in bones.

tines absorb less of the dietary sources of magnesium and eliminate the excess magnesium in feces. More powerfully, the renal tubules resorb less magnesium, and a greater amount of magnesium is excreted in the urine. If these physiologic responses are inadequate, hypermagnesemia results.

Most cases of hypermagnesemia are caused by advanced renal failure, with a decreased glomerular filtration rate and a resultant rise in the serum value of magnesium.

---

**Purpose of the Test**    The measurement of serum magnesium helps to evaluate electrolyte disorders, hypocalcemia, hypokalemia, and acid-base imbalance. It is also used to monitor patients who have a cardiac disorder, because low magnesium levels are dangerous. The test is also performed to monitor the pregnant patient with severe toxemia during the intravenous administration of magnesium sulfate.

---

**Procedure**    A red-topped tube is used to obtain 10 mL of venous blood.

**Quality Control**

> The tourniquet should be applied for no longer than 1 minute to avoid venous stasis. Venipuncture technique must be smooth, with a blood flow that fills the vacuum tube readily. If there is venous stasis, or if the blood has excessive turbulence because of flawed venipuncture technique, the hemolysis of erythrocytes will cause a false elevation of the results.

| **Findings** | **Elevated Values** | | |
|---|---|---|---|
| | Advanced renal failure | Excessive ingestion of magnesium-containing antacids | Magnesium sulfate infusion therapy |
| | Addison's disease | | |
| | Administration of multiple magnesium sulfate enemas | | |

| | **Decreased Values** | | |
|---|---|---|---|
| | Early renal disease | Diabetic ketoacidosis (during treatment) | Severe burns |
| | Chronic glomerulonephritis | Inadequate dietary intake | Hypoparathyroidism |
| | Chronic alcoholism | Malabsorption | Hyperaldosteronism |
| | Hypercalcemia | Prolonged nasogastric drainage | Cisplatin therapy |
| | Pancreatitis | | Prolonged intravenous therapy |
| | Hemodialysis therapy | | |
| | Pregnancy | | |
| | Prolonged hyperalimentation | | |

**Interfering Factors**

- Venous stasis
- Hemolysis

**Nursing Implementation**

Nursing care also includes the venipuncture site.

**Pretest**

Instruct the patient to fast from food and fluids for 8 hours before the test.

**Posttest**

Send the specimen to the laboratory without delay.

**Quality Control**

To avoid clumping of erythrocytes and invalid test results, the blood must be centrifuged quickly. The serum must then be refrigerated until it is analyzed.

**Critical Values**

**<1.2 mg/dL (SI <0.5 mmol/L) *or* >4.9 mg/dL (SI >2.0 mmol/L)**

With either extreme of magnesium values, the nurse must notify the physician immediately.

Severe hypomagnesemia causes neuromuscular changes that include weakness, irritability, tremors, tetany, convulsions, and cardiac arrhythmias. The nurse assesses for these symptoms, takes vital signs, institutes seizure precautions, and prepares for cardiac monitoring (Gaedeke, 1995).

*Continued on following page*

*Continued*

> The effects of hypermagnesemia include a slowing of cardiac conduction, heart block, hypotension, muscle flaccidity, loss of deep tendon reflexes, and muscle paralysis. At values greater than 14.6 mg/dL (SI >6 mmol/L), respiratory failure, general anesthesia, and cardiac arrest can occur (Tietz, 1996). The nurse takes vital signs, connects the patient to the cardiac monitor, and assesses for symptoms of cardiac, muscle, and nervous system impairment.

## Phosphorus, Serum

**(Serum)**    Synonyms: $P_i$, inorganic phosphate, $HPO_4^{--}$

**Normal Values**    Adult (12–60 years): 2.7–4.5 mg/dL *or* SI 0.87–1.45 mmol/L
(male, >60 years): 2.3–3.7 mg/dL *or* SI 0.74–1.2 mmol/L
(female, >60 years): 2.8–4.1 mg/dL *or* SI 0.90–1.32 mmol/L
Child (2–12 years): 4.5–5.5 mg/dL *or* SI 1.45–1.78 mmol/L
(10 days–2 years): 4.5–6.7 mg/dL *or* SI 1.45–2.16 mmol/L
(0–10 days): 4.5–9 mg/dL *or* SI 1.45–2.91 mmol/L

## Background Information

Phosphorus is a mineral element present in bone cells and extracellular fluid, including serum. The dietary sources of phosphorus are partially absorbed by the small intestine and provide renewal of the mineral. The homeostatic balance of the mineral in the extracellular fluid is maintained by the actions of parathyroid hormone, calcitonin, and vitamin D. Excess phosphorus is excreted in the feces and urine.

An inverse relationship exists between the serum levels of phosphorus and calcium. If the serum level of either mineral falls, the serum level of the other mineral rises.

The homeostatic regulation of serum phosphorus is based on the body's ability to detect alterations in the level of serum phosphorus and adjust accordingly. In hypophosphatemia, the kidneys possess the most rapid and best ability to raise the serum level by an increase of tubular resorption and a reduction of urinary excretion of the mineral. The small intestine also responds by absorbing more phosphorus.

In the extracellular fluid, most phosphorus is present in the form of free phosphate ions, and the small remainder is bound to plasma proteins. Most of the body content of phosphorus is not in the plasma, however, but is stored in bone as a component of the bone matrix. The mineral is stored and used as part of new bone formation. As bone resorption or bone turnover occurs, the phosphorus is rereleased into the extracellular fluid.

Serum phosphorus concentrations have a diurnal rhythm. The level is highest in the morning and lowest in the evening. The normal values also vary over a life span, with the highest serum values occurring in infants and children and the lowest values occurring in elderly individuals.

**Hyperphosphatemia.**    A fasting serum phosphorus level greater than 4.7 mg/dL (SI >1.5 mmol/L) in the adult is called hyperphosphatemia (Speicher, 1998). Severe hyperphosphatemia produces no symptoms but does cause hypocalcemia. With a rapid elevation of serum phosphorus to a level of >6 mg/dL (SI >1.94 mmol/L), the serum calcium declines and causes symptoms of hypotension and tetany from the calcium depletion. The most common cause of the hyperphosphatemia is severe renal insufficiency. Other causes include increased tubular resorption in the kidneys and diseases that cause increased bone turnover, releasing more phosphorus into the extracellular fluids.

**Hypophosphatemia.**   A serum value less than 2.7 mg/dL (SI 0.87 mmol/L) is called hypophosphatemia. Causes include inadequate food intake, impaired intestinal absorption, increased phosphate storage in bones, and increased renal excretion of phosphate (Speicher, 1998). This condition is of serious consequence because it can affect neuromuscular, neuropsychiatric, skeletal, gastrointestinal, and cardiopulmonary function.

## Purpose of the Test

Serum phosphorus helps diagnose kidney disorders and acid-base imbalance. It is also used to detect disorders of calcium, bone, or endocrine origin.

## Procedure

A red-topped tube is used to collect 10 mL of venous blood. For infants and small children, a heelstick puncture and capillary tube are used to collect a blood sample.

### Quality Control

Venipuncture technique must be smooth, with a blood flow that fills the vacuum tube readily. If the blood has excessive turbulence because of flawed technique, the hemolysis of the erythrocytes will elevate the results falsely.

## Findings

### Elevated Values

| | | |
|---|---|---|
| Renal failure | Postanesthesia | Vitamin D toxicity |
| Hypovolemia | hyperthermia | Respiratory acidosis |
| Dehydration | Cirrhosis of the liver | Sarcoidosis |
| Milk-alkali syndrome | Pulmonary embolism | Lactic acidosis |
| Acromegaly | Diabetic ketoacidosis | Hypoparathyroidism |
| Osteolytic metastatic bone cancer | | |

### Decreased Values

| | | |
|---|---|---|
| Osteomalacia | Vomiting, diarrhea | Prolonged nasogastric drainage |
| Osteoblastic bone cancer | Sepsis | Renal tubular disease |
| Acute gout | Acute respiratory infection | Severe malabsorption |
| Vitamin D deficiency | Prolonged intravenous glucose therapy | Starvation |
| Renal tubular disease | | Respiratory alkalosis |
| Hyperparathyroidism | | |
| Serum calcium elevation | | |

## Interfering Factors

- Hemolysis
- Carbohydrate-rich meals
- Recent phosphate enema

## Nursing Implementation

Nursing care includes care of the venipuncture site.

### Pretest

Schedule the test for early morning.

Instruct the patient to discontinue all food and fluids for 8 hours before the test.

**Quality Control**

It is best to obtain a fasting specimen, because carbohydrate intake and recent food intake tend to decrease the serum phosphate level. Blood is obtained in the early morning hours to avoid diurnal fluctuations.

Do not administer a phosphate enema just before the test, because some of the phosphate is absorbed by the colonic mucosa.

### Posttest

Arrange for prompt transport of the specimen.

**Quality Control**

A delay in centrifuge of the specimen results in a false rise in the serum value.

**Critical Value**

**<1 mg/dL (SI <0.32 mmol/L)**

The physician must be notified immediately when the phosphorus level falls to this extreme. Symptoms of cardiac and central nervous system dysfunction include decreased cardiac contractility and cardiac output, respiratory failure, tremor, weakness, convulsions, slurred speech, coma, and myopathy. About 20% of patients with this critical level of hypophosphatemia will die (Jacobs et al., 1996).

The nurse takes vital signs, initiates seizure precautions, and prepares for cardiac monitoring as initial interventions.

## Potassium, Serum

**(Serum)**                      Synonym: K+

**Normal Values**

Adult: 3.5–5.1 mEq/L *or* SI 3.5–5.1 mmol/L
Child: 3.4–4.7 mEq/L *or* SI 3.4–4.7 mmol/L
Infant: 4.1–5.3 mEq/L *or* SI 4.1–5.3 mmol/L
Newborn: 3.7–5.9 mEq/L *or* SI 3.7–5.9 mmol/L
Premature (48 hours): 3.0–6.0 mEq/L *or* SI 3.0–6.0 mmol/L

## Background Information

Potassium is an electrolyte that is present in all body fluids. Most of the potassium is concentrated in the intracellular fluids, with only 2% of the total potassium concentrated in the extracellular fluids, including the blood (Henry, 1996).

The renewable source of potassium is the daily food intake. About 90% of the potassium intake is absorbed by the intestinal tract, and the unabsorbed portion is excreted in the feces. Once the absorbed portion enters the blood and extracellular fluids, it is distributed throughout the body, primarily within the cells (Fig. 5–3).

In normal physiology, the extracellular potassium level remains within a relatively narrow range. The regulation of the extracellular potassium concentration is performed by the kidneys, with excretion of excess potassium in the urine.

Considerable danger is associated with either a depletion or an excess of potassium. The abnormal potassium concentration causes disturbances in the membrane potential and altered function of neuromuscular tissue, including the loss of cardiac contractility. With depletion or excess of this cation, the patient is at risk for the development of shock, respiratory failure, or cardiac arrhythmias, including ventricular fibrillation.

**Hypokalemia.**    A decreased amount of potassium in the extracellular fluid is called hypokalemia.

It can occur with fluid losses from the gastrointestinal tract, skin, or kidneys.

Injury to the gastrointestinal tissue can cause large losses of extracellular fluid, and it can also prevent the absorption of potassium from dietary intake. Potassium can be lost in sweat from the skin or from the secretion of extracellular fluid in areas denuded of skin. When the kidneys excrete high volumes of fluid, the potassium is washed out without opportunity for the renal tubules to resorb the needed electrolyte. Diuretic therapy is the most common cause of urinary potassium loss. Potassium can also be lost in conditions that cause renal tubular acidosis and excessive mineralocorticoid hormone levels.

Hypokalemia can also result from a decreased dietary intake or from alkalosis. In alkalosis, the potassium has increased entry into the cells, and the intracellular concentration of the cation increases.

**Hyperkalemia.**    An elevated level of potassium in the extracellular fluid and blood is called hyperkalemia. The most common source of hyperkalemia is renal disease. The potassium value also rises with mineralocorticoid deficiency or metabolic acidosis. Additionally, the damage to tissue and cells causes a release of intracellular potassium into the extracellular fluids.

In renal disease, the glomeruli may be unable

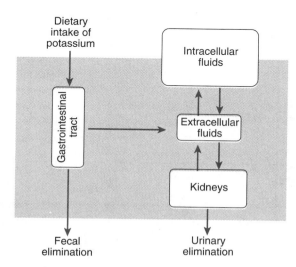

**Figure 5–3**
Homeostatic balance of potassium. Once the potassium is absorbed from the small intestine, most of it is stored within cells, and a small amount remains in the extracellular fluids, including blood. Excess potassium is excreted from the body in feces and urine. The kidneys are the best regulators of potassium homeostasis.

to filter the blood, causing a rise in the serum value and a decrease in the excretion of potassium in the urine. In acute renal failure, the potassium level begins to rise with the onset of oliguria. In chronic renal failure, the potassium level does not begin to rise until there is a 75% reduction in the glomerular filtration rate.

With the slower onset of chronic renal failure, the body is able to adapt its control of the potassium level. In the compensation, the renal tubules do not resorb potassium, and so greater excretion of potassium in the urine occurs. Additionally, the intestinal tract absorbs less dietary potassium and excretes more of the cation in the feces.

### Purpose of the Test

Serum potassium is used to evaluate electrolyte balance, acid-base balance, hypertension, renal disease or renal failure, and endocrine disease. It is used to monitor the patient receiving treatment for ketoacidosis as well as those receiving hyperalimentation, dialysis, diuretic therapy, or intravenous therapy.

### Procedure

A green- (heparin) or red-topped tube is used to collect 5 or 10 mL of venous blood.

#### Quality Control

Venipuncture technique must be smooth, with a blood flow that fills the tube readily. If the blood has excessive turbulence because of flawed technique, hemolysis of erythrocytes causes a false rise in the serum value.

### Findings

**Elevated Values**

Rapid or excessive intravenous potassium replacement
Dehydration
Acute renal failure

Chronic renal failure
Potassium-sparing diuretics
Massive hemolysis
Acidosis
Diabetic ketoacidosis

Traumatic crush injury
Severe burns
Addison's disease

**Decreased Values**

Diuretic therapy
Intravenous fluid therapy without potassium replacement
Vomiting or diarrhea

Severe burns
Renal tubular acidosis
Excessive sweating
Fistula drainage
Bartter's syndrome

Alkalosis
Primary aldosteronism
Secondary aldosteronism

### Interfering Factors

- Hemolysis

### Nursing Implementation

**Pretest**

In drawing the blood, it is preferable to avoid the use of a tourniquet. If the tourniquet is applied loosely, the fist should not be clenched. These measures prevent hemolysis of erythrocytes and a false elevation of the potassium value.

### Posttest

Arrange for transport of the specimen to the laboratory as quickly as possible, because a clotted specimen causes a false elevation of the serum value. Monitor the test results and immediately notify the physician of any changes into an abnormal range. Untreated hyperkalemia or hypokalemia can cause changes in the myocardium and the neuromuscular system, including very serious cardiac arrhythmias (Rutecki & Whittier, 1996; Speicher, 1998; White, 1997) (Table 5–1).

■
*Critical Thinking 5–3*
For the patient who receives thiazide diuretics, create a teaching plan with a focus on prevention of hypokalemia.

## Critical Values

**Adult: <2.5 mEq/L (SI <2.5 mmol/L) *or* >6.5 mEq/L (SI >6.5 mmol/L)**
**Newborn: <2.5 mEq/L (SI <2.5 mmol/L) *or* >7 mEq/L (SI >7 mmol/L)**

Once the values reach either critical level, the patient is in a life-threatening condition, with danger of severe cardiac arrhythmia, cardiac arrest, and death. Immediately notify the physician of the abnormal test value.

Assess the patient for manifestations of potassium imbalance. With hyperkalemia, the manifestations include muscle weakness, decreased reflexes, ascending paralysis, respiratory arrest, and a slow or irregular heartbeat (Perez, 1995a; White, 1997). In hypokalemia, the manifestations include weakness, cramps of the legs or body, tetany, anorexia, nausea, tachycardia, bradycardia, premature atrial contractions, and premature ventricular contractions (Perez, 1995b; Speicher, 1998; Tsuji et al., 1994).

Prepare for an electrocardiogram (ECG) (Fig. 5–4) or for cardiac monitoring and for the administration of prescribed medication or intravenous therapy to correct the potassium imbalance. Specific treatment will depend on the type and severity of the imbalance and its cause.

## Sodium, Serum

(Serum)    Synonym: Na+

## Normal Values

Adult: 136–145 mEq/L *or* SI 136–145 mmol/L
Child: 138–145 mEq/L *or* SI 136–145 mmol/L
Infant: 139–146 mEq/L *or* SI 139–146 mmol/L
Newborn: 133–146 mEq/L *or* SI 133–146 mmol/L
Premature (48 hours):  128–148 mEq/L *or* SI 128–148 mmol/L

## Background Information

Sodium is an electrolyte found in all body fluids. As the major extracellular cation, sodium is responsible for osmolarity and intravascular osmotic pressure.

With the change of sodium concentration in the blood, resultant changes occur in the water content into or out of cells. Thus, the alteration of sodium content is responsible for dehydration or overhydration within cells or in extracellular fluids.

**Table 5–1 ECG* Changes Associated with Critical Values of Serum Potassium**

**Hyperkalemia**

| Serum Potassium Level | ECG Manifestations |
|---|---|
| >6.5 mEq/L (SI >6.5 mmol/L) | Peaked T waves |
| 7–8 mEq/L (SI 7–8 mmol/L) | Prolonged P-R interval<br>Loss of P waves<br>Widening of the QRS complexes |
| >8–10 mEq/L (SI >8–10 mmol/L) | Sine wave pattern<br>Cardiac standstill; asystole |

**Hypokalemia**

| Serum Potassium Level | ECG Manifestations |
|---|---|
| 2–2.5 mEq/L (SI 2–2.5 mmol/L) | Sagging of the S-T segment<br>Flattened or depressed T wave<br>Elevation of the U wave |
| <2 mEq/L (SI <2 mmol/L) | Smaller T waves<br>Increased height (amplitude) of U waves |

*ECG = Electrocardiogram

In normal physiology, the level of serum sodium remains within a relatively narrow range. The homeostatic balance of sodium, water, and osmolarity is regulated by renal, posterior pituitary, and hypothalamic functions.

The daily intake of sodium is balanced by an equivalent amount of sodium excretion. The glomeruli of the kidneys filter the sodium from the extracellular fluids freely, with renal tubular resorption of isotonic concentrations of the electrolyte. The excess sodium is excreted in the urine. The amount of urinary excretion depends on the daily intake of sodium and the hydration status of the individual.

**Hyponatremia.** A low level of serum sodium is called hyponatremia. The cause is usually excessive sodium loss or excessive water retention. The origin of the problem is frequently renal, including renal tubular defects, advanced renal failure, or loop diuretic therapy. Each of these conditions alters the excretion of sodium and water in the proper concentrations. Metabolic alkalosis, ketonuria, or endocrine deficiency may also cause hyponatremia. In all these conditions, excessive loss of sodium or excessive resorption of water by the kidneys occurs.

Nonrenal causes of sodium loss include fluid and electrolyte losses from the gastrointestinal tract, "third space" losses, and severe thermal injury. The hyponatremia may also be a result of an increase in total body water, such as in conditions that cause water retention and edema. Although some sodium retention also occurs in the extracellular fluids, the amount of water retention is much greater, and the serum is diluted.

**Hypernatremia.** An elevation of serum sodium that is caused by sodium retention or an excessive loss of water is called hypernatremia. When a loss of water occurs, the concentration of sodium and the osmolarity of the blood increase.

In nonrenal causes of hypernatremia, a loss of body fluid occurs without adequate replacement. This can occur in diuresis, profuse sweating, diarrhea, burns, and respiratory infection. Renal losses of fluid may result from advanced renal failure.

The fluid loss can also be a result of the failure of the kidneys to secrete antidiuretic hormone because of a central nervous system disturbance. In some cases, the kidneys do not respond to antidiuretic hormone because of disease that affects the renal tubules. In the case of a lack of antidiuretic hormone, the tubules cannot resorb water. The urine is diluted and of high volume as the water is excreted.

## Purpose of the Test

Serum sodium levels are used to monitor electrolyte balance, water balance, and acid-base balance. They are also used in the evaluation of disorders of the central nervous system, musculoskeletal disorders, or diseases of the kidneys or adrenal glands.

## Procedure

A green- or red-topped tube is used to obtain 5 to 10 mL of venous blood. For infants and small children, a heelstick or finger puncture and a capillary tube are used to obtain capillary blood.

### Quality Control

Venipuncture technique must be smooth, with a blood flow that fills the tube readily. If the blood has excessive turbulence because of poor technique, the hemolysis of the erythrocytes will falsely elevate the test results.

## Findings

### Elevated Values

Dehydration
Cushing's syndrome
Primary aldosteronism
Secondary aldosteronism

Inadequate thirst
Diabetic acidosis
Azotemia
Excessive saline
 infusion

Profuse sweating
Vomiting or diarrhea

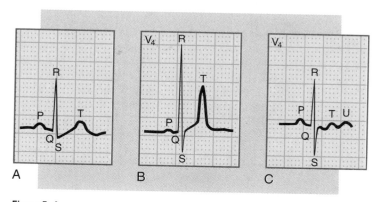

**Figure 5–4**
ECG changes in potassium imbalance. *A,* Normal ECG pattern. *B,* Moderate hyperkalemia with tall, peaked T waves. *C,* Moderate hypokalemia with a flattened T wave and elevation of the U wave.

### Decreased Values

Addison's disease
Hypopituitarism
Vomiting or diarrhea
Burns
Acute water intoxi-
cation
Cirrhosis
Congestive heart
failure

Nephrotic syndrome
Central nervous
system disturbance
(trauma, tumor)
Diuretic therapy
Salt-wasting nephritis
Hypothyroidism
Glucorticoid defi-
ciency

Syndrome of inappro-
priate antidiuretic
hormone
Acute or chronic
renal failure
Ketonuria
Bicarbonaturia

---

**Interfering Factors**

- Hemolysis

---

**Nursing Implementation**

Venipuncture technique and care of the puncture site are included in the nursing component.

### Pretest

The blood should be drawn without a tourniquet to avoid clotting and hemolysis.

### Posttest

To prevent clotting and hemolysis, arrange for prompt transport of the specimen to the laboratory.

---

**Critical Values**

**<120 mEq/L (SI <120 mmol/L) *or* >160 mEq/L (SI >160 mmol/L)**

Once the values reach either critical level, the patient can have significant dysfunction of the brain and nervous system. Immediately notify the physician of the abnormal test value.

Assess the patient for manifestations of sodium imbalance. With severe hypernatremia, the manifestations include somnolence, confusion, coma, and respiratory paralysis (Speicher, 1998). When the sodium value reaches the elevated critical level in less than 24 hours, the mortality rate is greater than 70% (Mandal, Saklayan, Hillman, & Harkert, 1997). In moderate hyponatremia, the patient is asymptomatic. Once the sodium value declines to the critical level or lower, the manifestations include lethargy, weakness, somnolence, seizures, and coma. Death can occur from this very severe hyponatremia (Jacobs et al., 1996; Speicher, 1998).

Notify the physician of the laboratory data and the assessment findings. Specific treatment will depend on the type and severity of the imbalance and its cause.

---

### References

Burtis, C.A., & Ashwood, E. R. (Eds.).(1994). *Tietz text-book of clinical chemistry* (2nd ed.). Philadelphia: W. B. Saunders.

Gaedeke, M. K. (1995). Evaluating serum magnesium levels. *Nursing 95, 25*(8), 75.

Good, C. B., McDermott, L., & McClosky, B. (1995). Diet and serum potassium in patients on ACE inhibitors [Letter]. *Journal of the American Medical Association, 274*, 538.

Henry, J. B. (1996). *Clinical diagnosis and management by laboratory methods* (19th ed.). Philadelphia: W. B. Saunders.

Higgans, C. (1996). Laboratory measurement of sodium and potassium. *Nursing Times, 92*(12), 40–42.

Jacobs, D. S., Demott, W. R., Grady, H. J., Horvat, R. T., Huestis, D. W., & Kasten, B. L. (Eds.). (1996). *Laboratory test handbook* (4th ed.). Baltimore: Williams & Wilkins.

Lab results: Nurses have the duty to notify the physician of rising potassium levels. (1996). *Legal Eagle Eye Newsletter for the Nursing Profession, 4*(6), 1.

Lehmann, C. A. (1998). *Saunders manual of clinical laboratory science.* Philadelphia: W. B. Saunders.

Locker, F. G. (1996). Hormonal regulation of calcium homeostasis. *Nursing Clinics of North America, 31,* 797–803.

Mandel, A. K., Saklayan, M. G., Hillman, N. M., & Markert, R. J. (1997). Predictive factors for high mortality in hypernatremic patients. *American Journal of Emergency Medicine, 15*(2), 130–132.

Morse, M., & Dix, D. (1995). Determining reference ranges by linear analysis: Serum electrolyte concentrations. *Laboratory Medicine, 26*(4), 282–285.

Perez, A. (1995a). Electrolytes: Restoring the balance. Hyperkalemia. *RN, 58*(11), 32–37.

Perez, A. (1995b). Restoring electrolyte balance: Hypokalemia. *RN, 58*(12), 33–36.

Rutecki, G. W., & Whittier, F. C. (1996). Hyperkalemia: How to identify and correct—The underlying cause. *Consultant, 36,* 564–566, 569–573.

Sonnenblick, M., Friedlander, Y., & Rosin, A. J. (1993). Diuretic-induced severe hyponatremia. *Chest, 103,* 601–606.

Speicher, C. (1998). *The right test* (3rd ed.). Philadelphia: W. B. Saunders.

Tietz, N. W. (Ed.). (1995). *Clinical guide to laboratory tests* (3rd ed.). Philadelphia: W. B. Saunders.

Tsuji, H., Venditti, F. J., Evans, J. C., Larson, M. G., & Levy, D. (1994). The associations of levels of serum potassium and magnesium with ventricular premature complexes. *American Journal of Cardiology, 74*(8), 232–235.

White, V. M. (1997). Hyperkalemia. *American Journal of Nursing, 97*(6), 35.

# CHAPTER 6

# Coagulation Screen

This chapter addresses the laboratory tests and diagnostic procedures that evaluate the coagulation processes. These processes include clot formation and clot lysis or the degradation of thrombus.

When bleeding occurs, the coagulation process involves the activation and function of platelets and the activation and interaction of coagulation factors to seal the injured blood vessel with a thrombus. Once the vascular tissue heals, the fibrinolytic response dissolves the thrombus so that blood flow can resume (Fig. 6–1).

Some of the blood tests and procedures measure the time that it takes for a clot to form. Others measure the presence or function of the components of coagulation and fibrinolysis. Disorders of coagulation can result in bleeding or hemorrhage because of an inability or a delayed ability to form a clot. Excessive or rapid formation of a thrombus can also occur because of abnormal coagulation processes.

The disorders that affect coagulation ability can be hereditary, as in hemophilia, or acquired, as in malignancy or pregnancy. Some diseases affect the coagulation system directly, for example, through the loss of platelets or abnormal platelet function. A number of other systemic illnesses affect a primary organ, such as the liver or kidney, with an alteration in coagulation as a secondary effect.

The laboratory tests and diagnostic procedures identify the existence of a coagulation disorder and also determine the part of the coagulation system that is affected. In this way, the treatment is specific and more likely to restore clotting ability.

## Laboratory Tests

## Activated Clotting Time

**(Whole Blood)**          Synonyms: Activated coagulation time, ACT

| Normal Values | 70–120 seconds |
| --- | --- |

## Background Information

The activated clotting time (ACT) test measures the amount of time that is needed to form a clot, particularly during heparin therapy. As a bedside test, the ACT test has the advantages of con-

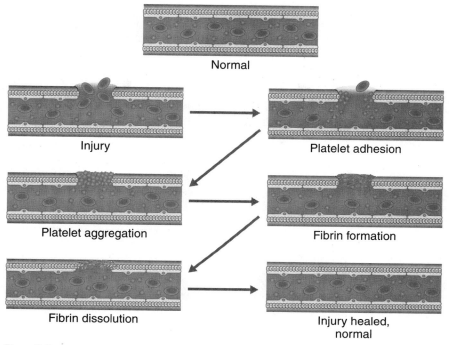

Normal

Injury

Platelet adhesion

Platelet aggregation

Fibrin formation

Fibrin dissolution

Injury healed,
normal

**Figure 6–1**

Vascular injury and hemostasis—An overview. (Reproduced with permission from Lehmann, C. A. [1998]. *Saunders manual of clinical laboratory science* [p. 962]. Philadelphia: W. B. Saunders.)

venience, low cost, and rapidity of results in monitoring the effects of heparin therapy.

Among individuals, response to heparin therapy varies widely. Also, a narrow therapeutic range exists that is not much higher than the normal range. It is essential to monitor the effect of the heparin in the blood so that a therapeutic level of anticoagulation is attained without progressing to the excessive level that can result in a hemorrhage.

The analysis of the test results can be performed in the laboratory, but the use of an automated analyzer permits the activated clotting time test to be performed at the patient's bedside and in other locations near the patient, including in the operating room during cardiopulmonary bypass and percutaneous transluminal angioplasty procedures (Noureddine, 1995). Only the medical technologist performs the test, because it involves precise technology, quality control practices, and variations in procedure according to

differences in analyzers (Jacobs et al., 1996; Stepp & Woods, 1998).

The ACT test is often used during and after cardiovascular surgery, coronary angioplasty, and hemodialysis. Because this test measures overall coagulation ability and not only the effect of heparin, the patient's baseline ACT level is established before heparin therapy is started.

With heparin therapy, the therapeutic range is 180 to 240 seconds for the activated clotting test. During cardiopulmonary bypass procedures, the suggested therapeutic value is much higher, with a range of 300 to 500 seconds (Jacobs et al., 1996). The reference values vary among manufacturers and laboratories because of variations in equipment and procedure, tube activator substances, and the size and source of the blood sample. For interpretation of the patient's results, the nurse should refer to the laboratory reference values of the institution.

**Purpose of the Test**

This test is used to monitor the effects of heparin anticoagulation. It can also be used to screen for coagulation deficiencies.

**Procedure**

A 5-mL, special, nonheparinized syringe with a 22- to 23-G needle is used to draw a sample of venous blood. Two milliliters of the blood is placed into a special tube that contains an activator of silica or siliceous-diatomaceous earth, and the tube is agitated vigorously to mix the blood and activator substance. The tube of blood is then placed into an automated analyzer that has warmed to 37°C. As the tube is rotated, the blood begins to form a clot that can be detected by the analyzer. At the finish of the clot formation, the machine emits an audible signal and displays the time needed for the clot formation. The test result is measured in seconds.

**Quality Control**

The amount of blood placed in the tube must be accurate. If too little blood is used, the proportion of activator to blood will be greater than it should be and will cause a false elevation of the test results.

A double-tube technique must be used to prevent specimen contamination with tissue thromboplastin. In the double-tube technique, a 1- to 2-mL blood sample is obtained and discarded; the special syringe is then used to collect the test sample.

Venipuncture technique must be smooth and accurate to avoid hemolysis of the erythrocytes.

**Findings**

**Elevated Values**

Heparin therapy            Severe coagulation
                               disorder

**Interfering Factors**

- Inadequate volume of blood in the test sample
- Hemolysis
- Coagulation of the specimen

**Nursing Implementation**

**Pretest**

Explain to the patient that the purpose of frequent testing is to monitor the effect of the anticoagulant medication.

When heparin is given in intermittent doses, ensure that the specimen is drawn 1 hour before the next dose. If the specimen is obtained less than 3 hours after a heparin dose is given, the ACT result will be excessively elevated.

When heparin is given in a continuous infusion, special timing of the test is unnecessary.

**Posttest**

For the patient receiving anticoagulants, assess the venipuncture site for signs of bleeding or ecchymosis.

To promote clotting, use sterile gauze to apply pressure to the site or raise the arm above the head while maintaining pressure on the site.

When the patient receives heparin anticoagulation therapy, monitor each ACT result for a value in the therapeutic range. If the result is very elevated or prolonged, notify the physician. It is common for the dosage of heparin to be adjusted to achieve and maintain the desired therapeutic range of clotting time (Lilley, 1995).

| **Critical Value** | **Two to three times the patient's baseline value (Lilley, 1995)** |
|---|---|
| | The nurse must notify the physician of a therapeutic value that is elevated or prolonged into the critical value range. The risk of a spontaneous bleeding episode or hemorrhage is high. Possible medical interventions include postponing or withholding the next heparin dose, discontinuing the continuous heparin infusion, or prescribing the administration of protamine sulfate, the antidote to heparin. |

## Activated Partial Thromboplastin Time

**(Blood)**  Synonyms: aPTT, partial thromboplastin time, PTT

| **Normal Values** | Average value: | 25–35 seconds |
|---|---|---|
| | Newborn: | <90 seconds |
| | Premature infants: | <120 seconds |

## Background Information

The activated partial thromboplastin time (aPTT) measures the number of seconds needed for a clot to form. In the laboratory, the patient's plasma is mixed with a reagent that includes excess calcium. If the plasma has all the intrinsic coagulation factors present, all the extrinsic factors present, and a normal component of inhibitors of coagulation present (Table 6–1), the aPTT is within normal limits. The aPTT is shortened when the patient's coagulation system is already activated. The test value is prolonged, and clotting ability is also impaired when there is a 30% to 40% deficiency of one or more clotting factors or when inhibitors of these factors are active.

The test results include the patient's value and the control value. The control value varies according to the reagent used, and it varies from test to test. To correct for the variation, the control value of the test is the reference or normal value that is used to evaluate the patient's test result.

The aPTT test is used to monitor the results of anticoagulation therapy with heparin. The goal of heparin anticoagulation is to maintain the aPTT in a therapeutic range about two times the normal value (Jacobs et al., 1996). With a prolonged aPTT, the patient takes longer to make a clot, and a thrombus or embolus is less likely to develop.

If the patient has an impairment of the intrinsic coagulation system that causes a prolonged aPTT, the medical treatment may be a transfusion of whole blood or plasma so that the clotting factors are increased and the aPTT value returns to normal (Gibbar-Clements, Shirrell, & Free, 1997).

**Table 6–1   Coagulation Factors–Activators and Inhibitors**

| Category | Factor | Synonym |
|---|---|---|
| *Activators* | | |
| | I | Fibrinogen |
| | II | Prothrombin |
| | | Tissue factor |
| | | Calcium |
| | V | Proaccelerin, labile factor |
| | VII | Prothrombin, proconvertin accelerator, stable factor |
| | VIII | Antihemophiliac factor |
| | IX | Christmas factor, plasma thromboplastin component (PTC) |
| | X | Stuart-Prower factor |
| | XI | Plasma thromboplastin antecedent (PTA) |
| | XII | Hageman coagulation factor |
| | XIII | Fibrin stabilizing factor |
| | Prekallikrein | Fletcher factor |
| | HMWK | High-molecular-weight kininogen, Fitzgerald factor |
| *Inhibitors* | | |
| | Antithrombin III | AT-III |
| | Protein C | PC |
| | Protein S | PS |

**Purpose of the Test**

The aPTT test is used to evaluate the intrinsic coagulation system and the function of factors I, II, V, VIII, IX, X, XI, and XII (Lehmann, 1998). The test helps identify bleeding or clotting disorders that are hereditary or acquired conditions. It is used to monitor the effect of heparin anticoagulant therapy and to adjust the dosage of the drug based on the test results.

**Procedure**

A blue-topped tube with sodium citrate is used to obtain 4.5 mL of venous blood. As an alternative, a heelstick, earlobe, or finger puncture may be used to collect capillary blood in siliconized sodium citrate micropipettes.

**Quality Control**

The tube must be filled with blood. If too little blood is used, the proportion of sodium citrate to blood will be greater than it should be and will result in a false elevation of the test results.

To mix the anticoagulant with the blood, the specimen tube is tilted gently from side to side 5 to 10 times. When multiple specimens are drawn, the aPTT test specimen is obtained last. When this is the only test specimen taken, a double-tube technique must be used to prevent specimen contamination with tissue thromboplastin. In the double-tube technique, a 1- to 2-mL blood sample is obtained and discarded; the blue-topped tube is then used to collect the test sample.

Venipuncture technique must be smooth, with a blood flow that fills the vacuum tube readily. If the blood has excessive turbulence because of flawed venipuncture technique, the hemolysis greatly shortens the aPTT result in normal individuals.

**Findings**

**Elevated Values**

Excess administration of heparin

Deficiency of one or more coagulation factors

Excessive inhibition of the coagulation system

Hemophilia

Disseminated intravascular coagulation (DIC)

Specific and nonspecific circulatory anticoagulants such as lupus anticoagulants

Liver failure

Vitamin K deficiency

**Decreased Values**

Hypercoagulable states (with arterial or venous thrombus formation)

**Interfering Factors**
■

*Critical Thinking 6–1*
The laboratory informs you that the most recent aPTT result is 72 seconds for a patient receiving an intravenous infusion with heparin. What nursing assessments are needed immediately?

- Hemolysis
- Inadequate blood sample
- Prolonged delay before analysis is performed

**Nursing Implementation**

**Pretest**

When heparin is given in intermittent doses, ensure that the aPTT specimen is drawn and the results known before the next dose. With subcutaneous administration of the heparin, some physicians request the test halfway between the scheduled heparin doses. Others request the test 30 minutes before the next injection, in time to adjust the heparin dose as needed. If the specimen is obtained less than 3 hours after a heparin dose is given, the aPTT result is excessively elevated (Samama, 1995).

When a continuous infusion of heparin is started, equilibrium occurs after 4 hours with a valid aPTT test result. Thereafter, testing is done to monitor the treatment, but special timing of the test is unnecessary.

**During the Test**

Ensure that a heparinized tube is not used to obtain the blood specimen.

Venipuncture is the preferred method of obtaining the specimen.

If an indwelling line, such as an arterial line or double-lumen (Hickman) catheter, is used to obtain blood for coagulation studies, special measures must be taken. These lines are flushed with heparin to maintain patency, and the presence of heparin would alter the aPTT test results (Jacobs et al., 1996). The line must be cleared of the contamination of heparin by drawing off and discarding an amount of fluid and blood before the actual specimen is collected. The amount of blood draw (waste) varies with the type and length of the catheter or with the dead space volume of that catheter. For aPTT studies, the discard amount is six times the dead space volume. Laboratory policy defines the amount of blood waste that must be discarded (Baer, 1995; Hancock, 1993; Henry, 1996).

### Posttest

For the patient receiving anticoagulants, assess the venipuncture site for signs of bleeding or ecchymosis.

To promote clotting at the venipuncture site, use sterile gauze to apply pressure to the site or raise the patient's arm above the head while maintaining pressure on the site.

Arrange for prompt transport of the specimen to the laboratory.

#### Quality Control

Specimens received more than 2 hours after collection will be rejected by the laboratory.
When the patient receives heparin anticoagulation therapy, monitor each aPTT result for a value in the therapeutic range. If the result is very elevated, notify the physician. The dose of heparin may be adjusted, or the intravenous infusion with heparin may be discontinued for a short time. Protamine sulfate is kept available to be used as prescribed. It can be prescribed for intramuscular injection as an antidote to heparin.

| Critical Value | >70 seconds |
| --- | --- |
| | If the aPTT value is in the critical value range, the physician must be notified. The patient is at risk for spontaneous bleeding or hemorrhage. |

## Clot Retraction Time

| (Blood) | Synonyms: None |
| --- | --- |

| Normal Values | Retraction of the clot starts in 1 hour and is complete in 24 hours. |
| --- | --- |

### Background Information

There is no single test that fully reflects the complex activities of platelets. Clot retraction is one of the tests of coagulation that is used to study the function of platelets in clot formation.

Following a vascular injury, platelets adhere to the vascular endothelium and aggregate. With the activation of the coagulation system, fibrin is formed to reinforce the platelet aggregation. A clot or thrombus is formed to provide a firm seal at the injury site. Once the clot has formed, the normal process of clot retraction or clot contraction begins within 1 hour and is completed in 24 hours.

In the test analysis of a person with normal quantity and quality of platelets, the clot forms in a test tube and retracts from the sides of the tube, changing its characteristics over a measured period of time. As the serum and some red blood cells leak out of the clot, the clot should retract by 40% to 50%. With this consolidation, the clot should finally appear to be dry, firm, and intact, with only 5% of the serum remaining within the clot.

Clot retraction is dependent on a normal platelet count and normal platelet function. In addition, the blood must have a normal hematocrit and fibrinogen level.

**Abnormal Values.**   Inadequate platelet count and platelet function affect the ability to form a clot. In thrombocytopenia, a reduced number of platelets exist. With thrombasthenia, also known as Glanzmann's disease, poor or abnormal platelet function occurs. Abnormal clot retraction resulting from platelet abnormality is described as delayed, incomplete, or poor. The clot remains soft, soggy, and friable, with excess retention of serum.

Abnormal clot retraction that is not related to platelets can also occur. If no clot formation occurs, as in disseminated intravascular coagulation (DIC) and hemophilia, no clot retraction can occur. With excess fibrinolysis, the clot forms initially but then dissolves. In other examples of abnormality, a decrease in fibrinogen inhibits both clot formation and clot retraction, and in severe anemia, the clot retraction time is prolonged or increased (Stepp & Woods, 1998).

---

**Purpose of the Test**

The clot retraction time investigates the function of platelets, particularly in the diagnosis of Glanzmann's disease, which is an inherited condition.

---

**Procedure**

A red-topped tube is used to collect 10 mL of venous blood. The tube must be filled. In some laboratories, the blood is drawn with a syringe and then transferred into a graduated centrifuge tube immediately.

**Quality Control**

With venipuncture, the tourniquet should be tied lightly for a brief time to prevent pooling of cells in the vein at the site of blood collection. Venipuncture technique must be smooth, with a blood flow that fills the vacuum tube or syringe readily. If the blood has excessive turbulence because of flawed venipuncture technique, the hemolysis of the erythrocytes will alter the test results.

---

**Findings**

**Abnormal Values**

| | | |
|---|---|---|
| Thrombocytopenia | Hyperfibrinogenemia | DIC |
| Anemia | Thrombasthenia | Secondary fibrinolysis |

---

**Interfering Factors**

- Aspirin therapy
- Hemolysis
- Coagulated specimen

---

**Nursing Implementation**    **Posttest**

Particularly for the patient with suspected clotting problems, assess the venipuncture site for signs of bleeding or ecchymosis.

To promote clotting at the venipuncture site, use sterile gauze to apply pressure to the site or raise the patient's arm above the head while maintaining pressure on the site.

Ensure that the specimen tube is labeled correctly. Arrange for prompt transport of the specimen to the laboratory.

**Quality Control**

| The blood must arrive at the laboratory and be prepared for the test within 1 hour. |
| --- |

## Coagulation Factor Assay

**(Plasma)**                    Synonym: Factor assay

| **Normal Values** | General values: | 0.50–1.50 µ/mL or 500–1,500 U/L |
| --- | --- | --- |
| | | 50%–150% of normal activity |
| | Factor II: | 0.6–1.5 U/mL |
| | | 60%–150% of normal activity or |
| | | SI 0.60–1.50 fraction of normal activity |
| | Factor V: | 0.5–1.5 U/mL |
| | | 50%–150% of normal activity or |
| | | SI 0.50–1.50 fraction of normal activity |
| | Factor VII: | 0.65–1.35 U/mL |
| | | 65%–135% of normal activity or |
| | | SI 0.65–1.35 fraction of normal activity |
| | Factor VIII: | 0.5–1.5 U/mL |
| | | 50%–150% of normal activity or |
| | | SI 0.50–1.50 fraction of normal activity |
| | Factor IX: | 0.5–1.5 U/mL |
| | | 50%–150% of normal activity or |
| | | SI 50–150 fraction of normal activity |
| | Factor X: | 0.6–1.3 U/mL |
| | | 60%–130% of normal activity or |
| | | SI 60–130 fraction of normal activity |
| | Factor XI: | 0.65–1.35 U/mL |
| | | 65%–135% of normal activity or |
| | | SI 0.65–1.35 fraction of normal activity |
| | Factor XII: | 0.65–1.5 U/mL |
| | | 65%–150% of normal activity or |
| | | SI 0.65–1.50 fraction of normal activity |
| | Factor XIII: | Clot is stable for 24 hours |

## Background Information

To achieve hemostasis, with the formation of a clot to arrest the bleeding, a series of highly ordered and complex chemical interactions occurs. The process of coagulation consists of three interacting components: platelet aggregation, activation of the intrinsic pathway, and activation of the tissue factor pathway.

Platelets form the initial plug and then aggregate to seal the bleeding vessel. Simultaneously, coagulation factors are activated via the intrinsic and tissue factor pathways and ultimately form fibrin (Fig. 6–2). Once fibrin fibers are integrated into the clot, the clot becomes stable and firm. This seals off the injured blood vessel so that no more blood is lost. Beneath the clot, the injured wall of the blood vessel can heal.

The tissue factor pathway is activated in a rapid

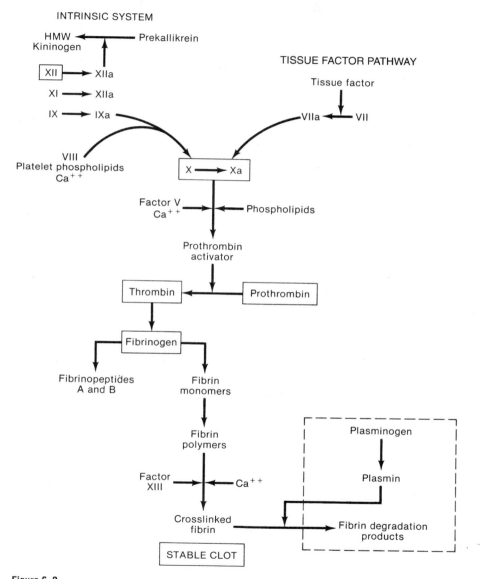

**Figure 6–2**

The coagulation pathways. Two interdependent pathways form a common pathway for clot formation. Once plasminogen is activated, the process of fibrinolysis or the dissolving of the clot begins. (Modified with permission from Clochesy, J. M., Breu, C., Cardin, S., Rudy, E. B., & Whittaker, A. A. [1993]. *Critical care nursing* [p. 1052]. Philadelphia: W. B. Saunders.)

response by tissue trauma and the escape of blood from the vasculature. The release of tissue factor then activates factor VII prothrombin. Prothrombin stimulates the intrinsic pathway by activation of factor X.

The intrinsic pathway is activated more slowly by vascular trauma, with the contact of collagen, prekallikrein, and high-molecular-weight kininogen at the site of injury. These contact factors initiate the conversion of factor XII. The intrinsic pathway proceeds by activation of additional coagulation factors in a series of events until fibrin is formed.

Although the activation of coagulation factors is in a cascade pattern for both the tissue factor and the intrinsic pathways, the coagulation response is not totally linear. There are additional crossover reactions and feedback loops that also occur at multiple levels of the cascade. These actions produce interdependence between the pathways, further enhancing the response of the coagulation system (Henry, 1996; Lehmann, 1998).

The coagulation factors are circulating plasma proteins (see Table 6–1). Once they become activated, each has a specific function in the coagulation process. The coagulation factor assay identifies one or more of the factors that are responsible for impaired coagulation ability. The coagulation factors that are part of the assay are factors II, V, VII, VIII, IX, X, XI, XII, and XIII.

## Purpose of the Test

This test is used to detect the deficiency of one or more coagulation factors in coagulation disorders that are hereditary or of acquired origin.

## Procedure

A blue-topped tube with sodium citrate is used to obtain 4.5 mL of venous blood. As an alternative, a heelstick, earlobe, or finger puncture may be used to collect capillary blood in siliconized sodium citrate micropipettes.

### Quality Control

The tube must be filled with blood. If too little blood is used, the proportion of sodium citrate will be greater than that of blood and result in a false elevation of the test results.

To mix the anticoagulant with the blood, the specimen tube is gently tilted from side to side 5 to 10 times. When multiple specimens are drawn, the coagulation factor assay specimen is obtained last. When this is the only test specimen, a double-tube technique must be used to prevent specimen contamination with tissue thromboplastin. In the double-tube technique, a 1- to 2-mL blood sample is obtained and discarded, and the blue-topped tube is then used to collect the test sample.

## Findings

### Elevated Values

Oral contraceptive therapy (elevation of factors II, VII, VIII, IX, X, and XII)

DIC (elevation of factor VIII)

### Decreased Values

Hemophilia A (deficiency of factor VIII)
Hemophilia B (deficiency of factor IX)

Hereditary deficiency of factor XI
Parahemophilia (deficiency of factor V)

von Willebrand's disease (decrease of factor VIII)

Lupus erythematosus (deficiency of factor II)

Liver disease (deficiencies of factors II, V, IX, X, and XIII)

Vitamin K deficiency (deficiencies of factors II, IX, and X)

DIC (deficiencies of factors V and VIII)

Factor V inhibitors

Gaucher's disease (deficiency of factor IX)

Nephrotic syndrome (deficiency of factor IX)

Amyloidosis (deficiency of factor X)

Renal or adrenocortical malignancy (deficiency of factor X)

---

**Interfering Factors**

- Anticoagulant therapy
- Inadequate blood sample
- Hemolysis
- Coagulation
- Pregnancy
- Time delay before analysis
- Warming of the specimen

---

**Nursing Implementation**

**Pretest**

Schedule this test for 2 weeks after coumarin therapy is discontinued or 2 days after heparin therapy is discontinued.

A specialized coagulation laboratory may be needed to perform the test. Coordinate with the local laboratory facility regarding the scheduling and transport of the specimen.

On the requisition slip, list any history of medication that interferes with coagulation, including a history of oral contraceptive use or anticoagulant therapy.

**Posttest**

Ensure that the venipuncture site has sealed and that the patient is not bleeding. Use sterile gauze to apply pressure to the puncture site as needed. Keeping pressure on the site, instruct the patient to raise the arm over the head. The combination of pressure and elevation should help coagulation occur and stop the bleeding.

Place the specimen in a cup of iced water immediately after the blood is drawn.

Arrange for prompt transport of the chilled specimen to the laboratory. With refrigeration, the coagulation factors are stable for about 2 hours.

---

## Coagulation Inhibitors

(Serum, Plasma)

Synonyms: Antithrombin III, protein C, protein S

---

**Normal Values**

| Antithrombin III | 21–30 mg/dL *or* SI 210–300 mg/L |
| | 85%–115% of normal activity *or* |
| | SI 0.85–1.15 (fraction of normal activity) |

*Continued on following page*

*Continued*

| | |
|---|---|
| Protein C | 2.82–5.65 µg/mL *or* SI 2.82–5.65 mg/L<br>70%–140% of normal activity *or*<br>SI 0.70–1.40 (fraction of normal activity) |
| Protein S | 21–42 µg/mL *or* 21–42 mg/L<br>67%–140% of normal concentration *or*<br>SI 0.67–1.40 (fraction of normal concentration) |

## Background Information

The regulation or control of the coagulation cascade consists of a balance between the activation and the inhibition of coagulation factors. Antithrombin III, protein C, and protein S all are natural inhibitors of coagulation. By neutralizing the actions of the coagulation factors, the formation of a thrombus or blood clot is inhibited. A patient may have deficiencies of one or more of these coagulation factors. The reference values vary according to the method of analysis that is used.

**Antithrombin III.**   The primary inhibitor of the activated form of factor X (factor Xa) and thrombin (factor IIa) is antithrombin III. It also inhibits the activity of factors XII, XI, and IX. In the presence of adequate antithrombin III, the anticoagulant action of heparin is increased. With low or inadequate levels of antithrombin III, patients can experience a resistance to heparin, but they respond to anticoagulant therapy with coumarin. The deficiency of antithrombin III can result in the formation of recurrent or extensive thrombus formation or a thromboembolic disorder.

The deficiency of antithrombin III can be hereditary or acquired. The abnormality can be decreased production of antithrombin III, normal production but impaired function of the protein, or a decreased amount because of excessive consumption (Halfman & Berg, 1993).

**Protein C.**   Protein C is synthesized by the liver and is a natural inhibitor of coagulation. It is activated by thrombin. It functions to inhibit activated factors V and VIII and prolongs the conversion of prothrombin to thrombin. These activities delay or reduce thrombus formation. In addition, protein C enhances the activity of tissue plasminogen activator (t-PA) in the lysis or dissolving of the thrombus.

Reduced levels of protein C cause recurrent or extensive thrombus formation. When the cause is hereditary, homozygous protein C deficiency usually results in death from massive clot formation in infancy. Heterozygous protein C deficiency is less severe. Either too little of the protein exists, or it is not completely functional. These patients often experience thrombus formation in adulthood in the form of a deep vein thrombosis, thrombophlebitis, pulmonary embolus, or a hypercoagulable state (Esmon, 1992). Acquired deficiency is associated with the decreased synthesis of protein C in liver disease.

**Protein S.**   Like protein C, protein S is a vitamin K–dependent coagulation protein that is synthesized by the liver. It is a cofactor of protein C, accelerating and enhancing the effect of protein C. In combination, proteins C and S inhibit the formation of a thrombus. The patient who has a deficiency of protein S also has the tendency to form recurrent thrombi in the form of a deep vein thrombosis, thrombus, embolus, or hypercoagulable state. The condition may be of hereditary or acquired origin.

## Purpose of the Tests

The three tests are used to investigate the underlying cause of a thrombus, particularly in young adults or in patients who have a family history of thrombus formation. These tests are also used to assess the cause of a hypercoagulable state and a fibrinolytic state. Antithrombin III is used to evaluate the response to heparin or to investigate the cause of heparin failure.

**Procedure**

**Antithrombin III.** Two blue-topped tubes with sodium citrate are used to collect 4.5 mL of blood in each tube.

**Protein C.** One blue-topped tube with sodium citrate is used to collect 4.5 mL of venous blood.

**Protein S.** One blue-topped tube with sodium citrate is used to collect 4.5 mL of venous blood. As an alternative, a heelstick, earlobe, or finger puncture may be used to collect capillary blood in siliconized sodium citrate micropipettes.

**Quality Control**

The tube must be filled with blood. If too little blood is used, the proportion of sodium citrate will be greater than that of blood, and a false elevation of the test results will occur.

To mix the anticoagulant with the blood, the specimen tube is tilted gently from side to side 5 to 10 times.

When multiple specimens are drawn, the coagulation inhibitor specimen is obtained last. When this is the only test specimen, a double-tube technique must be used to prevent specimen contamination with tissue thromboplastin. In the double-tube technique, a 1- to 2-mL blood sample is obtained and discarded, and the blue-topped tube is then used to collect the test sample.

Venipuncture technique must be smooth, with a blood flow that fills the vacuum tube readily. If the blood has excessive turbulence because of flawed venipuncture technique, the hemolysis alters the test results.

**Findings**

**Elevated Values**

ANTITHROMBIN III

| | | |
|---|---|---|
| Acute hepatitis | Obstructive jaundice | Inflammatory |
| Renal transplant | Vitamin K deficiency | disorder |

**Decreased Values**

ANTITHROMBIN III

| | | |
|---|---|---|
| Congenital deficiency | Pregnancy or postpar- | Hepatectomy |
| DIC | tum condition | Cirrhosis |
| Nephrotic syndrome | Liver transplant | Chronic liver failure |

PROTEINS C AND S

| | | |
|---|---|---|
| Congenital deficiency | DIC | Cirrhosis |

**Interfering Factors**

- Hemolysis
- Coagulation of the specimen
- Warming of the specimen
- Heparin
- Time delay in analysis of the specimen

**Nursing Implementation**

### Pretest

Schedule the test 2 to 4 weeks after anticoagulation therapy has been discontinued.

If the patient is currently receiving anticoagulant therapy, include the name and dosage of the drug on the requisition slip. Coumarin therapy lowers the patient's protein C value and may increase the antithrombin III value. Heparin can cause erroneous results for the antithrombin III and protein C tests.

### During the Test

Do not allow the blood to be collected from the arm with an intravenous line or a heparin lock device. The heparin flush procedure that is used to keep a venous catheter patent would contaminate the specimen and cause erroneous test results (Jacobs et al., 1996).

### Posttest

Place the antithrombin III tubes on ice immediately and arrange for prompt transport of all specimens to the laboratory.

### Quality Control

These three tests become invalid if a delay of more than 2 hours occurs before the blood is prepared for analysis. The coagulation inhibitors are more stable in cold temperatures.

## D-dimer Test

**(Plasma)**  Synonym: Fibrin degradation fragment

**Normal Values**

| | |
|---|---|
| Latex beads method: | <0.25 mg/mL *or* SI <250 µg/L |
| ELISA method: | Negative; no D-dimer fragments are present |

### Background Information

D-dimer is a fragment of fibrin that is formed as a result of fibrin degradation and clot lysis. The enzyme-linked immunosorbent assay (ELISA) method is a highly specific method that is used for emergency screening to exclude the presence of a deep vein thrombus. Deep vein thrombus is not present when the results are less than the normal values.

Elevated test results or the presence of D-dimer fragments is evidence that thrombus formation and lysis of the thrombus by the enzyme activity of plasmin occurred. The combination of elevated levels of fibrin split-products and D-dimer fragments >0.5 mg/L is highly predictive of DIC.

**Purpose of the Test**

The D-dimer test is used as a screening test for deep vein thrombosis. It helps determine whether a clot is present in the diagnosis of DIC, an acute myocardial infarction, and unstable angina. It is also used in the diagnosis of hypercoagulable conditions that cause recurrent thrombosis.

| Procedure | A plastic syringe and a special plastic tube with sodium citrate and aprotinin additives are used to collect 4.5 mL of venous blood. |
|---|---|

**Findings**

**Elevated (Positive) Values**

| | | |
|---|---|---|
| Thrombotic disease | Thrombolytic-defibrination therapy | Pregnancy (postpartum phase) |
| Deep vein thrombosis | | Malignancy |
| Pulmonary embolism | DIC | Surgery |
| Arterial thromboembolism | Sickle cell anemia crisis | |

**Interfering Factors**

• None

**Nursing Implementation**

Nursing care includes care of the venipuncture site.

**Posttest**

Arrange for immediate transport of the specimen to the laboratory. The patient is acutely ill, and the test results are needed as quickly as possible.

## Euglobulin Clot Lysis

(Blood)          Synonyms: Fibrinolysis time, euglobulin clot lysis time

**Normal Values**

Lysis time:          2–4 hours

## Background Information

Fibrinolysis is the dissolution of a formed clot. Once the injured blood vessel is sealed, the clot or thrombus begins to dissolve as a normal process that permits the blood flow to resume. In the function of the fibrinolytic system (Fig. 6–3), plasminogen is converted to the enzyme plasmin. The activation of plasminogen and its conversion to plasmin are aided or accelerated by t-PA, urokinase, and streptokinase. Plasmin degrades the bonds of fibrin, and clot lysis occurs. In normal fibrinolytic activity, it takes 2 to 4 hours to achieve euglobulin clot lysis, with the release of fibrin degradation products.

When the euglobulin clot lysis time is short-

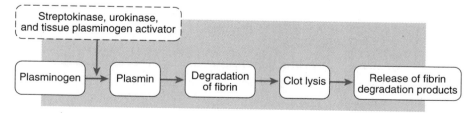

**Figure 6–3**
Simplified diagram of the process of fibrinolysis.

ened, increased fibrinolysis occurs. Shortened lysis time means that a clot dissolves rapidly. This problem is usually associated with increased activity of the plasminogen activators. Clot lysis time can be as short as 5 to 10 minutes. If 100% clot lysis occurs in less than 1 hour, the patient is at risk for bleeding.

## Purpose of the Test

The euglobulin clot lysis test assesses systemic fibrinolysis and abnormality that result in the rapid dissolution of a thrombus. It may be used to monitor fibrinolytic therapy with urokinase, streptokinase, or t-PA to dissolve a thrombus.

## Procedure

A blue-topped tube with sodium citrate is used to obtain 4.5 mL of venous blood. As an alternative, a heelstick, earlobe, or finger puncture may be used to collect capillary blood in siliconized sodium citrate micropipettes.

### Quality Control

The tube must be filled with blood. If too little blood is used, the proportion of sodium citrate will be greater than that of blood and will result in a false elevation of the test results.

To mix the anticoagulant with the blood, the specimen tube is tilted gently from side to side 5 to 10 times. When multiple specimens are drawn, the euglobulin lysis test specimen is obtained last. When this is the only test specimen, a double-tube technique must be used to prevent specimen contamination with tissue thromboplastin. In the double-tube technique, a 1- to 2-mL blood sample is obtained and discarded, and the blue-topped tube is then used to collect the test sample.

Venipuncture technique must be smooth, with a blood flow that fills the vacuum tube readily. If the blood has excessive turbulence because of flawed venipuncture technique, the hemolysis alters the test results.

## Findings

### Decreased Values (Shortened Lysis Time)

| | | |
|---|---|---|
| Circulatory collapse, shock | Pyogenic reactions | DIC |
| Pulmonary or pancreatic surgery | Epinephrine injection | |
| | Obstetric complications | |

## Interfering Factors

- Hemolysis
- Coagulation of the specimen
- Flawed venipuncture technique
- Inadequate amount of specimen
- Hemodilution
- Warming of the specimen
- Exercise

## Nursing Implementation

Nursing care includes care of the venipuncture or capillary puncture site.

### Pretest

For the patient who is physically active, exercise is avoided for 1 hour before the collection of the specimen.

### During the Test

Ensure that the specimen is not collected from the arm that has a catheter or intravenous line. The intravenous solution would dilute the specimen of blood.
After the tourniquet is applied, instruct the patient to relax the hand and refrain from clenching the fist. This will help prevent hemolysis of red blood cells.

### Posttest

Immediately place the specimen on ice.
Arrange for immediate transport of the chilled specimen to the laboratory.

### Quality Control

The specimen must be delivered to the laboratory within 15 to 20 minutes. The plasma will be tested within 30 minutes after obtaining the specimen.

## Fibrinogen

(Plasma)                                    Synonyms: Factor I, fibrinogen level

| Normal Values | | |
|---|---|---|
| Adult: | 200–400 mg/dL *or* SI 2–4 g/L | |
| Newborn: | 125–300 mg/dL *or* SI 1.25–3 g/L | |

### Background Information

Fibrinogen is a coagulation protein that is manufactured by the liver. It is a precursor of fibrin and a vital contributor to the meshwork that binds platelets into an aggregation and ultimately clot formation. When an acute vascular injury or tissue injury with inflammation or necrosis occurs, fibrinogen levels increase in the early phase of coagulation. Within 24 hours of the injury, the fibrinogen level rises dramatically.

At the site of vascular disruption, adhesive proteins and fibrinogen bind the platelets together and plug the break in the vascular wall (Fig. 6–4). As the clotting process progresses, the fibrinogen releases two pairs of peptide and converts to fibrin. The fibrin threads provide stability for the clot.

**Elevated Levels.** Elevated levels of fibrinogen normally occur during acute injury and in pregnancy. In abnormal conditions, the fibrinogen level rises, and an unwanted thrombus or embolus can occur.

**Decreased Levels.** Decreased levels of fibrinogen result in a prolonged time for conversion of fibrinogen to fibrin. Excess bleeding occurs until the clot is formed. Newborns have a different form of fibrinogen that requires a longer time to form a clot. The fibrinogen of the newborn converts to the adult form during the first few months of life. Thereafter, the infant has the same reference value as that of the adult.

### Purpose of the Test

The fibrinogen test is used to help diagnose bleeding disorders, including afibrinogenemia, DIC, and fibrinolysis.

### Procedure

A blue-topped tube with sodium citrate is used to obtain 4.5 mL of venous blood. As an alternative, a heelstick, earlobe, or finger puncture may be used to collect capillary blood in siliconized sodium citrate micropipettes.

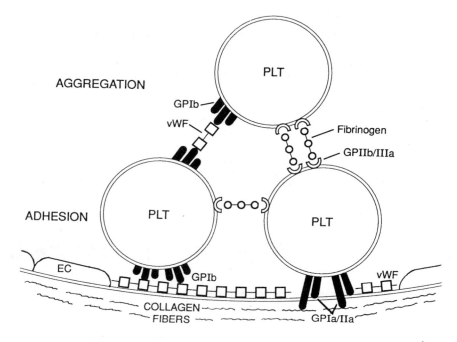

**Figure 6–4**
Platelet adhesion and aggregation. (Reproduced with permission from Berg, D. E. [1992].
Components and defects of the coagulation system. *Nurse Practitioner Forum, 3,* 65.)

**Quality Control**

The tube must be filled with blood. If too little blood is used, the proportion of sodium citrate will be greater than that of blood and will result in a false elevation of the test results.

To mix the anticoagulant with the blood, the specimen tube is tilted gently from side to side 5 to 10 times. When multiple specimens are drawn, the fibrinogen test specimen is obtained last. When this is the only test specimen obtained, a double-tube technique must be used to prevent specimen contamination with tissue thromboplastin. In the double-tube technique, a 1- to 2-mL blood sample is obtained and discarded, and the blue-topped tube is then used to collect the test sample.

Venipuncture technique must be smooth, with a blood flow that fills the vacuum tube readily. If the blood has excessive turbulence because of flawed venipuncture technique, hemolysis alters the test results.

**Findings**

**Elevated Values**

| | | |
|---|---|---|
| Sepsis, infection Inflammation | Malignancy | Traumatic injury |

**Decreased Values**

| | | |
|---|---|---|
| Hereditary afibrino-genemia | Hypofibrinogenemia Severe liver disease | DIC |

| | |
|---|---|
| **Interfering Factors** | • Heparinization<br>• Pregnancy (third trimester)<br>• Recent surgery<br>• Inadequate amount of specimen<br>• Hemolysis<br>• Coagulation of the specimen |

**Nursing Implementation**

### Pretest

For the patient who receives intermittent doses of heparin, schedule the test at least 1 hour after the heparin dose is administered. In some methods of analysis, a recent heparin dose alters the test result.

### During the Test

Do not use the intravenous catheter line with a heparin lock to obtain the specimen, because the heparin flush procedure and residual heparin can invalidate the test.

### Posttest

For the patient with a suspected bleeding disorder, assess the venipuncture site for signs of bleeding or ecchymosis.
To promote clotting, use sterile gauze to apply pressure to the site, or raise the arm above the head while maintaining pressure on the site.
Arrange for prompt transport of the specimen to the laboratory.

### Quality Control

If the specimen is clotted, or if a time delay greater than 1 hour occurs before test analysis is started, the specimen must be rejected by the laboratory.

**Critical Value**

**<100 mg/dL (SI <1.00 g/L)**

The nurse must notify the physician of this severely decreased value. The patient is at risk for abnormal bleeding.

## Fibrin Breakdown Products

(Serum, Urine)  Synonyms: FBP, fibrin(ogen) degradation products, FDP, FSP, fibrin split-products

**Normal Values**

| | |
|---|---|
| Serum: | <10 µg/mL *or* SI <10 mg/L |
| Urine: | <0.25 µg/mL *or* SI <0.25 mg/L |

## Background Information

Fibrinolysis is the normal body process that breaks down and dissolves a formed clot. In this process, the fibrin bonds are split, and fragments called breakdown products, split-products, or degradation products are released. The blood level of fibrin breakdown products rises in proportion to the amount of fibrinolysis activity.

The level of urinary fibrin breakdown products does not correlate with the serum values. When proteinuria is present, the elevation of fibrin breakdown products is an indicator of clotting and lysis in the renal tissues. After renal transplantation, the elevated urinary level can be a predictor of rejection of the transplant.

| | |
|---|---|
| **Purpose of the Test** | This test is used to help diagnose DIC and may be useful in monitoring fibrinolytic treatment. It also may be used in the study of disorders that produce clot formation and lysis of the clot. |

**Procedure**

**Blood.** A special tube for fibrin breakdown products is used to collect 2 mL of venous blood. The tube is obtained from the coagulation laboratory and contains thrombin and an antifibrinolytic agent.

**Quality Control**

The tube must not be overfilled. Once the blood is drawn, the tube is tilted from side to side 5 to 10 times to mix the blood with the clotting agents. The blood will coagulate.

**Urine.** A special tube for fibrin breakdown products is used to collect 2 mL of urine.

**Findings**

**Elevated Values**

SERUM

| | | |
|---|---|---|
| DIC | Liver disease | Malignancy |
| Myocardial infarction | Primary fibrinolysis | Infection or inflammation |
| Pulmonary embolus | Secondary fibrinolysis | |

URINE

Kidney disease
Renal transplant
   rejection

**Interfering Factors**

**Serum**

- Improper collection procedure

**Urine**

- Menstruation
- Hematuria

**Nursing Implementation**

**Pretest**

**Serum**

Nursing care includes care of the venipuncture site. No specific patient instruction or intervention is needed.

### Urine

The presence of hematuria, particularly from menstrual flow, invalidates test results. If blood is present, postpone the test and notify the physician.

### Posttest

Arrange for prompt transport of the specimen to the laboratory.

| Critical Value | **>40 µg/mL** |
| --- | --- |
| | The physician must be notified of this very elevated level. The critical value is associated with DIC. |

## Platelet Aggregation

(Plasma)                    Synonyms: Aggregometer test, platelet function studies

| Normal Values | Platelet aggregation occurs in 3–5 minutes. |
| --- | --- |

### Background Information

After an injury to a blood vessel, platelets initiate action in a coagulation response. The platelets adhere to the vascular endothelium and form a plug that prevents additional blood loss. At the same time that the coagulation system is activated, the platelets are stimulated in a second wave of activity to continue the coagulation process. The platelets change shape, develop pseudopods, contract, and release substances from their cytoplasmic granules. Ultimately, the platelets become sticky and are capable of binding plasma proteins, including fibrinogen. The platelets adhere to each other in platelet aggregation (Fig. 6–5).

In the patient with a coagulation disorder, platelet function is studied to help determine the cause of the problem. This test uses platelet-rich plasma and several chemical reagents to stimulate the platelets' ability to aggregate. In the presence of each of the chemical reagents, normal plasma specimens demonstrate rapid aggregation of the platelets. In patients who have *thrombocytopathy,* the abnormal function of platelets, platelet aggregation is decreased or absent. The disorder can be hereditary or acquired.

With abnormal platelet function and a decreased value of this test, the patient has deficient clotting ability and a tendency to bleed. The nurse should observe for characteristic bleeding, as evidenced by easy bruising, spontaneous bruising, epistaxis, and bleeding from mucous membranes, particularly the gingiva of the oral cavity, intestine, or bladder. With trauma or surgery, the patient may bleed profusely (Bick, 1995a).

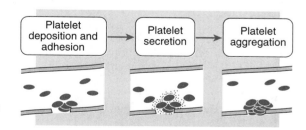

**Figure 6–5**
Platelet response to vascular injury.

**Purpose of the Test**

The platelet aggregation test is used to evaluate platelet function and to detect a hereditary or acquired platelet bleeding disorder.

**Procedure**

A plastic or siliconized glass syringe and a plastic tube with sodium citrate are used to obtain 10 mL of venous blood.

### Quality Control

During venipuncture, the tourniquet should be tied lightly for a brief time to prevent pooling of the platelets in the vein at the site of blood collection. Venipuncture technique must be smooth, with a blood flow that fills the syringe readily. If excessive turbulence occurs because of flawed venipuncture technique, the hemolysis of the erythrocytes will alter the test results. After the blood is put in the tube, the tube is gently tilted 5 to 10 times to mix the anticoagulant and prevent clotting.

**Findings**

### Elevated Values

Raynaud's
  phenomenon

### Decreased Values

| | | |
|---|---|---|
| Uremia | Macroglobulinemia | Wiskott-Aldrich |
| Liver disease | Myeloproliferative | syndrome |
| Leukemia | disorder | von Willebrand's |
| Bernard-Soulier | Hypothyroidism | disease |
| syndrome | | |

**Interfering Factors**

- Clotting of the specimen
- Hemolysis
- Chilling of the specimen
- Lipemia
- Caffeine
- Thrombocytopenia
- Aspirin

**Nursing Implementation**

### Pretest

Schedule this test for 10 days after medications that disrupt platelet function have been discontinued. Aspirin, antihistamines, and anti-inflammatory and psychotropic drugs all interfere with platelet aggregation and can cause a bleeding disorder.

Instruct the patient to fast from food or to eat only low-fat foods for 8 hours before the test. Caffeine intake must be avoided on the day of the test.

## Posttest

Ensure that the venipuncture site has sealed and that the patient is not bleeding. Use sterile gauze to apply pressure to the puncture site as needed. Keeping pressure on the site, instruct the patient to raise the arm over the head. The combination of pressure and elevation should help the process of coagulation and stop the bleeding.

Arrange for immediate transport of the specimen to the laboratory.

### Quality Control

After the blood is drawn, the platelets are stable at room temperature for a limited time only. The specimen cannot be chilled, and the test must be performed within 2 hours.

## Prothrombin Time

**(Plasma)**                    Synonyms: PT, protime

### Normal Values

| | |
|---|---|
| Average: | 10–13 seconds |
| Newborn to 6 months: | 13–18 seconds |
| INR: | 1.00–1.30 |

## Background Information

The prothrombin time test measures the amount of time needed to form a clot. The clot formation is dependent on the functional integrity of coagulation factors II, V, VII, and X. A deficiency of any of these factors prolongs the prothrombin time.

Each test includes the control time in the report of the patient's value. The control time is the normal reference value to be used in the evaluation of the patient's test result. Some variation in the control value always occurs from test to test, depending on the type of reagent and test method used.

Healthy newborns and healthy premature newborns have normal values that are 2 to 3 seconds longer than the adult value. Once the infant reaches about 6 months of age, the reference value is the same as that of an adult.

One use of the prothrombin time test is to monitor the effect of anticoagulant warfarin (Coumadin) therapy. This anticoagulant prolongs the prothrombin time. The response to oral anticoagulation varies among individuals and is unpredictable. If an excessive level exists, the risk is for hemorrhage. If the level is inadequate, the risk is for thrombus formation. The goal of anticoagulation is to maintain the blood level of the prothrombin time in a narrow therapeutic range of 1.5 to 2.5 times the normal (Gibbar-Clements et al., 1997; Lehmann, 1998).

**Internationalized Normalized Ratio.** Today, the Internationalized Normalized Ratio (INR) is the recommended laboratory measurement system for monitoring the effect of oral anticoagulants. For the patient with a mechanical heart valve, the therapeutic range of the INR is 2.5 to 3.5. For all other patients taking oral anticoagulants, the therapeutic range of the INR is 2.0 to 3.0. These conditions include prevention of deep vein thrombosis, pulmonary embolism, myocardial infarction, mitral valve disease, and other conditions with potential for clot formation.

## Purpose of the Test

The prothrombin time test is used to evaluate the extrinsic coagulation system; to help screen for coagulation deficiency of factors I, II, V, VII, and X; and to monitor oral anticoagulant therapy. It is also used to investigate the effects of liver failure and DIC and to screen for vitamin K deficiency.

| | |
|---|---|
| **Procedure** | A blue-topped tube with sodium citrate is used to obtain 4.5 mL of venous blood. As an alternative, a heelstick, earlobe, or finger puncture may be used to collect capillary blood in siliconized sodium citrate micropipettes. |

■

*Critical Thinking 6–2*
How do you teach a patient with anticoagulated blood to evaluate for and avoid nonprescription drugs that contain aspirin?

### Quality Control

The tube must be filled with blood. If too little blood is used, the proportion of sodium citrate will be greater than that of blood and will result in a false elevation of the test results.

To mix the anticoagulant with the blood, the specimen tube is tilted gently from side to side 5 to 10 times. When multiple samples are drawn, this test specimen is obtained last. When this is the only test specimen, a double-tube technique must be used to prevent specimen contamination with tissue thromboplastin. In the double-tube technique, a 1- to 2-mL blood sample is obtained and discarded, and the blue-topped tube is then used to collect the test sample.

Venipuncture technique must be smooth, with a blood flow that fills the vacuum tube readily. If the blood has excessive turbulence because of flawed venipuncture technique, the hemolysis alters the test result.

---

**Findings**

### Elevated Values

Fibrinogen deficiency
Prothrombin deficiency
Liver disease
Abnormal bleeding

Excess anticoagulant therapy
Deficiency of factor V, VI, or X

Vitamin K deficiency
DIC

---

**Interfering Factors**

- Lipemia
- Hemolysis
- Inadequate blood sample
- Prolonged delay before analysis is performed

---

**Nursing Implementation**

### Pretest

Instruct the patient to discontinue intake of alcohol and caffeine for 24 hours before the test. Lipemia from these substances interferes with the accuracy of the test.

If the patient receives intermittent doses of heparin, ensure that the blood is drawn at least 2 hours after the last dose. Recent heparin administration prolongs the prothrombin time excessively.

### Posttest

Ensure that the venipuncture site has sealed and that the patient is not bleeding. Use sterile gauze to apply pressure to the puncture site as needed. Keeping pressure on the site, instruct the patient to raise the arm over the head. The combination of pressure and elevation should help promote coagulation.

Arrange for prompt transport of the specimen to the laboratory. Any prothrombin time specimen received more than 2 hours after the blood is drawn is rejected by the laboratory.

Encourage the patient to maintain a routine, prescribed schedule of blood testing to monitor the anticoagulant effect. The nurse should also teach the patient to recognize early signs of bleeding that could indicate excessive anticoagulation and advise the patient to notify the physician of the problem.

| | |
|---|---|
| **Critical Values** | **(Nonanticoagulated) PT: >20 seconds**<br>**(Anticoagulated) PT: >3 times the control value**<br>**INR: >4.0–5.0**<br><br>The physician should be notified immediately of a severe elevation of the PT or INR result, because a high risk of hemorrhage exists. If the patient receives anticoagulant medication, the nurse should withhold the next dose until the physician responds. The physician may reduce or discontinue the medication temporarily. The physician also may prescribe vitamin K to reduce the anticoagulation effect. |

## Thrombin Time

**(Plasma)**    Synonyms: TT, thrombin clotting time, TCT

| | |
|---|---|
| **Normal Values** | Control value: 7–12 seconds<br>Patient's normal value: Less than 1½ times the control value |

## Background Information

This test measures the time it takes to form a clot by measuring the time of fibrinogen conversion to fibrin in a late phase of the coagulation process. The normal value of the thrombin time varies with the type of reagent and test equipment used. For analysis of the results, the nurse refers to the reference and control values provided by the laboratory of the institution.

The thrombin time is elevated (prolonged) when the fibrinogen level is decreased or absent. It is also prolonged when the fibrinogen is nonfunctional. When fibrin breakdown products generated by DIC or heparin are present in the plasma, the thrombin time is prolonged.

The thrombin time test is the best test to monitor fibrinolytic treatment to dissolve a clot (for example, a pulmonary embolus, myocardial infarction, or deep vein thrombus). The patient's baseline value is measured before treatment begins. In response to intravenous streptokinase or other thrombolytic agent, the clot begins to dissolve, and fibrin breakdown products are produced. The presence of the fibrin breakdown products causes the thrombin time to be elevated. During this treatment, the therapeutic goal is to maintain the thrombin time at 1.5 to 5 times the baseline value (Bell, 1995).

## Purpose of the Test

The test is used to determine hypofibrinogenemia or dysfibrinogenemia. It may be used to help diagnose and monitor disseminated intravascular coagulation and fibrinolysis and to monitor heparin therapy. It is also used to monitor fibrinolytic therapy.

**Procedure**

A blue-topped tube with sodium citrate is used to obtain 4.5 mL of venous blood.

**Quality Control**

The tube must be filled with blood. If too little blood is used, the proportion of sodium citrate will be greater than that of blood and will result in a false elevation of the test results.

To mix the anticoagulant with the blood, the specimen tube is tilted gently from side to side 5 to 10 times.

When multiple samples are drawn, this test specimen is obtained last. When this is the only test specimen, a double-tube technique must be used to prevent specimen contamination with tissue thromboplastin. In the double-tube technique, a 1- to 2-mL blood sample is obtained and discarded, and the blue-topped tube is then used to collect the test sample.

Venipuncture technique must be smooth, with a blood flow that fills the vacuum tube readily. If the blood has excessive turbulence because of flawed venipuncture technique, the hemolysis alters the test result.

**Findings**

**Elevated Values**

Hypofibrinogenemia
Dysfibrinogenemia

Afibrinogenemia
DIC

Primary fibrinolysis
Heparin therapy

**Interfering Factors**

- Hemolysis
- Coagulated specimen
- Insufficient volume of the specimen
- Delay in the analysis of the specimen

**Nursing Implementation**

**Pretest**

With fibrolytic therapy, establish the testing schedule to include a baseline test before therapy begins, 4 to 6 hours after therapy begins, and every 12 hours thereafter until therapy is finished (Bell, 1995).

**During the Test**

Ensure that a heparinized tube is not used to obtain the blood specimen. Venipuncture is the preferred method of obtaining the specimen.

If an indwelling line, such as an arterial line or double-lumen (Hickman) catheter, is used to obtain blood for coagulation studies, special measures must be taken. These lines are flushed with heparin to maintain patency, but the presence of heparin would alter the aPTT test results (Jacobs et al., 1996). The line must be cleared of the contamination of heparin by drawing off and discarding an amount of fluid and blood before the actual specimen is collected. The amount of blood drawn (waste) varies with the type and length of the catheter or the dead space volume of the catheter.

For coagulation studies, the discard amount is six times the dead space volume. Laboratory policy defines the amount of blood waste that must be discarded (Baer, 1995; Henry, 1996).

## Posttest

For the patient with a suspected bleeding disorder, assess the venipuncture site for signs of bleeding or ecchymosis.

To promote clotting, use sterile gauze to apply pressure to the site or raise the arm above the head while maintaining pressure on the site.

With thrombolytic therapy, apply a pressure dressing to any venipuncture site (except the infusion site) until the therapy is completed. During the treatment, the patient will not be able to maintain a clot, and potential exists for bleeding from other venipuncture sites.

Arrange for prompt transport of the specimen to the laboratory.

### Quality Control

If the specimen is clotted, or if a time delay greater than 2 hours occurs before test analysis is started, the specimen is rejected by the laboratory.

---

## Diagnostic Procedures

Bleeding Time    131
Capillary Fragility Test    132

---

## Bleeding Time

(Blood)                    Synonyms: None

---

### Normal Values

| | |
|---|---|
| Bleeding time (Mielke): | 2.5–10 minutes |
| Bleeding time (Ivy): | 2–7 minutes |
| Bleeding time (Duke): | 5 minutes |

---

### Background Information

The bleeding time test is used for the patient who is suspected of having a clotting abnormality, particularly one that involves capillaries or platelet function. The bleeding time can be performed by one of three methods: the Mielke, Ivy, or Duke bleeding time. Each of these methods involves skin punctures or cuts, followed by blotting of the drops of blood until the bleeding stops. The test is measured in the time (minutes) it takes for a clot to form. The elevated level or prolonged time needed for clot formation indicates a vascular problem or disorder of platelet function. Other coagulation disorders usually result in normal values.

The tests differ in method. Mielke uses a standardized cutting device; Ivy uses a sterile lancet, freehand; and the Duke method uses a lancet to puncture the earlobe. The Duke method is used with patients who cannot have an incision on either arm, for example, when bilateral casts or skin eruptions are present. In all three methods, the timing starts with the cut of the skin and stops when the bleeding ceases.

---

### Purpose of the Test

The bleeding time test is used to screen for platelet malfunction or for a vascular defect that interferes with clotting.

**Procedure**

**Mielke Bleeding Time.** A blood pressure cuff is applied to the arm and inflated to 40 mm Hg of pressure. This compresses the capillary circulation. Once the volar aspect of the skin is cleansed with alcohol, two cuts are made in the skin. Filter paper is used to blot the drops of blood every 30 seconds until the bleeding ceases (Fig. 6–6).

**Ivy Bleeding Time.** A blood pressure cuff is applied to the arm and inflated to 40 mm Hg of pressure. Once the skin is cleansed with alcohol, two puncture wounds are made on the volar aspect of the forearm. The blood drops are blotted with filter paper every 30 seconds until the bleeding ceases.

**Duke Bleeding Time.** Once the skin is cleansed with alcohol, a sterile lancet is used to puncture the earlobe. The blotting procedure is the same as for the other two methods.

**Findings**

**Elevated Values**

| | | |
|---|---|---|
| Thrombocytopenia | Macroglobulinemia | Hereditary afibrinogenemia |
| Glanzmann's thrombasthenia | von Willebrand's disease | Myeloproliferative diseases |
| DIC | Gray platelet syndrome | |
| Severe metabolic acidosis | Renal failure | |

**Interfering Factors**

- Laceration of a small vein
- Recent aspirin ingestion
- History of keloid formation
- Platelet count <100,000 cells/mm$^3$

**Nursing Implementation**

**Pretest**

Schedule this test at least 7 days after the last dose of aspirin has been taken (Steppe & Woods, 1998).

Explain the procedure to the patient. The patient should understand that a small scar can result from the puncture or incision. Some laboratories require a written consent.

For the Mielke or Ivy method, inspect the volar aspect of the forearm for rash, infection, or skin eruption. None should be present.

The nurse may assist with the test, but the test is performed by a medical laboratory technologist.

**Posttest**

For the Mielke method, apply a butterfly dressing to the skin site.

As it heals, inspect the skin site daily for signs of infection.

## Capillary Fragility Test

**(Pressure Measurement)** Synonyms: Rumpel-Leede test, tourniquet test, negative pressure suction cup capillary fragility test

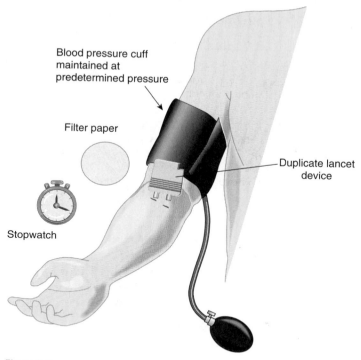

Blood pressure cuff
maintained at
predetermined pressure

Filter paper

Duplicate lancet
device

Stopwatch

**Figure 6–6**
Bleeding time test. (Reproduced with permission from Stevens, M. L. [1997].
*Fundamentals of clinical hematology* [p. 267]. Philadelphia: W. B. Saunders.)

| **Normal Values** | Male:<br>Female and child: | Fewer than 5 petechiae within a 2-in diameter circle<br>Fewer than 10 petechiae within a 2-in diameter circle |
|---|---|---|

## Background Information

The capillary fragility test is a procedure that gives a general estimate of the integrity or fragility of the capillary vascular tissue. When capillaries are healthy, they have effective capillary resistance. In abnormal conditions, the capillaries have increased vascular permeability and are described as fragile.

The test applies pressure on the tissue. The blood pressure cuff method applies positive pressure, and the suction cup method applies negative pressure. With the application of pressure, healthy capillaries produce few petechiae or bruises. Fragile capillaries produce many petechiae or a bruise as the capillaries bleed or leak small amounts of blood.

Generally, the number of petechiae is an indicator of the severity of the vascular permeability. A large number of petechiae or a large bruise is associated with thrombocytopenia, a clotting disorder caused by too few platelets. A petechiae count of greater than 50 indicates a severe abnormality. A petechiae count of up to 20 indicates a mild to moderate abnormality.

Positive results can occur after menstruation or in postmenopausal women because of the lower estrogen level. The normal value is higher in women and children than in men. This test should not be performed on a patient with known DIC or a known bleeding disorder.

## Purpose of the Test

The capillary fragility test is used to assess the fragility of the capillary walls, to evaluate spontaneous bruising or bleeding, and to identify one of the symptoms of thrombocytopenia.

## Procedure

**Positive Pressure Method.** A sphygmomanometer cuff is placed on the upper arm and inflated to a predetermined pressure for 5 minutes. On deflation, the skin is inspected for petechiae or bruises.
**Negative Pressure Method.** A special suction cup is applied to the skin of the arm for 1 minute. On removal of the device, the skin is inspected for petechiae or bruises.

## Findings

**Positive Values**

| | | |
|---|---|---|
| Thrombocytopenia | Factor VII deficiency | Vitamin K deficiency |
| Polycythemia vera | Hereditary vascular | von Willebrand's |
| Purpura senilis |   abnormality |   disease |
| DIC | Vitamin C deficiency | |

## Interfering Factors

- Skin that already has petechiae or bruising
- Known, active bleeding disorder

## Nursing Implementation

### Pretest

Ensure that the patient does not have a diagnosis of DIC or an active bleeding disorder, because these conditions can result in severe bruising.
Explain the procedure to the patient.
Inspect the skin of the arms and hands for petechiae or bruises. Select the extremity that has none. The selected extremity cannot have an intravenous line.

### During the Test

Apply the sphygmomanometer cuff to the upper arm. Inflate it to a pressure that is halfway between the systolic and diastolic pressures but no more than 100 mm Hg. For example, when the patient's blood pressure is 110/70, the cuff pressure is set at 90 mm Hg.
Maintain the pressure for 5 minutes and then deflate the cuff.
With the suction cup technique, apply the cup to the volar aspect of the forearm for 1 minute and then release the suction.

### Posttest

After releasing the pressure, instruct the patient to open and close the hand several times to restore the circulation.

With the blood pressure method, inspect the skin for petechiae and bruises. They can cover the entire forearm and hand.

For either method, count the petechiae within a 2-in diameter circle.

Describe the size and location of any bruises.

Record the findings in the patient's chart.

If the test is to be repeated, it should not be performed on the same arm within a 7-day period.

## References

Alving, B. M., & Griffin, J. H. (1995). Venous thrombosis: How to make the best use of the laboratory to guide therapy. *Consultant, 35*(1), 64–71.

Baer, D. M. (1995). Blood waste in draws. *Medical Laboratory Observer, 27*(7), 12.

Bell, W. R. (1995). Laboratory monitoring of thrombolytic therapy. *Clinics in Laboratory Medicine, 15*(1), 165–178.

Bick, R. L. (1994). Oral anticoagulants and the INR: Confusion, controversy, fiction and fact. *American Chemical Laboratory, 13*, 36–38.

Bick, R. L. (1995a). Laboratory evaluation of platelet dysfunction. *Clinics in Laboratory Medicine, 15*(1), 1–29.

Bick, R. L. (1995b). Oral anticoagulants in thrombolic disease. *Laboratory Medicine, 26*, 188–193.

Boyer-Neumann, C., Bertina, R. M., Tripodi, A., D'Angelo, A., Wolf, M., Vigano D'Angelo, S., Mannucci, P. M., Meyer, D., & Larrieu, M. J. (1993). Comparison of functional assays for protein S: European collaborative study of patients with congenital and acquired deficiency. *Thrombosis and Haemostasis, 70*(6), 946–950.

Cembrowski, G. S., Anderson, P. G., & Steeber, D. G. (1994). INR reporting of prothrombin time . . . Internalized normalized ratio (INR). *Medical Laboratory Observer, 26*(5), 51–54.

Davis. G. L. (1997). Hemostatic inhibitors. Fibrinolysis inhibitors. *Clinical Laboratory Science, 10*, 212–216.

Davis, G. L. (1997). Introduction to hemostatic inhibitors. *Clinical Laboratory Science, 10*, 210–211.

Diefenderfer, S., Matula, P., & Niznik, C. H. (1994). Protein S deficiency: A case study. *Journal of Vascular Nursing, 12*(2), 68–72.

Ellenger, P., & Peterson, P. (1995). Demonstrating proficiency for the bleeding time test. *Laboratory Medicine, 26*, 776–777.

Esmon, C. T. (1989). The roles of protein C and thrombomodulin in the regulation of blood coagulation. *Journal of Biological Chemistry, 264*, 4743–4746.

Esmon, C. T. (1992). Protein S and protein C. Biochemistry, physiology, and clinical manifestation of deficiencies. *Trends in Cardiovascular Medicine, 2*, 214–219.

Gewirtz, A. S., Miller, M. L., & Keys, T. F. (1996). The clinical usefulness of the preoperative bleeding time. *Archives of Pathology and Laboratory Medicine, 120*, 353–356.

Gibbar-Clements, T., Shirrell, D., & Free, C. (1997). PT and APTT: Seeing beyond the numbers, *Nursing 97, 27*(7), 49–51.

Halfman, M., & Berg, B. E. (1993). Venous thrombosis: Antithrombin III deficiency. *Critical Care Clinics of North America, 5*, 499–509.

Hancock, R. D. (1993). Venipuncture vs. arterial catheter activated partial thromboplastin times in heparinized patients. *Dimensions of Critical Care Nursing, 12*, 238–245.

Henry, J. B. (Ed.). (1996). *Clinical diagnosis and management by laboratory methods* (19th ed.). Philadelphia: W. B. Saunders.

Jacobs, D. S., Demott, W. R., Grady, H. J., Horvat, R. T., Huestis, D. W., & Kasten, B. L. (Eds.). (1996). *Laboratory test handbook* (4th ed.). Baltimore: Williams & Wilkins.

Jensen, R., & Ens, G. E. (1997). Hemostatic inhibitors. Resistance to activated protein C: A major cause of inherited thrombophilia. *Clinical Laboratory Science, 10*, 219–221.

Johnston, M., Harrison, L., Moffat, K., Willan, A., & Hirsh, J. (1996). Reliability of the internationalized normalized ratio for monitoring the induction phase of warfarin: Comparison with the prothrombin ratio. *Journal of Laboratory and Clinical Medicine, 128*(2), 214–217.

Koepke, J. A. (1994). D-dimer test. *Medical Laboratory Observer, 26*(9), 12.

Laxon, C. J., & Titler, M. G. (1994). Drawing coagulation studies from arterial lines: An integrative literature review. *American Journal of Critical Care, 3*(1), 16–24.

Lehmann, C. A. (1998). *Saunders manual of clinical laboratory.* Philadelphia: W. B. Saunders.

Lilley, L. (1995). A cautious look at heparin. *American Journal of Nursing, 95*(9), 14–15.

Mayo, D. J., Dimond, E. P., Kramer, W., & Horne, M. K. (1996). Discard volumes necessary for clinically useful coagulation studies from heparinized Hickman catheters. *Oncology Nursing Forum, 23*, 671–675.

McKeown, E. S. (1995). Undiagnosed hypercoagulable state: A case study. *Journal of Vascular Nursing, 13*(4), 117–127.

Noureddine, S. N. (1995). Research review: Use of activated clotting time to monitor heparin therapy in coronary patients. *American Journal of Critical Care, 4*, 272–277.

Oertel, L. B. (1995). Internationalized normalized ratio (INR): An improved way to monitor oral anticoagulant therapy. *Nurse Practitioner: American Journal of Primary Health Care, 20*(9), 15–16, 21–22.

Redei, I., & Rubin, R. N. (1995). Techniques for evaluating the cause of bleeding in the ICU. Diagnostic clues and keys to interpreting hemostatic tests. *The Journal of Critical Illness, 10*(2), 133–137.

Samama, M. M. (1995). Laboratory monitoring of unfractionated heparin treatment. *Clinics in Laboratory Medicine, 15*(1), 109–117.

Selig, P. M. (1996). Management of anticoagulation therapy with the international normalized ratio. *Journal of the American Academy of Nurse Practitioners, 8*(2), 77–80.

Severson, A., Baldwin, R., & DeLoughery, T. G. (1997). Internationalized normalized ratio in anticoagulant therapy: Understanding the issues. *American Journal of Critical Care,* 6(2), 88–92.

Simmons, A. (1996). Stability of plasma for fibrinogen assays. *Medical Laboratory Observer,* 28(8), 12, 88.

Stepp, C. A., & Woods, M. A. (1998). *Laboratory procedures for medical office personnel.* Philadelphia: W. B. Saunders.

Tietz, N. W. (Ed.). (1995). *Clinical guide to laboratory tests* (3rd ed.). Philadelphia: W. B. Saunders.

# CHAPTER 7

# Microbiologic Tests

Numerous microorganisms can cause infection in an individual, including bacteria, viruses, fungi, and parasites. Most infectious agents are transmitted from person to person or from an environmental source to a person via an intermediate vector, such as an insect or a rodent. Additionally, many microorganisms normally reside on the skin or in the mucous membranes of the individual. They are considered the *normal flora* of the body. If these bacteria and other organisms enter sterile tissue, they multiply and cause an infection.

Laboratory tests are used to identify the presence of a current or past infection. Serologic tests identify the patient's activated immunologic response. The presence of specific antibodies indicates a past or present exposure to the infectious agent. Microscopy may be used to count the number of organisms and to identify the organisms on slide preparations. A third method is to culture the specimen. Cultures are used to incubate and grow the infectious agent under controlled conditions. Once the source of infection is estab-

lished in the culture medium, the organism can be examined by microscope and identified. Susceptibility or sensitivity tests are performed to determine the antibiotics or antimicrobial drugs that are effective in killing the organism.

Specimen collection is a vital part of the microbiologic testing process. Measures are taken to obtain an adequate specimen, avoid external sources of contamination, and deliver the sample to the laboratory without delay. Improper technique or failure to apply quality control measures can result in false-positive or false-negative findings.

Specimen collection and specimen handling are of particular importance for all health care workers because of the risk of transmission of infection. Handwashing and the use of latex or plastic gloves are essential. Care is taken to avoid needle-stick injury. Specimen containers or tubes are closed tightly and secured before they are transported. To protect health care workers, standard precaution guidelines must be followed in handling blood and body fluids.

## Laboratory Tests

## Epstein-Barr Virus Serology

**(Serum)**                    Synonym: Epstein-Barr titer

**Normal Values**

| | |
|---|---|
| Antibodies to viral capsid antigen (IgM anti-VCA): | <1:10 |
| (IgG anti-VCA): | <1:10 |
| Antibody to Epstein-Barr nuclear antigen (anti-EBNA): | <1:5 |
| Antibodies to early antigen (anti-EA): | <1:10 |

### Background Information

As presented in Table 7–1, the Epstein-Barr virus is a herpesvirus that is responsible for most cases of infectious mononucleosis. Infectious mononucleosis causes fever, swollen lymph glands, and an inflamed oropharynx. In the blood, an increase in the number of B lymphocytes and a transient rise in the heterophil antibodies occur. The virus is transmitted via infected saliva.

The Epstein-Barr virus infects the B lymphocytes and stimulates DNA synthesis to form several new antigens. These antigens include viral capsid antigen (VCA), Epstein-Barr nuclear antigen (EBNA), and early antigen (EA). As the body develops its immunologic response to combat the infection, antibodies are formed against the specific antigens.

**Antibody Formation.**   The antibody VCA immunoglobulin M (IgM) appears in the blood before and during the acute phase of illness. It remains in the blood for 1 to 2 months and then disappears. The antibody VCA-IgG also elevates and peaks in the blood at an early stage of illness. In the convalescent stage, it declines but then persists for life at a lower, positive value. This antibody is the most often used test and is reported as the standard Epstein-Barr virus titer. It is the marker for current or prior infection.

**Table 7–1    Herpes Group of Viruses**

| Virus Type | Infection |
|---|---|
| Herpes simplex type 1 | "Cold sores"; infection of the mouth, lips, eyes, or skin; encephalitis (adult) |
| type 2 | Genital herpes, neonatal infection, encephalitis (newborn) |
| Epstein-Barr virus | Infectious mononucleosis, Burkitt's lymphoma, nasopharyngeal carcinoma |
| Cytomegalovirus | Cytomegalovirus, infectious mononucleosis, congenital infection<br>In immunocompromised patients: interstitial pneumonia, gastroenteritis, retinitis |
| Varicella-zoster virus | Chickenpox (varicella), shingles (herpes zoster) |

The anti-EA antibody appears a few weeks after the onset of symptoms and then gradually disappears from the blood. The IgG type, however, may persist for several years after an acute infection.

The anti-EBNA antibody appears in the blood several weeks after the onset of symptoms of infection. It remains elevated for life.

Several of the Epstein-Barr antibody titers also are elevated in certain malignant disorders, but a tissue biopsy must confirm the presence of malignancy.

| | |
|---|---|
| **Purpose of the Tests** | These serologic tests are used to diagnose Epstein-Barr viral infection in patients with infectious mononucleosis in whom heterophil antibody titers are negative. |

| | |
|---|---|
| **Procedure** | A red-topped tube is used to collect 10 mL of venous blood. |

**Findings**

**Elevated Values**

| | | |
|---|---|---|
| Infectious mononu-cleosis | Nasopharyngeal cancer | Hodgkin's disease |
| Burkitt's lymphoma | | |

**Interfering Factors**

- None

**Nursing Implementation**

Nursing measures include care of the venipuncture site.

**Pretest**

Schedule this test to be performed at the onset of illness and again after 2 to 3 weeks. This scheduling provides data during the acute and convalescent phases of illness.

**Posttest**

On the requisition slip, write the date of the onset of illness. Arrange for prompt transport of the specimen to the laboratory.

## Histoplasmosis Antibody Tests

(Serum)     Synonyms: None

| | | |
|---|---|---|
| **Normal Values** | Complement fixation titer: | <1:4 |
| | Immunodiffusion test: | Negative |

### Background Information

Histoplasmosis is a fungal disease caused by the *Histoplasma capsulatum* organism. The histoplasmosis infection results from the inhalation of spore-laden dust in the infected excreta of birds, bats, chickens, or turkeys. In the acute form, the spores usually cause pulmonary infection. The infection can also become chronic in the lungs and chest or disseminated in the reticuloendothelial system or any organ of the body.

The *complement fixation titer* is used to diagnose all forms of the disease. A complement fixation titer of greater than or equal to 1:8 to 1:16 is highly suspicious of infection. A higher titer (>1:32) is even more indicative of infection in an active state. In follow-up testing, a rising titer indicates the progression of infection, and a decreasing titer indicates a regression of the infection.

The *immunodiffusion test* demonstrates M and H bands as an indication of infection. The M band alone indicates early or chronic infection. The presence of an H band also indicates active infection. The immunodiffusion test may be used as a screening tool or as a supplement to the complement fixation test.

| | |
|---|---|
| **Purpose of the Test** | These serologic tests are used to help diagnose histoplasmosis and to monitor the response to therapy. |
| **Procedure** | A red-topped tube is used to collect 10 mL of venous blood. |
| **Findings** | **Elevated Values**<br><br>Histoplasmosis |
| **Interfering Factors** | • A recent skin test for histoplasmosis |
| **Nursing Implementation** | **Pretest**<br><br>Plan to obtain the first blood tests early in the infectious process and before the histoplasmosis skin test is performed. A recent skin test can cause a positive serologic result in 20% of patients (Tietz, 1995).<br><br>**Posttest**<br><br>Schedule repeat blood tests in 2 to 3 weeks to evaluate the convalescent phase of the infection. |

## Human Immunodeficiency Virus Tests

(Serum)   Synonyms: HIV tests, acquired immunodeficiency syndrome (AIDS) tests

| | | |
|---|---|---|
| **Normal Values** | **HIV Antibody Tests** | |
| | ELISA method: | Negative |
| | Western blot method: | Negative |
| | Immunofluorescent assay (IFA) method: | Negative |
| | p24 antigen test: | Negative |
| | DNA-PCR amplification: | No HIV viral DNA detected |
| | CD4$^+$ (T4) lymphocytes: | 800–1,100 cells/mm$^3$<br>40% of total lymphocytes |

| CD4+:CD8+ (T4:T8) ratio: | 1.0–3.5 |
| HIV-RNA concentration: | No HIV viral RNA copies detected |
| Home testing: | Negative for HIV antibodies |

## Background Information

The human immunodeficiency virus (HIV) is from the retrovirus family of RNA viruses. The two types of HIV are HIV-1 and HIV-2. HIV-1 is the more prevalent type, and it is the one presented here. HIV infection is transmitted by contaminated blood; by contaminated needles, as in intravenous drug use; by intimate sexual contact with an infected person; and from an infected pregnant woman to her fetus (Jacobs et al., 1996; Speicher, 1998).

HIV invades and infects targeted cells of the immune system, particularly the CD4+ lymphocytes (T4 lymphocytes), B lymphocytes, monocytes, and macrophage cells. The virus contains an RNA genome that incorporates into the host's DNA as proviral DNA, resulting in lysis of the infected cells and loss of the body's immune defenses. If the viral load increases considerably, or if the immune system is compromised by the HIV infection, the condition is diagnosed as acquired immunodeficiency syndrome (AIDS). Without an adequate immune system, the person is susceptible to opportunistic infections.

HIV has a characteristic, identifiable structure (Fig. 7–1). The proteins (P) and glycoproteins (GP) are the target antigens used in the HIV antigen and antibody tests. Within days after infection is initiated, the RNA virion of HIV can be detected in lymphocytes. Within 16 days after exposure HIV antigens can be identified in the blood and HIV DNA can be found in lymphocytes using polymerase chain reaction (PCR) amplification. Antibodies to HIV have been manufactured by the immune system and are detected in the blood by the 23rd day after exposure to the virus (Gore, 1996; Jacobs et al., 1996).

The diagnosis of HIV infection is carried out by testing for viral markers. Some tests detect specific antibodies that are present in response to the antigen. Others detect one or more HIV antigens. New test methodologies detect the DNA of HIV.

To monitor the response to treatment and evaluate the patient's condition, CD4+ lymphocytes are counted, and the viral load is measured.

**HIV Antibody Tests.**    Several tests are available that detect antibodies to HIV antigen in the patient's serum. HIV antibody tests also are used to screen blood donors, applicants for life insurance, and individuals entering the armed forces.

Enzyme immunoassay (EIA) or enzyme-

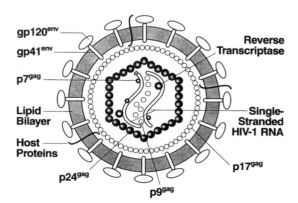

**Figure 7–1**
Basic structure of the human immunodeficiency virus. (Reproduced with permission from Sande, M. A., & Volberding, P. A. [1995]. *The medical management of AIDS* [4th ed., p. 24]. Philadelphia: W. B. Saunders.)

linked immunosorbent assay (ELISA) methodology is widely used to detect HIV antibodies, and test results are available in 2 to 4 days (Farzadegan, 1994). The test is positive when the patient's antibodies bind to the HIV antigen of the test reagent, changing the color of the solution. When HIV antibodies are identified in the blood, it is inferred that HIV antigen and the virus are present. Positive results are verified by a repeat ELISA test and an additional antibody test done by an alternate method.

The newest EIA method to screen for HIV antibodies is a rapid HIV-1 antibody screening test (single-use diagnostic HIV-1 [SUDS] assay, Murex Corporation). This test takes 10 to 15 minutes to perform, compared with several hours for conventional methods. As a test for a single individual, it can be used in small laboratories, physicians' offices, or clinics but cannot be used to screen for blood donor testing (Carter, Carter, & James, 1995; Speicher, 1998).

The Western blot test demonstrates antibodies to specific viral proteins. In this procedure, the different HIV antigens (proteins and glycoproteins) of the test reagent are separated electrophoretically. The patient's serum is placed over each of the antigens. If antibodies are present in the serum, they will bind to the test antigens and form colored bands. The formation of various bands of the viral proteins is considered a positive result, because the bands confirm the presence of specific HIV antibodies in the patient's blood (Warner, 1996) (Fig. 7–2). Because the Western blot test is technically difficult and expensive, it is used to confirm a positive ELISA test. Western blot test results are available in 1 to 2 weeks.

Indirect immunofluorescence assay (IFA) uses a different methodology to detect HIV antibodies and confirm a positive ELISA test. In the test, a dilute sample of the patient's serum is placed on a glass slide that contains HIV cells. After treatment with a fluorescent chemical, the slide is examined under ultraviolet light. When antigen-antibody complexes are present, the material glows with an apple-green fluorescence. When no antibodies are present, there is no fluorescence (Warner, 1996).

**HIV Antigen Tests.**   Several different methods are available to detect the presence of the p24 core antigen that is present in every HIV virion (see Fig. 7–1). The antigen test may be used for diagnosis in the early stage of acute infection, before an antibody response has occurred, or it may be used in cases in which diagnosis is difficult and alternate types of testing are needed (Lehmann, 1998). The HIV-1 antigen test is now used as one of the screening tests performed on donated blood (Gore, 1996).

**DNA-PCR Amplification.**   The PCR is an amplification technique used to detect the proviral DNA molecules in the infected nuclei of lymphocytes from the peripheral blood. The tiny amount of original proviral DNA is greatly increased (amplified) and then identified by using an HIV-specific DNA probe. The test can be used to identify the infected DNA when antibody tests are not conclusive. It is currently used to test neonates born to seropositive mothers (Barrick & Vogel, 1996; Jacobs et al., 1996; Warner, 1996).

**CD4+.**   CD4+ (T4) lymphocytes are cells that are killed by HIV. This was once the primary test to monitor the disease and to determine when to initiate treatment. The rationale was that the CD4+ count and its percentage of the total lymphocytes decreased as the infection increased. A newer and more reliable method to monitor the disease is to measure the amount of virus directly in the testing for HIV-RNA levels in the plasma (Carpenter et al., 1996; Speicher, 1998; Ungvarski, 1997).

The CD4+ measurement is still used as a way to monitor the patient's immune status and immune system response to antiviral therapy (Lehmann, 1998). The CD4+ cell count is measured at the time of diagnosis and is monitored at intervals thereafter.

If the CD4+ level is less than 200 cells/mm$^3$ or less than 14% of the total lymphocytes, the low value indicates severe immunosuppression, and the person is at risk to develop opportunistic infections (Barrick & Vogel, 1996; Ungvarski, 1997). Most patients with such a low value are diagnosed with full-blown AIDS (Jacobs et al., 1996) or are predicted to develop full-blown AIDS within 3 years (Lehmann, 1998).

**CD4+:CD8+ Ratio.**   This ratio compares two different subtypes of lymphocytes and their relation to each other in amount. In HIV infection, the CD4+ lymphocytes (T helper lymphocytes) decline because they are the primary target of the virus. They also decline in relation to the CD8+ lymphocytes (suppressor–cytotoxic T lymphocytes). One immunologic marker of AIDS is a CD4+:CD8+

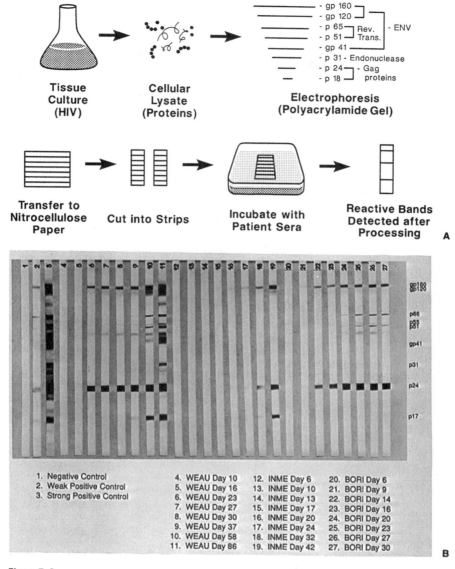

**Figure 7–2**

Western blot antibody test. *A,* Western blot test is performed by separating tissue culture–derived HIV-1 proteins (p) and glycoproteins (gp) via polyacrylamide gel electrophoresis, transferring (blotting) the separated proteins onto nitrocellulose paper, incubating the cut strips of nitrocellulose paper with patient serum, and detecting anti-HIV antibodies that have bound to the HIV-1–associated proteins at the precise point at which they migrated in the gel. Through this procedure, the antibody reactivity against specific antigens can be determined (e.g., anti-Gag, anti-Env, or anti-endonuclease antibodies). *B,* Examples of Western blot tests from three patients (*WEAU, BORI,* and *INME*) identified at the time of acute HIV-1 infection (seroconversion). Each lane represents a time point (in days) from the time of presentation with symptomatic acute HIV-1 disease or a positive or negative control (lanes 1 to 3). (Reproduced with permission from Sande, M. A., & Volberding, P. A. [1995]. *The medical management of AIDS* [4th ed., p. 71]. Philadelphia: W. B. Saunders.)

ratio that is less than 0.9 (Lehmann, 1998; Mahon & Manuselis, 1995).

**HIV-RNA Concentration.** This test measures the amount of HIV in the blood, or the viral load. The test measures ribonucleic acid (RNA), the genetic material of HIV. Each virion contains two copies of HIV-RNA, and the test measurements are reported as copies per millimeter. The virus can be detected and the amount of the virus measured at a very early stage of HIV infection, before symptoms appear and before AIDS develops. Once the diagnosis of HIV infection has been confirmed, the initial HIV-RNA test is done to establish a baseline value. The test is then repeated at 3- to 4-month intervals thereafter (Lehmann, 1998).

Currently, there are three test methods that can be used to measure the viral load. They are RT-PCR, branched DNA (bDNA), and nucleic acid sequence-based amplification (NASBA) (Lehmann, 1998; Ungvarski, 1997). A low risk for clinical progression is associated with an HIV-RNA count of less than 10,000 copies/mL. A moderate risk is in the range of 10,000 to 100,000 copies/mL, and a high risk is associated with an HIV-RNA count greater than 100,000 copies/mL (Ungvarski, 1997).

The change in the virus count is also a very important measurement. A rising count indicates worsening infection, and a falling level indicates improvement. The changes are used to predict risk for clinical progression and to guide the treatment of HIV infection (Carpenter et al., 1996; Speicher, 1998).

### Home Testing

There are a number of HIV test kits that can be purchased over the counter. These kits permit the person to do HIV antibody testing at home. The different types of kits analyze capillary blood, oral secretions, or urine (Speicher, 1998). Once the specimen is collected, the person sends it by mail to the designated laboratory. The person then calls to learn the test result. Particularly when the results are positive, a counselor provides the results, telephone support, information, guidance about repeat testing, and referral as needed.

## Purpose of the Tests

The HIV tests are used to diagnose the infection, to screen blood donated for transfusion purposes, and to monitor progression of the disease.

## Procedure

For most tests, a red-topped tube is used to collect 10 mL of venous blood.

For a $CD4^+$:$CD8^+$ test, a green-topped tube is used to collect 4.5 mL of venous blood.

For an HIV-DNA test, 2 yellow-topped, 2 lavender-topped, or 2 green-topped tubes are used to collect 10 to 20 mL of venous blood. For this test and the HIV-RNA test, the laboratory should specify the type of tube and the volume of blood that is required.

### Quality Control

With venipuncture, the tourniquet should be tied lightly for a brief time to prevent pooling of cells in the vein at the site of blood collection. Venipuncture technique must be smooth, with a blood flow that fills the vacuum tube readily. If the blood has excessive turbulence because of flawed venipuncture technique, the hemolysis of the erythrocytes will alter the test results. Standard precautions and careful handling of the syringe and blood must be done to avoid self-inoculation.

| **Findings** | **Positive Values** | | |
|---|---|---|---|
| | HIV infection | | AIDS |
| | **Decreased Values** | | |
| | CD4$^+$: AIDS | | CD4$^+$:CD8$^+$ ratio: AIDS |

---

**Interfering Factors**

- Hemolysis
- Insufficient volume of blood

---

**Nursing Implementation**

*Critical Thinking 7–1*
It takes 16 to 22 days after exposure before an HIV infection can be detected in the blood by antibody or antigen test. The newer tests using PCR technique can identify HIV genetic material in the blood 11 days after exposure (Gore, 1996). Should PCR methodology be used to screen the blood supply?

Nursing intervention includes care of the venipuncture site.

**Pretest**

Many states have requirements to preserve confidentiality of results. An informed consent is often required before an HIV test can be performed.

**Posttest**

For the patient with confirmed HIV infection

1. Inform the patient that he or she cannot donate blood.
2. Explain that safe sex practices or abstaining from sexual intercourse will help prevent transmission of the infection.
3. Instruct that intravenous needles must not be shared.
4. Instruct the patient to continue with regular periodic examinations and follow-up laboratory testing. In addition, the obstetrician of the pregnant female patient should be informed of the positive test results.
5. Teach the patient to seek health care assistance for symptoms of AIDS, including recurrent respiratory or skin infections, fatigue, diarrhea, weight loss, fever, lymphadenopathy, or a combination of these conditions.

**Home Testing**

The HIV antibody tests are likely to be accurate, although a nondecision can occur because of a lost or damaged specimen. Concerns exist that the patient may hear of a positive result without having face-to-face contact with a supportive person. A positive result is likely to upset the person and cause shock or deep emotional pain. Additionally, although a counselor can provide guidance or referral by phone, the person may not understand the information or may not follow through with additional testing and treatment at an early stage (Harris, 1994; Tamborlane & Kunz, 1996). Benefits of testing include ready access to the test, ease of testing, lower costs, anonymity, and potential for an early diagnosis.

The nurse can assist the patient with education, supportive counseling, encouraging repeat testing, and referral for prompt medical assistance (Burgess & MacGillis, 1995).

---

## Infectious Mononucleosis Tests

**(Serum)**              Synonyms: Monotest, monoscreen, heterophil antibody test

| Normal Values | Monotest: | Negative, nonreactive |
| | Heterophil titer: | <1:56 |

## Background Information

The Epstein-Barr virus is a herpesvirus that is responsible for most cases of infectious mononucleosis. This viral infection involves the reticuloendothelial system, including B lymphocytes, lymphoid tissues, and epithelial tissues of the oropharynx. The patient's immune response produces heterophil antibodies of the IgM class and Epstein-Barr antibodies. Six to 10 days after the symptoms appear, the heterophil antibodies can be detected or measured. The level peaks in 2 to 3 weeks and persists for months (Tietz, 1995).

The monotest detects the presence of heterophil antibodies. The sample of the patient's serum is mixed with horse erythrocytes. When the heterophil antibodies of infectious mononucleosis are present, the antibodies bind to the antigen of the horse cells (Fig. 7–3). With the visible agglutination or clumping that results from the antigen-antibody reaction, the test result is positive (Stepp & Woods, 1998). If the titer is to be measured, the heterophil antibody test is used. When the heterophil titer is 1:128 or higher, the test result is positive (Tietz, 1995).

The monotest is a rapid, simple, and effective test that identifies the presence or absence of infectious mononucleosis antibodies in the patient's serum. When the infectious mononucleosis-specific heterophil antibodies are present, the test result is positive.

## Purpose of the Test

These serologic tests help to diagnose infectious mononucleosis.

## Procedure

A red-topped tube is used to collect 10 mL of venous blood.

### Quality Control

With venipuncture, the tourniquet should be tied lightly for a brief time to prevent pooling of cells in the vein at the site of blood collection. Venipuncture technique must be smooth, with a blood flow that fills the vacuum tube readily. If the blood has excessive turbulence because of flawed venipuncture technique, the hemolysis of the erythrocytes will alter the test results.

## Findings

**Elevated Values**

Infectious mononucleosis

## Interfering Factors

- Hemolysis

## Nursing Implementation

### Pretest

Schedule this test a few days after the onset of illness. Until the antibodies have time to develop, the test results will remain negative.

### Posttest

On the requisition slip, include the date of the onset of illness.
Arrange for prompt transport of the blood to the laboratory.

Key:     △ Antigen    ⬤ Latex bead    ⋎ Antibody

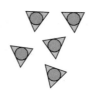

\+

\=

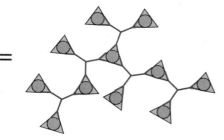

Antigen-coated latex beads

Patient's serum
containing antibodies

Results: Agglutination

**Figure 7–3**

Process of agglutination. If specific antibodies are present in the serum, they will bind to the antigen with which latex beads are coated. The visible clumping, or agglutination, of the antigen-antibody complexes provides positive proof that the antibodies are present in the serum. (Reproduced with permission from Stepp, C. A., & Woods, M. A. [1998]. *Laboratory procedures for medical office personnel* [Fig. 21–4, p. 282]. Philadelphia: W. B. Saunders.)

## Lyme Disease Tests

**(Serum, Cerebrospinal Fluid, Synovial Fluid, Tissue)**

Synonyms: Tests for *Borrelia burgdorferi*

### Normal Values

Negative for *Borrelia burgdorferi*

## Background Information

Lyme disease is an infection caused by the spirochete *Borrelia burgdorferi*. The infection is transmitted to the person by a bite from an infected tick of the *Ixodes* species.

The infection affects many body systems, and it progresses in two stages. In the early stage, most patients develop erythema migrans, a characteristic rash, and flulike symptoms. In the late stage, the spirochete infects different tissues of the body including the heart, joints, and brain. The patient develops symptoms of carditis, arthritis, and central nervous system disease, such as meningitis.

The infection is difficult to diagnose because the symptoms vary among individuals, and antibodies to the spirochete do not appear until 6 to 8 weeks after the tick bite (Speicher, 1998).

**Antibodies.**    In response to the infection, the immune system develops specific antibodies that can be detected by serologic testing of the blood. The IgM antibodies can be detected by ELISA method in the early stage of infection and by Western blot method in the late stage of the disease. In a two-stage process, these serologic blood tests are the diagnostic method of choice. If the patient has Lyme disease with meningitis, the cerebrospinal fluid may demonstrate IgM and IgG antibodies to *B. burgdorferi* (Speicher, 1998).

False-negative and false-positive results in antibody tests for this infection can occur. The antibody tests may detect only 40% to 60% of the cases in the early stage, because few organisms are present to initiate a strong antibody response (Jacobs et al.,

1996). By the late stage, however, the antibody detection rate is almost 100% (Speicher, 1998).

**Tissue Biopsy.**   The skin surrounding the rash or the synovial tissue of an inflamed joint may be biopsied. The tissue can be stained and examined by light microscopy or darkfield examination in efforts to visualize the *B. burgdorferi* spirochetes. In addition, these tissues may be cultured to encourage growth and multiplication of spirochetes for identification by microscopy (Jacobs et al., 1996; Tietz, 1995).

**DNA Identification.**   Using PCR amplification technology, fragments of the DNA of the *B. burgdorferi* spirochete can be detected and identified. In this laboratory method, the source of the specimen can be the patient's serum, cerebrospinal fluid, synovial fluid, or urine. This method is very specific and accurate in the identification of the spirochete at an early stage of infection (Jacobs et al., 1996; Mahon & Manuselis, 1995).

These tests should be done before antibiotic therapy is initiated.

---

**Purpose of the Tests**

These tests are used to help diagnose Lyme disease. They may also be used to investigate the cause of carditis, peripheral neuropathy, central nervous system changes, rash, or arthritis.

---

**Procedure**

**Serum.**   A red-topped tube is used to collect 10 mL of venous blood.
**Cerebrospinal Fluid.**   A sterile tube is used to collect cerebrospinal fluid during a lumbar puncture procedure.
**Synovial Fluid.**   A sterile tube is used to collect synovial fluid during an arthrocentesis procedure.
**Tissue Biopsy.**   A sterile dish with a cover is used to collect the skin biopsy or synovial tissue specimen during the biopsy procedure. No preservative or fixative can be used. If tissue examination (histology) and tissue culture are requested, two specimens are placed in separate containers.

---

**Findings**

**Abnormal Values**

*B. burgdorferi* infection

---

**Interfering Factors**

• Treatment with antibiotics before the testing is done.

---

**Nursing Implementation**

Nursing care includes care of the venipuncture site (see Chapter 2), lumbar puncture (see Chapter 23), arthrocentesis (see Chapter 24), or tissue biopsy (see Chapter 25).

### Pretest

In the nursing history, the patient may or may not remember a tick bite, which often occurs in late spring or summer. There may be travel or work history of exposure to ticks, particularly by walking through high grass in a field or at the edge of a forest. The exposure is often less than 1 month before the rash appears (Speicher, 1998).

### During the Test

If tissue or fluid specimens are obtained, label the requisition slip and the tube or container with the patient's name, the date, and the source of the specimen—such as, arthrocentesis, right knee.

### Posttest

Tissue specimens must be sent to the laboratory immediately to prevent drying of the specimen.

## Malaria Smear

**(Peripheral Blood)**  Synonym: Blood smear for malarial parasites

| **Normal Values** | No organisms identified |
|---|---|

### Background Information

There are four *Plasmodium* species. Humans become infected by the parasite via the bite from an infected *Anopheles* mosquito. Once the fertilized eggs penetrate the skin, they migrate to the liver within 1 hour. After 8 days of gestational development in the liver, the merozoite form enters the blood and penetrates the erythrocytes 2 days later. Depending on the species, the merozoites can cause the erythrocytes to become enlarged and distorted in shape. Additionally, each species causes distinct inclusions or markings within the cytoplasm. The organisms grow readily within the erythrocytes until they fill the red blood cells. With the simultaneous rupture of many infected erythrocytes, the patient spikes a fever.

All *Plasmodium* species can be seen on thin- or thick-stained blood films. The thin films are used to observe the change in characteristics of the infected erythrocytes and to identify the changes in cytoplasm that are characteristic of each species. The thick film is used when a low level of infection with fewer parasites exists or when the erythrocytes have already lysed and it is difficult to differentiate among the species.

| **Purpose of the Test** | The peripheral smear is used to detect and identify the specific *Plasmodium* species that has caused malaria. |
|---|---|

| **Procedure** | A fingerstick or earlobe puncture is used to obtain peripheral blood. Two or three of each of the thick and thin slides are prepared at the bedside. As an alternative, a lavender-topped tube with ethylenediaminetetraacetic acid (EDTA) is used to collect 7 mL of venous blood. |
|---|---|

### Findings

**Abnormal Values**

| | | |
|---|---|---|
| *P. vivax* *P. ovale* | *P. falciparum* | *P. malariae* |

### Interfering Factors

• Clotting of the specimen

### Nursing Implementation

**Pretest**

To establish the pattern of fever, monitor the temperature every 4 hours and document the results. Instruct the patient to tell you if chills and fever begin.

Notify the laboratory to draw the blood immediately before the time of the next anticipated fever spike.

**Quality Control**

In malaria, the cycle of fever occurs about every 48 hours, depending on the species. In the time just before the onset of fever, the erythrocytes are full of merozoites and have not yet caused hemolysis. More than one blood test may be needed to verify the diagnosis.

**Posttest**

On the requisition form, write any history of travel in endemic areas of the world, particularly in subtropical and tropical countries.

## Measles Antibody

**(Serum, Cerebrospinal Fluid)**  Synonym: Rubeola antibody

| Normal Values | | |
|---|---|---|
| | Antibody IgM: | <1:10; negative |
| | Antibody IgG: | <1:5; negative |

### Background Information

Measles (rubeola) is a viral infection that is transmitted by droplet and respiratory secretions from an infected person. The illness produces characteristic symptoms of cough, fever, congestion, and conjunctivitis; a maculopapular rash; and Koplik's spots. The infection is usually uncomplicated, but the disease can result in life-threatening pneumonia, postinfection encephalitis, or subacute sclerosing panencephalitis. Measles can be prevented by administration of the vaccine.

**Antibodies.**  At the time that the rash appears in acute measles infection, the levels of IgM and IgG measles antibodies rise. These values peak in about 10 days. Three months after the infection, the IgM antibodies disappear. The IgG antibodies decline somewhat, but the value remains positive for life.

The absence of the IgM and IgG antibodies indicates that no exposure to the measles virus occurred. It also indicates susceptibility to infection. Four weeks after vaccination, the antibodies appear in the blood.

With the neurologic complications of measles, encephalitis, and subacute sclerosing panencephalitis, the serum and cerebrospinal fluid show dramatic rises in antibodies. Neurologic damage and death can occur.

### Purpose of the Test

The test of the serum is sometimes used to diagnose the cause of a viral rash, particularly in the pregnant female. The IgG value is used to document measles immunization.

The test of the cerebrospinal fluid is used to diagnose the neurologic complications of measles.

### Procedure

**Serum.**  A red-topped tube is used to collect 10 mL of venous blood.
**Cerebrospinal Fluid.**  Lumbar puncture is performed to collect the fluid in a sterile tube.

| **Findings** | **Elevated Values** | | |
|---|---|---|---|
| | SERUM ANTIBODY IgM | | |
| | Measles infection | Giant cell pneumonia | Multiple sclerosis |
| | SERUM ANTIBODY IgG | | |
| | Immunity to future measles infection | | |
| | CEREBROSPINAL FLUID IgM ANTIBODY | | |
| | Measles encephalitis | Subacute sclerosing panencephalitis | |

---

**Interfering Factors**    • None

---

**Nursing Implementation**    Nursing care includes care of the venipuncture site and care related to lumbar puncture (see Chapter 23).

### Pretest

Teach the patient that the elevated or positive value of the IgG antibody indicates immunity to future measles infection. This occurs as a result of immunization or past infection.

### Posttest

If it has not been done, encourage the parents to have their children vaccinated. The vaccine is a combined measles, mumps, and rubella (MMR) vaccine, given at 15 months and again at 4 to 6 years. Despite vaccination programs, outbreaks of measles infection occur (Jacobs et al., 1996).

If the antibody titer is negative after vaccination, encourage the person to be revaccinated.

---

## Methylene Blue Stain, Feces

**(Feces)**    Synonym: Fecal leukocyte stain

---

**Normal Values**    No presence of leukocytes in the fecal matter

---

## Background Information

Intestinal bacterial infection can cause the abrupt onset of severe diarrhea, sometimes accompanied by the passage of blood and mucus in the feces. When the bacteria are invasive, they cause the release of polymorphonuclear leukocytes from the injured intestinal tissue. These white blood cells are released into the lumen of the intestine and are present in the feces. A fecal smear, stained with methylene blue, Gram's stain, or Wright's stain, reveals the presence and quantity of leukocytes in the stool.

Leukocytes are usually present in diarrheal infection that is caused by invasive bacteria including *Salmonella, Shigella, Campylobacter,* and *Yersinia.* Leukocytes usually are absent in diarrheal infection caused by the toxigenic bacteria *Escherichia coli, Vibrio cholerae,* and *Clostridium difficile.*

| | |
|---|---|
| **Purpose of the Test** | Methylene blue staining of a fecal smear is a rapid screening test that helps differentiate among the many causes of diarrhea and helps determine the need for a follow-up stool culture. |

| | |
|---|---|
| **Procedure** | About 2 g of fresh stool and mucus is placed in a clean plastic container with a lid. Although it is a less preferable alternative, a rectal swab may be used to obtain some fecal matter from the rectum (see also Chapter 2). |

**Findings**

**Elevated Values**

| | | |
|---|---|---|
| Infection with:<br>    *Campylobacter*<br>    *Yersinia*<br>    *Shigella*<br>    *Salmonella* | Antibiotic-associated<br>    colitis | Ulcerative colitis<br>Amebiasis |

**Interfering Factors**

- Barium in the fecal specimen
- Insufficient volume of fecal matter
- Delay or cooling of the specimen

**Nursing Implementation**

**Pretest**

Obtain the stool specimen before any barium studies are performed.
Wear gloves to obtain a fresh random stool sample.

**Posttest**

Place the lid securely on the collection container, discard gloves, and wash hands.
Send the specimen to the laboratory without delay.

**Quality Control**

Prolonged storage causes deterioration of the leukocytes and invalidates the test.

## Microfilaria Smear

**(Peripheral Blood)**    Synonym: Blood smear for *Trypanosoma* or *Filaria* parasites

| | |
|---|---|
| **Normal Values** | No parasites visualized |

## Background Information

Filarial worms of different species infect humans by insect bite from infected flies or mosquitoes. These parasites survive in warm climates, particularly in Africa, Mexico, Asia, India, Central and South America, the Philippines, and a few of the Caribbean islands. Once the filariae have infected a human, the ova mature to adult worms, reproduce, and reside in various tissues, including lymph glands and subcutaneous tissues.

The microfilariae are the larval stage of the parasite. They reside within erythrocytes and in the peripheral blood of the infected person. Their presence can be detected and the species identified by microscopic examination of the blood. Thick and thin blood films are prepared and stained to enhance the visualization.

The microparasites are often found in greater quantities in the blood in a diurnal rhythm. The optimal yield is often at noon and midnight, depending on the species and the geographic region. One negative result may not be conclusive, because it is difficult to isolate the microfilariae. They may or may not be in the blood at the time the blood sample is obtained. Biopsy of the skin or subcutaneous mass may also be needed.

## Purpose of the Test

A peripheral blood smear for filariae is performed in the diagnosis of elephantiasis, trypanosomiasis, or parasitic infection of the blood.

## Procedure

A fingerstick or earlobe puncture is used to obtain a peripheral blood sample for thick and thin films or smears.

As an alternative, a lavender-topped tube with EDTA may be used to collect 7 mL of venous blood.

## Findings

### Abnormal Values

| | | |
|---|---|---|
| *Wuchereria bancrofti* | *Mansonella ozzardi* | *Dipetalonema* |
| *Loa loa* | *Brugia malayi* | *perstans* |

## Interfering Factors

- None

## Nursing Implementation

### Pretest

Schedule the tests for noon and midnight to 2 AM, because these are the best hours for the diurnal rhythms of the parasites. If the patient experiences a fever spike, this is also an optimal time for the blood sample to be obtained.

Question the patient about any recent travel or residence in a tropical country or primitive region of the world. If the history is positive, include the date or dates of travel and the geographic exposure on the requisition slip.

### Posttest

Arrange for prompt transport of the slides or blood to the laboratory.

### Quality Control

For effective visualization, the blood or films must be fresh. As the microfilariae move around or flagellate, they will move the erythrocytes and can be located more easily.

## Mumps Antibody

**(Serum)** Synonym: Mumps serology

**Normal Values**

| | |
|---|---|
| Antibody IgM: | <1–10; negative |
| Antibody IgG: | <1–5; negative |

### Background Information

Mumps, or parotitis, is a viral infection, transmitted by droplets from an infected individual to the respiratory tract, gastrointestinal tract, or conjunctiva of a susceptible person. The infection produces classic inflammation of lymph glands, salivary glands, and one or both parotid glands. Complications can occur. Immunization with the MMR vaccine usually produces immunity to future infection.

**Antibodies.** Early in the acute infection, the IgM antibodies rise to a titer of 1:10 or higher. The rise of the IgG antibodies to a titer of 1:5 or higher indicates immunity, obtained by past infection or vaccination (Jacobs et al., 1996).

### Purpose of the Test

The IgM antibody test may be used to diagnose mumps infection. The IgG antibody test is used to document immunity.

### Procedure

A red-topped tube is used to collect 10 mL of venous blood.

### Findings

**Elevated Values**

ANTIBODY IgM:

Acute mumps infection

ANTIBODY IgG:

Past mumps infection
Mumps vaccination

### Interfering Factors

• None

### Nursing Implementation

Care of the venipuncture site is included in the nursing intervention.

**Pretest**

Teach the patient that the positive value of the IgG antibody titer indicates immunity to future mumps infection.

**Posttest**

If it is not done already, encourage the parents to have their children immunized for measles, mumps, and rubella at 15 months and again at 4 to 6 years. Despite immunization programs, outbreaks of mumps still occur in vaccinated and unvaccinated people (Lehmann, 1998).

If the IgG titer is negative or in the normal range, the person is susceptible to mumps infection. Encourage the person to be vaccinated or revaccinated to provide immunity.

## Ova and Parasites, Feces

(Feces)                                   Synonyms: Stool for ova and parasites, stool for O and P

**Normal Values**          No parasites or ova are found in the feces.

### Background Information

Numerous parasites can infect individuals and then live in the intestinal tract and other organs during parts of the parasitic life cycle (Fig. 7–4). Many ova, cysts, larvae, or spores from fecal-contaminated soil enter the person via a fecal-oral route. As these forms of the parasite reach the intestine, they mature to the adult stage of development and deposit new ova into the patient's intestinal tract.

Common methods of transmission are from unwashed hands, eating contaminated raw fruits and vegetables, and drinking from a fecal-contaminated water supply. Some intestinal parasites, such as *Schistosoma* and hookworms, invade the body through the skin and then migrate through body tissue to the intestinal lumen. Others, including tapeworms and flukes, are transmitted by eating undercooked meat, raw fish, or plants that are contaminated by the parasite.

As seen in Table 7–2, protozoa, nematodes, trematodes, and cestodes reside in different parts of the intestinal tract and have different methods of attachment or degree of tissue invasion. Some lodge primarily in the intestinal tract; others are in the intestinal tract for part of the time but also migrate to other body cavities or organs.

The schedule and procedure for stool collection are based on the type of parasite infection that is suspected. Because of the distinct life cycle of each species, the ova may or may not be present in the intestine at a particular time. Additionally, some species deposit many ova each day, and others deposit only a few at a time. Traditionally, the method of collection of fecal samples is to obtain three specimens on different days (Tietz, 1995). This maximizes the chance of identification of the ova in at least one of the samples.

Using microscopic examination of the feces, the specific parasite is identified by the presence of its ova, larvae, trophozoites, cysts, or oocysts. In some cases, the egg count per gram of feces helps to determine the intensity of infection. A patient may be infected with more than one type of parasite.

### Purpose of the Test

The microscopic examination of the feces is used to identify the presence of specific parasites in the intestinal tract.

### Procedure

**Stool Collection.**   Collect a small sample of feces directly into a clean, wide-mouthed container and close the lid. A common requirement is to collect one specimen each day for 3 days.

**Perianal Swab.**   Transparent tape is placed on a tongue depressor, sticky side out. Press the tape firmly on the perianal skin. Remove the tape and place it on a glass slide, sticky side down.

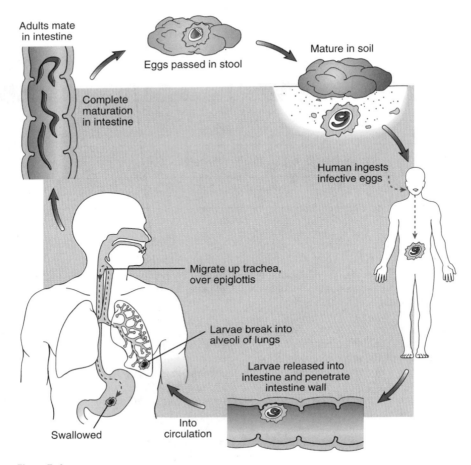

**Figure 7–4**
Life cycle of *Ascaris lumbricoides*. The eggs of this roundworm parasite enter the person via fecally contaminated soil, on food, or on unwashed hands. The eggs, larvae, and worms live in and migrate through the body. As the worms mature, new eggs are deposited in the colon and feces. (Reproduced with permission from Mahon, C., & Manuselis, G. [1995]. *Textbook of diagnostic microbiology*. Philadelphia: W. B. Saunders.)

| **Findings** | **Positive Values** | | |
|---|---|---|---|
| | Amebiasis | Pinworm | Hookworm |
| | Cryptosporidiosis | Giardiasis | Others (see |
| | Ascariasis | Tapeworm | Table 7–2) |

| **Interfering Factors** | • Antibiotic therapy in the 3- to 4-week pretest period |
|---|---|
| | • Soil, water, or urine contamination of the sample |
| | • Barium sulfate administration in the 2- to 3-week pretest period |

• Mineral oil, castor oil, antacids, or antidiarrheal medication in the week before the test

---

**Nursing Implementation**    **Pretest**

Schedule this test before any barium studies, because the barium obscures the microscopic visualization of the ova.

**Table 7–2    Gastrointestinal Location of Parasites**

| Name | Anatomic Sites | Characteristics of Residence |
|------|----------------|------------------------------|
| **Protozoa (Unicellular Parasites)** | | |
| Giardia lamblia | Small bowel | Mucosal attachment |
| Entamoeba histolytica | Colon, rectum | Lumen dweller, mucosal invasion |
| Balantidium coli | Colon, rectum | Lumen dweller, mucosal invasion |
| Isospora belli | Small bowel | Epithelial cell invasion |
| Dientamoeba fragilis | Small bowel, colon | Lumen dweller, mucosal invasion |
| Sarcocystis spp. | Small bowel | Epithelial cell invasion |
| Trypanosoma cruzi* | Esophagus, colon | Smooth muscle cells and autonomic nerve plexuses |
| Cryptosporidium parvum | Small bowel | Epithelial cell invasion |
| **Nematodes (Roundworms)** | | |
| Trichuris trichiura | Colon | Mucosal attachment |
| Ascaris lumbricoides | Small bowel | Lumen dweller |
| Ancylostoma (hookworm) | Small bowel | Mucosal attachment |
| Strongyloides stercoralis | Small bowel | Mucosal invasion |
| Trichostrongylus | Small bowel | Mucosal invasion |
| Enterobius vermicularis | Colon, rectum | Lumen dweller |
| Oesophagostomum* | Cecum | Mucosal invasion |
| Anisakis* | Stomach, small bowel | Mucosal invasion |
| Ternidens | Ileocecal region | Mucosal attachment and invasion |
| Capillaria philippinensis | Small bowel | Mucosal invasion |
| **Trematodes (Flukes)** | | |
| Opisthorchis (clonorchis) | Duodenum | Lumen dweller, epithelial attachment |
| Schistosoma spp. | Ileum, colon | Mesenteric veins, gut wall, mucosa, lumen |
| Fasciola hepatica | Small bowel | Mucosal attachment |
| Gastrodiscoides hominis | Colon | Mucosal attachment |
| Paragonimus westermani* | Small bowel, abdominal cavity, peritoneum | Peritoneal lesions |
| Echinostoma spp. | Small bowel | Mucosal attachment |
| **Cestodes (Tapeworms)** | | |
| Hymenolepsis nana | Small bowel | Mucosal attachment |
| Taenia spp. | Small bowel | Mucosal attachment |
| Diphyllobothrium latum | Small bowel | Mucosal attachment |
| Dipylidium caninum | Small bowel | Mucosal attachment |

*These parasites are not diagnosed by fecal examination.

Instruct the patient regarding correct collection procedure. The fecal matter should be evacuated directly into a clean, dry container or into a clean, dry basin and then transferred into the container. For this test, the feces should not be removed from the toilet bowl (Koontz & Weinstock, 1996; Stepp & Woods, 1998).

### Quality Control

The specimen must be free of contact with water or urine, because these liquids will kill any trophozoites that are present. The specimen must also be free of soil contamination, because amebae and other parasites of the soil will contaminate the specimen.

### Posttest

Place the lid on the specimen container. Remove gloves and wash hands thoroughly.

### Quality Control

Intestinal parasites are a highly transmissible source of infection via the fecal-oral route or via contact with the skin. Precautions are taken to prevent self-inoculation from poor hygiene practices.

*Critical Thinking 7–2*
To screen for ova and parasites, the nurse of a rural clinic is assigned to obtain one stool sample from each of 15 preschool-age children. What are important aspects of the project, and how can the nurse implement them effectively?

Include the time and date of the collection on the laboratory slip and the container. On the laboratory requisition form, record pertinent data regarding clinical history, such as immunosuppression or AIDS, or epidemiologic exposure, such as backpacking in the mountains or other travel (Koontz & Weinstock, 1996).

Send the specimen to the laboratory immediately, because the examination of the specimen must begin within 30 to 60 minutes.

### Quality Control

Time delay and exposure to heat or cold temperatures will result in the death of trophozoites and cysts.

## Ova and Parasites, Urine

(Urine)                    Synonym: Parasites, urine

| Normal Values | No ova or parasites are identified. |
| --- | --- |

## Background Information

*Schistosoma haematobium,* a parasitic fluke, dwells in fecal-contaminated water. It penetrates the skin of the person who comes into contact with the infective stage of the parasite during bathing or swimming in the polluted water. There are four species of *Schistosoma,* but the migration in the body and final destination of *S. haematobium* are somewhat different from those of the others. This difference is the basis for a different method of specimen collection for diagnostic testing.

After penetrating the skin and migrating to the lungs, all species of developing *Schistosoma* migrate to the portal vein and mesenteric veins. Three species of *Schistosoma* penetrate the intestinal wall and deposit ova in the lumen of the gastrointestinal tract. *S. haematobium* continues the vascular migration downward into the inferior mesenteric veins that surround the bladder and urethra. The female flukes deposit ova that penetrate the bladder wall and pass into the urine.

*Trichomonas vaginalis* and *Enterobius vermicularis* are other parasites that may be present in the urine. In the infected human female, the ova of *T. vaginalis* are located in the vagina and endocervix but may pass into the bladder and urine by localized contamination. In the human male, the *T. vaginalis* ova are located primarily in the urethra and exit from the body in the urine. The ova of the intestinal parasite *E. vermicularis* are deposited in the perianal area by the adult female. The ova enter the urinary tract through fecal contamination of the urinary meatus or by local migration of the gravid female parasite into the urinary tract.

---

**Purpose of the Test**

The urine is examined to detect the presence of the ova of *S. haematobium* and *T. vaginalis*.

---

**Procedure**

Daily urine specimens are obtained for 2 to 3 consecutive days.

---

**Findings**

**Positive Values**

| Schistosomiasis | Trichomoniasis | Enterobiasis |
|---|---|---|

---

**Interfering Factors**

- Refrigeration of the specimen
- Delay in transport of the specimen to the laboratory

---

**Nursing Implementation**

**Pretest**

Instruct the patient to use clean, dry containers to collect a specimen of urine each day for 2 to 3 days. When *S. haematobium* is suspected, instruct the patient to collect the urine at about noon each day. Additionally, the desired sample of the urine is collected toward the end of micturition. For unknown reasons, the ova deposits are heaviest at midday and are released in the greatest quantity in the terminal portion of the urinary stream.

**Posttest**

Wash the hands thoroughly after removing gloves or handling the urine container.

**Quality Control**

Parasites are highly infectious. The ova of *Schistosoma* burrow through the skin, and *Enterobius* is transmitted via a fecal-oral route.

Arrange for transport of each specimen to the laboratory within 3 to 4 hours after collection. Do not refrigerate the specimen.

**Quality Control**

When urine is cold or old, the yield of *Schistosoma* is reduced.

# Parasite Culture
**(Feces)**                    Synonym: Stool culture for parasites

| Normal Values | No parasites or their ova are present in the fecal culture. |
|---|---|

## Background Information

Many protozoa and helminths can live in the intestinal tract for part of the parasitic life cycle. Normally, the microscopic examination of the feces for ova and parasites is the best and easiest method for detection and identification of parasitic infection. Sometimes, however, the parasitic infection is light, and the ova remain elusive and undetected by routine microscopic analysis.

The stool sample can be cultured until the parasites and ova mature and multiply. Then sufficient numbers exist so that the ova can be located and identified. Only some of the parasites can yield positive results by stool culture method.

**Purpose of the Test**    This test detects light intestinal parasitic infections caused by amebae, nematodes, and schistosomes.

**Procedure**    A clean container with a tightly covered lid is used to collect about 2 g of fresh feces from a random stool. In most instances, three stool samples are required, one each day or one every other day (Mahon & Manuselis, 1995).

**Findings**

**Positive Values**

| | | |
|---|---|---|
| Amebiasis | *Trichostrongylus* | *Strongyloides* |
| *Giardia lamblia* | *Entamoeba histolytica* | *stercoralis* |
| *Ancylostoma* (hookworm) | *Schistosoma* spp. | |

**Interfering Factors**
- Barium administration
- Antibiotic or antiamebic medication
- Intestinal medications: bismuth, Metamucil, castor oil
- Refrigeration or delay in transport of the specimen

**Nursing Implementation**    **Pretest**

The stool culture must be obtained before the patient has any barium studies performed.

Instruct the patient to discontinue antibiotics, antihelmintics, and intestinal medications for 1 week before the fecal specimens are collected. These medications reduce the yield of ova or interfere with the microscopic view of the culture medium.

Teach the patient to evacuate a small sample of feces into a clean, dry container and then secure the container lid. If the patient requires assistance, use gloves to collect the specimen, and wash your hands immediately after removal of gloves.

### Quality Control

Intestinal parasites are highly infectious. Some are transmitted by fecal-oral spread and others by contact with the skin. Self-inoculation can be prevented by effective hygiene measures.

The fecal samples must not be contaminated by water, urine, or soil. The trophozoites of amebae are destroyed by water and urine. The soil introduces a new source of contaminants to the culture specimens.

### Posttest

Place the date and time of the specimen collection on each laboratory slip and container. Do not refrigerate the specimen. Arrange for prompt transport of the specimen to the laboratory (within 2 hours).

### Quality Control

The yield of trophozoites and other ova will be reduced by cooling or a time delay before the laboratory culture is started.

## Rotavirus, Feces

(Feces)      Synonyms: Rotavirus, EIA; rotavirus, direct examination; EIA

| Normal Values | No virus detected |
| --- | --- |

### Background Information

The rotavirus causes acute gastroenteritis with vomiting, dehydration, and moderate to severe diarrhea. This viral infection tends to affect infant and toddler age groups, particularly in the winter months.

The virus is maximally present in the feces during the first 3 days of illness. The shedding of the virus then gradually decreases until only minimal amounts are present in the feces by the eighth day of illness.

The virus cannot be cultured in vitro. The best method of identification of the rotavirus is by examination of the feces by EIA or radioimmunoassay. It is also possible to examine this virus by electron microscopy, but most laboratories do not have the equipment. If electron microscopic examination for enteroviruses is requested, the procedure and nursing implementation are the same as described for this test.

| | |
|---|---|
| **Purpose of the Test** | This test identifies the rotavirus in feces of patients in whom a viral cause of gastroenteritis is suspected. |
| **Procedure** | A sterile container is used to collect a random sample of diarrheal fecal matter. The timing of the collection is early in the course of illness or within 3 to 5 days after the onset of diarrhea. More than one specimen may be required to reduce the possibility of a false-negative result. |

**Findings**

**Positive Values**

Rotavirus infection          Viral gastroenteritis

**Interfering Factors**

- Delay in transport of the specimen
- Warming of the specimen

**Nursing Implementation**

**Pretest**

Because this virus is easily transmitted, use gloves when collecting the specimen.
Collect a small amount (4 to 8 g) of diarrheal stool in a sterile collection container or tube. A sterile tongue blade may be used to help in the collection.

**Posttest**

Close the container with the appropriate lid or stopper. After removing the gloves, wash your hands immediately.
Appropriately label the laboratory requisition slip and specimen container, including the time and date of the collection.
Arrange for immediate transport of the specimen to the laboratory.

**Quality Control**

Excessive delay contributes to warming and drying of the specimen, with a resultant loss of virion particles.

## Rubella Antibody

**(Serum)**          Synonym: German measles antibody

**Normal Values**

| IgM antibody: | Negative |
|---|---|
| IgG antibody: | <1:4; negative |

## Background Information

Rubella is an RNA viral infection that is characterized by a macular rash, lymphadenopathy, pharyn-

gitis, and conjunctivitis. It has an incubation period of 14 to 21 days. The virus is transmitted by droplet infection from the nasopharynx of the infected person to the susceptible individual. The virus can also cross the placental barrier of the infected pregnant woman. Rubella infection in the fetus has devastating consequences, particularly if it occurs in the first trimester of the pregnancy (Lehmann, 1998).

**Antibodies.** When the rubella IgM and IgG antibodies are negative, the person has not been exposed to the rubella virus. It also means that no immunity exists and that the person is susceptible to infection.

A positive value of IgM antibody is an indicator of acute infection. In rubella infection, this antibody titer stays positive for 4 to 5 weeks and then disappears. The IgG antibody also rises in infection but then remains elevated for life. The positive value of the IgG antibodies indicates post infection or post vaccination, with immunity to future rubella infection.

If the newborn infant is suspected of congenital rubella, rubella titers are performed. The presence of IgG antibodies in this infant is a strong indicator of the congenital infection.

| | |
|---|---|
| **Purpose of the Test** | Rubella antibody titer is used to determine the immunity status and to identify exposure to the rubella virus in the pregnant woman, fetus, or newborn child. |
| **Procedure** | A red-topped tube is used to collect 10 mL of venous blood. |
| **Findings** | **Elevated Values**<br><br>IgM ANTIBODY<br><br>Rubella infection, exposure<br>Rubella, acute infection<br><br>IgG ANTIBODY<br><br>Immunity to future rubella infection<br>Congenital rubella infection in the fetus or newborn |
| **Interfering Factors** | • None |
| **Nursing Implementation** | Intervention includes care of the venipuncture site.<br><br>**Pretest**<br><br>Recommend health screening for rubella susceptibility or immunity. If the young nonpregnant female does not have an elevated level of IgG antibodies, she should be vaccinated.<br>Teach that when IgG antibodies are elevated and positive, the person need not worry about future exposure to rubella infection (Jacobs et al., 1996).<br><br>**Posttest**<br><br>If the pregnant woman did not have previous immunity and now tests positive for IgG antibodies, the fetus has been exposed to rubella infection. The expectant parents will be advised of the risks for the fetus. The nurse pro- |

vides emotional support to the parents during this stressful time as they learn of the potential harm that can affect the fetus.

If it has not been done, teach parents to have their children immunized with the MMR vaccine at 15 months and again at 4 to 6 years.

## Stool Culture
(Feces)                              Synonym: Stool culture for enteric pathogens

| Normal Values | Negative for *Campylobacter, Salmonella,* and *Shigella* |
|---|---|

## Background Information

Stool culture may be used when the patient experiences severe, persistent, or recurrent bloody diarrhea with fever and tenesmus. The patient may have a history of travel to a developing country, a recent dietary intake of seafood, or exposure to a known bacterial agent.

The diarrhea is usually associated with one of three syndromes and indicates infection in a specific anatomic location. *Gastroenteritis* affects the stomach and causes vomiting. *Enteritis* affects the small bowel and causes fewer episodes of diarrhea. The fecal matter is profuse and very watery. *Dysentery* or *colitis* affects the colon and causes many episodes of diarrhea. The volume of fecal matter is small, and it is mixed with blood, mucus, and leukocytes.

Once the fecal specimen is brought to the laboratory, samples of the feces are inoculated into several types of culture media. Under incubation, enteric pathogens grow and multiply, whereas routine enteric pathogens are inhibited from growth. Routine microscopic examination is performed in 18 to 24 hours. When culture growth is negative, a final report is completed within 48 hours. When culture growth is positive, it will take several days to continue testing and identification of the microorganism.

In standard methodology, stool culture identifies *Salmonella* spp., *Shigella* spp., and *Campylobacter* spp. If specified on the requisition slip, other bacterial pathogens also can be identified by stool culture, including *Staphylococcus aureus, Clostridium difficile, Yersinia* spp., and *Vibrio* spp. (Mahon & Manuselis, 1995).

Stool culture is expensive. As a preliminary test, methylene blue staining of stool may be used to identify bacterial diarrhea and indicate the need for stool culture.

| Purpose of the Test | The stool culture is used to identify the bacterial organism that causes intestinal infection. |
|---|---|

| Procedure | **Random Stool Method.** A small amount of freshly passed feces is placed directly into a clean, dry container. |
|---|---|

**Rectal Swab Method.** The swab is inserted past the anal sphincter and into the rectum. The swab is gently rotated around the canal. To attain maximum absorption, the swab is kept in place for 15 to 20 seconds before it is withdrawn. Once the swab is placed in the culturette tube, the media compartment is crushed to moisten the specimen.

| Findings | Positive Values | | |
|---|---|---|---|
| | Shigellosis | Bacillary dysentery | Acute gastroenteritis |
| | *Salmonella* infection | Infant botulism | Typhoid fever |
| | Cholera | Enteric fever | Food poisoning |

**Interfering Factors**

- Contamination of the specimen with urine, detergent, or soap
- Improper technique of specimen collection
- Refrigeration or delay in transport of specimen
- Antibiotic therapy

**Nursing Implementation**

**Pretest**

Obtain the specimen before any antibiotic therapy is started.

Instruct the patient to evacuate a small amount of feces directly into the container. If a bedpan is used, it must be rinsed with water and dried thoroughly before use. No urine can be mixed with the feces.

**Quality Control**

Urine, soap, detergent, and drying of the specimen act to destroy the bacteria before they can be cultured.

■

*Critical Thinking 7–3*
The patient is acutely ill, with profound diarrhea, and a stool culture has been ordered. What other nursing assessments are indicated?

**Posttest**

Use gloves to handle the open container or culturette until it is sealed. Remove gloves and wash hands thoroughly.

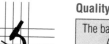

**Quality Control**

The bacteria are highly transmissible via a fecal-oral route.

Arrange for direct transport of the specimen to the laboratory without delay. If a delay of more than 2 to 3 hours is anticipated, the specimen should be placed in a laboratory-determined type of transport medium to maintain a moist environment.

**Quality Control**

Refrigeration of the specimen may be necessary when a delay in transport for more than 2 to 3 hours occurs. Cooling, however, will make the feces more acidic and destroy the *Shigella* spp.

## Syphilis Serology

**(Serum, CSF)**

Synonyms: Venereal Disease Research Laboratory test (VDRL), rapid plasma reagin test (RPR), fluorescent treponemal antibody absorption test (FTA-ABS), microhemagglutination assay–*Treponema pallidum* (MHA-TP).

| **Normal Values** | Negative; nonreactive |
|---|---|

## Background Information

*Treponema pallidum* is the spirochete that causes syphilis. The spirochete is usually transmitted as the result of sexual contact with an infected partner. In addition, a pregnant woman with primary- or secondary-stage syphilis can also transmit the spirochete to her fetus.

Syphilis in the primary stage causes a chancre or ulcerated lesion on the external genitals or cervix or in the vagina. It can also appear on the anus or any other mucosal or nonmucosal surface. In the secondary stage, the spirochete has become systemic. The patient has a rash, and the central nervous system, bones, eyes, and liver may be involved. In the latent phase, there are no clinical complaints. If the infection proceeds to the tertiary stage, the patient develops granulomatous inflammations, called gummas, in the organs and tissues of the body. Spirochete damage to the cardiovascular system and brain also occurs.

Several laboratory tests can be used to detect antibodies produced in response to the infection. Each blood test has distinct advantages and disadvantages at the various phases of the disease. The Venereal Disease Research Laboratory test (VDRL), rapid plasma reagin test (RPR), and automated reagin test (ART) are used to screen for the disease and monitor the responseto treatment. The fluorescent treponemal antibody absorption test (FTA-ABS) and microhemagglutination assay–*T. pallidum* (MHA-TP) are specific antibody tests used to confirm the diagnosis. The results are reported as reactive, weakly reactive, or nonreactive.

**Venereal Disease Research Laboratory Test.** The VDRL is an effective screening test for syphilis. In most cases, the blood becomes reactive 1 to 3 weeks after the chancre appears. It is 100% reactive in the secondary phase and remains reactive in most cases of latent syphilis. The VDRL results may convert back to a nonreactive state in tertiary- or late-stage syphilis. VDRL results are negative or nonreactive after effective treatment has eradicated the spirochete.

The VDRL is the only test used on cerebrospinal fluid to assess for neurosyphilis. The VDRL of the spinal fluid is very specific but not very sensitive. This means that positive results are highly accurate, but negative results are not always correct in the diagnosis of neurosyphilis (Jacobs et al., 1996).

There are a number of nontreponemal diseases that can cause a false-positive VDRL. These are infectious mononucleosis, infectious hepatitis, malaria, brucellosis, systemic lupus erythematosus, rheumatoid arthritis, typhus, atypical pneumonia, Hansen's disease, pregnancy, and drug addiction. Because of the possibility of a false-positive result, a reactive VDRL should be followed up by one of the specific treponemal tests to confirm the diagnosis.

**Rapid Plasma Reagin Test.** The RPR is an effective screening test for primary- and secondary-phase syphilis. Like the VDRL, it produces serum agglutinin (reagin) in the presence of the syphilis antigen. The agglutinin indicates a positive or reactive serum. When a positive result occurs, the test is often followed up with one of the specific treponemal laboratory tests to confirm the diagnosis. Like the VDRL, this test also produces false-positive results in patients with collagen disease, infection, pregnancy, and drug addiction.

**Automated Reagin Test.** The ART is similar to the RPR. Because the analysis is performed by automated equipment, the test is used to screen large numbers of serum samples. A positive test result should be followed up with one of the specific treponemal tests to confirm the diagnosis.

**Fluorescent Treponemal Antibody Absorption Test.** The FTA-ABS identifies the specific antibodies to *T. pallidum* that are present in the serum. This test is the most sensitive test for all stages of syphilis. It is used to confirm positive test results with the VDRL, ART, or RPR, but it cannot itself be used as a screening test. This test also cannot be used to monitor treatment, because once the results are reactive, they remain reactive for life (Lehmann, 1998). Because this test is highly sensitive and specific, even in detecting the third phase of syphilis, it is particularly useful for patients who have symptoms that suggest neurosyphilis. There are some false-positive results among the general population and in patients with collagen vascular disorders, pregnancy, and drug addiction.

**Microhemagglutination Assay–*Treponema pallidum.*** The MHA-TP also identifies specific antibodies to *T. pallidum* in the serum. The antibodies in the serum agglutinate when exposed to the antigen of this spirochete. The test is specific and sensitive in identification of all phases of syphilis except the primary stage. It is somewhat less sensitive than the FTA-ABS in the detection of early-stage disease. The test is used to confirm a positive result on a reagin screening test. It is not used as a screening test itself and cannot monitor the results of treatment, because once the results are reactive, they remain reactive throughout life. False-positive results can occur in systemic lupus erythematosus, infections, mononucleosis, and Hansen's disease.

## Purpose of the Tests

These blood tests are used to screen for or confirm the diagnosis of syphilis. The VDRL is used to monitor the response to therapy.

## Procedure

**Serum.** A red-topped tube is used to collect 10 mL of venous blood.
**Cerebrospinal Fluid.** A sterile tube is used to collect a sample of cerebrospinal fluid during a spinal tap.

### Quality Control

With venipuncture, the tourniquet should be tied lightly for a brief time to prevent pooling of cells in the vein at the site of blood collection. Venipuncture technique must be smooth, with a blood flow that fills the vacuum tube readily. If the blood has excessive turbulence because of flawed venipuncture technique, the hemolysis of the erythrocytes will alter the test results.

## Findings

**Positive Values**

Syphilis

## Interfering Factors

- Lipemia
- Alcohol
- Hemolysis

## Nursing Implementation

### Pretest

Instruct the patient to avoid alcohol intake for 24 hours before the test. Fasting for 8 hours is also recommended to reduce the serum lipid content.

### Posttest

Arrange for prompt transport of the specimen to the laboratory. The MHA-TP specimen requires refrigeration when a delay occurs before analysis can be performed.
Instruct the patient to abstain from sexual contact until the results are known.
When the test results are positive for this sexually transmitted disease, instruct the patient to inform all sexual partners of the test results. Sexual partners are advised to undergo testing.
Positive test results are reported to the state health department.
Instruct the patient to refrain from sexual contact until the infection is treated and cured.

## Toxoplasmosis Serology

(Serum)     Synonym: Toxoplasmosis titer

| Normal Values | IgM antibody titer (IFA method): | <1:16; negative (Tietz, 1995) |
|---|---|---|
| | IgM antibody titer (ELISA, EIA method): | No antibody detected (Lehmann, 1998) |

### Background Information

*Toxoplasma gondii* is a sporozoan parasite that infects domestic and wild animals and feline animals, including household cats. The oocysts are excreted in feces and mature to the infective stage as sporozoites in the environment, such as in the soil or in cat litter. In addition, the cysts may be present in raw or undercooked meat. When the undercooked meat is eaten, the sporocytes are also ingested. This parasite produces infection of any nucleated cell (Fig. 7–5).

Most infections are asymptomatic or produce mild lymphadenopathy and may resemble infectious mononucleosis. When the primary infection is acquired by a pregnant woman, the sporozoites are transmitted to the fetus via an infected placenta or infected maternal blood. Congenital toxoplasmosis can have devastating consequences for the fetus. This damage can include intrauterine death, brain damage, central nervous system disturbance, or chorioretinitis. The disease is also devastating to the immunocompromised patient. This parasitic infection can cause central nervous system involvement or infection of many different organs.

**Antibody Titer.** In acute toxoplasmosis, antibodies of the IgM class appear in 1 to 2 weeks, and the titer peaks at 6 to 8 weeks. Many individuals already have antibodies from a previous asymptomatic infection, and the low or insignificant elevations persist for months to years. An IgM antibody titer of 1:1024 or more is considered positive for acute infection of the past 4 months or less (Tietz, 1995).

When the pregnant woman has acute toxoplasmosis, the parasite can pass through the placenta and infect the fetus, with devastating consequences. Testing may be performed on the fetus's blood, obtained by fetal blood sampling of the umbilical vein in utero (see also Chapter 22). An elevated IgM antibody or the newer IgA anti-*Toxoplasma* antibody test is considered diagnostic for congenital toxoplasmosis (Jacobs et al., 1996).

Infection in the immunocompromised patient or the neonate may produce a lower antibody titer or show a false-negative result (Lehmann, 1998). This is because the infection increases faster than antibodies can be produced.

**Polymerase Chain Reaction.** PCR assay testing is another new laboratory method that can be used to assess the fetal blood when the pregnant female has toxoplasmosis. This method has high specificity and sensitivity in detecting toxoplasmosis. This test method is not yet widely available (Lehmann, 1998).

| Purpose of the Test | The antibody tests help in the diagnosis of toxoplasmosis. They identify antibody formation that results from exposure to the sporozoan parasite *Toxoplasma gondii*. |
|---|---|

| Procedure | A red-topped tube is used to collect 10 mL of venous blood. |
|---|---|

| Findings | **Elevated Values** |
|---|---|
| | Toxoplasmosis |

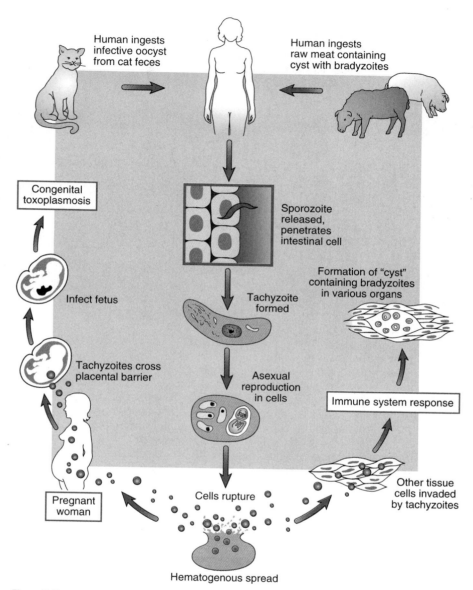

**Figure 7–5**

Life cycle of *Toxoplasma gondii*. The person ingests the infective stage of the parasite from infected feline fecal contamination on the hands or by eating raw or undercooked meat of an infected animal. In the person, the parasite passes through several maturation stages and infects cells and organs of the body. If the person is pregnant, the infection passes from the mother to the fetus. (Reproduced with permission from Mahon, C., & Manuselis, G. [1995]. *Textbook of diagnostic microbiology* [Fig. 24–35, p. 761]. W. B. Saunders.)

| **Interfering Factors** | • None |
|---|---|

| **Nursing Implementation** | **Pretest** |
|---|---|
| | Schedule the test to be performed at the onset of illness and 2 to 3 weeks later during the convalescent phase. |

## Varicella-Zoster Viral Antibody

(Serum)                    Synonyms: Chickenpox serology, VZV serology

| **Normal Values** | IgM antibodies: | Negative |
|---|---|---|
| | IgG antibodies: | <1:4; negative |

### Background Information

Varicella-zoster virus is a herpesvirus that causes two types of infection (see Table 7–1). The primary type is chickenpox infection, spread by droplet infection from an infected person. This form of illness usually occurs in children under the age of 10, causing the characteristic macular and crusted skin eruptions. In adults, pregnant women, newborn babies, and those who are immunocompromised, the infection can be very severe. The second type of infection, shingles, occurs as the varicella-zoster virus is reactivated. The painful, blistering skin reaction erupts along the lines of the dorsal root ganglia.

**Antibodies.** A negative test result means that the person was never exposed to the varicella-zoster virus and has no immunity. The person is susceptible to infection.

If the person has positive IgG antibodies or a high IgG titer, there is lifetime immunity to future chickenpox infection, but no immunity to shingles.

The varicella-zoster virus can cross the placental barrier. If a pregnant female with no immunity becomes infected with chickenpox in the first trimester or in the last 3 weeks of the pregnancy, the fetus may acquire the infection. The newborn baby remains at risk for the first 5 to 10 days after birth because of exposure in the last few days or weeks of the pregnancy. To reduce the severity of the infection in this newborn, varicella immunoglobulin is given to the baby (Lehmann, 1998).

To prevent chickenpox, vaccination with the live attenuated vaccine is recommended for all children and for patients who are immunocompromised (Jacobs et al., 1996).

| **Purpose of the Test** | The IgG antibody test is used to confirm past infection or vaccination that provides immunity from future chickenpox infection. The IgM antibody test is used to identify congenital infection in the newborn baby. |
|---|---|

| **Procedure** | A red-topped tube is used to obtain 10 mL of venous blood. |
|---|---|

| **Findings** | **Elevated Values** |
|---|---|
| | Past or present varicella-zoster infection |

| **Interfering Factors** | • Infection with another type of herpesvirus |
|---|---|

**Nursing Implementation**    Nursing intervention includes care of the venipuncture site.

### Pretest

Teach the patient that a positive IgG antibody titer indicates immunity from future chickenpox infection.

### Posttest

If the newborn baby has recent exposure to the varicella-zoster virus, keep the infant in isolation in the newborn nursery. To determine the presence of congenital infection, the infant's blood is tested for IgM antibodies.

## Diagnostic Procedures

## Blood Culture

(Blood)                    Synonyms: None

| **Normal Values** | Negative; no growth of organisms |
|---|---|

## Background Information

Septicemia, an infection of the blood, can be caused by almost any bacterial organism. The blood is cultured to detect and identify the organism and to determine effective antibiotic treatment. The indications of sepsis and the need for a blood culture include fever, a change in pulse rate, and hypotension or prostration. Shaking chills may or may not be present. The patient may also have a history of intermittent or persistent fever and a heart murmur, creating suspicions of bacterial endocarditis.

In sepsis, the bacteria are often present in the blood on an intermittent basis only. Specimen collection is timed to try to obtain the blood when the bacteria are present. The best time to collect the specimen is just before a chill or temperature spike, with two additional specimens taken at hourly intervals thereafter. Generally, after the bacteria enter the blood an onset of chills or fever occurs about 1 hour later. By the time the fever begins, the bacteria may have moved out of the blood. It can take several blood culture attempts before the bacteria are identified.

There are variations in the timing of specimen collection in an effort to isolate the elusive organism. Sometimes, instead of three hourly specimens on 1 day, two consecutive blood culture specimens are obtained on 1 day, and two more are obtained 24 hours later. The maximum total number of specimens, however, is four. Each blood culture specimen must be collected at a different vascular site with a separate venipuncture. There must be at least a 1-hour interval between collections of specimens.

These guidelines help one obtain at least one successful culture, and they prevent blood loss that results from excessive specimen collection.

False-positive results will occur when the normal flora of the skin contaminate the specimen. The microorganisms can be introduced into the specimen during the venipuncture procedure. The skin bacteria then grow in the culture medium and appear to be the cause of the sepsis. To prevent this confusion, careful antiseptic skin preparation must be done before the venipuncture is performed.

False-negative results can also occur. This means that pathogens are in the blood but that they did not grow in the culture medium. The causes include an inadequate sample of blood and the administration of antibiotics before the specimen was drawn.

A preliminary culture report is available in 48 hours or more. To avoid any further delay in treatment, the report is usually delivered verbally, by phone, or by computer. The written confirmation follows by mail. A final report is available in 7 to 10 days.

## Purpose of the Test

The blood culture confirms the presence of an infection in the bloodstream and identifies the causative organism. Susceptibility testing measures the sensitivity of the pathogen to various antibiotics.

## Procedure

For each blood culture specimen, preliminary careful skin antisepsis is done. Sterile technique is used to cleanse the skin and collect the blood.

For the adult, a needle and syringe, a transfer set, or a special set of blood tubes with culture media is used to collect 20 mL of venous blood.

For infants and small children, the procedure is the same, but 1 to 5 mL of blood may be obtained from pediatric patients.

For the neonate, 0.5 to 1 mL of blood is sufficient for each specimen (Brown, Kutler, Rai, Chan, & Cohen, 1995). The heelstick method and capillary tube blood sample are used only as a last resort because of the problem of contamination (Paisley & Lauer, 1994).

### Quality Control

With venipuncture, the tourniquet should be tied lightly for a brief time to prevent pooling of cells in the vein at the site of blood collection. Venipuncture technique must be smooth, with a blood flow that fills the syringe or tube readily. If excessive turbulence occurs because of flawed venipuncture technique, the hemolysis of the erythrocytes will alter the test results.

## Findings

### Positive Values

| | | |
|---|---|---|
| Bacterial endocarditis | Brucellosis | Bacterial pneumonia |
| Bacterial meningitis | Sepsis or septicemia | Toxic shock |
| Septic arthritis | Osteomyelitis | syndrome |
| Typhoid fever | | |

## Interfering Factors

- Contamination of the specimen
- Hemolysis
- Antibiotic therapy

## Nursing Implementation

■

*Critical Thinking 7–4*
On the same day, four different physicians order blood cultures for an acutely infected patient. How does the nurse respond to these multiple requests?

### Pretest

Inform the patient about the procedure, including the series of blood specimens and the skin asepsis. Ask the patient about any history of skin sensitivity to iodine.

Schedule the tests before antibiotic therapy is administered.

To assist with the timing of the blood sampling, monitor the patient's temperature, pulse, respiration, and blood pressure at frequent and regular intervals. Record the results in the patient's chart.

### During the Test

The nurse assists the physician or lab technician as needed. The skin of the venipuncture site is scrubbed in concentric circles in an outward direction with 80% to 95% alcohol and then allowed to dry. The second scrub is done in the same pattern using povidone-iodine solution. This solution remains on the skin for at least 1 minute. By using this method, most of the normal flora are killed, and dirt and debris are removed from the pores. If the patient has a sensitivity to iodine, green soap may be substituted, or the alcohol preparation alone can be used (Mahon & Manuselis, 1995).

The tops of the culture bottles or tubes are cleansed with alcohol or povidone-iodine before the blood is injected into them. If a blood collection system is used, only alcohol may be applied to clean the stoppers.

Using sterile gloves and aseptic technique, the blood is drawn from the vein. The blood is then divided among the different bottles or tubes.

### Quality Control

If an *intravenous* catheter is in place, the specimen is obtained from a venous site *below* the catheter or from the opposite extremity. This prevents hemodilution with intravenous fluids. Blood is never drawn from the intravenous line or the heparin-lock device because of the risk of external contamination. Additionally, heparin can inhibit bacterial growth.

### Posttest

Ensure that each requisition slip and all collection containers or tubes are correctly identified. The time, date, and venous site are included.

In the patient's chart, record each blood culture specimen collection, the time, the date, and the venous site. These data help keep track of the number and timing of the blood culture specimens and ensure that alternative venous sites are used.

Arrange for prompt transport of the specimens to the laboratory.

## Critical Value

The physician must be notified of a positive blood culture result immediately. Septicemia is very serious, and effective antibiotic treatment should be started promptly.

## Darkfield Examination, Syphilis

(Cell Scrapings)                   Synonym: *Treponema pallidum* darkfield examination

| **Normal Values** | Negative |
| --- | --- |

## Background Information

*Treponema pallidum* is the spirochete that causes syphilis, which is a sexually transmitted disease. During the primary stage of infection, an ulcerated lesion called a chancre appears on a mucosal or nonmucosal surface. The spirochete is present in the cell scrapings and in the moist exudate at the base of the lesion. In the secondary stage of disease, it is also present in the rash and the enlarged lymph nodes.

The best specimen of cell scrapings is obtained from a young, moist lesion. If present, dried serum must be removed before the scrapings are obtained. Oral and rectal lesions are not used because of the inevitable contamination from the normal flora and other organisms present.

Using darkfield microscopy, the slides of the cells and secretions reveal the absence or presence and characteristic movements of the syphilis spirochete. *T. pallidum* is a corkscrew-shaped organism that has rapid bending, flexing, and rotational movements.

A positive darkfield examination reveals syphilis at an early stage. Syphilis serologic tests are used to confirm the diagnosis, but these blood tests do not produce positive results until several weeks after the spirochete has caused infection.

## Purpose of the Test

The microscopic examination of infected cells and exudate is used to diagnose the syphilis infection.

## Procedure

**Pipette Method.**    After the surface of the chancre is cleansed with a saline-moistened swab, a sterile pipette is used to aspirate cells and exudate from the base of the ulcer. The secretions are placed on a sterile glass slide.

**Slide Method.**    After cleansing the surface of the chancre with a saline-moistened swab, a sterile glass slide is pressed directly on the ulcerated lesion.

**Quality Control**

Once the specimen is obtained, a coverslip is placed over the slide to prevent drying of the secretions and cells.

## Findings

**Positive Values**

*T. pallidum* infection

## Interfering Factors

- Contamination of the specimen
- Drying of the specimen
- Antibiotic therapy
- Healed lesion
- Ointment on the lesion

**Nursing Implementation**    **Pretest**

Schedule this test before antibiotic therapy is started.
Instruct the patient to avoid placing lotions or creams on the lesion before the
test is performed.

**During the Test**

Wear gloves during the test and when handling the specimen slide. If the test
result is positive, the lesion and secretions are contaminated.

**Posttest**

Ensure immediate transport of the specimen to the laboratory. The darkfield
examination must be performed within 15 minutes of collection. The
secretions must not become dry before the examination is completed.
Instruct the patient to abstain from sexual contact until the results are known.
When the test result is positive for this sexually transmitted disease, instruct the
patient to inform all sexual partners of the test results. Sexual partners are
advised to undergo testing.
Positive test results are reported to the state health department.
Instruct the patient to refrain from sexual contact until the infection is treated
and cured.

## Genital Culture

(Secretions)

Synonyms: Genitourinary culture, cervical culture, endocervical culture, prostatic fluid culture, vaginal culture, *Candida* culture, gonorrhea culture

**Normal Values**    Negative; normal flora present

## Background Information

A genital infection in the female is indicated by vaginitis, vulvovaginitis, or vaginal secretions. In the
male, it is indicated by urethritis and urethral
discharge. The infection may be caused by a sexually transmitted disease, or it may be the result
of other causes that are not related to sexual
contact. There are numerous pathogens that can be
responsible for a sexually transmitted disease, as
presented in Table 7–3. The culture of the secretions or tissue scrapings is used to identify the
causative organism.

**Nonspecific Vaginitis.**    This infection is common
in women. The cause is often a yeast organism
called *Candida albicans*, which is normally present in
the flora of the vagina. The infection may be sexually transmitted, but it is often caused by a change

in the host's resistance or by changes in the combination of bacteria in the normal flora of the vagina.
Bacterial vaginosis can also produce the vaginal discharge. When the balance of bacterial flora changes
because of antibiotic therapy or hormonal therapy,
some of the normal flora increase. These normal
flora include *Gardnerella vaginalis*, *Bacteroides*, and
*Mycoplasma hominis*.

**Gonorrhea.**    This infection is caused by the
organism *Neisseria gonorrhoeae*. It has a high incidence in young adults of both sexes. Two drug-
resistant strains of gonococcus are increasing in
incidence: penicillinase-producing and tetracycline-
resistant strains.

The initial infection involves the urethra of the
male or the vagina and endocervix of the female.

**Table 7–3   Diseases That May Be Transmitted Sexually and the Organisms Responsible**

| Disease | Organism(s) |
|---|---|
| Acquired immunodeficiency syndrome (AIDS)* | Human immunodeficiency virus (HIV) |
| Bacterial vaginosis | Gardnerella vaginalis |
|  | Bacteroides |
|  | Mycoplasma hominis |
| Chancroid | Haemophilus ducreyi |
| Chlamydial infection† | Chlamydia trachomatis |
| Cytomegalovirus infections | Cytomegalovirus |
| Enteric infections |  |
| Hepatitis A | Hepatitis A virus |
| Amebiasis | Entamoeba histolytica (protozoan) |
| Giardiasis | Giardia lamblia (protozoan) |
| Shigellosis | Shigellae (bacteria) |
| Genital herpes† | Herpes simplex virus |
| Genital Mycoplasma infections | Mycoplasma hominis |
|  | Ureaplasma urealyticum |
| Genital (venereal) warts† | Human papillomavirus |
| Gonorrhea† | Neisseria gonorrhoeae |
| Granuloma inguinale (donovanosis) | Calymmatobacterium granulomatis |
| Group B streptococcal infections | Group B-hemolytic streptococcus |
| Molluscum contagiosum | Molluscum contagiosum virus |
| Pubic lice | Phthirus pubis |
| Scabies | Sarcoptes scabiei |
| Syphilis† | Treponema pallidum |
| Trichomoniasis | Trichomonas vaginalis |

*U. S. Public Health Service fact sheet "Facts about AIDS" is available from the National Institute of Allergy and Infectious Disease (NIAID).

†Discussed in individual fact sheets available from NIAID.

From National Institute of Allergy and Infectious Disease. (1987). *Miscellaneous STDs* (NIH Publication No. 87–909H). Washington, DC: U. S. Department of Health and Human Services, National Institutes of Health.

The gonococcus is capable of ascension to the upper pelvic organs, causing pelvic inflammatory disease. Because the infection can exist in other zones of sexual activity, cultures of the anus and throat may be needed in addition to a genital culture.

**Genital Herpes.**   This condition is caused by the herpes simplex virus (HSV). It is transmitted by contact with the infected secretions or during asymptomatic shedding of the virus. Of the two different types of HSV, type 1 is transmitted by oral secretions, and type 2 is transmitted by genital secretions. The neonate may experience HSV-2 infection during delivery when he or she is in contact with the virus of the infected mother.

The viral culture is used to confirm the diagnosis of genital herpes, but current test methods are not fully effective. To obtain the best chance for an accurate diagnosis, more than one urogenital or anorectal site should be cultured.

**Chlamydia.**   This infection is the leading sexually transmitted disease in the United States (Stepp & Woods, 1998). Caused by *Chlamydia trachomatis*, the infection is transmitted by vaginal or anal sexual contact with an infected partner. Transmission can also occur during delivery from the infected mother to the neonate. Culture of genital secretions is one way to diagnose this infection, but the bacteria do not always grow under laboratory conditions. Alternative methods include screening the first voided urine by various laboratory methods.

**Chancroid.** This is a soft chancre or genital ulcer that is caused by *Haemophilus ducreyi* and is spread by sexual contact with an infected partner.

**Trichomoniasis.** This disorder is the most common sexually transmitted parasitic infection. It usually involves the vagina, vulva, and urethra and is caused by the protozoan parasite *Trichomonas vaginalis* (Fig. 7–6). In addition to culture of the genital area, the protozoan can be identified by microscopic examination of the urine sediment (Brunzel, 1994).

**Toxic Shock Syndrome.** This condition is caused by *Staphylococcus aureus*. Commonly, the bacteria are present on the skin and may also be present in other locations, including the vagina. Certain strains of the organism can produce toxins that enter the bloodstream. When this occurs, the septic infection is severe.

Preliminary reports of a genital culture are usually available in 24 hours. When the culture is negative, the report is final in 48 hours. For a positive culture, a minimal wait of 48 hours is necessary before the report is completed.

---

**Purpose of the Test**

The genital culture is used to identify the pathogenic organism that causes abnormal discharge and inflammation of the vagina or urethra.

---

**Procedure**

**Female.** With the assistance of a speculum, a sterile swab or wire loop is inserted into the cervical canal to obtain secretions or endocervical cell scrapings.

**Male.** A sterile cotton swab is used to collect secretions from the penile discharge. The physician may insert a wire loop into the urethra to obtain cell scrapings or a swab to obtain urethral secretions (Fig. 7–7).

**Chancroid.** The base of the genital ulcer is irrigated with saline. The fluid is aspirated with a sterile pipette or a moist, sterile cotton swab.

**Herpes Simplex.** A sterile cotton swab is used to remove epithelial cells from the base of fresh lesions. Fluid from vesicles may also be obtained by aspiration with a sterile pipette.

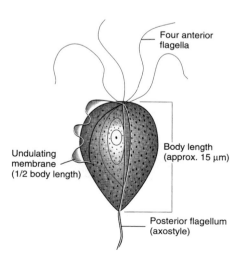

**Figure 7–6**
Schematic diagram of *Trichomonas vaginalis*. (Reproduced with permission from Brunzel, N. A. [1994]. *Fundamentals of urine and body fluid analysis* [p. 258]. Philadelphia: W. B. Saunders.)

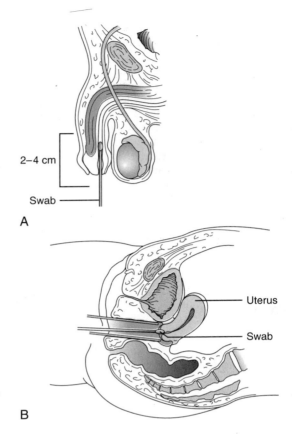

**Figure 7–7**
Specimen collection for genital culture. *A*, Sterile swab in male urethra. *B*, Sterile swab in female endocervical canal. (Reproduced with permission from Stepp, C. A., & Woods, M. A. [1998]. *Laboratory procedures for medical office personnel* [p. 364]. Philadelphia: W. B. Saunders.)

For any of these procedures, a sterile culture tube is used to receive the specimen of cell scrapings or fluid aspirate.

| Findings | Positive Values | | |
|---|---|---|---|
| | *Neisseria gonorrhoeae* | *Gardnerella vaginalis* | *Chlamydia trachomatis* |
| | *Candida albicans* | *Giardia lamblia* | Human papillomavirus |
| | *Staphylococcus aureus* | Herpes simplex virus | *Haemophilus ducreyi* |
| | Group B streptococcus | *Trichomonas vaginalis* | |

| Interfering Factors | |
|---|---|
| | • Recent urination |
| | • Recent douching |
| | • Improper collection technique |
| | • Contamination of the specimen |
| | • Antibiotic administration |

**Nursing Implementation**

### Pretest

Instruct the patient regarding pretest conditions as follows:

*Male:* Do not urinate within 1 hour of the test, because there will be fewer organisms available for culture.

*Female:* Do not douche for 24 hours before the test, because douching results in fewer organisms available for culture.

Inquire about any current use of antibiotics. The culture should be performed before any antibiotic therapy is started.

### During the Test

Place the male in the supine position. The female is placed in the lithotomy position, as for gynecologic examination.

Provide emotional support to the patient during the collection of the specimen. For the female, the procedure may produce mild apprehension or discomfort, but it is not painful. The male may experience nausea, sweating, fainting, or weakness as the wire loop or swab is inserted into the urethra. These discomforts are temporary.

To avoid contamination, place the swab or tissue specimen into the culture tube carefully.

### Posttest

The requisition slip should include information regarding the source of the specimen, the patient's name and age, the clinical diagnosis, the time and date of the specimen collection, and any current antibiotic therapy.

Arrange for transport of the specimen to the laboratory within 2 hours.

### Quality Control

The specimen must not be refrigerated, because cooling would reduce the microbial count.

Instruct the patient to abstain from sexual contact until the results are known.

When the culture is positive for a sexually transmitted disease, counsel the patient to inform all sexual partners of the test results. Sexual contacts are advised to undergo testing.

Positive test results for gonorrhea are reported to the state health department.

Instruct the patient to refrain from sexual contact until the infection is treated and cured. With gonorrheal infection, instruct the patient to have the culture repeated 1 week after the completion of antibiotic therapy.

As part of follow-up nursing care for a sexually transmitted disease, the nurse discusses ways to reduce risk for repeat infection. From the patient's sexual history, the nurse can identify the individual's practices that resulted in infection and make suggestions for future safe practices. The best protection from sexually transmitted disease is achieved through abstinence, a long-term monogamous relationship, or the use of condoms (Sharts-Hopko, 1997).

## Herpes Simplex Virus Antigen Test

(Cell Scrapings, Tissue Biopsy, Cerebrospinal Fluid)

Synonyms: None

**Normal Values**

Negative; no cells infected with herpes simplex virus are noted.

### Background Information

In the herpes family of viruses, there are several types of the virus that cause different infections (see Table 7–1). The HSV infection is caused by one of two viral types. In general, type 1 causes characteristic lesions in and around the mouth, and type 2 causes lesions of the genitalia. HSV-1 can also cause HSV encephalitis in adults, and HSV-2 infection can cause disseminated HSV neonatal disease. Once a primary infection has occurred, the individual is a carrier of the virus, and antibodies are present throughout life.

Using direct fluorescent antibody methodology, the antigen of HSV can be detected in cell preparations and inflammatory exudate. Using specific anti-bodies, the two serotypes of HSV can be differentiated. Possible tissue sources include scrapings of a lesion or vesicle from the conjunctiva, throat, bronchus, or genitalia. Tissue biopsy, brain biopsy, cornea scrapings, or spinal fluid specimens can also be tested.

Although this test is not as sensitive as a viral culture, it is faster. it It takes only hours to obtain this test result, as compared with several days to obtain culture results. Because of the rapid results, this test is used in urgent situations such as when there is brain involvement or when chemotherapy must be started and a herpes infection could erupt as the patient becomes immunocompromised.

**Purpose of the Test**

The herpesvirus antigen direct fluorescent antibody test identifies HSV-1 or HSV-2.

**Procedure**

A sterile swab, curette, or scalpel is used to collect cells and secretions from the base of a fresh ulcerated eruption. The specimen is then placed on a slide and air-dried. Universal precautions are used in the presence of an open, weeping lesion.

**Findings**

**Positive Values**

Herpes simplex virus type 1 (HSV-1)

Herpes simplex virus type 2 (HSV-2)

**Interfering Factors**

• Delay in the analysis of the specimen

**Nursing Implementation**

**Pretest**

If an operative biopsy specimen or spinal fluid specimen is obtained, it must be processed immediately. Notify the laboratory beforehand when the specimen is to be analyzed for immunofluorescence.

### During the Test

Label the slide and requisition slip with the patient's identification data and the tissue source of the specimen.

### Posttest

Arrange for prompt transport of the specimen to the laboratory.

**Quality Control**

The analysis must be performed on a fresh or frozen specimen.

---

## Mantoux Skin Test

**(Intradermal Skin Test)**    Synonyms: PPD skin test, tuberculosis skin test

---

**Normal Values**    Negative; induration <5 mm

---

## Background Information

*Mycobacterium tuberculosis* is the bacillus responsible for tuberculosis infection. By means of coughing, sneezing, or talking, an actively infected person spreads the bacilli by airborne droplet nuclei. If an individual has been exposed to the bacilli and infected, the infection is classified as latent, active, or reactivated. The Mantoux skin test detects the infection. If the Mantoux response is positive, an additional diagnostic workup, a chest x-ray, and microbiologic culture of the sputum are done to determine if the tuberculosis is in an active or reactivated state (Mahon & Manuselis, 1995).

Purified protein derivative (PPD) is a protein substance extracted from dead tuberculosis bacilli. In the Mantoux skin test, the PPD extract is injected intradermally to observe for a delayed hypersensitivity reaction. A positive reaction means that an infection with *M. tuberculosis* exists. The stage of the infection (latent, active, old disease, or reactivated infection) cannot be determined by this method of testing.

**Interpretation of the Result.**    Evaluation of the test result is done by observation, palpation, and measurement of the skin site. A negative result is indicated by no change in the skin site or by the presence of erythema, a reddened area that is not raised. There is no need for measurement. A positive result is a *raised* reddened area called an induration. A vesicle or a blackened necrotic area in the center may exist. The diameter of the induration is measured in millimeters from one edge of the raised area to the edge on the opposite side.

Previously, an induration of 10 mm or more was called a positive result. Today, different categories of a positive result exist, based on the person's risk to develop tuberculosis (Table 7–4) (Leiner & Mays, 1996; Maguire, 1997). To interpret the result accurately, the nurse or physician must identify the person's risk factors from the health history.

As seen in Table 7–4, the person with no risk factors is positive with an induration of 15 mm or more. For the individuals or population groups who have a high incidence of tuberculosis infection, an induration of 10 mm or more is positive. Individuals who are in close contact with a person who has newly active tuberculosis, individuals with the fibrotic scar visible on chest x-ray, and those with known or suspected HIV infection are considered positive when the PPD reading is 5 mm or more. Once the PPD is positive, it remains positive for life.

**BCG Vaccination.**    Bacille Calmette-Guérin (BCG) vaccine is used in underdeveloped countries

---

### Table 7–4   Definition of a Positive Tuberculin Skin Test*

**5 mm**

HIV infection (known or suspected)
Close contact with patients with newly diagnosed active tuberculosis (TB)
Radiographic fibrotic scars suggestive of old disease

**10 mm**

Immigrants from high-prevalence countries
U. S.-born, low-income, and medically underserved city dwellers
Staff and residents of nursing homes, mental institutions, correctional facilities, homeless shelters,
    and other high-prevalence settings (e.g., health care workers in particular hospitals)
Intravenous drug users
Patients with medical conditions that increase the risk of active TB (diabetes, chronic immunosup-
    pressive therapy, silicosis, renal failure, hematologic malignancies, chronic illnesses predisposing
    to undernutrition)†
Residents of urban areas where TB is prevalent
Children younger than 4 years

**15 mm**

No identifiable risk of TB‡

---

*Defined in millimeters of palpable induration.
    †For some of these persons who are immunocompromised by virtue of advanced disease, 5 mm may be considered positive.
    ‡Tuberculin skin testing is not usually recommended.
    Used with permission from Leiner, S., & Mays, M. (1996). Diagnosing latent and active pulmonary tuberculosis: a review for
clinicians. *Nurse Practitioner, 21*(2), 86–106. © Springhouse Corporation.

---

and some eastern European countries to prevent complications of tuberculosis infections. For 6 to 12 months or more after the BCG vaccination, the PPD test is positive, but that response abates thereafter. The Centers for Disease Control and Prevention (CDC) and the American Thoracic Society (ATS) both recommend that the PPD test be used for these individuals, ignoring the past history of BCG vaccination. The positive PPD result is far more likely a result of infection with tuberculosis bacilli (Leiner & Mays, 1996).

In most cases, a result of 4 mm or less is considered negative. There are, however, some qualifiers to this interpretation. False-negative results may occur for up to 10 weeks after exposure as the body activates its cell-mediated immunity response to the bacilli. The cell-mediated immunity is the response that causes the PPD reaction. Viral infection and the measles vaccine also delay or suppress the sensitivity. Anergy, the failure to react to the skin test, can occur. Those individuals who are immunocompromised, as with HIV, AIDS, various other chronic illnesses, or use of corticosteroids or immunosuppressive medications, may have a negative PPD with active tuberculosis (Jones, 1996; Maguire, 1997).

---

**Purpose of the Test**

The Mantoux test screens for tuberculosis exposure, latent infection, old tubercular infection, or active tuberculosis.

---

**Procedure**

PPD solution, 0.1 mL, is injected intradermally, with an assessment of the skin site 48 to 72 hours later.

| | |
|---|---|
| **Findings** | **Positive Values** |
| | Tuberculosis infection |

**Interfering Factors**

- Corticosteroid medication
- Immunosuppressive disorder
- Previous tuberculosis infection
- Previous vaccination with BCG vaccine
- Other recent vaccinations

**Nursing Implementation**

**Pretest**

High-risk population groups include the urban poor and ethnic minority groups such as Hispanics, Native Americans, and African Americans (Maguire, 1997). The nurse should choose a culturally sensitive approach to gain cooperation and community participation. The goal is not to discriminate but rather to screen those who are at risk (Denison & Shum, 1995).

Ask the patient if he or she has a known history of a positive skin test result or a history of tuberculosis. If the answer is yes, do not administer the Mantoux test.

To interpret the test results, ask the patient about risk factors (see Table 7–4) and in particular about any recent exposure to a person with active tuberculosis.

Explain that the test is mildly uncomfortable while the needle is inserted and the solution injected but that the sensation is temporary.

**During the Test**

Ensure that the PPD solution is kept refrigerated at all times, except when a dose is to be drawn up in the syringe. Administer the solution immediately to prevent warming by room temperature (Leiner & Mays, 1996).

Inspect the inner aspect of the forearm. The site of the skin test should be free of skin eruption, infection, and excess hair.

Draw up 0.1 mL of the PPD solution in a tuberculin syringe.

Cleanse the skin at the test site with alcohol.

Hold the skin taut and introduce the needle between the layers of skin until the bevel of the needle is fully enclosed.

Inject the PPD solution. When the needle is positioned correctly, an intradermal blisterlike formation occurs.

**Quality Control**

The test is invalid if the solution is placed in the subcutaneous tissue beneath the layers of skin.

**Posttest**

Record the Mantoux test administration in the patient's record, including the site of the injection, the dose and strength of the solution, the time, and the date.

Instruct the patient that normal activities, including bathing, can be resumed. If the test site itches, it must not be scratched or rubbed.

Instruct the patient to return for a reading of the test result in 48 to 72 hours. To read the test result, inspect and palpate the test site for a red, raised area of tissue reaction. If induration exists, use a millimeter tape to measure the diameter of the induration from the edge of one side to the edge of the other.

Record the measurement result in the patient's record.

## Nasopharyngeal Culture

(Secretions)     Synonyms: None

| Normal Values | Normal nasopharyngeal flora |
|---|---|

## Background Information

A variety of normal flora exists in the nose and nasopharynx, including *Staphylococcus aureus, Streptococcus pneumoniae, S. pyogenes, Branhamella catarrhalis, Neisseria* spp., and *Haemophilus influenzae*. These normal organisms may multiply and cause illness, particularly in children, the elderly, immunocompromised individuals, or individuals in a weakened condition. A nose culture positive for one of these organisms may indicate infection in the nasopharynx, sinuses, oropharynx, or tonsils. Infection can also occur elsewhere in the body, with the source of the infection being in the nose or throat. Additionally, some individuals are asymptomatic carriers of *S. aureus* or *N. meningitidis*.

***Staphylococcus aureus.*** The anterior nasal cavity is a major reservoir of *S. aureus*. In drug addicts with bacterial endocarditis, or in renal dialysis patients with septicemia, the nasal passageway may be the source of infection. This bacteria is also implicated in postoperative wound infection and in bacterial infection of the skin (furunculosis).

A large number of normal individuals harbor this organism, and the incidence is higher in hospital personnel and hospitalized patients. When an outbreak of this infection occurs, the nasopharyngeal culture may be performed as a screening test to identify asymptomatic carriers.

***Bordetella pertussis* and *Bordetella parapertussis.*** These organisms cause pertussis or whooping-cough. This respiratory tract infection usually occurs in infants and school-age children who are not vaccinated or who are incompletely vaccinated and are in close contact with an infected individual.

The nasopharyngeal culture is performed early in the course of the illness to verify the diagnosis. Once the specimen is obtained, the pathogens are placed in a culture medium. After growth of the organism in the culture occurs, microscopic examination can identify the cause of infection. Preliminary reports are usually available in 24 hours, and reports of no growth are complete in 48 hours. In a positive culture, the bacterial and fungal causes can be identified in 48 hours, but viral cultures require 1 to 2 weeks to complete.

| Purpose of the Test | The nasopharyngeal culture is performed to identify the bacteria that cause upper respiratory tract infection and to detect carriers of the organism. |
|---|---|

| Procedure | A special sterile, flexible nasopharyngeal wire swab is used to collect a specimen from the posterior nasopharynx. For the pertussis culture, the swab is placed near the septum and floor of the nose (Jacobs et al., 1996). The swab is carefully rotated and then withdrawn. Once collected, the swab is placed in the culture tube. The specific culture medium is designated by the laboratory. |
|---|---|

| **Findings** | **Positive Values** | | |
|---|---|---|---|
| | Pharyngitis | Thrush | *N. meningitidis* carrier |
| | Scarlet fever | Pertussis | |
| | Diphtheria | *S. aureus* carrier | |

| **Interfering Factors** | • Antibiotic therapy |
|---|---|
| | • Improper technique in specimen collection |

## Nursing Implementation

### Pretest

If possible, obtain the specimen before antibiotics are started.

Inform the patient that the sterile wire swab will be put into the back of the nose and throat. Any mild discomfort disappears after the swab is removed.

Instruct the patient to cough before the swab is inserted.

### During the Test

Help the patient sit up and tilt the head back.

Use a light or sterile nasal speculum, or both, to visualize the posterior nasal passage and nasopharynx.

*Nasopharyngeal culture:* Insert the sterile wire through the nasal passage into the nasopharynx. Allow the wire to remain for about 15 to 30 seconds. The patient may gag.

*Pertussis culture:* Insert the sterile wire 1 in into the nares and rotate it against the nasal mucosa.

### Posttest

Place the swab or wire in the sterile culture tube.

On the requisition slip, write the time, date, specific site used to obtain the culture specimen, and patient's name and age. Include the suspected clinical diagnosis and any current antibiotic therapy.

Arrange for prompt transport of the specimen to the laboratory. Do not refrigerate the specimen, because the yield of organisms would be reduced.

## Sputum Culture and Sensitivity

(Sputum)                Synonym: Sputum C and S

| **Normal Values** | No growth |
|---|---|

## Background Information

Sputum is a product of the lower respiratory tract, not a product of the oropharynx, such as saliva. Sputum cultures are obtained to identify pathogenic organisms in patients with suspected pulmonary infections. If bacteria are present, a sputum *Gram's* stain is performed to classify the bacteria as gram positive or gram negative. This knowledge may be used to initiate appropriate antibiotic therapy until the bacterial sensitivity portion of the test is completed. The sensitivity results identify which antibiotics are effective against the organism that is present in the sputum and which antibiotics are not effective because the organism is resistant.

The results of the acid-fast bacteria (AFB) smear for tuberculosis should be available within 24 hours (Woods, 1994). Sputum culture reports for other pathogens should be available in 24 to 48 hours. The sputum report for Gram's stain and the sensitivity study will follow the culture report. The mycobacterial culture to detect and identify *M. tuberculosis* takes 2 to 3 weeks for the results (Woods, 1994).

## Purpose of the Test

Sputum culture and sensitivity testing are performed to diagnose respiratory infections, identify the pathogenic organism responsible for the infection, and determine the appropriate antibiotic therapy. They are also performed to evaluate the effectiveness of the antibiotic or antibiotics.

## Procedure

**Expectoration Method.** A sputum specimen may be obtained by the patient's coughing up the sputum into a wide-mouthed sterile container with a cap.

**Aspiration Method.** A bronchial sputum specimen may be obtained by aspiration. If a bronchial specimen is needed, suctioning equipment and a sterile sputum trap are used.

**Bronchoscopy or Transtracheal Method.** A sputum specimen may also be obtained during a bronchoscopy or via transtracheal aspiration. The nurse may assist with these procedures but does not perform them.

## Findings

**Positive Values**

| | | |
|---|---|---|
| Pneumonia | Diphtheria | Parasitic infection of the lungs |
| Influenza | Tuberculosis | |
| Gonorrhea | | |

## Interfering Factors

- Contamination of the specimen
- Antibiotic therapy

## Nursing Implementation

**Pretest**

Perform this test before antibiotic therapy is started. This timing helps prevent a false-negative result.

Assess the patient's ability to follow instructions in coughing up the sputum as well as his or her ability to expectorate.

Provide a sterile container with a cap.

Instruct the patient to do the following:

1. Collect the specimen on arising in the morning before eating or drinking.
2. Take several deep breaths.
3. Cough up the sputum from deep within the lungs.
4. Expectorate into the sterile container.

### Quality Control

Demonstrate the procedure and have the patient perform a return demonstration to ensure that the container and lid are not contaminated during the collection procedure. A major problem with the expectoration method is contamination of the specimen by the normal flora, the microorganisms normally found in the mouth and throat (DeGroot-Kosolcharoen, 1996; Havlik & Woods, 1995).

## During the Test

Support and encourage the patient's attempts to produce sputum. If it is not contraindicated, postural drainage, clapping the back, and vibration may assist in raising the sputum. If the sputum is very tenacious, aerosol therapy may be necessary.

Approximately 1 tsp of sputum is necessary for a sputum culture and sensitivity test. When the patient is unable to produce this amount in one attempt, the container should be capped between attempts to expectorate.

If the patient is extubated, a sputum trap is used to obtain the specimen (Fig. 7–8). In this case, suctioning is performed as usual, except that the sputum trap is inserted between the sterile suction catheter and the suction tubing attached to the wall suction regulator.

Use the sputum trap as follows:

1. Tighten the cap to obtain an airtight seal.
2. Attach the wall suction tubing to the plastic "chimney" on the cap.
3. Connect the distal end of the sterile container to the latex tubing.
4. Suction as usual, but do not flush the catheter while the trap is in place.
5. After suctioning, disconnect the suction tubing and catheter.
6. Connect the latex tubing to the chimney of the cap.

## Posttest

Ensure that the lid is tightly sealed and that the container is labeled correctly. Send the specimen to the laboratory as soon as possible.

Do not refrigerate the specimen.

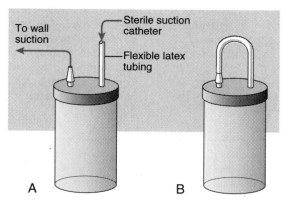

**Figure 7–8**
Sputum aspiration. *A*, Sputum trap. *B*, Closed sputum trap.

| | |
|---|---|
| **Complications** | There are no specific complications in obtaining a sputum culture and sensitivity test. The nurse should be cognizant of the complications of endotracheal suctioning, however, if that method is used to obtain the specimen. |

## Throat Culture
(Secretions)  Synonyms: None

| | |
|---|---|
| **Normal Values** | Negative; normal organisms in the oropharynx |

### Background Information

A variety of flora is found in the normal oropharynx. These flora do not cause respiratory illness unless some change occurs in the patient's health. When acute pharyngitis occurs, or when a clinical illness indicates an oropharyngeal source of infection, a throat culture may be indicated. The routine throat culture is used to screen for group A beta-hemolytic streptococcus. Another reason to perform a throat culture is to identify specific bacteria or fungi that cause infection of the oropharynx. When a specific organism is suspected because of the clinical condition of the patient, the laboratory is notified so that an appropriate and specific culture medium can be prepared. A routine throat culture may be ordered simultaneously with the specific throat culture.

**Routine Throat Culture.** This is used to screen for group A beta-hemolytic streptococcus— *Streptococcus pyogenes*. This bacterial cause of acute pharyngitis can result in the sequelae of rheumatic fever, scarlet fever, glomerulonephritis, wound infection, and sepsis. With early identification of the bacteria and effective antibiotic therapy, the potential for development of a serious complication is diminished or eliminated. The colonization of the bacteria is in the pharynx and tonsils.

**Throat Culture for *Corynebacterium diphtheriae.*** This test is used to screen for the bacterium that causes diphtheria. In diphtheria, a gray pseudomembrane appears on the tonsils and oropharynx. It spreads upward to the palate and nasopharynx and downward toward the larynx and trachea. Under the membrane are ulcers in the tissue. Culture results of no growth of these bacteria require 72 hours to report. A culture positive for *C. diphtheriae* requires at least 4 days for a complete report. Generally, a routine throat culture and a nasopharyngeal culture are performed simultaneously to identify or eliminate other possible organisms that may be the cause of respiratory disease.

**Throat Culture for *Neisseria gonorrhoeae.*** This gonorrheal throat culture is used to identify the gonococcal organism that has infected the oropharynx. The infection may be asymptomatic or may cause tonsillitis and acute pharyngitis. The throat is a primary site of sexually transmitted infection in homosexual males. Often, cultures of the genitalia and anal canal are performed at the same time. In children, a throat culture positive for this pathogen is indicative of child sexual abuse. The throat culture requires a minimum of 48 hours to identify this organism.

| | |
|---|---|
| **Purpose of the Test** | The throat culture identifies the bacteria that cause infection of the oropharynx, pharynx, and tonsils. It is also used to screen for an asymptomatic carrier of the infection. |

| | |
|---|---|
| **Procedure** | Two sterile Dacron swabs are used to obtain a specimen of exudate from the throat. The swab is then placed in a culture tube and capped tightly. |

| Findings | Positive Values | | |
|---|---|---|---|
| | Group A beta-hemolytic streptococcus throat infection | Scarlet fever Pertussis Pharyngitis Thrush | Diphtheria Gonococcal infection |

| Interfering Factors | • Antibiotic therapy<br>• Contamination of the specimen |
|---|---|

**Nursing Implementation**

**Pretest**

Obtain the culture specimen before antibiotic therapy is started.

Inform the patient that the test involves swabbing the throat. The swabbing may cause a brief gagging sensation. The discomfort disappears as soon as the procedure is finished.

In cases of acute epiglottitis or suspected diphtheria, do not perform this test unless prepared to establish an alternate airway, as needed. The nurse would not perform this throat culture, but would assist the physician.

If diphtheria is suspected, notify the laboratory in advance so that a special isolation medium can be prepared.

**During the Test**

Instruct the patient to tip the head back.

Use a tongue blade to depress the tongue.

The two sterile swabs are used together to rub the inflamed sites and areas of exudate in the oropharynx and tonsils (Fig. 7–9).

The swabs from a routine culture are placed in a regular culture tube. Throat culture for suspected diphtheria or gonococcal infection requires a special swab and culture-transport medium.

**Quality Control**

During the swabbing of the throat, ensure that the tongue, cheeks, and uvula are not touched. Many organisms are commonly present in the oropharynx. Poor technique will cause a false-positive result.

**Posttest**

Ensure that the specimen is placed in the sterile culture tube or transport medium as appropriate for the specific test.

On the requisition slip, identify the source of the specimen, the name and age of the patient, the clinical diagnosis, and any antibiotic therapy that the patient is currently undergoing.

Arrange for prompt transport of the specimen to the laboratory.

■

*Critical Thinking 7–5*
The throat culture report for a 5-year-old male patient is positive for *Neisseria gonorrhoeae*. What nursing response is indicated?

| Complications | There are no complications from a routine throat culture. In cases of acute epiglottitis or suspected diphtheria, however, assess the patient for a possible |
|---|---|

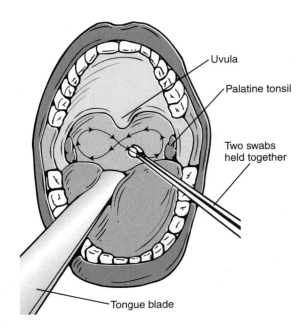

**Uvula**

**Palatine tonsil**

**Two swabs held together**

**Tongue blade**

**Figure 7–9**

Technique for obtaining a throat culture. (Reproduced with permission from Stepp, C. A., & Woods, M. A. [1998]. *Laboratory procedures for medical office personnel* [Fig. 25–12, p. 339]. Philadelphia: W. B. Saunders.)

laryngospasm immediately after the specimen is obtained. In such cases, prepare to support oxygenation and assist with the establishment of an airway as needed. Record the results of the respiratory assessment in the patient's chart.

## Urine Culture

**(Urine)**   Synonyms: Midstream urine culture; urine culture, midvoid specimen; urine culture, clean catch; urine culture, indwelling catheter

| **Normal Values** | No growth; $<10^4$ colony-forming units/mL |
| --- | --- |

### Background Information

The normal urinary tract and the urine are sterile except for the normal flora that reside in the distal urethra and at the urinary meatus. Bacteriuria is the presence of bacteria in the urine. A lower urinary tract infection consists of an infection in the bladder or urethra, or both. An upper urinary tract infection involves the renal pelvis or renal interstitial tissues, or both. Any bacterial or fungal organism can cause a urinary tract infection, but the most common pathogens are those that are present in normal feces (Brunzel, 1994). An infec-

tion in the urinary tract produces bacteria in the urine.

A bacterial count of $10^5$ colony-forming units per milliliter (CFU/mL) or more is considered positive and indicates significant bacteriuria. The count of the organism is evaluated together with the patient's symptoms, predisposing factors, and the type of organism(s) isolated (Mahon & Manuselis, 1995).

In the female patient, the test may be repeated once or twice to ensure the accuracy of the diagnosis, because contamination of the specimen could cause a false-positive result. In the male patient, only one specimen is needed for a correct diagnosis.

Routine culture methodology identifies the organism or organisms, and the sensitivity study identifies the antimicrobial medications that are effective or ineffective against the pathogen. Culture results with no growth are available after 24 hours. Positive cultures require 24 to 48 hours to complete, and identification of fungi requires 2 to 5 days or more (Mahon & Manuselis, 1995).

## Purpose of the Test

Culture of the urine is used to diagnose a urinary tract infection and to monitor the number of microorganisms in the urine. Sensitivity testing identifies the appropriate antibiotics and antimicrobials that are effective.

## Procedure

**Midstream Catch.** A clean-voided midstream technique is used to obtain 15 mL or more of urine in a sterile container. A first voided specimen of the day is used, because it has the highest colony count after an overnight incubation period.

**Indwelling Catheter.** A sterile needle and syringe are used to obtain 4 mL or more of urine from the urine sample port of the catheter. The urine is then placed in a sterile container.

***Mycobacterium* Culture.** For a tuberculosis culture of the urine, first voided morning specimens are collected on 3 separate days.

**Suprapubic Puncture.** Occasionally, suprapubic puncture is used to obtain the specimen. Using sterile technique, a needle is inserted into a full bladder, and the urine is aspirated with a syringe. The nurse may assist with the procedure but does not perform a suprapubic aspiration.

## Findings

### Positive Values

| | | |
|---|---|---|
| *Escherichia coli* | *Staphylococcus aureus* | *Pseudomonas* |
| *Enterobacter* spp. | *Mycobcterium* spp. | *Streptococcus faecalis* |
| *Klebsiella* spp. | *Proteus* spp. | *Candida albicans* |

## Interfering Factors

- Contamination of the specimen
- Antimicrobial therapy
- Inadequate volume of urine

## Nursing Implementation

### Pretest

Instruct the patient regarding the proper procedure for collection of a clean-catch midstream urine sample. Hands must be washed with soap before the specimen is collected. As described later, the perineum and urinary meatus must be cleansed carefully.

### Quality Control

Contamination of the specimen from the external genitalia, hair, vagina, or rectum would introduce microbes into the urine sample and cause a false-positive result.

### During the Test

#### Midstream or Clean-Catch Method

*Female:* Instruct the female patient that after spreading the labia, the perineum, vulva, and urinary meatus are cleansed with three soapy sponges, using one downward stroke for each sponge. Each sponge is used only once and is discarded, and then a sponge with water is used to remove the soap. The same single downward stroke is used, and the sponge is discarded. After the cleansing is completed, the labia must be maintained in that separated position until after the urine is collected.

*Male:* Instruct the male patient to cleanse the urethral meatus with the three soapy sponges and then rinse with the water sponge. Each sponge is used once and discarded. If the patient is uncircumcised, the prepuce must be retracted and the glans cleansed.

*Collecting the urine:* Instruct the patient to begin the urinary stream and void about 1 oz and then, as the urine flow continues, collect the urine by catching it midstream into the container. The first and last parts of the urinary stream are not used for the collection of the specimen. During the collection process, the container must not touch the perineal skin or hair. Once the specimen is obtained, the patient places the lid on the container without touching the inner surfaces.

#### Indwelling Catheter Method

When the catheter is already in place, the urine is removed from the catheter port. The urine in the collection bag is never used, because it is old.

Clamp the tubing below the urine collection port for 10 minutes. Cleanse the port with an alcohol sponge.

Use a sterile needle and syringe to collect the urine sample through this port. Place the urine in a sterile container. Unclamp the tubing.

#### Quality Control

Urine must not be collected from the drainage bag, because bacteria can be present on the outside of the bag. Additionally, the urine is not fresh, and bacteria have had an opportunity to colonize while the specimen remained at room temperature.

### Posttest

The specimen and requisition slip are labeled, including the patient's name, the time of collection, and the date. On the requisition slip, include the method of collection and any antibiotic therapy that may have been initiated already.

## Wound Culture
(Secretions, Cell Scrapings)

Synonym: Bacterial culture, wound

| Normal Values | No growth |
| --- | --- |

## Background Information

Soft-tissue infections affect various depths of tissue layers, including the epidermis, dermis, subdermis, fascial planes, and muscle tissue. The infectious organism may be enclosed or contained, such as in an abscess. The pathogens may also be in an open, ulcerated, or necrotic wound or fistulous tract that is exposed to the external environment. In addition, there may be foreign debris in a wound that promotes the infection.

Surgical microbes may include *Streptococcus pyogenes, Staphylococcus aureus,* or numerous other possible bacteria. The organisms may be aerobic or anaerobic.

One of the problems in culturing the infected wound is that many normal flora grow in an open, draining wound, fistula, or opened abscess. In the case of an ulcerated or necrotic infection, the wound must be cleansed and debrided to remove many of the surface bacterial flora. After exploring the wound, the culture is performed on the underlying tissue or sinus tract at the base of the wound.

The preliminary report from a wound culture is usually available in 24 hours. The isolation of the pathogen requires 48 hours or more, and a final negative result takes 72 hours to complete.

| | |
|---|---|
| **Purpose of the Test** | The wound culture is used to determine the presence of infection and to identify the causative organism. |

| | |
|---|---|
| **Procedure** | A syringe and needle can be used to aspirate purulent material from a wound. The liquid can be placed in a sterile tube. Tissue samples from a biopsy or scraping of the wound may also be done. For transport, the tissue sample is protected from drying by the addition of a small amount of sterile saline. |
| | Swabs and a culture tube can be used, but this is not the best choice because the swab often fails to absorb sufficient material from the wound. If this method is used, two swabs are needed, one for culture and one for a smear (Mahon & Manuselis, 1995). |

| | |
|---|---|
| **Findings** | **Positive Values** |

| | | |
|---|---|---|
| *Staphylococcus aureus* | *Escherichia coli* | *Clostridium* spp. |
| *Streptococcus pyogenes* | *Proteus* spp. | Group D streptococci |
| *Staphylococcus epidermidis* | *Pseudomonas* spp. | *Klebsiella* spp. |
| | *Bacteroides* spp. | |

| | |
|---|---|
| **Interfering Factors** | • Antibiotic therapy<br>• Contamination of the specimen |

| | |
|---|---|
| **Nursing Implementation** | **Pretest** |
| | If possible, schedule this procedure before antibiotic therapy is started. |
| | Explain that only minor discomfort occurs as an open wound is swabbed. If an abscessed area must be opened surgically, or a tissue biopsy, debridement, or scraping is required, a local anesthetic may be used. A written consent is needed for these surgical procedures. |

### During the Test

The nurse may assist but does not collect the wound culture specimen. For an open wound, the physician may irrigate it with sterile saline. For cleansing of the open wound to kill the surface bacteria, a 3% solution of hydrogen peroxide is useful.

### Quality Control

The goal is to culture the infecting organism and avoid contamination with flora and colonizing organisms (Mahon & Manuselis, 1995). The contamination of the specimen with surface organisms produces invalid results.

### Posttest

Ensure that the requisition slip indicates the patient's name and age, specific culture site, time, date, clinical diagnosis, and any current antibiotic therapy.
Arrange for prompt transport of the specimen to the laboratory.

### Quality Control

A delay in starting the culture growth can produce a reduced yield of microorganisms.

## References

AIDS Alert. (1996). New era makes viral load testing an important tool. *AIDS Alert, 11*(8), 1–2.

Avalos-Bock, S. (1994). Getting a rise out of tuberculosis with the PPD skin test. *Nursing 94, 24,* 51–53.

Barrick, B., & Vogel, S. (1996). Application of laboratory diagnostics in HIV nursing. *Nursing Clinics of North America, 31*(1), 41–56.

Bayer, R. (1995). Home testing for HIV: Has its time come? *Patient Care, 29*(16), 66–69.

Brown, D. R., Kutler, D., Rai, B., Chan, T., & Cohen, M. (1995). Bacterial concentration and blood volume required for a positive blood culture. *Journal of Perinatology, 15*(2), 157–159.

Brunzel, N. A. (1994). *Fundamentals of urine and body fluid analysis.* Philadelphia: W. B. Saunders.

Burgess, J., & MacGillis, A. (1995). HIV antibody testing. Comments on home test kits. *Connecticut Nursing News, 68*(5), 2.

Carpenter, C. J., Fischi, M. A., Hammer, S. M., Hirsch, M. S., Jacobsen, D. M., Katzenstein, D. A., Montaner, J. S., Richman, D. D., Saag, M. C., Schooley, R. T., Thompson, M. A., Vella, S., Yeni, P. G., & Volberding, P. A. (1996). Antiretroviral therapy for HIV infection. *Journal of the American Medical Association, 276*(2), 146–152.

Carter, S., Carter, J. B., & James, K. (1995). Rapid HIV-1 antibody screening. *Laboratory Medicine, 26,* 339–342.

Clague, J. E., & Horan, M. A. (1994). Urine culture in the elderly: Scientifically doubtful and practically useless? *Lancet, 344,* 1035–1036.

Cozad, J. (1996). Infectious mononucleosis. *Nurse Practitioner: American Journal of Primary Health Care, 21*(3), 14, 16, 23, 27–28.

De Groot-Kosolcharoen, J. (1996). Solving the infection puzzle with culture and sensitivity testing. *Nursing, 26*(9), 33–35, 38.

Denison, A. V., & Shum, S. Y. (1995). The evolution of targeted populations in a school-based tuberculin testing program. *Image, 27,* 263–266.

Farzadegan, H. (1994). HIV-1 antibodies and serology. *Clinics in Laboratory Medicine, 14,* 257–269.

Gore, M. J. (1996). What's new in blood banking? Plenty. *Clinical Laboratory Science, 9*(1), 5–9.

Harris, H. R. (1994). Home testing for HIV. *Surgical Technologist, 26*(6), 14.

Havlik, D., & Woods, G. L. (1995). Screening sputum specimens for mycobacterial culture. *Laboratory Medicine, 26,* 411–413.

Henry, J. B. (1996). *Clinical diagnosis and management by laboratory methods* (19th ed.). Philadelphia: W. B. Saunders.

Jacobs, D.S., Dermott, W. R., Grady, H. J., Horvat, R. T., Huestis, D. W., & Kasten, B. L. (Eds.). (1996). *Laboratory test handbook* (4th ed.). Baltimore: Williams & Wilkins.

Jones, S. G. (1996). Tuberculin testing in patients with human immunodeficiency virus/acquired immune deficiency syndrome. *AACN Clinical Issues: Advanced Practice in Acute and Critical Care, 7,* 378–379.

Koontz, F., & Weinstock, J. V. (1996). The approach to stool examination for parasites. *Gastroenterology Clinics of North America, 25,* 435–449.

Lehmann, C. A. (1998). *Saunders manual of clinical laboratory science.* Philadelphia: W. B. Saunders.

Leiner, S., & Mays, M. (1996). Diagnosing latent and active pulmonary tuberculosis: A review for clinicians. *Nurse Practitioner: American Journal of Primary Health Care, 21*(2), 86, 88, 91–92, 95–96, 98–100, 102–104, 106.

Maguire, M. C. (1997). Primary care approaches. Tuberculosis skin testing at the end of the century. *Pediatric Nursing, 23,* 209–211.

Mahon, C., & Manuselis, G. (1995). *Textbook of diagnostic microbiology.* Philadelphia: W. B. Saunders.

Markel, E. K., Voge, M., & John, D. T. (1992). *Medical parasitology* (7th ed.). Philadelphia: W. B. Saunders.

Michael, R. S., Hayden, G. F., & Hendly, J. O. (1995). Pharyngitis in children: When to culture, when to treat. *Consultant, 35,* 1469–1472, 1476–1477, 1482–1484.

Novak, R., Sandowski, L., Klespies, S. L. (1995). How useful are fecal neutrophil determinations? *Laboratory Medicine, 26,* 743–745.

Onderdonk, A. B., Winkelman, J. W., & Orni-Wasserlauf, R. (1996). Eliminating unnecessary urine cultures to reduce coughs. *Laboratory Medicine, 27,* 829–832.

Paisley, J. W., & Lauer, B. A. (1994). Pediatric blood cultures. *Clinics in Laboratory Medicine, 14,* 17–30.

Prandoni, D., Boone, M. H., Larson, E., Blane, C. G., & Fitzpatrick, H. (1996). Assessment of urine collection technique for microbial culture. *American Journal of Infection Control, 24,* 219–221.

Regan, T. C., & Pahira, J. J. (1995). UTI in men: How to recognize, how to treat. *Consultant, 35,* 1162–1166.

Rust, D. (1996). FDA approves HIV home-testing system. *Oncology Nursing Forum, 23,* 1489.

Schutze, G. E., Rice, T. D., & Starke, J. R. (1993). Routine tuberculin screening of children during hospitalization. *Pediatric Infectious Disease Journal, 12*(1), 29–32.

Sharts-Hopko, N. C. (1997). STDs in women: What you need to know. *American Journal of Nursing, 97*(4), 46–53.

Smith, L. A. (1997). Still around and still dangerous: *Giardia lamblia* and *Entamoeba histolytica. Clinical Laboratory Sciences, 10,* 279–285.

Speicher, C. E. (1998). *The right test* (3rd ed.). Philadelphia: W. B. Saunders.

Stepp, C. A., & Woods, M. A. (1998). *Laboratory procedures for medical office personnel.* Philadelphia: W. B. Saunders.

Tamborlane, T. A., & Kunz, D. A. (1996). Home HIV tests: The need for regulation. *Caring, 15*(8), 52–55.

Texas Nursing. (1996). TDH issues explanation of new state HIV laws . . . Texas Department of Health. *Texas Nursing, 70*(1), 7, 9, 14.

Tietz, N. W. (Ed.). (1995). *Clinical guide to laboratory tests* (3rd ed.). Philadelphia: W. B. Saunders.

Ungvarski, P. J. (1997). Update on HIV infection. *American Journal of Nursing, 97,* 1, 44–51.

Warner, N. A. (1996). In practice: Microbiology. Clinical detection and diagnosis of human immunodeficiency virus. *Clinical Laboratory Science, 9,* 276–281.

Washington, J. A. (1994). Collection, transport and processing of blood cultures. *Clinics in Laboratory Medicine, 14,* 59–68.

Woods, G. L. (1994). T. B. testing: Methods and time targets . . . Tuberculosis (TB). *Medical Laboratory Observer, 26*(3), 25–28.

Wright, M. S., & Collins, P. A. (1997). Waterborne transmission of *Cryptosporidium, Cyclospora,* and *Giardia. Clinical Laboratory Science, 10,* 287–290.

# PART III

# Multisystem Diagnostic Procedures

# CHAPTER 8

# Ultrasonography

Ultrasonography, or ultrasound, sends pulsed, high-energy sound waves into the body and records the pattern of the echo as the sound waves bounce back from the tissues and organ structures. The echoes are converted to images that are seen on a monitor and photographed for later analysis.

Ultrasound has many advantages as a diagnostic procedure. Because it is noninvasive and does not use ionizing radiation, it is very safe for the patient. The scanning can be performed on the coronal, sagittal, or transverse planes or in a combination of planes to give a complete visualization of the targeted tissue (Fig. 8–1). When compared with the cost of computed tomography (CT) or magnetic resonance imaging (MRI), ultrasonography is inexpensive (Tempkin, 1993).

General information about ultrasound is presented in this chapter. Specific applications of ultrasound in different body systems are presented in the appropriate chapters in Part IV of this text.

## Ultrasound
**(Sound Wave Imaging)**    Synonyms: Sonogram, diagnostic sonography

| Normal Values | No anatomic or functional abnormalities exist. The organs are normal in size, shape, contour, and position. The internal structures of the organs and nearby tissues are within normal limits. |
| --- | --- |

## Background Information

Sound waves are transmitted through fluid, and they bounce back, or "echo," off more solid substances. In ultrasound, the sound waves are transmitted from the tissue surface through the body tissues in a directed path. Parts of the beam are reflected back quickly when they encounter a structure or substance of different acoustic character (Fig. 8–2). The remaining parts of the beam continue to a greater depth and are also reflected back as they ultimately encounter tissues of differing densities. The sound waves transmit through fluid but do not transmit through air, bone, or barium.

Many different ultrasound scans are used to examine organs, tissues, lymph nodes, and the vascular circulation. The more common scans are listed in Table 8–1.

**Transducers.** The transducer, sometimes called the probe or the scan head, converts electric energy to high-frequency ultrasound energy. The ultrasound waves are sent by the transducer and also are received as they are reflected back. Once the transducer receives the echoes, they are converted back to electric impulses and are then converted to audio signals or visual images.

In the ultrasound procedures that are performed externally, the handheld transducer moves over the skin in defined directions. The patterns of movement are determined by the anatomic location of the target organ (Fig. 8–3). Before the

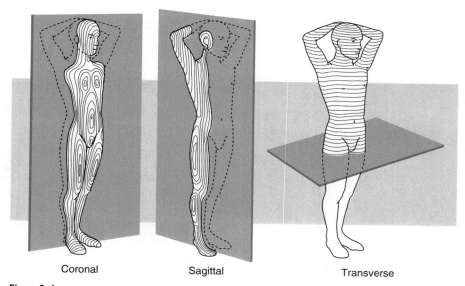

Coronal      Sagittal      Transverse

**Figure 8–1**

Scanning planes for ultrasound examination. (Reproduced with permission from Tempkin, B. B. [1993]. *Ultrasound scanning: Principles and protocols.* Philadelphia: W. B. Saunders.)

procedure begins, acoustic gel is applied to the skin. This creates an air-free surface for the transducer and eliminates the interference caused by air (Kremkau, 1998).

Some transducers are designed as specialized probes that enter the body. These probes are used in the esophagus, vagina, rectum, or lumen of a blood vessel. The internal application is useful because the sound waves are placed nearer the particular organ or tissue. The procedure reduces or eliminates the interference of other tissues and of the air of the lungs or bowel.

**Technologic Variations.** In ultrasound technology, there are several modes of examination available. The selection is based on the qualities and physiologic functions of the target tissues. *Diagnostic ultrasound* produces cross-sectional anatomic images of tissues or organs. *Doppler ultrasound* is used to detect and measure the movement of body fluids as it applies to blood flow. *Duplex Doppler ultrasound* combines the cross-sectional view of the blood vessel with the Doppler measurement of the movement of the blood (Zwiebel & Sohaey, 1998).

Diagnostic ultrasound produces a wedge-shaped cross-sectional image of tissues or organs.

The ultrasound pulsations pass through all tissues in their path until they reflect off solid structures. Some of the pulses echo quickly, and others pass through fluid-filled structures until they encounter firm structure or high-density tissue at a more distant point. In diagnostic ultrasound, there are three variations or characteristics of the displayed images.

One way of displaying the ultrasound image is called a *B-scan* because of the intensity of *brightness* of the image. The image is made of white dots on a black background, and the human eye sees tones of white, gray, and black. The strength of the echo produces varying intensities of brightness. The image of a strong echo is white and bright, as produced by sound impulses passing through fatty tissue. The absence of an echo is black, as produced by sound impulses passing through fluid. A second characteristic is that homogeneous tissues appear in shades of gray. This variation is called the *gray scale*. The third variation in the image display is called *real-time* scanning. Real-time refers to the ability to display two-dimensional (2-D) images of tissues that are in motion. For example, in echocardiography, the heart valves can be seen as they open and close (Kremkau, 1998).

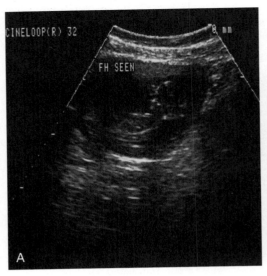
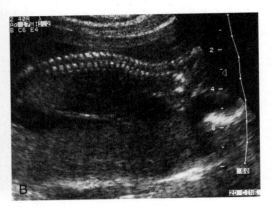

**Figure 8–2**

Pregnancy ultrasound. The varying densities and compositions of tissue allow visualization of the uterine contents. *A*, A normal 4-month-old fetus. The fetal heart (FH) is identified. *B*, The normal spinal structure of a 4-month-old fetus.

Doppler ultrasound detects the presence, direction, speed, and character of arterial or venous blood flow within the vascular lumen. The Doppler pulses echo off the moving erythrocytes in the blood in patterns that correlate with the flow of the blood. The echoes are converted to an audio signal or a linear graphic reading on a paper strip, similar to an electrocardiogram strip.

The audio signal changes according to the character of the blood flow. The blood flow may be characterized as *normal; disturbed,* as at the bifurcation of a blood vessel; or *turbulent,* as encountered beyond the point of a partial obstruction (Fig. 8–4).

Severely obstructed circulation produces a weak signal or silence. In the graphic printout, the changes in circulation produce characteristic patterns in the linear tracings. Additional discussion of Doppler ultrasound in peripheral vascular disease is presented in Chapter 16.

Duplex Doppler ultrasound combines the measurement of blood flow with the imaging of the lumen of the blood vessel or a cross-sectional, anatomic view of a particular structure or organ. The disturbance and turbulence of blood flow is located and visualized. It may be used to assess the circulation within an artery or vein or to

| Table 8–1 | Ultrasound Procedures | |
|---|---|
| Popliteal artery scan | Pelvic scans |
| Inferior vena cava scan | Female pelvic scan |
| Abdominal aorta scan | Obstetric scan |
| Carotid artery scan | Endovaginal scan |
| Abdominal scan | Male pelvic scan |
| Liver scan | Thyroid scan |
| Gallbladder, biliary tract scan | Scrotum scan |
| Pancreas scan | Breast scan |
| Renal scan | Neonatal brain scan |
| Spleen scan | Transesophageal echocardiography |

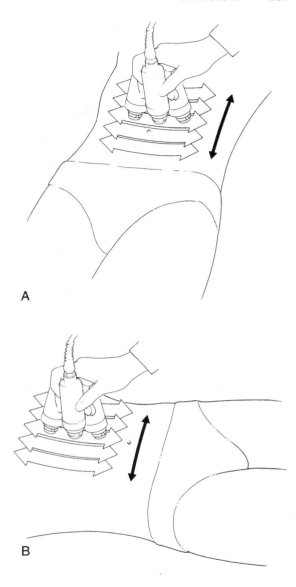

A

B

**Figure 8–3**

Technique of ultrasound examination of the abdomen. *A,* The transducer moves in a "rock-and-slide" motion in transverse planes. *B,* Using the same motion, the transducer scans the abdominal organs in sagittal planes. (Reproduced with permission from Tempkin, B. B. [1993]. *Ultrasound scanning: Principles and protocols* [p. 11]. Philadelphia: W. B. Saunders.)

detect the vascular or avascular characteristics of a tumor. It may also be used to evaluate the blood flow before or after a kidney or liver transplant.

When a color flow instrument is used with the duplex Doppler ultrasound, the images provide a color map or 2-D view of the blood flow and its characteristics. The colors indicate the direction, speed, and turbulence of the flow. In the image, red indicates blood flow that moves toward the transducer, and blue indicates blood flow that moves away from the transducer. Green indicates a wide range of velocities that are present in the blood flow. Yellow, white, or mosaic patterns indicate high-velocity or complex blood flow patterns.

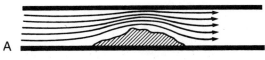

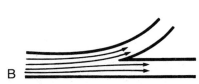

**Figure 8–4**
Patterns of blood flow detected by ultrasound. *A,* Disturbed blood flow at a stenosis. *B,* Disturbed flow at a bifurcation. (Reproduced with permission from Kremkau, F. W. [1998]. *Diagnostic ultrasound: Principles and instruments* [5th ed., p. 223]. Philadelphia: W. B. Saunders.)

---

**Purpose of the Test**

Ultrasound examines organs, blood vessels, and structures of the body to identify malposition, malformation, malfunction, or the presence of a foreign body.

---

**Procedure**

High-frequency sound waves are directed into an area of the body in a specific pattern. The echoes of the ultrasound are converted to visual images (Fig. 8–5), linear tracings, or audible sounds.

---

**Findings**

■

*Critical Thinking 8–1*
A pregnant woman wants to stay with her confused, elderly mother during the ultrasound examination but explains that she is afraid of "exposure to radiation." How do you respond, and what arrangements can be made?

**Abnormal Values**

| | | |
|---|---|---|
| Cyst (Fig. 8–6) | Aneurysm | Abscess |
| Tumor | Foreign body | Congenital anomaly |
| Hypertrophy | Vascular occlusion | Hematoma, bleeding |
| Obstruction or | Venous thrombosis | Pregnancy, fetal |
|   stricture | Atherosclerotic |   development |
| Calculus |   plaque | |

---

**Interfering Factors**

- Air
- Overlying bones
- Bowel gas
- Barium
- Obesity

---

**Nursing Implementation**

**Pretest**

Obtain a written consent for any ultrasound procedure that involves insertion of a transducer into a body cavity or blood vessel. No consent is needed for the routine ultrasound examination that uses an external transducer and a noninvasive method of examination.

Schedule the ultrasound examination before or several days after any barium studies.

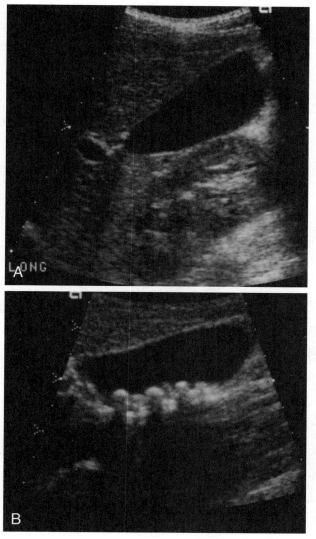

**Figure 8–5**
Abdominal ultrasound, gallbladder. *A,* Normal gallbladder. *B,* Gallbladder with gallstones.
(Reproduced with permission from Godderidge, C. [1995]. *Pediatric imaging* [p. 193]. Philadelphia:
W. B. Saunders.)

**Quality Control**

> Barium is an opaque substance that would block the transmission of ultrasound impulses. Residual barium causes an ultrasound problem for about 24 hours after a barium x-ray examination.

Instruct the patient about any dietary restrictions or modifications. Any abdominal ultrasound examination requires fasting from food for 12 hours. If the

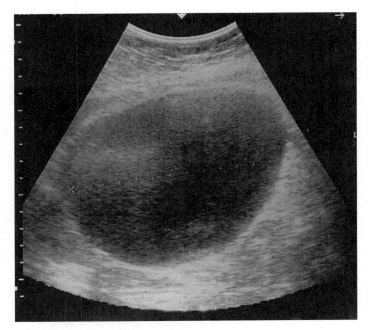

**Figure 8–6**
Abdominal ultrasound, liver. A hepatic cyst was the cause of the patient's pain in the right upper quadrant. The core of the cyst appears black because it is filled with fluid. (Reproduced with permission from Schlager, D. [1997]. Ultrasound detection of foreign bodies and procedure guidance. *Emergency Medicine Clinics of North America, 15*[4], 910.)

patient has a tendency toward bowel gas, a low-residue diet is implemented for 24 to 36 hours, followed by a 12-hour fast from all foods.

Some abdominal ultrasound protocols require an enema before the examination. Schedule the abdominal tests for the early morning, before breakfast.

Gynecologic ultrasound procedures often require drinking 40 oz of water without voiding before the test. This fills the urinary bladder and moves it upward and away from the uterus.

### Quality Control

Intestinal gas must be removed from the colon, because ultrasound impulses cannot pass through air. In addition, visualization of the abdominal organs and vasculature would be impaired by the overlying colon and its contents.

Inform the patient that the examination is safe and painless. To alleviate anxiety, provide reassurance before and during the test.

The older child or adult responds well to explanations. These patients may like to see the screen with the ultrasound image. An explanation of the anatomy that is seen on the monitor may help make the experience more interesting.

A small child or an agitated, anxious adult patient may be accompanied by a calming parent or other adult.

■
*Critical Thinking 8–2*
Just before the abdominal ultrasound examination begins, a
5-year-old patient sees the transducer and becomes visibly
apprehensive. Which approaches
can be effective in helping the
child cope with the experience?

Assist the patient in removing all clothes, jewelry, and metallic objects. A hospital gown is worn.

## During the Test

Position the patient on the examining table.
Instruct the patient to remain still during the examination.
Apply the acoustic gel to the skin surface in the area to be examined. The gel
serves as a conducting agent and eliminates the thin layer of air that causes
a barrier to the transmission of impulses.
Neonates and infants are kept warm during the examination. Neonates are particularly prone to hypothermia, so a warming lamp may be used. The dark
room, a pacifier, and gentle touch help keep the infant calm (Sorensen &
Godderidge, 1995).

## Posttest

Remove the acoustic gel to prevent the soiling of the patient's clothes.

## References

Craig, M. (1993). *Introduction to ultrasonography and patient care.*
    Philadelphia: W. B. Saunders.
Godderidge, C. (1995). *Pediatric imaging.* Philadelphia: W. B.
    Saunders.
Hayden, C. K. (1996). Ultrasonography of the acute pediatric
    abdomen. *Radiologic Clinics of North America, 34,* 791–806.
Kremkau, F. W. (1998). *Diagnostic ultrasound: Principles and in-
    struments* (5th ed.). Philadelphia: W. B. Saunders.
Schlager, D. (1997). Ultrasound detection of foreign bodies and
    procedure guidance. *Emergency Medicine Clinics of North
    America, 15,* 910.
Sorensen, L., & Godderidge, C. (1995). Pediatric ultrasound.

In C. Godderidge (Ed.), *Pediatric imaging.* Philadelphia:
    W. B. Saunders.
Snopek, A. M. (1992). *Fundamentals of special radiographic proce-
    dures* (3rd ed.). Philadelphia: W. B. Saunders.
Tempkin, B. B. (1993). *Ultrasound scanning: Principles and proto-
    cols.* Philadelphia: W. B. Saunders.
Torres, L. S. (1993). *Basic medical techniques and patient care
    for radiologic technologists* (4th ed.). Philadelphia: J. B.
    Lippincott.
Zwiebel, W. J., & Sohaey, R. (1998). *Introduction to ultrasound.*
    Philadelphia: W. B. Saunders.

# CHAPTER 9

# Radiography

Many different radiographic methods use a source of radiation for imaging the patient's tissues. These include x-ray studies, computed tomographic (CT) scans, radioisotope scans, and contrast studies. Although these methods vary in complexity of technique and equipment, all are based on the same principle. Electromagnetic energy passes partially through opaque tissues of varying radiodensities. The radio waves that pass through the patient's body are captured by the photographic film and produce a corresponding image of the tissues. The radio waves that are absorbed by body tissues do not affect the photographic film.

Discussions of radioisotope scans, contrast studies, and CT scans are presented in different chapters in Part III. This chapter concentrates on conventional x-ray studies, which are used to image many tissues and organs of the body.

## X-Ray Studies

**(Radiography)** Synonyms: Plain film, conventional x-ray, simple radiography

| **Normal Values** | The size, shape, appearance, thickness, and position of the organs and tissues are within normal limits for the patient's age. No anatomic or functional abnormalities are noted. |
|---|---|

## Background Information

The source of the x-ray emissions is a high-voltage electric current that passes through a special vacuum tube in the x-ray machine. Within the vacuum tube, the electric current is converted to x-ray waves. As the x-ray beams are emitted from the machine, they pass through the patient and onto a photographic plate called an x-ray film (Fig. 9–1).

In the imaging process, the x-ray beam passes freely through air and almost as freely through fatty tissue. Because all or most of the x-ray beam strikes the radiographic film, the resultant film image is black or very dark. As an example, the air cavities of lung tissue appear very dark to black on the chest x-ray film.

In soft tissue that is somewhat dense, some of the x-ray beam is absorbed by the tissue, and the remainder passes through the tissue and strikes the photographic plate. The resultant images are in soft gray tones that vary in intensity of shading. Thus, blood, muscles, organs, and other soft tissues are seen in shades of gray and are lightly visible on the x-ray film (Fig. 9–2).

Most x-ray emissions are absorbed or blocked by bone because of the calcium content of osseous tissue. Thus, the film image of bone is white, particularly for dense, healthy bone tissue that has a high concentration of calcium. In bones that are fractured, the crack, break, or displacement of bone is quite visible. In the patient with osteoporosis, the bones have less calcium content, and the film image of the bone is more gray and porous.

The radiographic image is affected by several other variables in addition to tissue composi-

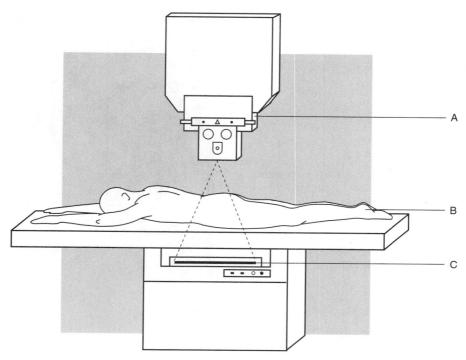

**Figure 9–1**

Simple radiograph. *A*, X-ray machine. *B*, Patient. *C*, X-ray film.

tion. Some tissues are thicker and more dense or radiopaque. Others are thinner and therefore more radiolucent. The size, shape, and position of the organs or tissues are accurately reproduced because of the differences in the densities of the tissues.

All metals absorb x-rays. Because the x-ray beam is absorbed or blocked, metal objects appear totally white on the film. For example, x-rays easily locate a metallic foreign body that has been aspirated or swallowed (Fig. 9–3). Because metal objects block the x-rays and any tissue behind the metal objects, the patient must remove all jewelry and metal objects from the area that is to be imaged.

The radiopacity of metals also works to benefit the patient and personnel. X-ray beams cannot pass through lead of a particular thickness. Thus, a lead shield or apron is worn to protect reproduc-

**Figure 9–2**

The four basic densities on an x-ray. A lateral view of the forearm shows that bone is most dense, or white; soft tissue is gray; fat is somewhat dark; and air is very dark. The abnormality in this case is the fat in the soft tissue of the forearm, which is due to a lipoma. (Reproduced with permission from Mettler, F. A. [1996]. *Essentials of radiology* [p. 2]. Philadelphia: W. B. Saunders.)

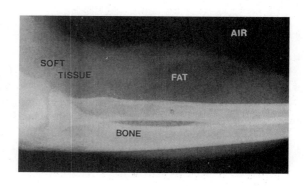

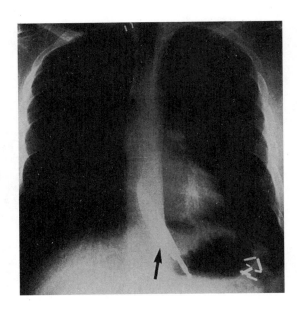

**Figure 9–3**

Steak knife lodged at the esophagogastric junction. This mentally ill patient claimed to have swallowed his steak knife at dinnertime. The chest x-ray shows the metallic blade (arrow) at the gastroesophageal junction. The wooden handle of the knife, which is down in the stomach, is not seen because wood typically is not visible on an x-ray. Metallic surgical clips are seen to the left of the stomach air bubble. These are from previous surgery to remove other swallowed objects. (Reproduced with permission from Mettler, F. A. [1996]. *Essentials of radiology* [p. 185]. Philadelphia: W. B. Saunders.)

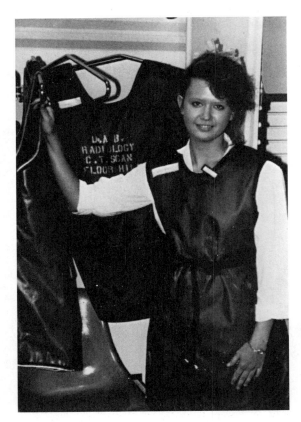

**Figure 9–4**

Protection from radiation exposure. Lead aprons should be handled carefully and stored on special holding racks when not in use. Film badges should be worn at the collar level, outside the lead apron. (Reproduced with permission from Thompson, M. A., Hall, J. D., Hattaway, M. P., & Dowd, S. B. [1994]. *Principles of imaging science and protection* [Vol. 2, Slide 371]. Philadelphia: W. B. Saunders.)

tive organs and other radiosensitive tissue from undesired exposure to radiation (Fig. 9–4). Radiography rooms have lead-lined walls to prevent the passage of radiation into offices and corridors. This protects workers and others from inadvertent exposure.

Three-dimensional (3-D) views of the tissue are obtained by filming from the front to the back of the body as well as from the side. In radiology, these views are called *anteroposterior* and *lateral* (AP and lateral) (Fig. 9–5). If the patient is imaged from the back-to-front and side views, the positions are called *posteroanterior* and *lateral* (PA and lateral). Other positions, such as oblique views, may be requested to image a particular section of anatomy that is less visible from a traditional position.

All AP x-ray films are viewed as if the patient were facing you. This means that the patient's left side is on your right side. Conversely, the PA x-ray film is viewed as if you were behind the patient facing his or her back. To prevent confusion and possible error in the interpretation of the film, the technician places the letters R and L on the film to indicate the *patient's* right and left sides.

**Chest X-Ray.** This film is obtained routinely for hospitalized and preoperative patients to screen for tuberculosis and other serious pulmonary or cardiac diseases. It also provides a preoperative comparison film for the postoperative patient in whom a pulmonary or cardiac complication develops, and it is a basic radiologic procedure for the patient with a suspected pulmonary disorder.

The film produces images of the lungs, trachea, bronchi, diaphragm, mediastinum, part of the heart, bony thorax, and pulmonary vasculature. It reveals characteristic patterns of opacity that help differentiate pneumonia from other conditions of similar symptomatology, such as atelectasis, pulmonary embolism, heart failure, or pneumothorax. The opacities may also reveal the presence and location of a pulmonary tumor, a lesion of the rib, enlarged mediastinal lymph nodes, a cavitation, or an abscess of the lung. The chest x-ray film does not always produce a definitive diagnosis, but it can identify abnormal findings that are suggestive of or compatible with a particular pulmonary disorder.

The chest x-ray also provides data about the heart, including its size and shape. In congenital and acquired cardiac disease, the enlargement of the heart and its atria or ventricles provides in-

formation about the improper function of the cardiac valves, pulmonary or aortic arterial hypertension, and venous pulmonary conditions that affect heart size.

**Abdominal X-Ray.** Various abnormal findings on the abdominal film are useful in obtaining a diagnosis. The patterns of air and gas appear light and bright on the abdominal film. In normal findings, the air remains contained within the intestinal tract. With a perforation of either the stomach or the intestines, the gas escapes into the abdominal cavity. When the patient is seated or in an erect position, the air rises and gathers under the diaphragm, where it is visible on the abdominal x-ray film. In intestinal obstruction, air and fluid collect above the area of obstruction, distending the lumen of the intestine. The abnormal width of the intestinal tissue and the air within the lumen are visible and diagnostically significant.

In the biliary tract, opaque stones or calculi produce a white, bright image on the abdominal film. The location of the stone is identified in the gallbladder or the cystic or common duct. Cholesterol stones are nonopaque, however, and cannot be seen on the abdominal film. This type of stone is visualized only on x-ray examination using contrast medium.

**Kidney-Ureter-Bladder X-Ray.** This x-ray film is also known as a flat plate of the abdomen. It images the structure, size, and position of the kidneys, ureters, and bladder, screening for abnormality in these organs and nearby tissues. Calcification of the renal calyces or renal pelvis is visible, as are any radiopaque calculi that are present in the upper urinary tract.

**Bone and Joint X-Ray.** X-ray studies are a vital tool in the assessment of bones and joints. In cases of trauma, the x-ray film is used to identify the presence, location, and type of fracture; the potential for injury to the surrounding soft tissue; and the healing activity after the fracture has been treated. Dislocation of a joint, a bone tumor, a bone infection, and a loss of bone mass are also visible radiographically. In arthritic disorders or metabolic diseases such as gout, x-ray studies are used to visualize the size and structure of the joints and soft tissues and the alignment of the bones that articulate at the joints (Fig. 9–6).

**Child Abuse.** When child abuse is suspected as the cause of a skeletal injury, multiple x-ray studies of all parts of the skeleton are performed.

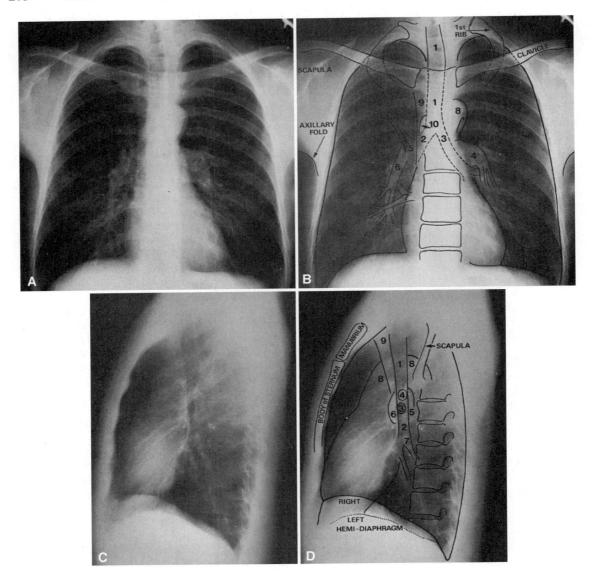

**Figure 9–5**

Normal chest roentgenograms—posteroanterior and lateral projections. *A,* Chest roentgenogram in an asymptomatic 26-year-old man taken in the erect position. *B,* Diagrammatic overlay shows the normal anatomic structures numbered or labeled: 1, trachea; 2, right main bronchus; 3, left main bronchus; 4, left pulmonary artery; 5, right upper lobe pulmonary vein; 6, right interlobar artery; 7, right lower and middle lobe vein; 8, aortic knob; and 9, superior vena cava. *C,* Chest roentgenogram in an asymptomatic 26-year-old man taken in the erect position. *D,* Diagrammatic overlay shows the normal anatomic structures numbered or labeled: 1, tracheal air column; 2, right intermediate bronchus; 3, left upper lobe bronchus; 4, right upper lobe bronchus; 5, left interlobar artery; 6, right interlobar artery; 7, confluence of pulmonary veins; 8, aortic arch; and 9, brachiocephalic vessels. (Reproduced with permission from Fraser, R. G., Paré, J. A. P., Paré, P. D., Fraser, R. S., & Genereux, G. P. [1988]. *Diagnosis of diseases of the chest* [3rd ed., Vol. 1, pp. 287–290]. Philadelphia: W. B. Saunders.)

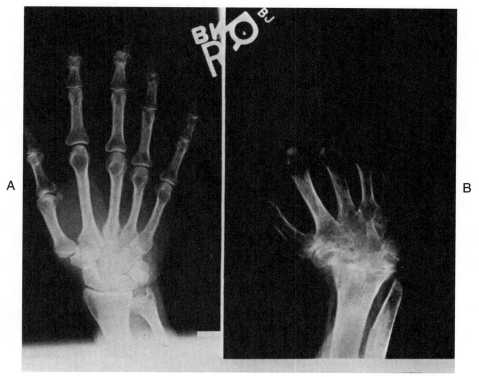

**Figure 9–6**
Effects of calcium on bone density. *A,* Hand radiograph of a 28-year-old patient with good calcium deposits in bone. *B,* Hand radiograph of a 72-year-old patient whose bones appear transparent as the result of calcium loss. This radiographic appearance is also attributed to pathologic changes caused by rheumatoid arthritis. (Reproduced with permission from Thompson, M. A., Hall, J. D., Hattaway, M. P., & Dowd, S. B. [1994]. *Principles of imaging science and protection* [Vol. 2, Slide 290]. Philadelphia: W. B. Saunders.)

In cases of child abuse, the incidence of bone fracture is high, and the sites of skeletal injury are often multiple, particularly in children younger than 18 months (Kao & Smith, 1997). The skeletal views include those of the skull, cervical spine, chest, and thoracolumbar spine and views of the entire length of arms and legs. To differentiate between abuse and other causes of the trauma, the radiologist looks for correlation or noncorrelation by comparing the history of how and when the injuries occurred with the x-ray findings.

**Skull-Vertebral X-Ray.** The x-ray films of the skull can detect abnormality of shape, size, and contour, including skull fractures. The skull series can be used to help identify changes in the skull that cause increased intracranial pressure, bleeding into the brain, bleeding within the skull cavity, or infection of the bone. Usually, a CT scan or magnetic resonance imaging (MRI) is used instead of skull radiographs, because tomography is more accurate and detailed in the imaging of both skull and brain tissue.

The vertebral x-ray films provide visualization of a fracture, dislocation, or deformity of the spine. They demonstrate degeneration or faulty alignment of the spinal vertebrae that causes a disorder in the intervertebral discs (Kathol, 1997).

**Findings**

**Abnormal Values**

CHEST AND HEART

| | | |
|---|---|---|
| Pneumothorax | Atherosclerosis | Chronic obstructive |
| Atelectasis | Cor pulmonale | pulmonary disease |
| Pleural effusion | Cardiac hypertrophy | Mediastinal nodes |
| Pleurisy | Pneumonia | Aortic aneurysm |
| Cystic fibrosis | Tuberculosis | Congestive heart |
| Pulmonary fibrosis | Pulmonary abscess | failure |
| Tumor or cyst | Fracture | Adult respiratory |
| Silicosis | Scoliosis | distress syndrome |

INTESTINAL TRACT

| | | |
|---|---|---|
| Intestinal tract | Volvulus | Foreign body in the |
| perforation | Intussusception | abdomen |
| Intestinal tract | Subphrenic abscess | Gastroenteritis |
| obstruction | Swallowed foreign | Biliary tract calculus |
| Paralytic ileus | body | |

URINARY SYSTEM

| | | |
|---|---|---|
| Renal abscess | Hematoma | Renal or ureteral |
| Renal tuberculosis | Congenital mal- | calculus |
| Pyelonephritis | formation | Hydronephrosis |
| Glomerulonephritis | Tumor or cyst | Amyloidosis |
| Polycystic renal | | |
| disease | | |

BONES AND JOINTS

| | | |
|---|---|---|
| Fracture | Vitamin D deficiency, | Gout |
| Dislocation | rickets | Osteomyelitis |
| Subluxation | Paget's disease | Osteoporosis |
| Bone cyst or tumor | Osteoarthritis | Osteomalacia |
| Congenital mal- | Rheumatoid arthritis | |
| formation | | |

SKULL

| | | |
|---|---|---|
| Congenital anomaly | Osteomyelitis | Paget's disease |
| Neoplasm, skull | Fracture | Acromegaly |

SPINAL VERTEBRAE

| | | |
|---|---|---|
| Ankylosing spon- | Tuberculosis | Osteoarthritis |
| dylitis | Pott's disease | Osteoporosis |
| Lordosis | Fracture | Paget's disease |
| Scoliosis | Subluxation | |
| Kyphosis | Ruptured disc | |

**Interfering Factors**

- Excessive movement
- Failure to remove jewelry or other metal from the x-ray field
- Improper positioning

- For abdominal and kidney-ureter-bladder films: retained barium or contrast medium, feces, ascites, gas, obesity

---

## Nursing Implementation

■

*Critical Thinking 9–1*
In the waiting room, an elderly patient complains to you that every time that she has an x-ray, she becomes stiff and cold. What nursing measures can help relieve or prevent the discomfort?

### Pretest

For the patient who requires an abdominal or kidney-ureter-bladder film, schedule the x-ray study before any radiologic study that uses barium or contrast medium. The contrast medium is radiopaque, and the residual contrast interferes with the visualization of the underlying tissues.

For most imaging procedures, instruct the patient to remove all clothes and put on a hospital gown. The exceptions are skull radiographs and x-ray films of the distal extremities.

Instruct the patient to remove all jewelry and metal objects from the area that is to be imaged.

Provide reassurance to the patient. Young children often fear the equipment, strange room, isolation, and separation from their parents. Adults may also feel somewhat apprehensive.

### During the Test

Ensure the patient's safety at all times, particularly when there is a risk of the patient's falling. The radiography table has no siderails. A Velcro waist restraint may be used, but sometimes the restraint interferes with the positioning and imaging needed (Torres, 1993).

Position the patient for the specific views needed.

Instruct the patient to remain motionless during the imaging. Sometimes the patient is instructed to inhale deeply and hold the breath until the image is taken.

■

*Critical Thinking 9–2*
The x-ray finding of a 68-year-old woman describes mild osteoporosis of the hips. What health care teaching measures can help to lessen the risk of a fractured hip in her future?

The patient must often wait in the imaging area as the decision is made concerning whether to take additional x-ray films. Provide a blanket or extra gown for the patient who is chilled in the cool room.

### Posttest

Assist the patient in dismounting from the radiography table and getting dressed, as needed.

---

## References

Adler, A. M., & Carlton, R. R. (1994). *Introduction to radiography and patient care.* Philadelphia: W. B. Saunders.

Cummings, S. R. (1998). Prevention of hip fractures in older women: A population-based perspective. *Osteoporosis International, 8*(Suppl. 1), S8–S12.

Kao, S. C., & Smith, W. L. (1997). Skeletal injuries in the pediatric patient. *Radiologic Clinics of North America, 35,* 727–744.

Kathol, M. H. (1997). Cervical spine trauma. What is new? *Radiologic Clinics of North America 35,* 507–529.

Mettler, F. A. (1996). *Essentials of radiology.* Philadelphia: W. B. Saunders.

Snopek, A. M. (1992). *Fundamentals of special radiographic procedures* (3rd ed.). Philadelphia: W. B. Saunders.

Sturman, M. F. (1993). *Effective medical imaging: Signs and symptoms approach.* Baltimore: Williams & Wilkins.

Torres, L. S. (1993). Basic medical techniques for patient care for radiologic technologists. Philadelphia: J. B. Lippincott.

# 10

# Nuclear Imaging

Nuclear imaging consists of several radiologic methods that are used to visualize the functions of particular organs or tissues. In comparison with other radiologic procedures, nuclear imaging is less precise in providing anatomic information, but it is helpful in demonstrating physiologic function and activity.

Most nuclear scans provide full-thickness images of organs. Two nuclear scans, positron emission tomography (PET) and single photon emission computed tomography (SPECT), produce tomographic views that locate the abnormal function more precisely. The images of a PET or SPECT scan may be merged with a computed tomographic (CT) scan or a magnetic resonance imaging (MRI) scan to provide additional information about the physiologic function and biochemical processes of a particular organ or region of the body.

Nuclear scanning can locate the site of abnormal physiologic function. It often detects the abnormality at an earlier stage than is possible with other radiologic techniques. It is a minimally invasive procedure, with a high degree of safety, accuracy, and sensitivity (Godderidge, 1995).

## Diagnostic Procedures

## Nuclear Imaging
**(Radionuclide Study)**                Synonyms: Nuclear scan, isotope scan, scintigraphy

## Normal Values

Normal uptake, distribution, and excretion of the radionuclide is done by the targeted organ or tissue.

## Background Information

In most radiologic procedures, the source of the radiation is in a machine that emits radio waves aimed to pass through the patient from the external source. In the nuclear scan, the process is different, because the radiation source is placed within the patient. Once in the patient's body, the radionuclide is taken up, concentrated, and distributed in the targeted organ or tissue. For a short time, it emits gamma rays in the pattern and concentration that correspond to the physiologic uptake of that tissue.

A gamma camera or scintillation scanner detects and records the emission of the gamma rays as the equipment rotates around the patient. The data are converted into a visual image by the computer and its special software. The image appears on a monitor and is reproduced on film. This allows additional study of the images after the procedure is completed (Fig. 10–1).

**Radionuclides.** Radionuclides are artificially produced, unstable, radioactive isotopes that emit small amounts of gamma rays. The radionuclides in nuclear medicine have a short half-life, which is the time needed for the nuclear material to decay and the radioactivity to become reduced to half its origi-nal strength. By the end of the half-life period, the radioactive emissions of the radionuclide are considerably reduced or negligible.

Technetium 99m is one of the most common radionuclides used in nuclear scans. It emits a low level of gamma rays and has a half-life of 6 hours. After it is released from the target organ or tissues of the body, most of it is filtered out of the blood by the kidneys and excreted in the urine. Some of the ion is secreted directly into the colon and excreted in the feces.

Other common radionuclides include the iso-

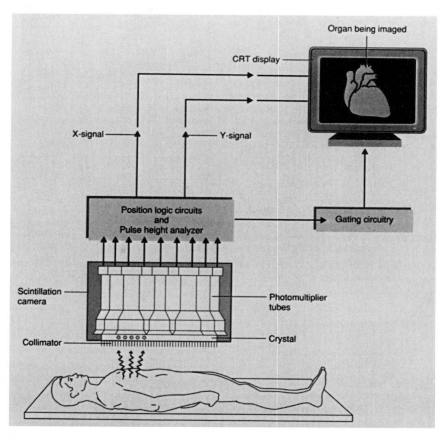

**Figure 10–1**

Diagram of the nuclear medicine scanning process. After administration of the radionuclide, the nuclear imaging is performed with a scintillation scanner and sensitive radiation detector. The nuclear emissions are computer converted to produce an image of the targeted organ on the monitor. (Reproduced with permission from Thompson, M. A., Hall, J. D., Hattaway, M. P., & Dowd, S. B. [1994]. *Principles of imaging science and protection* [Vol. 2, Slide 391]. Philadelphia: W. B. Saunders.)

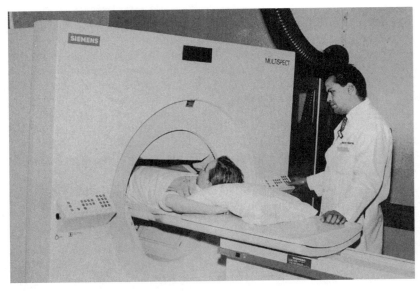

**Figure 10–2**

SPECT scan. A pediatric patient undergoing a multidetector single photon emission computed tomography (SPECT) examination. (Reproduced with permission from Godderidge, C. [1995]. *Pediatric imaging.* [Fig. 12–3, p. 174]. Philadelphia: W. B. Saunders.)

topes of iodine, xenon, gallium, indium, and thallium. They all vary in their characteristics, including their radioactive strength and half-life. Each radionuclide has a binding capacity that allows it to work as a radiopharmaceutical.

**Radiopharmaceuticals.** The radionuclide is the radiation source needed for imaging, but it cannot enter the target tissue by itself. A radiopharmaceutical is a combination of a radionuclide and the specific element, compound, or cellular component that it is bound to. The bound substance is taken up by specific target tissues, and the radionuclide is absorbed with it.

In one example of how a radiopharmaceutical works, technetium 99m is bound to phosphorus or calcium to form the radiopharmaceutical that is used in a bone scan. Active bone cells absorb the calcium or phosphorus as part of bone metabolism, and the radioactive isotope is absorbed at the same time. Concentrations of active bone cells are identified because they emit the gamma rays that are recorded in the scan. Nonactive bone cells, such as those in a bone cyst or a nonhealing fracture, do not absorb the mineral element or radiopharmaceutical, and the deficit is seen on the scan.

In other examples, the radiopharmaceutical

that contains heat-damaged erythrocytes is used in the spleen scan, because the spleen collects and destroys damaged red blood cells. The radiopharmaceutical that contains leukocytes is used in the gallium scan, because white blood cells will sequester in areas of infection. When human cells are used, the cells are obtained from the patient's own blood to prevent problems of incompatibility.

Most radiopharmaceuticals are injected intravenously. Exceptions are those used in the lung ventilation scan, which requires a radiopharmaceutical that is inhaled as a gas, and those used in upper gastrointestinal scans, which require orally ingested radiopharmaceuticals.

**Imaging Process.** The gamma camera or scintillation scanner moves in an orbit around the patient, detecting the concentrations of gamma rays from all angles. The scanner never touches the patient, and the equipment is relatively quiet. The patient is positioned appropriately so that the scanner can detect the emissions from the targeted organ clearly. When a whole body scan is performed, such as a bone scan or gallium scan, the patient is placed on a moving table that gradually passes through the arcs of the scanner (Fig. 10–2).

Imaging begins as soon as the radiopharmaceutical is absorbed by the targeted tissue. The images become more clearly defined as a greater amount of radioisotope is concentrated in the targeted tissue. In some scans, the imaging is rapid and begins as soon as the radiopharmaceutical is injected. In other scans, it takes hours for the radiopharmaceutical to be taken up by the target organ, so the imaging is performed after a specific interval.

**Emissions Computed Tomography.** The process of emissions computed tomography (ECT) combines the use of special radionuclides with the use of a gamma camera or scintillation camera and a computer to produce tomographic images of specific tissues or body organs. As with traditional nuclear scans, the radiopharmaceutical is injected intravenously and localizes in the target tissue or organ. The gamma camera or scintillation scanner rotates around the patient, detecting the concentration and pattern of the radioactive material (Fig. 10–3). The emissions data are collected and converted to numeric (digital) data and then into visual images by the computer.

One advantage of the ECT process is that the computer and software can produce many thin slices or tomographic views of the targeted area. The views can be produced from any angle and provide clear localization and visualization of an abnormality. Nearby tissues that overlie or underlie the targeted area are less likely to obscure the view.

The ECT process is differentiated by the type of radioactive isotope used. The two types of ECT are the PET scan and the SPECT scan. Each of these processes has benefits and limitations.

PET uses cyclotron-produced isotopes such as fluoride 18, carbon 11, oxygen 15, and rubidium 82 for the radiopharmaceuticals. These radioisotopes produce excellent contrast for specific tissues and measure glucose metabolism. Glucose provides the energy for the cells to function. The measurement of glucose metabolism in a specific area or organ reflects the functional activity of the cells. Simply stated, PET can image the metabolic functioning of the targeted organ or tissue. The images demonstrate pathophysiology "at work" by showing decreased or increased metabolism and perfusion, distinctly different responses than those of normal tissue (Fig. 10–4).

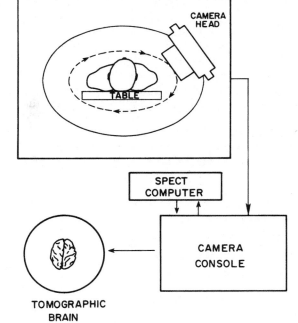

**Figure 10–3**

Single photon emission computed tomography (SPECT) nuclear scan. A schematic representation of a SPECT system. The camera detector rotates around the patient in an orbital path while acquiring data to be fed into the computer. Reconstructed tomographic images are created by the SPECT computer and are then displayed on the monitor. (Reproduced with permission from Mettler, F. A., & Guiberteau, M. J. [1991]. *Essentials of nuclear medicine imaging* [3rd ed., p. 38]. Philadelphia: W. B. Saunders.)

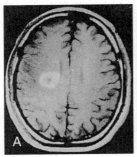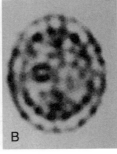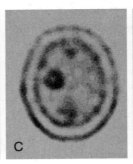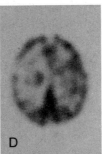

**Figure 10–4**

Comparison of brain images from magnetic resonance imaging (MRI) and positron emission tomography (PET) scan. *A,* MRI of a cross section of the brain. *B, C, D,* Fluorodeoxyglucose positron emission tomography (FDG-PET) images in a 27-year-old patient with glioblastoma of the brain. In the PET scan, there is markedly increased glucose metabolism in the tumor, shown in three levels of the brain (*B, C, D*). The middle image (*C*) shows a cold area, which corresponds to the necrotic area on the MRI scan. (Reproduced with permission from Wagner, H. N., Szabo, Z., & Buchanan, J. W. [1995]. *Principles of nuclear medicine* [2nd ed., Fig. 46–1, p. 1047]. Philadelphia: W. B. Saunders.)

In an early stage of Alzheimer's disease, this new technology is able to demonstrate the characteristic hypoperfusion and hypometabolism in the temporoparietal lobes of the brain. It also provides images of the altered brain metabolism of Parkinson's disease. Before cardiac surgery, the PET myocardial perfusion study is used to identify viable myocardial tissue and nonviable tissue that would not benefit from improved coronary artery circulation. In oncology, PET imaging can differentiate a malignant, highly metabolic tumor from a benign, low-metabolic growth. In oncology, PET is used for diagnosing and monitoring the tumor response to treatment (Tan & Pomeroy, 1995).

The major limitations of this diagnostic modality are the limited number of PET scanners and their cyclotron laboratories, the short half-life of the radioactive material, and the costs of the test. The cyclotron is a sophisticated machine that splits atoms to make the isotopes. Then, additional work is needed to process these isotopes into material that is ready to use. A few health insurers cover this procedure in selected cases, but most do not (Wagner, Szabo, & Buchanan, 1995). Despite these obstacles, PET scans are becoming more common because of the quality of information that the imaging can provide (Tan & Pomeroy, 1995; Winchester, Dhekne, Moore, & Murphy, 1994).

SPECT uses radioisotopes, such as technetium 99 or iodine 123, with a SPECT camera for the imaging process. Two major advantages are the use of standard radiopharmaceuticals and the use of standard scanning equipment to perform the procedure. Thus, the procedure is more readily available and has lower costs. Other advantages are faster imaging time and the ability to magnify and clarify the image in the detection of tissue abnormality (Godderidge, 1995). There are some limitations, because the radiopharmaceuticals vary in their depth of activity and have a more scattered distribution that can interfere with the imaging. See Chapter 23 for additional discussion of SPECT imaging of the brain.

**Abnormal Findings.**   In a nuclear scan, the pathologic condition that affects the target organ or tissue results in abnormal uptake and distribution of the radionuclide. The abnormality may be a space-occupying lesion or tumor, nonfunctioning tissue such as scar tissue, a loss of structural integrity such as a fracture, or another abnormality. The types of abnormalities include deficiency of uptake, excessive uptake, localization of activity in focal areas of tissue, disseminated activity throughout the organ, and asymmetry when the results should be bilateral and symmetrical.

When little to no uptake occurs, the image appears faint gray or clear. With the diminished uptake of radioactive material in the tissue, there is a limited emission of gamma rays or photons to transmit the image.

With normal or excessive uptake, the image appears dark or black because of the concentration of the radionuclide and the strength of the emissions.

**Nonvisualization.** When the targeted organ or tissue is not visualized, no uptake of the radionuclide has occurred. One possible cause is that vascular or ductal obstruction blocks the radionuclide from reaching the target site. Another possible cause is that the organ is nonfunctional. For example, nonvisualization can occur in the spleen scan of a patient with advanced sickle cell anemia. The lack

of uptake of the radionuclide can be caused by organ atrophy from repeated infarct or mechanical obstruction of the splenic blood flow by sickled, clumped erythrocytes.

**Decreased Activity.** An area of decreased activity in the target organ is called a *defect* or a *cold spot*. One or more focal areas of tissue are nonfunctional because of the pathologic change in the tissue. For instance, an abnormal liver scan can demonstrate a defect because of a cyst or abscess that has formed a space-occupying lesion. Multiple focal defects are often the result of metastatic disease. As seen in Figure 10–5, a defect in the image of the head of the right femur is in-

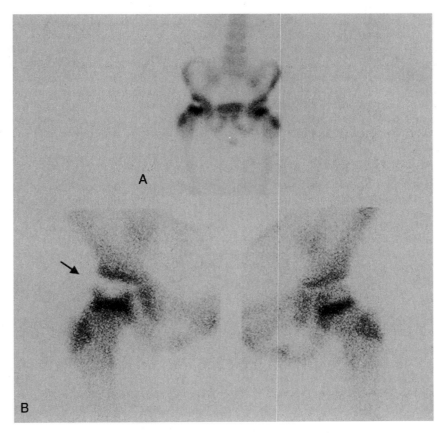

**Figure 10–5**
Bone scan of the hip joint. *A,* Composite (planar) imaging was performed on a patient to evaluate the hip joint. Without magnification, the decrease in uptake of the radionuclide may be missed. *B,* In the same patient, the enlarged images show a lack of perfusion to the right femoral head *(arrow),* consistent with avascular necrosis. (Reproduced with permission from Godderidge, C. [1995]. *Pediatric imaging* [Fig. 12–5, p. 177]. Philadelphia: W. B. Saunders.)

dicated by the lack of uptake of the radiopharmaceutical by necrotic bone tissue.

**Increased Activity.** An area of increased activity in the target organ is called a *focal abnormality* or *hot lesion* in otherwise normally functional tissue. The excess activity may also involve the entire organ. For instance, the thyroid scan of the patient with Graves' disease demonstrates increased activity throughout the gland (Fig. 10–6). All the thyroid tissue is hyperactive and absorbs a maximum amount of the iodine radionuclide.

In evaluation of the healing of a bone fracture 24 to 48 hours after the fracture occurs, a bone scan reveals excess activity at the fracture site. The increased focal activity correlates with the osteogenic changes that are needed for normal bone repair and healing.

**Loss of Tissue or Vascular Integrity.** In cases of trauma or tissue damage, blood can become pooled or compartmentalized and remain undetected for a period of time. In particular, slow or intermittent bleeding may be difficult to diagnose (O'Hara, 1996). When the radionuclide is tagged to red blood cells, the radionuclide pools in the area where the blood has collected. The pooled blood has a high concentration of the radionuclide, with the emission of many gamma rays or photons in an abnormal pattern. In trauma, the scan can demonstrate a linear defect, peripheral indentation, or displacement of the injured organ or tissue. A frank rupture, a subcapsular hematoma, and a bleeding episode are also examples of losses of tissue integrity that produce excessive radioactivity at the site of the tissue injury.

In gastrointestinal bleeding, the source can be anywhere in the lengthy gastrointestinal tract. To locate the source of the bleeding, a gastrointestinal scan can be done (Winchester et al., 1994). The bleeding is detected when the injected radionuclide leaves the circulation and enters the lumen of the intestine. Over time, the pooled radionuclide in the intestine demonstrates movement by peristalsis.

**Pediatric Nuclear Scans.** Nuclear imaging can be used to provide early diagnosis and to evaluate the function of particular organs. An example of function and dynamic imaging is the imaging of a left-to-right shunting of blood within the chambers of the heart. A second example is vesicoureteral reflux, with a backflow of urine in a ureter because of partial obstruction or malformation. In the imaging process of children, low-dose radionuclides are used, and short-time imaging procedures are best.

Psychosocial approaches based on the child's age and maturity are used to help the child cope

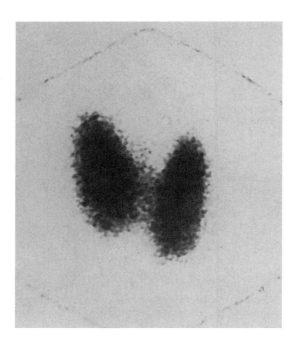

**Figure 10–6**
Thyroid scan. Diffusely enlarged thyroid gland in Graves' disease. The scintiscan was made 3 hours after an oral dose of $^{123}$ I. (Reproduced with permission from Wagner, H. N., Szabo, Z., & Buchanan, J. W. [1995]. *Principles of nuclear medicine* [2nd ed., Fig. 30–91, p. 611]. Philadelphia: W. B. Saunders.)

with the procedure. When the child is old enough to cooperate and remain motionless for brief periods of time, sedation is not used. The technologist helps by providing brief explanations to promote understanding and cooperation. The parents can participate in helping the child during the imaging. The child is never left alone (Godderidge, 1995).

To help the child remain motionless, restraints may be used. These include a Velcro strap, contour pillow, sandbags, or, for infants, a "mummy" wrap. Sedation or general anesthesia may be used for the infant or small child who cannot remain motionless for a long imaging procedure or for the child with a behavior or seizure disorder who cannot be immobile.

**Versatility of Nuclear Scans.** Many different nuclear scans can be used to visualize the function of different organs or tissues. A variety of radionuclides also exist that can be used to identify the area of abnormality. Some of these scans, their purposes, and the pertinent patient care information are presented in Table 10–1. Scans that are used more frequently are presented in greater detail throughout Part IV of this text.

| **Purpose of the Test** | A nuclear scan is used to assess the physiologic function and assist in the localization and diagnosis of abnormality in a designated organ or tissue. |
| --- | --- |

| **Procedure** | A radiopharmaceutical is administered to the patient, and a gamma camera or scintillation scanner records the radioactive emissions. These emissions are then converted to images that correspond to the location, distribution, and concentration of the radionuclide in the targeted organ or tissue. |
| --- | --- |

**Findings**

**Abnormal Values**

| Organ atrophy or fibrosis | Hyperactivity of organ function | Vascular obstruction |
| --- | --- | --- |
| Congenital defect | Hematoma | Obstruction of a duct |
| Tumor or cyst | Traumatic disruption of tissue | Ischemia or necrosis of tissue |
| Metastatic lesions | | |
| Inflammation or abscess | | |

**Interfering Factors**

- Failure to follow specific pretest dietary or medication restrictions
- Recent intake of iodine
- Pregnancy

**Nursing Implementation**

**Pretest**

If the patient is female and of childbearing age, ask if she is pregnant, the date of the last menstrual period, and if she is breastfeeding. Pregnancy is a contraindication because of the patient's exposure to radiation. If she is breastfeeding, she will have to avoid breastfeeding for a period of time until the radioisotope clears out of her body (Winchester et al., 1994). Record the patient's responses, and inform the physician of any interfering factors.

Provide the pretest patient instructions, which vary for each scan. Some scans have dietary restrictions to prevent an increase in the circulation to the liver or intestines. Many medications interfere with the absorption of the radio-

**Table 10–1  Nuclear Scans**

| Name of Scan | Purpose | Patient Position during Scan | Special Measures |
|---|---|---|---|
| Brain and cerebral flow scan (PET scan) | To evaluate brain tissue, internal carotid arteries, and their intracranial branches for the detection of cerebrovascular abnormality such as stroke or atherosclerosis<br><br>To identify brain tissue abnormality such as tumor, hematoma, cyst, atrophy, or edema | Supine | During imaging, the head must be motionless<br><br>Fasting is required for at least 4 hr before the test<br><br>To document the circulation in the arteries and brain, initial views are taken immediately after the radiopharmaceutical is administered<br><br>Additional images of the brain tissue are taken after 45 min |
| Brain imaging scan (SPECT) | To visualize the function of brain tissue, particularly in the evaluation of dementia, cerebrovascular disease, and the location of foci of seizure activity | Supine | In the pretest and test periods, the patient must remain in an unstimulated state<br><br>The room is kept dark, quiet, and without traffic |
| Cerebrospinal fluid imaging scan (cisternogram) | To investigate the passageway and flow of cerebrospinal fluid in the ventricular system of the brain<br><br>To help diagnose hydro-cephalus<br><br>To investigate brain trauma, with leakage of cerebrospinal fluid | Supine and possibly Trendelenburg | If there is suspected leakage of cerebrospinal fluid from the ears or nose, packing is placed in these orifices<br><br>A lumbar puncture is performed to instill the radiopharmaceutical intrathecally<br><br>For adults, images are taken at 2, 6, 24, and 48 hr<br><br>For children, images are taken at 1, 2, 4, 6, 8, and 24 hr |
| Thyroid scan with technetium 99m | To rapidly assess thyroid function and structure | Supine, with neck in hyper-extension | This test is preferred for patients who receive propylthiouracil, because the radiopharmaceutical contains no iodine |

**Table 10–1    Nuclear Scans** (continued)

| Name of Scan | Purpose | Patient Position during Scan | Special Measures |
|---|---|---|---|
| Thyroid scan with technetium 99m continued | To help diagnose hypothyroidism, thyroid nodule, cancer, and Graves' disease | | The radiopharmaceutical is injected intravenously |
| | | | The patient should not swallow during the imaging stage |
| Thyroid scan with iodine 123 | To assess thyroid function and structure | Supine, with neck in hyperextension | Thyroid medications and iodine interfere with iodine uptake in the test; these are discontinued in the pretest period, as per physician's orders and test protocol |
| | To help diagnose hypothyroidism, thyroid tumor or nodule, and Graves' disease | | Pretest, no solid foods are permitted for 4–6 hr |
| | | | The radiopharmaceutical is given orally, 4–24 hr before imaging begins |
| Liver-spleen scan | To assess the physiologic functions of the liver and spleen | Supine | The patient should fast for at least 4 hr before the test |
| | To identify focal or diffuse areas of deficit, caused by tumor, fibrosis, circulatory abnormality, or trauma | | The radiopharmaceutical is injected intravenously |
| Hepatobiliary scan | To assess for patency of the hepatic ducts, biliary ducts, and gallbladder | Supine | Nothing by mouth for 6–8 hr, pretest (some protocols require nothing by mouth for a minimum of 2 hr) |
| | To identify defects, abnormal function, and blockage | | Scanning time is 4 hr, with possible additional images for up to 24 hr |

(continued on the following page)

**Table 10–1 Nuclear Scans** *(continued)*

| Name of Scan | Purpose | Patient Position during Scan | Special Measures |
|---|---|---|---|
| Thallium scan with thallium 201, resting or exercise | To determine the blood flow to the myocardium, at rest or after maximal stress or exercise | Upright before and during administration of the radiopharmaceutical<br><br>Supine and lateral for the imaging | Nothing by mouth for 4–6 hr pretest to reduce radiopharmaceutical uptake in nearby organs<br><br>Blood pressure and electrocardiogram are monitored during treadmill exercise and imaging phases<br><br>Exercise is performed to the maximal heart rate, using the treadmill<br><br>After injection of the radiopharmaceutical, imaging is performed immediately and after 3–4 hr |
| Myocardial infarction scan | To assess the cardiac tissue for damage caused by acute myocardial infarction, particularly when other tests are inconclusive | Supine | Scan is performed 10–72 hr after a possible myocardial infarction or cardiac insult<br><br>Imaging is performed 2–3 hr after the radiopharmaceutical is injected |
| Gated blood pool ventriculography (ventriculogram) | To measure cardiac ventricular performance at rest and during stress or exercise<br><br>To evaluate coronary artery disease, acute cardiomyopathy, valvular disease, and intracardiac shunting | Supine | The patient's erythrocytes are tagged to form the *blood pool;* the image sequence is *gated* (timed or triggered by the R wave of the electrocardiogram)<br><br>Stress or exercise studies may be performed<br><br>The patient has nothing by mouth for 4–8 hr before the test<br><br>The imaging is performed immediately after the injection of the radiopharmaceutical |
| Pulmonary perfusion scan | To assess the integrity of the pulmonary circulation and to identify obstruction as from pulmonary embolus | Seated or supine | The radiopharmaceutical is given intravenously, and the imaging is performed immediately thereafter |

**Table 10–1    Nuclear Scans** *(continued)*

| Name of Scan | Purpose | Patient Position during Scan | Special Measures |
|---|---|---|---|
| Pulmonary ventilation scan | To assess the ventilatory ability of the lungs, particularly in chronic obstructive pulmonary disease and inflammatory lung disease | Seated or upright | After the rapid imaging begins, the patient exhales deeply and inhales xenon 133 gas delivered by mask for 15 sec; the patient then rebreathes oxygen for 2–3 min followed by normal air for 2–3 min, to clear the lungs |
| Meckel's diverticulum scan | To assess for bleeding in the ilium, the distal part of the small intestine | Supine or left posterior oblique | Nothing by mouth for 3–4 hr before the test<br><br>After administration of the intravenous radiopharmaceutical, scanning of the lower abdomen is carried out every 5 min for 30 min, and then scanning of the right lateral midabdomen is performed for 30 min |
| Gastrointestinal scan | To identify and locate the source of lower gastrointestinal bleeding; the causes include diverticulitis, vascular abnormality, neoplasm, and inflammatory bowel disease | Supine | After intravenous injection of the radionuclide, images are obtained at 1–5 min intervals for 30–45 min |
| Testicular scan | To differentiate among the causes of a painful, swollen testicle<br><br>To assess for the vascular integrity of the testicle | Supine | After intravenous administration of the radiopharmaceutical, the imaging is performed immediately and again in 15 min |
| Bone marrow scan | To identify malignant tumor or abnormal distribution of bone marrow<br><br>To locate active sites for biopsy | Supine, prone, or sitting | 20 min after intravenous administration of the radiopharmaceutical, imaging begins and lasts for 1 hr<br><br>Shield the liver and spleen during imaging |

pharmaceutical. Often, after consultation with the patient's physician, medications are withheld and the patient remains under medical supervision during the period of the test.

If the scan involves the uptake of radioactive iodine (iodine 123, iodine 125, or iodine 131), instruct the patient to avoid the intake of iodine from food (shellfish, kelp preparations) and medication sources (some cough medicines, some multivitamin-with-mineral tablets, Lugol's solution) for 3 to 5 days before the test.

On the day of the test, assist the patient in removing all clothing, jewelry, and metal objects. A hospital gown is worn.

Provide reassurance regarding the scanning process. Other than the venipuncture, the procedure is painless.

If the patient is anxious, a family member or friend can plan to be in the room during the scanning procedure. Unlike x-ray imaging, no external source of radiation exposure, and therefore no risk, exists.

Sedatives are avoided for the older child or adult. Sedation is sometimes used for the infant or child younger than 3 years, particularly when the scan requires an extended period of immobility. A nurse often administers the prescribed sedative and remains readily available to monitor and assist the patient during and after the imaging procedure. The medication is usually chloral hydrate, nembutal, or phenobarbital.

### During the Test

If sedatives are administered, monitor vital signs on a regular basis. This ensures early detection of any untoward response to the medication.

Instruct the patient to remain in the preestablished position while a bolus dose of radionuclide is administered intravenously and during the scanning process, which may begin immediately after the injection.

### Posttest

As with the handling of all body fluids or waste products, wear gloves to dispose of any urine or feces, and then wash your hands. The radionuclide is excreted in urine and feces for several days, although the radioactivity level is minimal after a few hours. The body wastes can be disposed of in the toilet.

Instruct the patient to wash his or her hands after voiding or a bowel movement. Parents and others should wash their hands after changing the diapers of an infant who has had a nuclear scan. Reassure the patient that the amount of radioactivity is negligible but that it can remain on the hands unless they are washed.

■
*Critical Thinking 10–1*
A young male college student's bone scan reveals a nonhealing fracture of a bone in the foot. Surgical repair is planned, with postoperative cast and crutches. To help him cope with these additional problems, what nursing assessments should be part of your interview?

### References

Bernier, D. R., Christian, P. E., & Langan, J. K. (1994). *Nuclear medicine technology and techniques* (3rd ed.). St Louis: C. V. Mosby.

Castronovo, P., & Vielleux, N. M. (1996). Diagnostic radiopharmaceutical exposure of nurses in health care units at a large research hospital. *Journal of Nuclear Medicine Technology, 24*(1), 45–48.

Corley, J., Yoder, J., Raibon, S., (1995). Nuclear medicine's new role in peptic ulcer disease management. *Journal of Nuclear Medicine Technology 23,* 299–300.

Cronin, V., Galantowicz, P., & Nabi, H. A. (1997). Development of oncology protocol using fluorine-18FDG: One center's experience. *Journal of Nuclear Medicine Technology, 25*(1), 66–69.

Davidhizar, A. R., & Dowd, R. B. (1996). Fear in the patient with undiagnosed symptoms. *Journal of Nuclear Medicine Technology, 24,* 325–328.

Godderidge, C. (1995). *Pediatric imaging.* Philadelphia: W. B. Saunders.

MacIntyre, W. J., & Harris, C. C. (1995). The decline and fall of the rectilinear scanner: Nuclear medicine instrumentation (1970–1995). *Journal of Nuclear Medicine Technology, 23*(4), 16S–20S.

Mettler, F. A., & Guiberteau, M. J. (1991). *Essentials of nuclear medicine imaging* (3rd ed.). Philadelphia: W. B. Saunders.

O'Hara, S. M. (1996). Pediatric gastrointestinal imaging. *Radiologic Clinics of North America, 34,* 845–862.

Snopek, A. M. (1992). *Fundamentals of special radiographic procedures* (3rd ed.). Philadelphia: W. B. Saunders.

Sturman, M. F. (1993). *Effective medical imaging: Signs and symptoms approach.* Baltimore: Williams & Wilkins.

Tan, T. X. L., & Pomeroy, S. J. (1995). PET: A new frontier in diagnosis and patient care . . . Positron emissions tomography. *Applied Radiology, 24*(12), 6–8, 11–15, 18.

Torres, L. S. (1993). *Basic medical techniques and patient care for radiologic technologists* (4th ed.). Philadelphia: J. B. Lippincott.

Wagner, H. N., Szabo, Z., & Buchanan, J. W. (1995). *Principles of nuclear medicine* (2nd ed.). Philadelphia: W. B. Saunders.

Winchester, C. B., Dhekne, R. D., Moore, W. H., & Murphy, P. H. (1994). Clinical applications of nuclear medicine in gastroenterology. *Gastroenterology Nursing, 17*(1), 20–26.

# 11

# Angiography

*Angiography* refers to the radiographic visualization of blood vessels. This chapter addresses the visualization of the lumens of arteries and the arterial blood flow throughout many areas of the body. Additional discussions, such as those of coronary and cerebral angiography and angiography in the assessment of peripheral vascular disease, are presented in detail in subsequent chapters in Part IV of this text.

| **Angiography** | |
|---|---|
| **(Radiology)** | Synonym: Arteriography |

| **Normal Values** | No anatomic or functional abnormalities of the arteries are noted. No stenosis, occlusion, aneurysm, or bleeding is visualized. |
|---|---|

## Background Information

Angiography is an invasive test that uses an arterial injection of contrast medium to visualize the lumens of arteries. Multiple radiographic images are taken with fluoroscopy and x-rays to illustrate the arterial abnormality.

**Digital Subtraction Angiography.** This procedure consists of angiography combined with digital subtraction to enhance the radiographic image. The system compares the images taken before and after the arrival of the contrast medium and subtracts the images of bone, soft tissue, and surrounding structures (Fig. 11–1). It can be performed to visualize the whole arterial tree, the arteries of the upper extremities, or those of the lower extremities. Additionally, the computer application can focus and sharpen the image, alter the shades of gray, and provide diagnostic information that the human eye is unable to see without computer system assistance (Kim & Orron, 1992). Digital subtraction angiography has an additional advantage over conventional angiography because it uses a smaller, safer dosage of the contrast medium.

**Intravenous Digital Subtraction Angiography.** This procedure uses an intravenous route for administering the contrast medium. Once the contrast material is in the venous circulation, it flows through the heart and enters the arterial circulation. Despite the advantage of easier and safer venipuncture technique with a reduced risk of hemorrhage, this method is used infrequently. It has a higher rate of nondiagnosis and requires a larger bolus of contrast material to obtain the images. It is occasionally used in selected circumstances, such as when aortic occlusion is suspected (Kim & Orron, 1992).

**Pathophysiology of Arterial Disease.** *Atherosclerosis* is a common cause of arterial disease. The atheromas, or deposits of fibrofatty plaque, grow on the tissue surfaces of the lumens of arteries, impeding the blood flow. Thrombus formation can also develop at the site of the atherosclerotic deposit, increasing the size of the blockage and causing further restriction of the circulation.

In severe atherosclerotic disease, the athero-

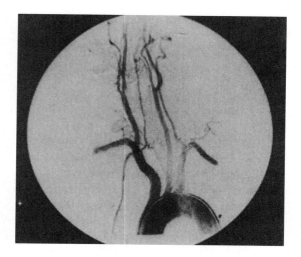

**Figure 11–1**

Digital angiogram of the thoracic aorta and the main arteries it supplies. Vessels appear dark because of the computer manipulation that is used in digital subtraction angiography. (Reproduced with permission from Adler, A. M., & Carlton, R. R. [1994]. *Introduction to radiography and patient care* [Vol. 1, Slide 208C]. Philadelphia: W. B. Saunders.)

mas are greater in number and also larger. In atherosclerosis, many arteries of the body contain the atheromatous deposits, although some arteries may be more occluded than others. The arteries affected most commonly are the aorta, renal arteries, coronary arteries, femoropopliteal arteries, internal carotid arteries, and arteries of the circle of Willis.

Arteriography provides visualization of the atherosclerotic deposits and the stenosis or occlusion of the artery. It also demonstrates the diminished circulation to the distal tissue beyond the site of the obstruction and the presence of any collateral circulation that helps provide blood flow to the distal tissue.

**Emboli.**   Emboli may also cause stenosis or obstruction in the arterial circulation. Commonly, the original cause of the clot is atrial fibrillation with the formation of a mural thrombus. As particles of the clot break off, they move into the arterial circulation and lodge in a distal part of the arterial tree (Fig. 11–2). Emboli also may originate from the thrombus that develops on atheromatous plaque. Particles of thrombus or fibrofatty plaque break off and travel to a more distal arterial site. Angiography demonstrates the location of the embolus or emboli and the extent of the circulatory impairment caused by embolic activity.

**Aneurysms.**   Aneurysms are often caused by atherosclerosis, although in some instances they result from infection or trauma. An aneurysm is a dilation of the artery that results from the degeneration and weakening of the muscular layer in the wall of the artery. Once the aneurysm develops, it interferes with the arterial blood flow. It tends to enlarge over time, and a thrombus may develop on the luminal surface. The abdominal aorta is a common site for the development of an aneurysm; it can extend in size and involve the iliac arteries as well (Fig. 11–3). Other sites of aneurysmal disease are the femoral, popliteal, and cerebral arteries.

**Dissection of an Artery or Aneurysm.**   On the luminal surface, blood penetrates and separates the tissue layers of the artery (DeSilvey, 1996). As a result, hematoma formation, expansion of the tear, and creation of a false lumen or a blood-filled channel in the arterial wall occur. The dissection can occlude arteries (Fig. 11–4), and a dissecting aneurysm is prone to rupture. The aorta, particularly the ascending aorta just above the aortic valve, is a common site of dissection.

Angiography provides visualization of the size, type, and location of the aneurysm. It also defines the location of other arterial vessels that originate in or near the aneurysm or dissection. These arteries can be occluded or stenosed because of the aneurysmal defect. In the angiographic procedure, a risk of rupture of the aneurysm during the injection of the contrast material under high pressure always exists. Therefore, computed tomography (CT), with contrast medium, may be the preferred diagnostic procedure to identify the defect. This noninvasive technique provides a clear image of an aneurysm with less risk to the patient.

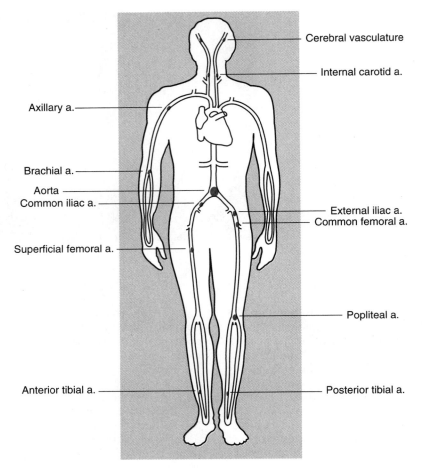

**Figure 11–2**
Common locations of arterial emboli. Eighty percent of all emboli lodge in the lower extremities.

The *aortogram* or *aortography* is angiography of the aorta. It is the best radiographic procedure for the diagnosis of a dissecting aneurysm. The false lumen fills with and empties of the contrast material more slowly than does the true lumen. While the false lumen remains filled with contrast material, the affected area of dissection is opacified and can be seen clearly.

**Arteriovenous Fistula and Arteriovenous Malformation.** These are false or abnormal communications between an artery and a vein. The fistula usually develops as a result of trauma, and the malformation is of congenital origin. Angiography is used to identify the condition and its precise loca-

tion. When embolization or surgery is planned for correction of the condition, angiography provides specific locations and landmarks. These conditions and their vascular sources can be difficult to locate visually.

**Technique of Angiography.** Angiography is performed using a 2% lidocaine solution for local anesthesia. The patient may also receive sedative-analgesia to promote relaxation. The procedure is performed under sterile conditions to minimize the risk of septicemia.

Arterial access is achieved by the use of a special needle or catheter that passes through the skin and is inserted directly into an artery. When a needle is used, the access is by puncture

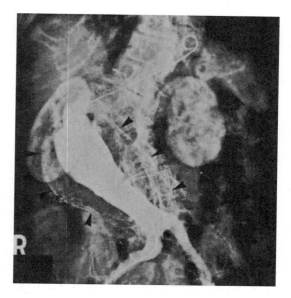

**Figure 11–3**

X-ray film of an abdominal aortic aneurysm. In addition to visualizing the aneurysm, the x-ray provides information about the size of the aneurysm and the possible involvement of the renal or femoral arteries. Calcification in the wall of an abdominal aortic aneurysm gives a good indication of the aortic size (*arrows*). (Reproduced with permission from Fahey, V. A. [1994]. *Vascular nursing* [2nd ed., p. 260]. Philadelphia: W. B. Saunders.)

technique. Once the needle has been properly placed in the lumen of the artery, the contrast medium is instilled by an automatic injection through the hollow core of the needle.

When a catheter is used, a small incision in the skin is made, and a needle is then used to enter the artery. Once the needle is in place, a specifically shaped guidewire is inserted through the core of the needle and is advanced into the artery. The needle is then removed, and an arterial catheter is inserted, gliding over the guidewire. The

combined guidewire and catheter, called a guided catheter, is carefully manipulated and advanced through the arterial structure until the tip reaches the area to be examined (Fig. 11–5). The guidewire is then removed, leaving the catheter in place. The contrast medium is injected by automated technique.

When the catheter is used to enter a specific branch of the aorta, the procedure is called a *selective arteriogram*. For example, *arch arteriography* means that the catheter is advanced to the aortic

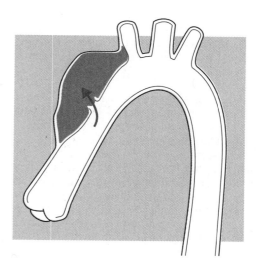

**Figure 11–4**

Dissection of the ascending aorta. Concerns include the size of the dissection and any occlusion of the main arteries that arise from the aortic arch.

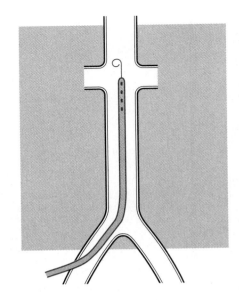

**Figure 11–5**
Transfemoral catheterization of the abdominal aorta. Once the
catheter is inserted into the femoral artery, it is advanced in
a retrograde direction through the aorta until it reaches the
desired level.

arch for arteriographic study. Selective arteriography
provides a view of the arterial circulation in specific
sites or organs, including the heart, brain, lung,
kidney, liver, spleen, and pancreas.

**Arterial Puncture Site.**   The selection of the
puncture site is based on several variables, including the goal or purpose of the study, the arterial
problem that exists, and the condition of the arteries. The common femoral artery is often used
because of its wide diameter and superficial location. In the transfemoral approach, the needle
puncture site is in the groin, usually on the side
with the best pulses.

When the femoral approach cannot be used
because of pulselessness or occlusion of the aorta or
iliofemoral arteries, an alternative route is selected.
The transaxillary and translumbar approaches may
be used as alternatives.

In the transaxillary approach, the catheter is
placed in the proximal brachial artery of the left
arm in the section that overlies the head of the
humerus. Once it is in the artery, it is advanced
into the descending aorta. In the translumbar approach, the needle or catheter is inserted through
the back, past the anterolateral edge of the vertebra,
and into the aorta. Translumbar aortography is
performed at the level of T12–L1 (high) for examination of the abdominal aorta. The level of L2–L3
(low) is used for examination of the peripheral

or pelvic arterial circulation (Snopek, 1992).

Knowing the location of the puncture site is
important, because in the postoperative period, the
nurse must assess for bleeding, neurologic deficit,
and the presence of distal pulses. The assessments vary based on the location of the possible
arterial obstruction or bleeding source. The
three sites generally used for arterial puncture are
presented in Figure 11–6.

**Contrast Medium.**   Numerous intravascular
agents are available, and some of them contain
iodine. The iodinated contrast material provides
the radiopacity and enhances the imaging of arteriography procedures. The different contrast
preparations vary in their osmolarity to the blood.
Those that are hyperosmolar provide the image
with the best contrast but also a higher degree of
toxicity. The noniodinated contrast medium is used
for patients who are at increased risk for a reaction to the contrast medium. The more minor
reactions (nausea, hives) have a lower incidence,
but no difference exists in the incidence of
severe cardiorespiratory complications.

The sensation of pain, heat, a warm feeling, or
burning on injection is related to the hyperosmolarity of the contrast medium. Contrast material with
high osmolarity will cause greater discomfort, and
low-osmolarity preparations cause markedly decreased sensations of pain. Problems of nausea and

vomiting are also related to the hyperosmolarity of the contrast medium.

All contrast media have the potential to affect the heart, including the myocardial cells, the coronary arteries, and the conduction system. As contrast material is injected into the heart or its coronary arteries, or as it passes through the heart in the circulatory route, potential exists for sudden hypotension, bradycardia, or altered conductivity. The changes are generally small or insignificant, but on rare occasions they can lead to cardiorespiratory arrest (Bettmann, 1996).

All iodinated contrast material is eliminated from the body by the kidneys. The contrast medium is somewhat nephrotoxic, however, and does alter the renal blood flow and filtration rate temporarily. In almost all cases, the contrast material is easily eliminated without damage, but occasionally renal failure occurs. The cause is not clearly understood, but it is important to maintain hydration before, during, and after angiography to promote complete excretion of the contrast medium.

Allergic reactions to the iodine can also occur. The mild form is a temporary urticaria and flushing that responds to the administration of an $H_1$ antagonist such as diphenhydramine (Benadryl). The more severe but uncommon reactions include bronchoconstriction, laryngeal edema, and cardiopulmonary arrest.

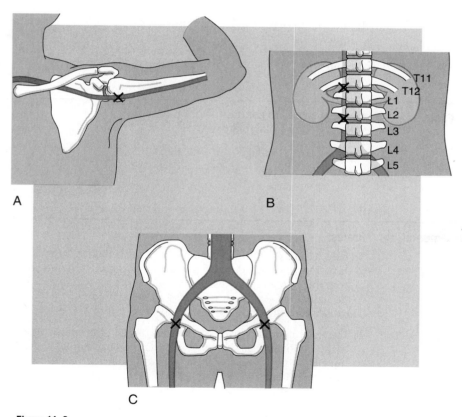

**Figure 11–6**
Arterial access sites for angiography. *A,* Transaxillary arterial puncture, frontal view. *B,* Translumbar aortography arterial puncture, dorsal view. *C,* Femoral arterial puncture, frontal view.

**Purpose of the Test**

Angiography is used to investigate arterial vascular disease, to provide visualization of the arteries during treatment procedures, and to evaluate the effectiveness of vascular surgery in the postoperative period.

**Procedure**

Iodinated contrast medium is injected into an artery using a percutaneous approach with a needle or an arterial catheter. Fluoroscopic images and serial x-ray films are taken to demonstrate the vasculature and any arterial abnormalities that are present. The procedure requires 30 to 90 minutes to complete.

**Findings**

**Abnormal Values**

Peripheral vascular disease
Arterial occlusion
Aneurysm
Vascular fistula
Traumatic arterial injury
Thromboangiitis obliterans

Fibromuscular dysplasia
Collagen vascular disease
Arterial spasm
Tumor
Pseudoaneurysm
Arteriovenous malformation

Inflammatory vasculitis
Giant cell arteritis
Raynaud's disease or phenomenon
Cystic medial necrosis

**Interfering Factors**

- Severe allergy to contrast medium (iodine)
- Recent myocardial infarction
- Coagulation disorder
- Renal failure
- Sickle cell disease
- Homocystinuria

**Nursing Implementation**

**Pretest**

To help reduce distress and anxiety, instruct the patient regarding the procedure. Most patients do not know much about the test and will benefit from information. The discussion can help with accurate expectations and reduction of the anxiety associated with the unknown.
The discussion should include the following information:

1. The patient should drink extra fluids on the days before the test and after the test. No food can be taken after midnight or 8 hours before the test, but clear liquids and medications (except heparin) can be continued during this time (Kandarpa & Gardiner, 1996). Intravenous fluids will be administered during the test. An intravenous line is established before the test begins.
2. Analgesic and sedative medication is usually given in the pretest period to help with relaxation.
3. A local anesthetic is injected to numb the tissue surrounding the arterial puncture site.

■
*Critical Thinking 11–1*
During the pretest assessment interview, what type of information makes you suspect that the patient is vulnerable to an allergic reaction during the procedure?

4. The patient will lie on the radiography table and will not be able to move during the test. A lot of equipment is in the room, used for imaging, computer calculations, and radiographs. The patient will hear clicking and whirring sounds during the procedure.
5. As the contrast medium is injected, the patient may feel a burning sensation or heat, pain, or nausea. Although momentary discomfort occurs, the sensations are normal and brief.

Identify and report any patient history of allergy to iodine or shellfish or of previous reaction to a radiologic procedure that used a contrast medium or dye.

Obtain written consent from the patient or the person legally responsible for the patient's health care decisions.

Ensure that recent laboratory test results are posted in the patient's chart. The nurse should notify the physician of abnormal values. Blood urea nitrogen and creatinine determinations are needed to verify adequate renal function. Activated partial thromboplastin time, prothrombin time, and platelet determinations are needed to verify adequate clotting ability (Kandarpa & Gardiner, 1996).

Begin the nothing-by-mouth status 8 hours before the test as prescribed. The time variable is based on the protocol of the physician or institution and the type of angiographic study planned. Continue with clear fluids and medications.

Monitor the vital signs and record the results in the chart. Hypertension should be under control before this test is performed.

On the morning of the test, assess the peripheral pulses and record the findings. A small ink mark should be placed on the skin to record the distal sites of pulsation.

When a cerebral angiogram is planned, an assessment of mental status is carried out.

Have the patient void to empty the bladder before going to the radiology department. The contrast medium acts like a diuretic and can cause the discomfort of a full bladder.

Assist the patient in removing all clothing and putting on a hospital gown. All metal objects, such as jewelry, must be removed from the area of the x-ray field.

Administer the on-call pretest sedation. This usually consists of an intramuscular injection of the narcotic-analgesic meperidine (Demerol) and a sedative-relaxant such as midazolam (Versed) or diazepam (Valium).

## Posttest

Place the patient on bedrest for 6 to 8 hours. The punctured extremity is to be kept straight. When the aorta has been used as the puncture site, the patient must remain in the supine position for the same amount of time.

Monitor vital signs and peripheral pulses every 15 minutes for 1 hour and every hour for 2 hours. With a femoral puncture site, the pertinent pulses are those of the popliteal, dorsalis pedis, and posterior tibialis arteries. With an aortic puncture site, the bilateral pulses include the femoral sites as well as those of the lower extremities. With an axillary puncture site, the brachial, radial, and ulnar pulses are significant.

Assess and compare the extremities bilaterally for signs of occlusion of the cir-

## Table 11–1    Complications of Angiography

| Complication | Nursing Assessment |
| --- | --- |
| Hematoma or hemorrhage | **Femoral Puncture Site**<br>Ecchymosis and swelling in the thigh or inguinal or abdominal area<br>Inability to void<br>Hypotension<br>Tachycardia<br><br>**Axillary Puncture Site**<br>Ecchymosis and swelling in the axilla and inner aspect of the arm<br>Paresthesias (numbness, tingling, "pins-and-needles" sensations)<br>Severe pain<br><br>**Translumbar Site**<br>Dorsal ecchymosis<br>Dyspnea<br>Hemoptysis<br>Hypotension<br>Tachycardia |
| Dissection or pseudoaneurysm | Pain<br>Obstruction of distal circulation<br>Diminished or absent pulses<br>Cyanosis of distal tissue<br>Palpable mass at puncture site |
| Thrombus or embolus | Diminished or absent pulses<br>Pain<br>Cool, dusky, cyanotic extremity<br>Loss of sensation in distal part of extremity |
| Neurologic deficits | **Peripheral**<br>Pain<br>Paresthesias (numbness, pins-and-needles sensation)<br>Loss of motor function distally<br><br>**Cerebral**<br>Hemiplegia<br>Confusion<br>Aphasia<br>Loss of consciousness<br>Pupillary changes<br>Contrast reaction<br>Urticaria (hives, itching)<br>Flushed skin<br>Wheezing, stridor, dyspnea<br>Hypotension<br>Cardiac arrhythmias<br>Cardiac arrest |
| Renal failure | Oliguria or anuria<br>Elevated blood urea nitrogen and creatinine levels |

culation and neurologic deficit. The data include color, warmth, movement, and the absence of neurologic signs such as pain or paresthesias.

Frequently observe the pressure dressing and the tissue surrounding the puncture site for signs of swelling or hematoma. Gentle palpation of the tissue near the puncture site also may be performed.

Extra fluid intake is essential to prevent nephrotoxicity from the contrast medium. The patient should drink extra fluids to achieve a 2,000- to 3,000-mL intake in the 24-hour posttest period.

Because of the high volume of fluids and the diuretic effect of the contrast material, the patient will experience a frequent need to urinate. Remind the patient that a urinal or bedpan must be used during the period of bedrest. Record intake and output measurements.

## Complications

The overall complication rate for the angiography procedure is 1% to 3%. The axillary approach has the most complications, and the femoral approach has the fewest (Kandarpa & Gardiner, 1996). Complications at the puncture site are the largest group of problems. Hemorrhage and hematoma are the most frequent complications, particularly when the axillary approach is used. During a translumbar puncture, a poorly placed needle can puncture the pleural lining or lung, causing a hemothorax. Hypertension, atherosclerotic disease, and coagulation problems are factors that contribute to the risk of bleeding.

Dissection, pseudoaneurysm, and perforation of the artery are usually caused by incorrect insertion of the needle, passage of the guidewire, or the high pressure of the contrast medium as it is injected.

Thromboembolic complications can develop because thrombi tend to form at the puncture site, on the catheter or guidewire, or at the area of arterial wall abnormality.

Neurologic complications are varied, depending on the underlying cause or location. In the axillary approach, the brachial nerve plexus is near the puncture site. If hemorrhage or hematoma occurs and the brachial nerve plexus is compressed, the compression can result in paralysis of the arm and hand. When cerebral angiography is performed, the patient can experience cerebral ischemia from a thrombus or embolus.

Complications from the contrast medium can range from mild to severe. They consist of an allergic response, cardiorespiratory complications, and renal failure. The complications of angiography and the nursing assessments are presented in Table 11–1.

## References

Bettmann, M. A. (1996). Angiographic contrast media. In K. Kandarpa, & J. E. Aruny (Eds.), *Handbook of interventional radiologic procedures* (2nd ed.). Boston: Little, Brown.

DeSilvey, D. L. (1996). Aortic dissection: Update on choosing the right diagnostic study promptly. *Consultant, 36,* 357–364.

Dowd, S. B., Wilson, B. G., Hall, J. D., Steves, A., & Benson, T. (1996). Review of techniques used to image aortic dissection. *Radiologic Technology, 67,* 223–232.

Fahey, V. A. (Ed.). (1994). *Vascular nursing* (2nd ed.). Philadelphia: W. B. Saunders.

Kandarpa, K., & Aruny, J. E. (1996). *Handbook of interventional radiologic procedures* (2nd ed.). Boston: Little, Brown.

Kandarpa, K., & Gardiner, G. A. (1996). Angiography. General principles. In K. Kandarpa & J. E. Aruny (Eds.), *Handbook of interventional radiologic procedures* (2nd ed.). Boston: Little, Brown.

Kim, D., & Orron, D. E. (1992). *Peripheral vascular imaging and intervention.* St. Louis: Mosby–Year Book.

Mettler, F. A. (1996). *Essentials of radiology*. Philadelphia: W. B. Saunders.

Snopek, A. M. (1992). *Fundamentals of special radiographic procedures* (3rd ed.). Philadelphia: W. B. Saunders.

Torres, L. S. (1993). *Basic medical techniques and patient care for radiologic technologists* (4th ed.). Philadelphia: J. B. Lippincott.

Vogelzang, R. L., & Methe, D. M. (1994). Percutaneous vascular intervention and imaging techniques. In V. A. Fahey (Ed.), *Vascular nursing* (2nd ed.). Philadelphia: W. B. Saunders.

# CHAPTER 12

# Tomography

Computed tomography (CT) and magnetic resonance imaging (MRI) are diagnostic scanning procedures that provide multidimensional images of an organ or body section. Each test provides many cross-sectional images that are called *tomographic slices* or *axial slices*. These slices give two-dimensional (2-D) detailed views of the anatomy and internal structure of the target area. Because axial slices can be obtained every few millimeters, the dimension of depth can also be achieved. The transverse, sagittal, coronal, and other planes can be selected to obtain the best view of the target tissue and its relationship to the surrounding tissues (Fig. 12–1). The different planes are selected by computer operations rather than by moving the patient into awkward positions.

CT uses ionizing radiation to produce the images, which are seen in black, white, and gray, depending on the density of the tissue. MRI uses a large magnet and radio waves to measure the rapidly changing magnetic fields of specific tissues. MRI is based on the biochemical and physical properties of different tissues, including the movements of hydrogen ions. The distinct movements of the electrons are converted to images in shades of gray.

Both procedures use the computer and specialized software to integrate the images, provide clear definition or focus, and assist in the selection of axial slices. The image quality is precise and accurate so that even the smallest abnormalities can be visualized.

## Diagnostic Procedures

The basic procedures of tomography are presented in this chapter. The uses of the procedures in specific body systems are summarized in Part IV of this text.

## Computed Tomography

**(Radiologic Scan)**        Synonyms: CT scan, computerized axial tomography, CAT scan

**Normal Values**        No structural or anatomic abnormalities are noted.

## Background Information

CT uses a fan of x-ray beams in a multidimensional scanning process to produce cross-sectional images of the body. As the x-rays pass through the body tissues, they fall on a circle of detectors

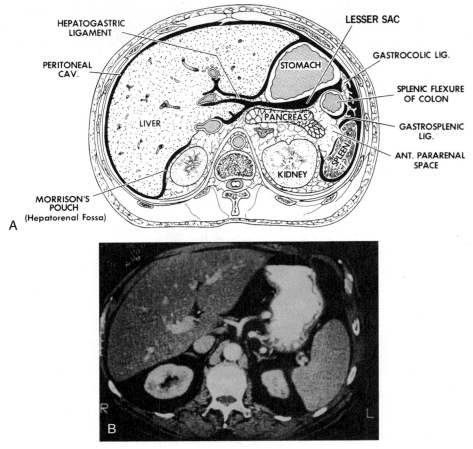

**Figure 12–1**

Cross-sectional views of the abdomen. *A,* Diagram of a transverse section of the upper abdomen showing the relationship of the organs and structures. *B,* A transverse computed tomographic (CT) image of the abdomen. (*A,* Reproduced with permission from Moss, A. A., Gansu, G., & Genant, H. K. [1992]. Computed tomography of the body with magnetic resonance imaging [2nd ed., Vol. 3, p. 1140]. Philadelphia: W. B. Saunders. *B,* Reproduced with permission from Thompson, M. A., Hall, J. D., Hattaway, M. P., & Dowd, S. B. [1994]. *Principles of imaging science and protection* [Vol. 2, Slide 390]. Philadelphia: W. B. Saunders.)

located in the scanner ring. In some models, the x-ray source remains stationary while the detectors rotate around the patient. In other models, the detectors remain stationary while the x-ray sources rotate (Fig. 12–2). The scanning process uses the images taken from many angles to form a 360-degree composite scan for each axial slice.

As the radiation passes through the body, some of the energy is absorbed, based on the density of the tissue that is examined. The detectors register the photons that are able to pass through the tissue. The impulses are converted to numeric data by computer operations. The computer then translates the numbers to specific images that reflect the cross-sectional views of the targeted tissue. The images appear on the monitor and are photographed for further study.

The differences in tissue density and composition are reflected clearly in the final images. As the x-ray photons pass through dense tissue such as bone, calcium, metallic implants, or thrombi, many of the photons are absorbed. Because few photons reach the detectors in the scanner ring, the image of this dense tissue appears whiter or brighter on the monitor or film. Conversely, less dense, more radiolucent tissue allows more photons to pass through the tissue to the detectors. These tissues appear in various shades of gray, according to their density and structure. Air and fat are very radiolucent and produce dark or black tones.

**Conventional CT.** In this standard slower technology, from 1 to 10 seconds is needed to obtain a single, 2-D axial slice. The patient lies on a movable table that gradually advances through the scanner ring. Every few seconds the table advances a small but precise distance, and another axial slice is imaged. Using the sum of many axial slices and the computer resolution of the views, the entire target organ or area of the body can be viewed. The computer rapidly integrates many images to provide the final views desired.

**Helical (Spiral) CT.** In this newest CT technology, used particularly for scanning the body, the imaging is more rapid and continuous. More than 100 images can be obtained in 30 seconds of helical scan exposure (Brink, 1995). The x-ray tube traces a helical or spiral pattern over the patient's body surface as the imaging is done rapidly. With computer software applications, reconstruction of the image can be done in various planes. With this faster imaging and the computer applications, the patient's motion from respiration or bowel peristalsis no lon-

ger interferes with the clarity of the images within the torso. The procedure requires a shorter imaging time, so this method of CT is very useful for the patient who is critically ill.

The helical CT scan can produce 2-D images (transaxial slices), similar to the conventional CT scan. In addition, helical CT can provide three-dimensional (3-D) images from the data, producing a different view and additional information for the physician or surgeon. For example, 3-D images of vascular abnormalities such as aneurysm, stricture, or stenosis are readily visible, and the size of the abnormality is measurable (Fig. 12–3). The 3-D images of a bone can reveal greater detail about a fracture, tumor, or metastasis (Fig. 12–4).

The CT scan can image the head with or without contrast medium. When it is used, the contrast medium provides a sharper, more enhanced view of the tissue. In the head, the CT scan clearly identifies the intracranial or extracerebral abnormalities that are present. In the torso, it is effective in its imaging of the liver, pancreas, kidneys, adrenal glands, lungs, heart, great vessels, abdominal lymph glands, retroperitoneal area, abdominal cavity, vertebrae, and spinal cord. It can differentiate between a cyst and a malignant tumor.

For abdominal or pelvic CT, iodinated contrast medium may be administered orally, intravenously, rectally, or vaginally, depending on the individual area of interest. For imaging of the gastrointestinal tract, liquid barium may be administered orally or instilled rectally. Air may also be used with the barium as a double contrast for imaging the upper or lower gastrointestinal tract (Brant, 1998).

**Figure 12–2**

Computed tomography that uses a stationary ring system. In this system, the detectors ($D_N$) are aligned in a stationary ring. The radiation sources are in a fanlike array that moves clockwise around the patient. Each source of radiation transmits photons through the patient so that they fall on a particular detector on the opposite side of the body. As the sources move circularly, new detectors receive the radiation signals and record the data until the entire circle and a single axial slice are completed. (Modified with permission from Moss, A. A., Gansu, G., & Genant, H. K. [1992]. Computed tomography of the body with magnetic resonance imaging [2nd ed., Vol. 3, p. 1365]. Philadelphia: W. B. Saunders.)

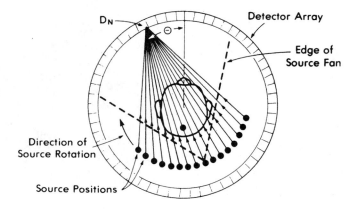

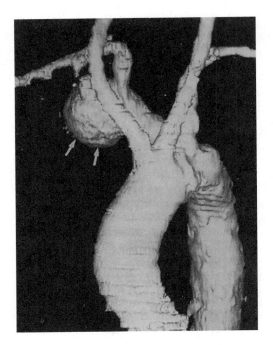

**Figure 12–3**
Helical (spiral) CT three-dimensional image of an artery. The image of the aneurysm of the subclavian artery (*arrows*) is generated from the data of a helical computed tomographic (CT) scan. The vascular image clearly shows the external surface of the artery and documents the abnormality. (Reproduced with permission from Touliopoulos, P., & Costello, P. [1995]. Helical [spiral] CT of the thorax. *Radiologic Clinics of North America, 33*[5], 848.)

**Psychologic Needs.**   The research of Peteet et al. (1992) investigated the psychologic needs of patients who undergo CT scanning. The data revealed that patients who had this diagnostic test for the first time appreciated the explanation of the procedure and information about what to expect. Patients who repeated the test demonstrated less need for explanations, because they were already experienced and knowledgeable. Both the "first-time" patients and the "repeaters" reported anxiety, discomfort, fear of the test results, fear of the machine, and some feelings of claustrophobia. Relaxation techniques were helpful in controlling the anxiety or discomfort.

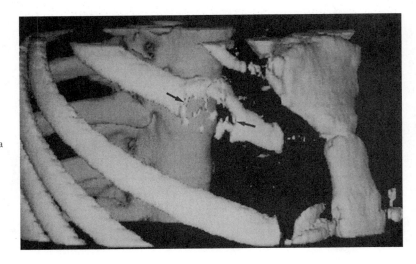

**Figure 12–4**
Helical (spiral) computed tomographic (CT) three-dimensional (3-D) image of a rib. The 3-D image shows the extent of a cancer metastasis (*arrows*) to the right fifth anterior rib from a primary synovial sarcoma. (Reproduced with permission from Touliopoulos, P., & Costello, P. [1995]. Helical (spiral) CT of the thorax. *Radiologic Clinics of North America, 33*[5], 858.)

**Purpose of the Test**

CT provides precise visualization of the structure, size, shape, and density of soft tissue, bone, major blood vessels, and organs of the head and torso. It distinguishes between benign and malignant tissue and is used in the staging of cancerous tumors. It can also be used to analyze the bone mineral content of the vertebrae in the assessment of osteoporosis.

**Procedure**

With or without the use of an iodinated contrast medium, the patient moves through a scanner ring, and multiple x-ray beams pass through the tissue (Fig. 12–5). As the x-ray photons fall on the scanner, data are acquired. Using the computer and special software, various 2-D or 3-D images of the tissue are produced from the data.

**Findings**

**Abnormal Values**

Tumor
Malignancy
Cyst
Stenosis
Thrombus
Embolus
Arteriosclerotic
  plaque

Calcification
Congenital malformation
Abscess
Calculus
Inflammation
Fluid collection

Bleeding or
  hemorrhage
Organ atrophy
Bone fracture

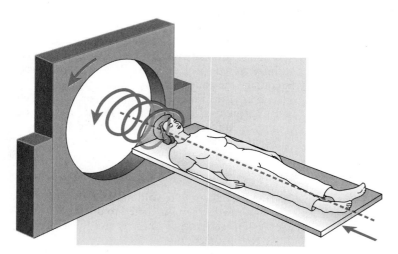

**Figure 12–5**
The scanning process in helical CT. The patient is moved on a table through the scanner. As the x-ray and detector system rotate, a helix or spiral of data is obtained. (Reproduced with permission from Brink, J. A. [1995]. Technical aspects of helical [spiral] CT. *Radiologic Clinics of North America, 33*[5], 826.)

| | |
|---|---|
| **Interfering Factors** | • Jewelry or metal in the x-ray field<br>• Uncooperative behavior<br>• Pregnancy<br>• Failure to maintain nothing-by-mouth status (as indicated)<br>• Allergy to iodine (with the use of contrast medium)<br>• Severe liver or kidney disease (with the use of contrast medium) |

**Nursing Implementation**

■

*Critical Thinking 12–1*
After a car accident, a 14-year-old boy is scheduled for a CT scan of the abdomen, stat. He is frightened and in moderate pain, but his vital signs are stable. What nursing interventions can help him follow instructions and complete the scan without delay?

### Pretest

Ask the patient if there is any history of allergy to iodine or shellfish or of allergic reaction to dye or contrast material used in a previous x-ray study.

Explain the procedure to the patient and obtain written consent from the patient or person legally designated to make health care decisions for the patient.

If contrast medium is to be used, instruct the patient to discontinue all food and fluids for 4 to 8 hours before the test.

In gastrointestinal CT imaging, instruct the patient to drink prescribed amounts of liquid contrast on the night before the test and again at timed intervals in the hours before the scan.

With the use of intravenous contrast medium, explain that the contrast agent is injected intravenously. The patient may feel warmth at the injection site, a salty taste, headache, or nausea as the agent is injected. These are temporary sensations that will disappear in a few minutes.

When no contrast material is used, reassure the patient that the procedure is painless.

Instruct the patient to remove all clothes, jewelry, and other metal objects. A hospital gown is worn.

Provide appropriate orientation and reassurance so that fear of the unknown is diminished. Many patients feel some degree of apprehension as they enter the enclosed space of the machine. The scan itself is painless.

Encourage the patient to relax during the scanning process by using techniques such as visual imagery, meditation, or prayer (Peteet et al., 1992).

Sedatives are usually used for the infant or child younger than 3 years, particularly when the scan requires an extended period of immobility. For these patients, general anesthesia may also be used and requires sedation before the administration of the anesthesia (Chin, 1995).

### During the Test

Instruct the patient to remain motionless while in the scanner and to hold his or her breath when instructed to do so.

Keep an emesis basin in a nearby area in case the patient vomits after receiving the contrast medium.

### Posttest

If sedatives were administered, monitor the vital signs on a regular basis until the patient is responsive and awake.

No other special nursing measures are needed.

## Magnetic Resonance Imaging

(Magnetic Field Scan)    Synonyms: MRI, nuclear magnetic resonance, NMR

| Normal Values | No structural or anatomic abnormalities are noted. |
|---|---|

### Background Information

MRI is a noninvasive imaging technique that uses a large, powerful magnet and a radiofrequency coil to obtain cross-sectional images of body tissues. The images of axial planes are similar to those produced by CT, but MRI has a greater ability to produce images of any plane (Fig. 12–6). This is particularly useful in imaging the head, neck, brain, and spinal cord.

MRI is based on the biochemical differences among cells. The nuclei of cells contain many atoms that have electric fields. For example, each hydrogen atom has one proton with a positive charge. These protons are distributed randomly in tissue and behave like tiny magnets. When in the presence of the strong magnetic field produced by the MRI magnet, the body protons spin and move to realign in a new axis formation. The machine then emits pulses of radio waves to stimulate and detect the magnetized protons. The pulsed signal first displaces the aligned protons, and then, on cessation of the radio wave stimulus, the machine detects the proton return to magnetized alignment (Fig. 12–7).

Different tissues have different densities, water contents, proton concentrations, and patterns of movement. Once these differences are identified by the radiofrequency coil, the messages are transmitted to the computer for number coding and translation into images of the tissue. In shades of black, white, and gray, the images are seen on the monitor and are photographed or taped for further diagnostic study. Fat and marrow produce high signal intensities and brighter images. Bone and air produce low-intensity, weak signals and dark images. For this reason, MRI cannot image bones, bone density, calcification, or calcium stones.

Some of the pulse sequences are used to detect anatomic differences among tissues, including the difference between cystic and solid tissues or the differences among muscle, ligament, and tendon. Other pulse sequences are used to detect pathologic changes. Fluid-filled growths, edema, inflammation, hematoma, and neoplasm all produce weak signals, and the images are darker than those of the surrounding tissue.

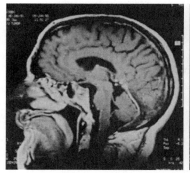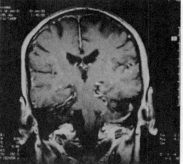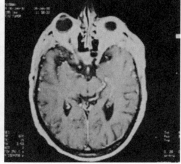

**Figure 12–6**

Magnetic resonance imaging (MRI) of the head. MRI can produce images in almost any body plane: *Left,* sagittal; *middle,* coronal; *right,* transverse. (Reproduced with permission from Thompson, M. A., Hall, J. D., Hattaway, M. P., & Dowd, S. B. [1994]. *Principles of imaging science and protection* [Vol. 2, Slide 393]. Philadelphia: W. B. Saunders.)

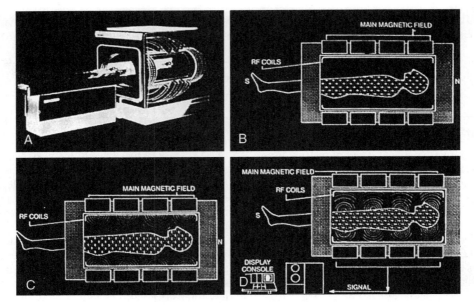

**Figure 12–7**

The process of MRI. *A,* Scanner consists of a cylinder (the magnet itself) into which the patient enters by a movable tabletop based on a large platform. *B,* The main magnetic field is oriented parallel to the long axis of the patient. The hydrogen nuclei of the patient's body water and fat point north in the direction of the main field. *C,* Radiofrequency (RF) coils acting as a radio transmitter send a radio signal of sufficient energy to tilt the nuclei 90 degrees, or at right angles to the main field. *D,* In the process of recovering alignment with the main field, the protons emit radio signals picked up by the RF coils and are transformed into an image. (Reproduced with permission from Nadolo, L. A., Easterbrook, J., McArdle, C. B., Mendelson, D. B., & Ponder, T. H. [1991]. The neuroradiology of visual disturbances. *Neurologic Clinics, 9,* 5.)

**Types of Magnetic Resonance Imaging Systems.**
The conventional MRI uses a *circumferential whole body* scanner. The entire body must be placed within the chamber and bore of the magnet. With an *open configuration* scanner, the patient is not completely enclosed in the cylindrical chamber but still has some discomfort from the noise.

The newest type of MRI is the *dedicated extremity MRI* (E-MRI). This system uses a special scanner to image the affected extremity only. The patient's extremity is placed within the bore of a small magnet, but the rest of the body remains outside the scanner. The noise can be heard, but in general, this process is more comfortable for the patient. The arm or the leg can be placed in the scanner to image the middle and lower joints of the extremity. The shoulder and the hip cannot be imaged in this manner (Peterfy, Roberts, & Genant, 1997).

**Safety Concerns.** Definite risks exist for the patient with a ferromagnetic metal implant. The magnetic forces of MRI are so great that they will twist, damage, or move the metallic object and cause injury. The implants or metallic items that are contraindications for this test are aneurysmal vascular clips, shrapnel located near the eyes or neurologic system, pacemakers, cochlear implants, joint implants, and intrauterine devices.

Also, a strong ambient magnetic force exists around the outside of the scanner. The examination room must be kept clear of all extraneous metal objects such as wheelchairs, canes, crutches, and vacuum cleaners. No person can enter the examination room with coins, keys, scissors, or hairpins. If these items are present, they become missiles that will be pulled into the scanner with force. The patient can be seriously injured by these objects (Saysell, 1997).

**Psychologic Needs.** The patient experiences no pain during MRI, but the whole body MRI scan is perceived as an unpleasant experience for many individuals. In the whole body MRI procedure, most patients report minor anxiety, but some have considerable apprehension and feelings of claustrophobia. Throughout the test, the patient hears loud, harsh noise that sounds like the crushing of metal, and it is difficult to remain still for the time that it takes to complete the imaging. In addition to the worry about the possible diagnosis, the patient feels uncertainty and sensory deprivation.

Because of acute anxiety and feelings of "panic," 5% to 10% of the patients are unable to complete the examination, and some others need sedation to help them cope with the procedure (MacKenzie, Sims, Owens, & Dixon, 1995; Peterfy et al., 1997).

## Purpose of the Test

MRI is used to assess anatomic structures, organs, and soft tissue, including visualization of any pathologic condition that is present. It can differentiate between benign and malignant growth and may be used to stage cancer or evaluate the response to treatment of a malignancy.

## Procedure

The patient enters the tube of the MRI machine, which contains a circular magnet and a radiofrequency coil. In the presence of the magnetic field and radio wave stimulation, changes in and movement of tissue protons occur. These movements are converted by computer to precise images of the tissue in any plane selected.

## Findings

**Abnormal Values**

| | | |
|---|---|---|
| Tumor | Malformation | Bleeding or |
| Stricture | Abscess | hemorrhage |
| Stenosis | Inflammation | Organ atrophy |
| Thrombus | Edema | |
| Embolus | Fluid collection | |

## Interfering Factors

- Jewelry or other metal in the magnetic field
- Metallic implant in the body
- Uncooperative behavior

## Nursing Implementation

**Pretest**

Ask the patient if there is a history of any metallic implant having been placed in the body.

Ensure that the patient and staff have removed all external metallic objects, such as jewelry, hairpins, and magnetized credit cards.

Explain the procedure and the sensations that the patient will experience. Obtain written consent from the patient or the person legally designated to make the patient's health care decisions.

To help minimize anxiety, encourage the patient to have a friend or relative stay during the procedure.

To help minimize the emotional discomfort, encourage the patient to use relaxation strategies such as mental imagery of landscapes or seascapes, closing the eyes, and breathing for relaxation.

■
*Critical Thinking 12–2*
Because of trauma to the joint, a promising young male athlete must have an MRI scan of the knee. He expresses anxiety and dismay about his future athletic ability and asks you how MRI can help him. How would you respond to his question and feelings?

Instruct the patient on how to obtain help while inside the machine.

Sedatives are usually used for the infant or child younger than 3 years, particularly when the scan requires an extended period of immobility. Administer the prescribed sedative.

### During the Test

Instruct the patient to remain motionless on the narrow table during the test.

### Posttest

If sedatives were administered, monitor the vital signs on a regular basis until the patient is responsive and awake.

No other special nursing measures are needed.

## References

Brant, W. E. (1998). Introduction to CT of the abdomen and pelvis. In W. R. Webb, W. E. Brant, & C. A. Helms (Eds.), *Fundamentals of body CT* (2nd ed.). Philadelphia: W. B. Saunders.

Brink, J. A. (1995). Technical aspects of helical (spiral) CT. *Radiologic Clinics of North America, 33,* 825–841.

Brown, R. H., & Zerhouni, E. (1998). New techniques and developments in physiologic imaging of airways. *Radiologic Clinics of North America, 36,* 211–229.

Chin, M. A. (1995). Preparation for computed tomography and magnetic resonance imaging. In C. Godderidge (Ed.), *Pediatric imaging.* Philadelphia: W. B. Saunders.

DeSilvey, D. L. (1996). Aortic dissection: Update on choosing the right diagnostic study promptly. *Consultant, 36,* 357–359, 363–364.

Eustace, S. (1997). MR imaging of acute orthopedic trauma to the extremities. *Radiologic Clinics of North America, 35,* 615–629.

Godderidge, C. (1995). *Pediatric imaging.* Philadelphia: W. B. Saunders.

Harisinghani, M. G., Saini, S., & Schima, W. (1996). Computed tomography and magnetic resonance imaging of focal hepatic masses. *Applied Radiology, 25,* 11, 15–16, 19–20, 25–26.

MacKenzie, R., Sims, C., Owens, R. G., & Dixon, A. K. (1995). Patients' perceptions of magnetic resonance imaging. *Clinical Radiology, 50,* 137–143.

Melendez, J. C., & McCrank, E. (1993). Anxiety-related reactions associated with magnetic resonance imaging examinations. *Journal of the American Medical Association, 270,* 745–747.

Mercader, V. P., Gateby, R. A., & Curtis, R. A. (1996). Radiographic assessment of genitourinary trauma. *Trauma Quarterly, 13*(1), 129–151.

Moss, A. A., Gansu, G., & Genant, H. K. (Eds.). (1992). Computed tomography of the body with magnetic resonance imaging (2nd ed., vol. 3, Abdomen and pelvis). Philadelphia: W. B. Saunders.

Nadalo, L. A. (1991). The neurology of visual disturbances. *Neurologic Clinics, 9,* 1–35.

Peteet, J. R., Stomper, P. C., Ross, D. M., Cotton, V., Truesdell, P., & Moczynski, W. (1992). Emotional support for patients with cancer who are undergoing CT: Semi-structured interviews of patients at a cancer institute. *Radiology, 182,* 99–102.

Peterfy, C. G., Roberts, T., & Genant, H. K. (1997). Dedicated extremity MR imaging: An emerging technology. *Radiologic Clinics of North America, 35*(1), 1–18.

Phillips, S., & Dreary, I. J. (1995). Interventions to alleviate patient anxiety during magnetic resonance imaging. *Radiology, 179*(1), 137–143.

Saysell, M. A. (1997). An introduction to paediatric magnetic resonance imaging. *Radiography (London), 3*(1), 31–41.

Webb, W. R., Brant, W. E., & Helms, C. A. (1998). *Fundamentals of body CT* (2nd ed.). Philadelphia: W. B. Saunders.

# 13

CHAPTER

# Genetic Testing

Laboratory techniques have expanded to include genetic testing. Genetic testing has moved from the research laboratories into mainstream medical practice. It has advanced from chromosomal analysis to almost daily recognition of genes that may put a person at risk for a medical disorder.

In 1989, Congress initiated the Human Genome Project (HGP). The HGP is an organized, collaborative, scientific endeavor to share genetic discoveries and information. The major goal of the HGP is to map the order of genes and the genetic distance between each of the chromosomes (Lea, Jenkins, & Francomano, 1998). It is believed that through our understanding of the structure and function of the human genome (all the genetic material contained in the chromosomes of a particular organism), we may eventually be able to diagnose, treat, and prevent genetic disease.

This chapter describes some common genetic tests. It attempts to present the information with a minimum of specialized vocabulary from the field of genetics. Because genetic testing is very complex, with tests having different levels of sensitivity and specificity, the nurse needs to work closely with a specialist in genetics. As Gilbert (1997) reported, misinterpretation of the results of genetic testing is common among doctors. The nurse is one member of a health team that should include a geneticist and a genetic counselor.

Genetic testing is technologically advanced. As genetic testing proliferates, a need exists for more education of health professionals about genetic disorders, predisposition to cancer and other diseases, genetic testing, and the psychosocial interventions needed to help the individual and his or her family members understand the implications of the test results. Most nurses do not have the educational background in genetics to answer all the questions raised by genetic testing, whether they

deal with decisions regarding procreation or with cancer risk management. However, nurses can concentrate on the individual and the family who are considering genetic testing and its implications in their lives. The person undergoing genetic testing is faced with critical decisions. The nurse supports the person at each step of the process. The nurse is frequently in a central position to coordinate and support the person through the testing procedures. The nurse initiates this support before the test begins, if possible, by helping the person to identify the risks versus the benefits of the testing, to understand the process of testing, and to be aware of the limitations of the test. The nurse should assess the patient's level of anxiety and his or her coping skills.

Some nurses are specializing in the field of genetics. The International Society of Nurses in Genetics has been formed and is a resource for all nurses. A nurse may also take a master's degree in genetic counseling and become a board-certified genetic counselor. Genetic counselors provide information and consultation to individuals and families regarding the occurrence and chances of occurrence of birth defects, developmental disabilities, hereditary disease, and cancer. Genetic counselors evaluate medical records of family members, review results of genetic screening and diagnostic tests, and perform an extensive family history. The genetic counselor provides emotional support during the decision-making process surrounding the procedures and treatment choices. The genetic counselor may refer the patient or family, or both, to support groups or social service agencies.

With the rapid advances in genetic testing and the public's demand for such testing, it is evident that the number of genetic counselors in the United States cannot meet the public need. In addition, the proliferation of information from the field of genetics has implications for all fields of nursing. Because of the nurse's role with patients and families and within society, all nurses need some understanding of genetics, its role in susceptibility to disease, and its limitations. Nurses have the unique responsibility to identify and treat the human responses to genetic testing. Nurses can provide short- and long-term support to patients and families who choose or choose not to have genetic testing.

## Background Information

Genetic testing is performed to confirm the diagnosis of a genetic disorder or to determine if a person is at risk for a particular inherited condition. Genetic testing may be requested by individuals with a strong family history of an inherited disorder to determine whether they are carriers of the affected gene. Genetic testing may be done before birth when genetic abnormality is suspected. Genetic predisposition testing is the newest advancement in genetic testing. A number of commercially available tests can identify gene mutations to specific cancers. Genetic predisposition testing is not limited to cancers, but this is the area that is expanding most rapidly.

Genetic testing includes cytogenetic analysis and biochemical and molecular genetics. Cytogenetic analysis involves careful examination of the chromosomes under a microscope and preparation of a karyotype from a photograph or by computer imaging (Fig. 13–1). Chromosomal disorders can occur from alterations in the number and structure of the chromosomes or from structural rearrangement within or between chromosomes. Common chromosomal disorders diagnosed by cytogenetic analysis are Down syndrome, Turner's syndrome, trisomy 13 syndrome, and trisomy 18 syndrome. Molecular genetics integrates molecular technology with chromosomal analysis. A single identified gene may be analyzed based on family history. This form of testing is appropriate for breast cancer, colon cancer, fragile X syndrome, Huntington's disease, Tay-Sachs disease, and sickle cell anemia. Indirect genetic molecular testing is done when the gene mutation itself has not been identified but the region of the chromosome on which the defect occurs is known. Disorders for which indirect testing is available include familial melanoma, hemophilia, neurofibromatosis, and adult onset polycystic kidney disease. Indirect testing is less precise than direct gene analysis.

Table 13–1 summarizes procedures used in prenatal testing. Selection of procedure is frequently determined by the gestational period. Prenatal testing may be used to detect possible birth defects. Testing can and often does lead to reassurance that no abnormality is present. If a defect is present, the parents have time to prepare to care for the child's special needs or may choose to terminate the pregnancy. Parents must be cognizant that current chromosomal testing identifies only a minority of birth abnormalities. A normal test result does not guarantee a healthy infant. Table 13–2 summarizes information on cytogenetic analysis.

Table 13–3 presents information on biochemical genetic tests. These tests are usually ordered as clinical problems evolve and confirmation of suspected diagnosis is needed.

Table 13–4 is a partial listing of disorders that can be diagnosed by molecular genetic testing. These tests are frequently carried out not only to diagnose but also to determine carrier status. Information provided by these tests may be used for life planning.

The study of genetics has identified genes that, when altered, substantially increase one's risk for certain forms of cancer. Note that the gene does not determine who will get cancer or what cancer a person will get, but rather determines a predisposition to a particular form of cancer. The etiology of cancer is believed to be a combination of factors including genetic predisposition and environmental and personal factors. The inherited basis for cancer predisposition is a multistep process of genetic mutation, which allows uncontrollable cellular growth. Some mutations cause inactivation of tumor suppressor genes. Table 13–5 is a partial listing of cancers for which predictive genetic tests are available. This list is expanding rapidly. The National Cancer Genetics Cooperative Network has been formed by the National Cancer Institute to centralize information gathered from clinical trials on genetic testing and make recommendations for its clinical application.

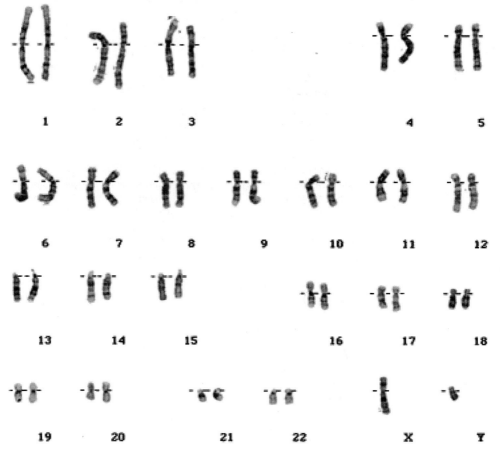

**Figure 13-1**

A karyotype of an amniotic fluid cell metaphase that has been cytogenetically banded. (Reproduced with permission from Lehmann, C. A. [Ed.]. [1998]. *Saunders manual of clinical laboratory science* [p. 1157]. Philadelphia: W. B. Saunders.)

As technology advances, bioethical and psychological issues emerge. Nurses, because of their relationship with patients and families, are in a strategic position to help patients and families work through ethical dilemmas, fears, uncertainty, and conflicts that may occur. The nurse can facilitate patient and family growth by listening, clarifying, and supporting. Patients and families need clarification not only of information but also of their emotional responses to the testing and its implications.

Unlike other laboratory testing, the implica-

tions of genetic testing apply to the other members of a family. An individual's genetic test results will affect other family members who may or may not want to know whether they are at risk genetically. Ethical issues may arise regarding having knowledge of a predisposition to a life-threatening, yet preventable, disease and not notifying family members at risk.

Another ethical issue is the question of genetic testing of children. A child cannot give informed consent. It is difficult to determine possible benefits versus risks that may occur if parents have knowl-

## Table 13–1 Prenatal Testing

**Name of the Test**

Amniocentesis (see pp. 702–708)

**Purpose of the Test**

To detect chromosomal abnormalities, such as gross abnormalities of the sex chromosomes, trisomies, monosomies, translocations, deletions, and duplications. Biochemical and molecular testing may also be carried out on amniotic fluid.

**Procedure**

Test is performed by a physician, usually between the 15th and 17th wk of gestation (may be done in the third trimester to confirm suspected defects before delivery). 20–30 mL of clear amniotic fluid is aspirated and placed in a sterile, clear, capped centrifuge tube. Keep at room temperature unless a delay occurs. Refrigerate if overnight delay is anticipated.

**Interfering Factors**

Less than 5 mL of amniotic fluid
Freezing of specimen
Contamination of specimen with maternal cells, blood, or meconium

**Findings**

Sex of fetus
Chromosomal abnormalities, such as Down syndrome, Turner's syndrome, trisomy 13 syndrome, or trisomy 18 syndrome

**Name of the Test**

Chorionic villus sampling (CVS)

**Purpose of the Test**

Same as an amniocentesis, but can be done earlier, in the 11th wk of gestation

**Procedure**

The physician removes a small sample of placental tissue by aspiration biopsy using a thin plastic catheter inserted via the cervix or transabdominally. The sample is placed in a centrifuge tube. Refrigerate if a prolonged delay in transporting the specimen to the laboratory occurs.

**Interfering Factors**

Samples that are older than 3 days or frozen
Less than 3 mg of specimen

**Findings**

Same as for an amniocentesis

**Table 13–1   Prenatal Testing** (continued)

**Name of the Tests**

Maternal serum markers
   Alpha-fetoprotein (AFP)
   Human chorionic gonadotropin (hCG)
   Unconjugated estriol (uE$_5$)

**Purpose of the Tests**

To determine fetal risk for neural tube defects and chromosomal abnormalities

**Procedure**

Markers can be determined from evaluation of amniotic fluid or from maternal serum after the 15th wk of gestation.

**Interfering Factors**

Test done before the 15th wk of pregnancy
Multiple fetuses
Diabetes mellitus

**Findings**

Increase in AFP can indicate the following:
   Neural tube defects, including anencephaly, encephalocele, and meningomyelocele
   Ventral wall defects including omphalocele and gastroschisis
Decrease in AFP, hCG, and uE$_5$ is suggestive of trisomy defects, including Down syndrome.*

*Must be followed up with a chromosome analysis.

edge of a genetic predisposition to a disorder. The American Society of Human Genetics and the American College of Medical Genetics recommend that predictive genetic testing of children be performed only when an immediate medical benefit to the child is evident.

Care must be taken at all times to ensure confidentiality of the test results. This may be difficult, especially if an insurance company is paying for the test. An individual's genetic makeup may be considered a pre-existing condition, and insurance companies may not pay for treatment. Employers may also discriminate against persons with genetic predispositions because of the potential increase in health care costs and sick leave.

Ethical issues exist in relation to genetics and society as a whole. Fears of using genetic testing to ensure "designer babies" or a "super race" exist. The role of government in genetic screening and individual rights to privacy need to be addressed. Nurses must be advocates for their individual patients but also need to be involved nationally to protect the rights of their patients.

---

**Nursing Implementation**   **Pretest**

Assess patient's baseline knowledge about the purpose and goals of the testing. Identify and correct any misconceptions.
Observe and validate psychological response to testing and its implications.
Prenatal testing is likely to create intense emotional responses. Couples

---

### Table 13–2    Cytogenetic Test

**Name of the Test**

Chromosomal analysis

**Purpose of the Test**

To determine the karyotype of individuals and parents for genetic diagnosis and determination of
carrier status
To assess chromosomal damage in persons exposed to environmental hazards

**Procedure**

Blood: 5 mL of venous blood is collected in a green-topped tube that contains sodium heparin.
In neonates, 1–2 mL of blood is adequate.
Amniotic fluid: 20–30 mL of clear amniotic fluid is collected in a capped centrifuged tube.
Chorionic villus sampling (CVS): Aspiration biopsy of placental tissue is performed.

**Interfering Factors**

Delay in transport to laboratory (more than 48 hr)
Refrigeration or freezing of blood

**Findings**

Chromosomal mosaicism
Monosomies
Structural abnormalities, such as abnormal translocations, inversions, and derivative chromosomes
Trisomies

---

**Name of the Test**

Microdeletion studies

**Purpose of the Test**

To confirm diagnosis of suspected genetic syndromes

**Procedure**

5 mL of venous blood is collected in a green-topped tube containing sodium heparin. In neonates,
1–2 mL of blood is adequate.

**Interfering Factors**

Blood that has been drawn more than 5 days before testing

**Findings**

Angelman's syndrome
DiGeorge syndrome
Cri du chat syndrome
Miller-Dieker syndrome
Smith-Magenis syndrome
Prader-Willi syndrome
Velocardiofacial syndrome
Williams syndrome
Wolf-Hirschhorn syndrome

---

## Table 13–3  Biochemical Genetic Testing

**Name of the Test**

Amino acid analysis

**Purpose of the Test**

To determine inborn errors of metabolism when genetic abnormality is suspected as the cause of developmental disability, digestive disorder, psychomotor retardation, or neurological symptoms

**Procedure**

10–20 mL of urine is collected randomly for the initial screening. A 24-hr urine specimen may be ordered. If plasma is used, 5 mL of venous blood is collected in a green-topped tube.

**Interfering Factors**

Pregnancy
Diet
Medications

**Findings**

Phenylketonuria (PKU)
Maple syrup urine disease (MSUD)

**Name of the Test**

Organic aciduria

**Purpose of the Test**

To diagnose inherited disorders of amino acid and organic acid metabolism

**Procedure**

10 mL of first-voided morning urine is required.

**Interfering Factors**

Most elevations in a sick child are considered nonspecific, and repeat analysis is recommended.

**Name of the Test**

Biotinidase deficiency

**Purpose of the Test**

To determine biotinidase insufficiency

**Procedure**

2 mL of venous blood is collected in a red-topped tube and sent to the lab immediately for centrifuging and freezing.

**Interfering Factors**

Sulfonamides

*(continued on the following page)*

**Table 13–3 Biochemical Genetic Testing** *(continued)*

### Findings

Biotin-dependent carboxylases

---

### Name of the Test

Carnitine cycle

### Purpose of the Test

To assist in the diagnosis of infants who fail to thrive and who have other metabolic abnormalities

### Procedure

Urine: 10 mL of randomly collected urine is taken. Sometimes a 12- or 24-hr urine specimen is ordered.
Blood: 2–3 mL of venous blood is collected in a red-topped tube.

### Interfering Factors

Dehydration of the patient

---

### Name of the Test

Tay-Sachs disease (TSD)*

### Purpose of the Test

To diagnose TSD or to determine if the person is a carrier of TSD

### Procedure

For men and for nonpregnant women not on birth control pills: 10 mL of venous blood is collected in a red-topped tube.
For pregnant women: 10 mL of venous blood is collected in two lavender-topped tubes.
For nonpregnant women on birth control pills: 10 mL of venous blood is collected in a red-topped tube and two lavender-topped tubes.

### Findings

Absence of the alpha subunit of hexosaminidase A gene is consistent with TSD.

---

### Name of the Test

Lysosomal storage diseases

### Purpose of the Test

To determine the cause of developmental delay or regression in infants and children under 10 yr.
For carrier testing for relatives of a person with a lysosomal storage disease.

## Table 13–3    Biochemical Genetic Testing *(continued)*

### Procedure†

Leukocytes (initial screening): 5–10 mL of venous blood is collected in a purple-topped tube.

Serum: 5–10 mL of venous blood is collected in a red-topped tube.

Skin fibroblasts: Biopsy of the skin, usually of the forearm, is performed.

### Findings

Low or absent enzyme activity is consistent with lysosomal enzyme disorders, such as fucosidosis, Gaucher's disease, Hunter's disease, mucolipidosis II and III, multiple sulfatase deficiency, Niemann-Pick disease, and Pompe's disease.

---

*TSD may be diagnosed by molecular testing.

†Specimen selection is based on suspected disorder.

---

may already have a child with a severe disability whom they love, yet may need to know the potential for and want to prevent the birth of another affected child.

Fear of passing on genes that could result in a serious disorder creates problems of guilt, decreased self-worth, and multiple losses.

Assess family dynamics. Do situational factors influence the decision for testing? Is the family supportive of the individual's decision to have testing done?

With predictive testing, clearly differentiate between being at risk and having a disease.

Identify supportive resources, such as skilled genetic counselors or support groups, or both.

Ensure that informed consent is given. Obtaining informed consent includes discussing the physical and psychological risks and benefits and discussing the limitations of the findings and possible discrimination by health insurance companies and employers.

If microdeletion studies are ordered (see Table 13–2), inform the laboratory before sending the specimen, because special techniques are needed.

### During the Test

Care is dependent on purpose and procedure, as well as the age of the patient.

### Posttest

As part of the health team, explain the results of the test in language the patient can understand. If several members of a family were tested, confidentiality should be maintained by giving the results separately.

Although the patient may want results to be given in absolutes, most results are given in degrees of risk. Assess how the person interprets the risks or probabilities.

Do not give false reassurances. Double messages will only confuse the patient.

Listen to clues from patients. How much information do they want, and how much can they absorb?

Assist the person through the decision-making process. Inform the patient of options. Refer the patient for genetic counseling if indicated.

■

*Critical Thinking 13–1*

Your pregnant neighbor, age 38 years, is told by her doctor to have an amniocentesis done. Knowing you are a nurse, she asks you why the doctor told her to do this, because she has no intention of aborting the child even if it is abnormal. What response would help your neighbor?

### Table 13–4   Molecular Genetics

**Genetic Disorder**

Alpha-antitrypsin deficiency

**Purpose of the Test**

To determine the cause of early onset emphysema and liver disease

**Procedure**

Blood: 2–5 mL of venous blood is collected in a purple-topped tube. Invert tube several times to mix blood with ethylenediaminetetraacetic acid (EDTA) in the tube. Store at room temperature.

**Interfering Factors**

Blood drawn more than 48 hr before testing

**Findings**

Confirmation of deficiency consistent with infantile cirrhosis and emphysema in a young person

**Genetic Disorder**

Cystic fibrosis

**Purpose of the Test**

To confirm diagnosis of cystic fibrosis (CF) and to determine the carrier status for the disease

**Procedure**

Blood: As above
Amniotic fluid: 10–15 mL of fluid is aspirated between 14th and 17th wk of gestation. Keep refrigerated. Do not freeze or ship in dry ice.

**Interfering Factors**

As above

**Findings**

CF mutations detected. CF cannot be excluded if no detectable CF mutation is found, because more than 500 CF mutations have been identified and may be unique to a family. For carrier testing, results should be compared with those of an affected family member.

**Genetic Disorder**

Fragile X syndrome

**Purpose of the Test**

To determine the cause of developmental disability or autism
To diagnose carrier status in those with a family history of fragile X syndrome

**Procedure**

As above

**Table 13–4    Molecular Genetics** (continued)

### Findings

Large expansion of a CGG triplet repeat region of the FMR-1 gene is consistent with the diagnosis of fragile X syndrome, also known as Martin-Bell syndrome.

### Genetic Disorder

Huntington's disease

### Purpose of the Test

To diagnose who will develop Huntington's disease

### Procedure

Blood: As above
Amniotic fluid: As above
Chorionic villi: Biopsy of the chorion frondosum during the 9th to 12th wk of gestation

### Interfering Factors

As above

### Findings

Huntington's disease

### Genetic Disorder

Gaucher's disease

### Purpose of the Test

To diagnose cause of splenomegaly with thrombocytopenia
To determine presence of mutation in those with a family history of the disorder

### Procedure

As above

### Interfering Factors

As above

### Findings

Mutation in the glucocerebrosidase gene consistent with Gaucher's disease

### Genetic Disorder

Mitochondrial DNA

### Purpose of the Test

To identify cause of painless bilateral vision loss

(continued on the following page)

**Table 13–4   Molecular Genetics** (continued)

**Procedure**

As above

**Interfering Factors**

As above

**Findings**

Mutation of mitochondrial DNA consistent with Leber's hereditary optic neuropathy and mitochondrial encephalomyopathies

**Genetic Disorder**

Muscular dystrophy

**Purpose of the Test**

To confirm diagnosis of muscular dystrophy and to determine carrier status in people with a family history of the disease

**Procedure**

Blood: As above

**Interfering Factors**

As above

**Findings**

Mutation of the dystrophin gene consistent with the diagnosis of Becker's muscular dystrophy or Duchenne type muscular dystrophy

**Genetic Disorder**

Tay-Sachs disease (TSD)

**Purpose of the Test**

To determine the cause of neurodegeneration and determine the carrier status of people with a family history of TSD

**Procedure**

As above

**Interfering Factors**

As above

**Findings**

Mutation in the hexosaminidase A gene is consistent with the diagnosis of TSD.

| Table 13–5 | Partial Listing of Cancers for Which Predisposition Testing Is Possible |
| --- | --- |

Ataxia telangiectasia
Breast cancer
    BRCA1
    BRCA2
Colon cancer
    Familial adenomatous polyposis
    Hereditary nonpolyposis
    Lynch's syndrome I and II
Endocrine cancers
    Multiple endocrine neoplasia (MEN)
Fanconi's syndrome
Li-Fraumeni cancer syndrome
Neuroblastoma
Ovarian cancer
    BRCA1
Retinoblastoma

With predictive genetic testing, results indicating no hereditary susceptibility will be reassuring, but educate the patient not to ignore other risk factors or to discontinue screening for the disease. For example, if the test for the BRCA gene, which indicates a genetic predisposition for breast cancer, is negative, the woman should continue performing monthly breast examinations and receiving periodic mammograms as recommended for all women. Listen for indications of "survivor guilt." Persons may feel guilty because they have not inherited a disease that is afflicting other members of their family.

If predictive genetic testing indicates a hereditary predisposition to a disease, assess the psychological response. Depression, distress, guilt, decreased self-worth, anxiety, and anticipation of loss may occur. Discuss with the patient his or her options, including aggressive surveillance for the disease and prophylactic measures, such as surgery to prevent the disease. Make appropriate referrals based on the patient's decisions.

## References

Ackerman, T. F. (1996). Genetic testing of children for cancer susceptibility. *Journal of Pediatric Oncology Nursing, 13,* 46–49.

ASHG/ACMG report: Points to consider: Ethical, legal, and psychological implications of genetic testing in children and adolescents. (1995). *American Journal of Human Genetics, 57,* 1233.

Baird, M. L. (1996). Use of DNA identification for forensic and paternity analysis. *Journal of Clinical Laboratory Analysis, 10,* 350–358.

Baron, R. H., & Borgen, P. I. (1997). Genetic susceptibility for breast cancer: Testing and primary prevention options. *Oncology Nursing Forum, 24,* 461–468.

Baroni, M. A., Anderson, Y. E., & Mischler, E. (1997). Cystic fibrosis newborn screening: Impact of early screening results on parenting stress. *Pediatric Nursing, 23,* 143–151.

Calzone, K. A. (1996). Information sources: Cancer genetics and genetic testing. *Cancer Practice, 4,* 346–349.

Calzone, K. A. (1997). Genetic predisposition testing: Clinical implications for oncology nurses. *Oncology Nursing Forum, 24,* 712–718.

Codori, A. (1997). Psychological opportunities and hazards in predictive genetic testing for cancer risk. *Gastroenterology Clinics of North America, 26,* 19–34.

Denton, J. (1997). Inheriting an ethical dilemma. *Nursing Standard, 11,* 22–23.

Dizikes, G. J. (1997). Update on the human genome project. *Clinics of Laboratory Medicine, 17,* 973–988.

Engelking, C. (1995). Genetics in cancer care: Confronting a Pandora's box of dilemmas. *Oncology Nursing Forum, 22,* (Suppl.), 27–34.

Friderici, K. H. (1997). Molecular diagnosis for cystic fibrosis. *Clinical Laboratory Medicine, 17,* 59–72.

Geller, G. (1995). Cystic fibrosis and the pediatric caregiver: Benefits and burdens of genetic technology. *Pediatric Nursing, 21,* 57–61.

Gilbert, S. (1997, March 26). Interpreting genetic tests. *New York Times,* C8.

Glassman, A. B. (1997). Cytogenetics: An evolving role in the diagnosis and treatment cancer. *Clinics in Laboratory Medicine, 17,* 21–38.

Jacobs, D. S. (Ed.). (1996). *Laboratory test handbook.* Cleveland: Lexi-Comp.

Kadlec, J. V., & McPherson, R. A. (1997). Ethical issues in screening and testing for genetic diseases. *Clinics of Laboratory Medicine, 17,* 989–1000.

Kiechle, F. L. (1996). Diagnostic molecular pathology in the twenty-first century. *Clinics of Laboratory Medicine, 16,* 213–226.

Lea, D. H., Jenkins, J. F., & Francomano, C. A. (1998). *Genetics in clinical practice.* Boston: Jones & Bartlett Publishers.

Lehmann, C. A. (1998). *Saunders manual of clinical laboratory science.* Philadelphia: W. B. Saunders.

Loescher, L. J. (1995). Genetics in cancer prediction, screening and counseling: Part II, the nurse's role in genetic counseling. *Oncology Nursing Forum, 22,* 16–19.

Mahon, S. M., & Casperson, D. S. (1995). Hereditary cancer syndrome: Part 1—clinical and educational issues. *Oncology Nursing Forum, 22,* 763–781.

Mahon, S. M., & Casperson, D. S. (1995). Hereditary cancer syndrome: Part 2—psychosocial issues, concerns, and screening—results of a qualitative study. *Oncology Nursing Forum, 22,* 775–780.

Merjavier, S. D., & Petty, E. M. (1996). Risk assessment and pre-symptomatic molecular diagnosis in hereditary breast cancer. *Clinics in Laboratory Medicine, 16,* 139–168.

Michie, S., McDonald, V., & Marteau, T. (1996). Understanding responses to predictive genetic testing: A grounded theory approach. *Psychology and Health, 11,* 455–470.

Penticuff, J. H. (1996). Ethical dimensions in genetic screening: A look into the future. *Journal of Obstetric, Gynecologic, and Neonatal Nursing, 25,* 785–789.

Raines, D. A. (1996). Fetal surveillance: Issues and implications. *Journal of Obstetric, Gynecologic, and Neonatal Nursing, 25,* 559–563.

Robinson, K. D., Abernathy, E., & Conrad, K. J. (1996). Gene therapy of cancer. *Seminars in Oncology Nursing, 12,* 142–151.

Skirton, J. (1995). Psychological implications of advances in genetics—3 predictive studies. *Professional Nurse, 10,* 644–646.

Small, G. W., Mazziotta, J. C., Collins, M. T., Baxter, L. R., Phelps, M. E., Mandelkern, M. A., Kaplan, A., La Rue, A., Adamson, C. F., & Chang, L. (1995). Apolipoprotein E type 4 allele and cerebral glucose metabolism in relatives at risk for familial Alzheimer disease. *Journal of the American Medical Association, 273,* 942–947.

Williams, J. K. (1995). Genetics and cystic fibrosis: A focus on carrier testing. *Pediatric Nursing, 21,* 444–448.

Williams, J. K., & Lessick, M. (1996). Genome research: Implications for children. *Pediatric Nursing, 22,* 40–45.

Williams, J. K., & Schutte, D. L. (1997). Benefits and burdens of genetic carrier identification. *Western Journal of Nursing Research, 19,* 71–81.

# PART IV

# Laboratory and Diagnostic Tests of Specific Body Systems

# 14

# Pulmonary Function

In the hierarchy of human needs, oxygen ($O_2$) is the primary basic need. Humans evolved to take in $O_2$ (pulmonary system) and deliver that $O_2$ (circulatory system) to meet cellular requirements. This chapter presents the laboratory and diagnostic tests used to evaluate an individual's ability to ventilate and oxygenate the blood. Older tests, which have been replaced by advanced technology such as computed tomography (CT) and magnetic resonance imaging (MRI), are not included.

Unfortunately, multiple environmental and personal habits place individuals at risk for pulmonary disorders. The experience of dyspnea, shortness of breath, breathlessness, and cough frequently brings the individual to the primary caregiver. Because many pulmonary disorders produce the same clinical manifestations, pulmonary laboratory and diagnostic testing is required for accurate diagnosis. This chapter presents many of the tests required to evaluate the patient with a respiratory dysfunction. Chapter 7 discusses tests related to respiratory infection.

The goal of the majority of tests included in this chapter is to identify the cause of the individual's distress so that appropriate therapy and relief may be provided. These tests are also used to evaluate the effectiveness of the therapies prescribed.

## Laboratory Tests

Angiotensin-Converting Enzyme   264
Anion Gap   265
Arterial Blood Gases   266
Lactic Acid   273
Mixed Venous Blood Gases   274

## Angiotensin-Converting Enzyme

**(Serum)**          Synonyms: ACE, serum angiotensin-converting enzyme, SACE

**Normal Values**

**Adult**
**Male:** 12–36 IU/L (SI same)
**Female:** 10–30 IU/L (SI same)

## Background Information

Angiotensin-converting enzyme (ACE) is found primarily in the pulmonary epithelial cells. ACE converts angiotensin I to angiotensin II. Angiotensin II stimulates the adrenal cortex to produce and secrete the hormone aldosterone and is also a powerful vasoconstrictor. Because angiotensin II is a vasopressor, ACE levels are determined as part of the diagnostic work-up for hypertension.

ACE levels increase with sarcoidosis, a disease that causes widespread granulomatous lesions that may affect any organ, including the lungs. When sarcoidosis is suspected, ACE levels are determined to diagnose the disorder, assess its severity, and evaluate its therapy.

### Purpose of the Test

ACE levels are determined to evaluate hypertension and to diagnose and treat sarcoidosis.

### Procedure

A venipuncture is performed to collect 5 mL of blood in a red-topped tube. If a delay is expected in sending the specimen to the laboratory, place the specimen on ice.

### Findings

■

*Critical Thinking 14–1*
After SACE results have been found to be elevated, how do you explain to your patient with hypertension why an ACE inhibitor has been prescribed for him or her?

**Elevated Values**

| | | |
|---|---|---|
| Cirrhosis | Hansen's disease | Myeloma |
| Gaucher's disease (familial disorder of fat metabolism) | Histoplasmosis | Pulmonary fibrosis |
| | Hodgkin's disease | Sarcoidosis |
| | Hyperthyroidism | Scleroderma |

**Decreased Values**

| | | |
|---|---|---|
| Adult respiratory distress syndrome | Diabetes mellitus | Tuberculosis |
| | Hypothyroidism | |

### Interfering Factors

• Steroids

### Nursing Implementation

The nursing actions are similar to those for other venipuncture procedures.

## Anion Gap

**(Serum)**                    Synonyms: None

### Normal Values

3–11 mEq/L *or* SI 3–11 mmol/L
Normal values in older automated systems are 10–15 mEq/L *or* SI 10–15 mmol/L.

## Background Information

The anion gap is the sum of unmeasured anions in the serum: phosphates, sulfates, ketones, proteins, and organic acids. It is used to distinguish among causes of metabolic acidosis. The anion gap is used to determine if the metabolic acidosis is a result of the accumulation of hydrogen ions or of a loss of bicarbonate. The major determinant of the anion gap is protein. A significant decrease in plasma protein, which is composed of anions, causes a large decrease in the anion gap.

In addition to disease states that cause an increase or decrease in anions or cations, or both, in the blood, fluid volume also affects the anion gap, because it may cause hemoconcentration (higher sodium and potassium concentration) or hemodilution (dilutional hyponatremia).

| | |
|---|---|
| **Purpose of the Test** | The anion gap is calculated to determine the cause of metabolic acidosis. |

| | |
|---|---|
| **Procedure** | The anion gap is determined by subtracting the sum of measured anions (bicarbonate [$HCO_3$] and chloride [Cl]) from the measured cations (sodium [Na] and potassium [K]). |

**Findings**

■

*Critical Thinking 14–2*
Calculate your patient's anion gap when the number of $Na^+$ cations is 140, $K^+$ is 5, $HCO_3^-$ is 30, and $Cl^-$ is 100. How would you interpret this result?

**Elevated Values**

| | | |
|---|---|---|
| Hypernatremia | Hypomagnesemia | Lactic acidosis |
| Hyperosmolar coma | Ketoacidosis | Starvation |
| Hypocalcemia | | |

**Decreased Values**

| | | |
|---|---|---|
| Hypercalcemia | Hypoalbuminemia | Multiple myeloma |
| Hypermagnesemia | Hyponatremia | |

**Interfering Factors**

■

*Critical Thinking 14–3*
Your patient is in severe hypovolemic shock. You, therefore, expect the patient to be in a state of lactic acidosis. However, you calculate the anion gap, and it is 10 mEq/L. How can you explain this finding?

- Dehydration
- Ingestion of licorice
- Excessive ingestion of antacids, ethylene glycol, methanol, paraldehyde, or salicylates
- Use of medications such as adrenocorticotropic hormones, antihypertensive agents, bicarbonates, chlorpropamide, diuretics, lithium, Na penicillin, phosphates, steroids, sulfates, and vasopressin

**Nursing Implementation**

After the results of blood electrolyte determinations are obtained, calculate the anion gap during the test with the following formula:

$$(Na + K) - (HCO_3 + Cl) = anion\ gap$$

## Arterial Blood Gases

**(Arterial Blood)**      Synonym: ABGs

**Normal Values**

| | |
|---|---|
| pH | 7.35–7.45 *or* SI 7.35–7.45 |
| $Pco_2$ | 35–45 mm Hg *or* SI 4.7–5.3 kPa |
| $HCO_3$ | 21–28 mEq/L *or* SI 21–28 mmol/L |
| $Po_2$ | **Adult:** 80–100 mm Hg *or* SI 10.6–13.3 kPa |
| | **Newborn:** 60–70 mm Hg *or* SI 8.0–10.33 kPa |
| $Sao_2$ | **Adult:** >95% *or* SI fraction saturated >0.95 |
| | **Newborn:** 40%–90% *or* SI fraction saturated 0.40–0.90 |
| Base excess | ±2 mEq/L *or* SI ±2 mmol/L |

## Background Information

Arterial blood gases (ABGs) provide valuable information about the acid-base balance, ventilatory ability, and oxygenation status of the individual. The data derived from blood gas determinations support clinical assessments and are invaluable in evaluating medical treatment and nursing interventions. ABG determinations provide the pH, partial pressure of carbon dioxide ($Pco_2$), partial pressure of oxygen ($Po_2$), bicarbonate ($HCO_3$), $O_2$ saturation ($Sao_2$), and base excess levels.

The pH (the partial pressure of hydrogen [$H^+$] ions in the blood) reflects the acid-base balance of the blood. A narrow normal range of pH reflects the body's need to maintain a relatively constant internal environment. An inverse relationship exists on the pH scale between $H^+$ concentration and pH. As the $H^+$ ion concentration goes up, the pH goes down. As the $H^+$ ion concentration increases in solution, $H^+$ ions can be given up. This is *acidosis*. As the $H^+$ ion concentration decreases in solution, $H^+$ ions may be taken on ($H^+$ ion receiver). This is *alkalosis*.

The pH of human blood is normally 7.35 to 7.45, which on the pH scale of 1 to 14 is above the neutral point of 7 and is therefore slightly alkaline. In the clinical setting, however, a pH of 7.35 to 7.45 is used as the neutral state. A pH below 7.35 is acidotic, and a pH above 7.45 is alkalotic. One must remember that other body fluids have a different normal pH.

To maintain a normal pH, the body has evolved several mechanisms, including its buffering system and its respiratory and renal systems. Within seconds, the body buffers respond to changes in pH. Within minutes, the respiratory system adapts to changes in $H^+$ ion concentration, and in days, the kidneys respond to the acid-base needs of the body. These changes reflect the body's ability to compensate for deviations in the acid-base balance and the need to maintain that balance within a narrow range.

$Pco_2$ reflects the ventilatory ability of the body to maintain a normal pH. Carbon dioxide ($CO_2$) in blood travels as an acid (carbonic acid) until it dissociates in the lungs to be exhaled as $CO_2$. When the blood becomes acidotic, the respiratory system increases its rate and depth of ventilation to blow off $CO_2$ and thus reduce the acid load in the blood. If

the blood is alkalotic, the respiratory system hypoventilates to retain $CO_2$ and thus move the pH toward normal. Pathologic conditions of the pulmonary system may interfere with this normal compensatory action. If an individual cannot adequately ventilate, $CO_2$ is retained, and acidosis occurs. Because this acidosis is due to a pulmonary cause, it is called respiratory acidosis. If the lungs blow off too much $CO_2$, respiratory alkalosis occurs. Table 14–1 presents causes of respiratory acid-base imbalances and the nursing assessments for the imbalances.

The bicarbonate ion concentration in the blood ($HCO_3$) reflects the renal system's response to the acid-base balance. $HCO_3$ is made by the kidneys, and its production is increased whenever acidosis is present. However, it takes several days for the kidneys to respond fully to changes in pH. If the kidneys are unable to make $HCO_3$ to buffer the acid in the blood, the patient will be in a state of metabolic acidosis. If the patient has too much $HCO_3$ or has lost acid from the gastrointestinal or genitourinary tract, a state of metabolic alkalosis occurs (see Table 14–1 for causes of metabolic acid-base imbalances and the nursing assessments for the imbalances).

The pulmonary and renal systems are constantly balancing and adapting to maintain a normal pH. An abnormality in pH initiates a compensatory mechanism to restore the pH to normal or to achieve at least a partial compensation. For example, a patient with chronic obstructive pulmonary disease retains $CO_2$ and thus experiences respiratory acidosis. The kidneys respond to the decrease in pH and increase their production of $HCO_3$. This response results in a normal pH and high $Pco_2$ and $HCO_3$ levels (see Fig. 14–1 for the process used to assess acid-base balance). A serious clinical problem occurs with mixed acid-base imbalances, in which the patient has both respiratory and metabolic acidosis or respiratory and metabolic alkalosis, because compensation cannot take place.

The partial pressure of oxygen in the blood ($Po_2$) is the amount of $O_2$ dissolved in the plasma. $Sao_2$ is the percentage of hemoglobin saturated with $O_2$. Together, the $Po_2$ and the $Sao_2$ form the $O_2$ *content,* the total amount of $O_2$ in the blood.

When interpreting the $O_2$ levels in the blood, barometric pressure must be considered. At sea

**Table 14–1    Causes and Assessments of Acid-Base Imbalances**

| Cause | Clinical Assessment |
| --- | --- |
| *Respiratory Acidosis* | |
| Respiratory center dysfunction | Dyspnea |
|    Opiates, anesthetics, sedatives | Tachycardia |
|    Oxygen-induced hypoventilation | Headache |
|    Central nervous system lesions | Confusion |
| Disorders of the respiratory muscles or chest wall | Pallor |
|    Myasthenia gravis, amyotrophic lateral sclerosis | Diaphoresis |
|    Kyphoscoliosis | Apprehension |
|    Pickwickian syndrome | Restlessness |
|    Splinting caused by pain | Lethargy |
| Disorders of gas exchange | Drowsiness |
|    Chronic obstructive pulmonary disease | Coma |
|    Acute pulmonary edema | Hypertension |
|    Asphyxia | Papilledema |
| Hypoventilation while on a mechanical ventilator | |
| *Respiratory Alkalosis* | |
| Hyperventilation | Restlessness |
|    Atelectasis | Dizziness |
|    Severe anemia | Agitation |
|    Pulmonary emboli | Tetany |
|    Anxiety | Numbness |
| Central nervous system disorders | Tingling |
|    Brain stem dysfunction | Muscle cramps |
|    Subarachnoid hemorrhage | Seizures |
| Salicylate poisoning | Increased deep tendon reflexes |
| Hypermetabolic states | |
|    Fever | |
|    Thyrotoxicosis | |
|    Sepsis | |
| Hyperventilation while on mechanical ventilation | |
| *Metabolic Acidosis* | |
| Diabetic ketoacidosis | Lethargy |
| Lactic acidosis | Nausea |
|    Cardiac arrest | Vomiting |
|    Anaerobic metabolism | Dysrhythmias |
| Ingestion of acid | Coma |
|    Salicylates | Hypotension |
|    Ethylene | Hyperventilation |
|    Methanol | |
|    Paraldehyde | |
| Loss of bicarbonate | |
|    Diarrhea | |
|    Fistulas | |
| Renal failure | |

**Table 14–1    Causes and Assessments of Acid-Base Imbalances** (continued)

| Cause | Clinical Assessment |
|---|---|
| *Metabolic Alkalosis* | |
| Loss of acid | Dullness |
|   Vomiting | Weakness |
|   Excessive gastric suction | Dysrhythmias |
| Urine loss | Tetany |
|   Diuretics | Hypokalemia |
|   Excessive corticosteroids | Hyperactive reflexes |
|     Exogenous | |
|     Endogenous | |
| Hypokalemia | |
| $HCO_3$ overload | |
|   Excessive ingestion of $NaHCO_3$* | |
|   Massive blood transfusions | |
| Excessive ingestion of licorice | |
| Nonparathyroid hypercalcemia | |

*$NaHCO_3$ = sodium bicarbonate.

level, barometric pressure is 760 mm Hg; at 5,000 ft above sea level, barometric pressure is 630 mm Hg; thus, the norms for $Po_2$, $Sao_2$, and $O_2$ content must be adjusted. Use the normal values of the laboratory doing the testing to interpret oxygen levels.

When one assesses the patient's oxygenating ability, there may be a need to determine the ability of the $O_2$ to diffuse from the alveoli into the blood. This cannot be measured directly but can be estimated with the *alveolar-arterial* difference in partial pressure of $O_2$ ($Pao_2 - Pao_2$), also known as the *alveolar-arterial (A-a) gradient*. The A-a gradient is the difference between the alveolar $Po_2$ and the $Po_2$ in the arterial blood. It is calculated by first estimating the alveolar $Po$, which is done by subtracting the water vapor pressure from the barometric pressure, multiplying the resulting pressure by the $Fio_2$ (percentage of oxygen the patient is breathing), and subtracting this from $1\frac{1}{4}$ times the arterial $Pco_2$. To obtain the A-a gradient, the patient's arterial $Po_2$ is subtracted from the calculated alveolar $Po_2$. Thus,

A-a gradient = (barometric pressure − water vapor pressure × $Fio_2$ − $1\frac{1}{4}$ × $Paco_2$) − $Pao_2$

The normal A-a gradient is less than 20.

An a:A ratio may also be calculated. The a:A ratio is the percentage of alveolar $Po_2$ that arterial $Po_2$ represents.

a:A ratio = measured arterial $Po_2$ : calculated alveolar $Po_2$

The normal a:A ratio is greater than 0.75. The A-a gradient normally increases as the $O_2$ concentration the patient breathes increases; the a:A ratio does not. Therefore, for patients on mechanical ventilation with a changing $Fio_2$, the a:A ratio is used to determine whether oxygen diffusion is improving.

The arterial $Po_2$ and $Sao_2$ are used to assess oxygen supply available to body tissue and also allow the nurse to calculate how well oxygen is delivered to the body tissue. Two formulas are available to calculate *oxygen delivery* ($DO_2$), the absolute and the approximate $DO_2$. The absolute formula for $DO_2$ is as follows:

Cardiac output (hemoglobin × 1.34 × $Sao_2$) + ($Po_2$ × .0031) 10

The approximate formula for $DO_2$ is as follows:

Cardiac output (hemoglobin × 1.34 × $Sao_2$) 10

The 1.34 in the formula is the oxygen capacity per gram of hemoglobin. 0.0031 is the solubility coefficient of oxygen per 100 mL of blood. To convert hemoglobin from g/dL to g/L, a constant of 10 is used. To adjust for body size, an *oxygen delivery index* ($DO_2I$) may be obtained by either substituting the cardiac index for the cardiac output in the above

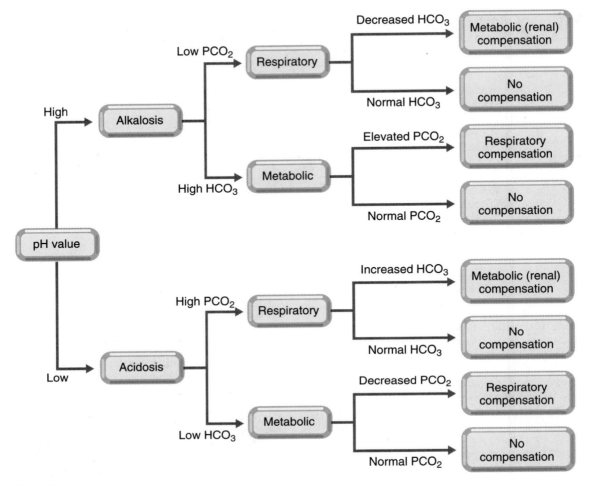

**Figure 14–1**
Evaluation of arterial blood gas results. (Reproduced with permission from Lehmann, C. A. [Ed.]. [1998]. *Saunders manual of clinical science* [p. 163]. Philadelphia: W. B. Saunders.)

formula or dividing the $DO_2$ by the patient's body surface area. The normal $DO_2$ in an adult is 800 to 1,200 mL/$O_2$/min. The normal $DO_2I$ is 520 to 720 mL/min/m². If oxygen delivery is inadequate for the body tissue needs, a greater percentage of oxygen will be extracted from the blood (see pp. 273–274 on assessing oxygen consumption).

The base excess or base deficit on the ABG determinations reflects the metabolic nonrespiratory contribution to the maintenance of normal pH. With a base excess, a positive balance greater than 2 correlates with metabolic alkalosis, and with a base deficit, a negative balance less than −2 correlates with metabolic acidosis.

**Purpose of the Test**    ABG determinations are obtained for a variety of reasons, including the diagnosis of chronic and restrictive pulmonary disease, adult respiratory failure, acid-base disturbances, pulmonary emboli, sleep disorders, central nervous system dysfunctions, and cardiovascular disorders such as congestive heart failure, shunts, and intracardiac atrial or ventricular shunts, or both.

ABG determinations are used in the management of patients on mechanical ventilators and during the weaning process from the ventilators.

## Procedure

An arterial blood sample of 5 mL is obtained via an arterial puncture or arterial line. The radial or femoral artery is usually used in adults, whereas the temporal artery is used in infants.

Continuous intra-arterial blood gas monitoring is a new technology that provides $Pao_2$, $Paco_2$, and pH levels to be displayed. In addition, derived parameters of $O_2$ saturation, bicarbonate, base excess, and total $CO_2$ content are calculated and displayed every 20 to 30 seconds. With continuous intra-arterial blood gas monitoring, a sensor is inserted into a radial or femoral artery via an 18- or 20-G arterial catheter. The tip of the sensor is advanced 1 to 2 inches beyond the tip of the catheter, so it is exposed to arterial blood that is not heparinized. The major benefit of continuous intra-arterial monitoring of blood gases is blood conservation (Szaflarski, 1996).

## Findings

Acid-base imbalances (see Table 14–1)
Hypoxia

## Interfering Factors

- Noncompliance with proper collection procedure, including air bubbles in syringe and hemolysis of sample
- Low hemoglobin level
- With continuous intra-arterial blood gas monitoring, clot formation at sensor tip, sensor lying against arterial wall, and transition periods, when a change in $Fio_2$ occurs

## Nursing Implementation

**Pretest**

Before a radial artery puncture is executed or a radial arterial line is inserted, perform an Allen test to ensure adequate collateral circulation to the hand. With the Allen test, occlude the radial and ulnar arteries with the fingertips while instructing the patient to tighten the fist (Fig. 14–2). Ask the patient to open the fist and remove pressure from the ulnar artery while maintaining pressure on the radial artery. If color returns to the palm and fingers within 5 seconds, adequate ulnar circulation exists.
Prepare ice and heparinized syringe.

*Critical Thinking 14–4*
What potential injury to a patient may occur if the Allen test is not performed before a radial artery puncture?

**Quality Control**

Excessive amounts of heparin or an air bubble in the syringe will cause inaccurate results. Draw 1 mL of heparin up into a 5- to 10-mL glass syringe or plastic syringe with vented plunger. The plunger is pulled back to coat the barrel of the syringe. Excess heparin is discarded, leaving the needle full of heparin. A 22- or 25-G needle is used.

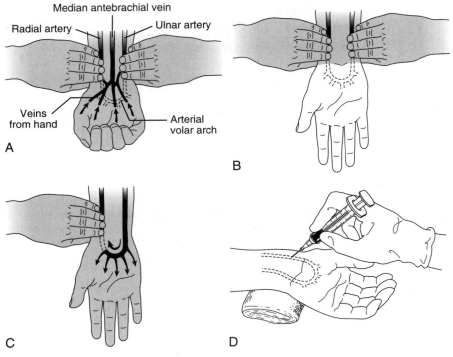

**Figure 14–2**
The Allen test.

### Quality Control

> The patient's temperature affects results because the ABG machines are calibrated using gases at 37°C. Note on the requisition slip the patient's temperature at the time the blood is drawn.

Instruct the patient about the arterial puncture; it is painful.
If the patient is anxious, hyperventilation may occur, giving false readings because $CO_2$ is blown off.
Do not obtain an ABG reading for 20 to 30 minutes after a procedure or event that does not reflect the patient's current status (e.g., suctioning).

### During the Test

Nurses in specialized units may perform arterial punctures. The procedure is usually performed by a physician or a respiratory therapist.
If a radial artery is used, the wrist is hyperextended and the arm is externally rotated.
Palpate the artery for the point of maximal impulse. Cleanse the site with an alcohol swab.
The needle is inserted at a 45- to 90-degree angle at the point of maximal pulsation.
Observe the syringe; the plunger will move upward under arterial pressure.
Withdraw the needle and cork the syringe with the airtight rubber stopper.

■
*Critical Thinking 14–5*
A patient with chronic obstructive pulmonary disease (COPD) presents with a pH of 7.34, a $P_{O_2}$ of 64, and a $P_{CO_2}$ of 68. How can the nurse plan to prevent $O_2$-induced hypoventilation in this patient?

Roll the syringe between your palms to mix the blood with the heparin.
Label the syringe and place it on ice.
Send the specimen to the laboratory immediately with a requisition slip marked with the patient's temperature, the $F_{IO_2}$ value, and the time.
Care of the continuous intra-arterial blood gas line is similar to care of any arterial line. The maximum duration of monitoring is usually 72 hours.

### Posttest

Immediately after the needle is withdrawn, exert pressure on the arterial site for a minimum of 5 minutes. If the patient is taking anticoagulants, pressure on the site should be maintained for at least 10 minutes.

**Complications**

Complications from ABG determination result from the trauma of arterial puncture. They include arterial occlusion from hematoma formation or thrombosis, bleeding, and infection (Table 14–2).

## Lactic Acid

**(Venous)**    Synonyms: Lactate, L-lactate

**Normal Values**    8.1–15.3 mEq/L *or* SI 0.9–1.7 mmol/L

### Background Information

Lactic acid levels may be used to assess cellular oxygenation. If the cells do not receive adequate oxygen, anaerobic metabolism will occur. Lactic acid is the byproduct of anaerobic metabolism. Rising lactate levels indicate a need to examine $O_2$ transport and consumption parameters.

**Purpose of the Test**    Lactate levels are used to support the diagnosis of cellular hypoxia. Lactate levels can also predict survival. High lactate levels (>4 mmol/L) indicate higher mortality rates.

| Table 14–2 | Complications of Arterial Puncture | |
|---|---|
| | **Complication** | **Nursing Assessment** |
| | Arterial occlusion | Loss of distal pulse |
| | | Distal parts: pale, cool, cyanotic |
| | Bleeding | Hematoma formation |
| | | Restlessness |
| | | Tachycardia |
| | | Hypotension |
| | Infection | Tachycardia |
| | | Fever |
| | | Elevated white blood cell count |

| | |
|---|---|
| **Procedure** | A venipuncture is performed to obtain 7 mL of blood, which is placed in a gray-topped tube. |

**Findings**

**Elevated Values**

| | | |
|---|---|---|
| Alcoholism | Liver failure | Peritonitis |
| Diabetic ketoacidosis | Malignancies | Shock states |
| Hyperthermia | | |

**Decreased Values**

Hypothermia

**Interfering Factors**

- Noncompliance with dietary and activity restrictions
- The drugs acetaminophen (large dose), ethanol (large dose), epinephrine, fructose, morphine, and sorbitol

**Nursing Implementation**

The nurse takes actions similar to those taken with other venipuncture procedures.

**Pretest**

Instruct the patient not to eat or drink for 12 hours before the test and to ingest no alcohol for 24 hours before the blood is drawn.
Instruct the patient to lie quietly for 2 hours before the blood is drawn.

**During the Test**

No tourniquet should be applied, and the patient should not clench the fist.
Send the specimen to the laboratory immediately.

■

*Critical Thinking 14–6*
When blood is drawn for a lactic acid level, why is the tourniquet omitted?

**Posttest**

Advise the patient to resume a normal diet and activity level.

## Mixed Venous Blood Gases

**(Venous)**    Synonyms: None

**Normal Values**

| | |
|---|---|
| pH | 7.33–7.43 *or* SI 7.33–7.43 |
| $Pco_2$ | 41–51 mm Hg *or* SI 5.3–6.0 kPa |
| $HCO_3^-$ | 24–28 mm Hg *or* SI 24–28 mmol/L |
| $Pvo_2$ | 35–49 mm Hg |
| $Svo_2$ | 60%–80% |

## Background Information

Mixed venous blood gases provide a method for evaluating the dynamic balance between $O_2$ supply and $O_2$ delivery to the body. Since the organs of the body use various amounts of $O_2$, mixed venous blood gases measure the blood in the pulmonary artery, which contains the venous return from all the body systems. ABGs reflect what is available for body use (supply), whereas venous blood gases tell how well the body used this supply.

With ABGs, the nurse can assess the oxygen supply available to the body tissues and determine oxygen delivery (see pp. 269–270). With mixed venous oxygen saturation ($Svo_2$), the nurse can assess oxygen consumption and whether the person has adequate venous reserves of oxygen.

*Venous reserve* is that amount of oxygen in the blood that returns to the right side of the heart after systemic circulation. If oxygen demand is greater than oxygen supply, the amount of oxygen in the returning blood decreases. This is seen at the bedside as a low $Svo_2$. The venous reserve is calculated as follows:

Cardiac output $\times$ hemoglobin $\times 1.34 \times 10$

1.34 is the oxygen capacity per gram of hemoglobin. Multiplying by 10 converts the hemoglobin units from g/dL to g/L.

Knowing the venous reserve, *oxygen consumption* ($VO_2$) can be calculated as follows:

$VO_2 = O_2$ delivery (see p. 269) $-$ venous reserve

To adjust for body size and obtain an *oxygen consumption index* ($Vo_2I$), use the following formula:

Cardiac index $\times 13.4 \times$ hemoglobin $\times$
(arterial $O_2$sat $-$ venous $O_2$sat)

The normal $Vo_2$ is 225 to 275 mL/$O_2$/min when the person is at rest. The normal $VO_2I$ is 120 to 160 mL/min/m².

Mixed venous blood gases may be obtained periodically, or the mixed venous oxygen saturation ($Svo_2$) may be monitored continuously.

$Svo_2$ monitoring has been made possible by the development of fiberoptic pulmonary catheters. It is measured by light emitted from the catheter and reflected onto red blood cells within the pulmonary artery. The wavelength of reflected light is interpreted by the $Svo_2$ computer and continuous readings of the $Svo_2$ in the blood *after* systemic circulation is provided. Because the hemoglobin normally unloads about 25% of its $O_2$ during systemic circulation, the normal $Svo_2$ is 75%, with a range of 60% to 80%.

No specific value for $Svo_2$ is correlated with anaerobic metabolism. A $Pvo_2$ of 28 mm Hg does correlate with lactic acidosis, however, and this $Pvo_2$ corresponds to an $Svo_2$ of 53%, which seems to be a critical value.

The $Svo_2$ is used to evaluate the response to nursing care. For an unstable patient, changes in position, bathing, suctioning, and so forth can increase $O_2$ consumption, resulting in a corresponding lowering of the $Svo_2$. If the $Svo_2$ falls to less than 60% or varies by 10% from the patient's baseline for longer than 3 minutes (10 minutes after suctioning), a full assessment of the patient is needed, including a cardiac output determination.

---

| | |
|---|---|
| **Purpose of the Test** | Mixed venous blood gases are obtained to assess the $O_2$ supply and tissue $O_2$ consumption. Changes in $Svo_2$ indicate a need to determine which factor in $O_2$ supply and delivery is abnormal: cardiac output, hemoglobin level, tissue $O_2$ consumption, or $Sao_2$. |

---

| | |
|---|---|
| **Procedure** | A mixed venous sample may be obtained in a heparinized syringe from the distal port of the pulmonary artery catheter, or continuous $Svo_2$ may be assessed from a fiberoptic pulmonary artery catheter attached to an oximeter. |

---

**Findings**

**Elevated Values**

$Svo_2$ OVER 80%

| | | |
|---|---|---|
| Anesthesia | Left-to-right shunt | Sepsis, early stages |
| Cyanide toxicity | Neuromuscular | Sleep |
| High $Fio_2$ | blockade | Vasodilation |
| Hypothermia | Relaxation | |

**Decreased Values**

$Svo_2$ UNDER 60%

| | | |
|---|---|---|
| Anemia | Hyperthermia | Position changes |
| Anxiety | Hypovolemia | Seizures |
| Bleeding | Inadequate $Fio_2$ | Severe pain |
| Cardiogenic shock | Large burns | Shivering |
| Congestive heart | Pain | Stress |
| failure | Pulmonary disease | Strenuous exercise |
| Fever | Multiple trauma | Suctioning |

■
*Critical Thinking 14–7*
As you turn a patient while giving a bath, the $Svo_2$ oximeter drops to 36%. What should you do?

**Interfering Factors**

• Inadequate perfusion
• Poorly positioned pulmonary artery catheter

**Nursing Implementation**

Care is based on the technique used. With a random mixed venous blood gas determination, use the procedures that follow.

**Pretest**

Explain the procedure to the patient.
Assess the hemodynamic monitoring system.
Gather the following equipment: a 3-mL syringe, two 10-mL syringes, a syringe cap, heparin, and ice.

**During the Test**

Wear gloves.
Draw up 1 mL of heparin into the 3-mL syringe and draw back to coat the barrel. Expel heparin, leaving heparin in the needle.
Attach an empty 10-mL syringe to the sampling stopcock at the distal port of the pulmonary artery catheter.
Turn the stopcock off to the infusion solution.
Aspirate 5 mL into the syringe to clear the distal line of solution. Close the stopcock to the infusion and syringe.
Remove the syringe and discard. In special situations, such as in neonates, the blood is saved and returned to the patient after the sample is drawn.
Attach the 3-mL heparinized syringe to the stopcock.
Open the stopcock to the syringe and aspirate the blood slowly.
Close the stopcock, remove the 3-mL syringe, and expel any air bubbles. Cap the syringe.
Gently roll the syringe in your hand to mix heparin and blood. Place on ice.
Attach a 10-mL syringe to the stopcock. Open the stopcock to the solution and flush to clear the stopcock of blood.
Turn solution off to the stopcock port used to obtain the sample and cap the sampling port.
Flush the line and ensure the patency of the distal port. Check the monitor for pulmonary artery waveform.
Send blood to the laboratory immediately; clearly indicate on the slip that the blood is a mixed venous sample.
Obtain and send an ABG sample, if ordered.

### Posttest

Compare ABG and mixed venous blood gas samples.

With continuous $Svo_2$ monitoring, a special pulmonary artery catheter is inserted with $Svo_2$ sampling capability.

### During the Test

Attach the $Svo_2$ port to the oximeter.

Calibrate the oximeter when the catheter is inserted and once a day while it is in the patient.

Calibration or recalibration is needed if a 4% or greater difference exists between the mixed venous sample sent to the laboratory and the $Svo_2$ reading on the oximeter.

Set alarm parameters at plus and minus 10% of the displayed $Svo_2$.

Adjust alarms as the patient's $Svo_2$ varies or when the oximeter is recalibrated.

If the intensity alarm signals, check catheter placement and patency. Check for air bubbles in the system or kinking of the catheter. Reposition the patient. Flush the catheter if needed.

Document hourly $Svo_2$ readings.

---

### Diagnostic Procedures

---

## Bronchoscopy

**(Endoscopy)**                    Synonyms: None

---

| **Normal Values** | No abnormalities visualized |
|---|---|
| | No growth in culture specimen |

---

### Background Information

Bronchoscopy is an endoscopic diagnostic procedure involving the inspection and observation of the trachea, larynx, and bronchi. Bronchoscopy is ordered when patients have unexplained pulmonary signs and symptoms or when nonspecific radiologic abnormalities exist.

A bronchoscope permits direct visualization of the tracheobronchial tree down to the subsegmental bronchi. A biopsy of lung tissue may also be performed via the bronchoscope (*transbronchial lung biopsy*). It is usually done under fluoroscopy to permit proper positioning and opening of the forceps. A *transcatheter bronchial brushing* may also be carried out to obtain a biopsy. A small brush is inserted through the bronchoscope, which is moved back and forth until cells adhere to the brush. Once the brush is removed, the cells are brushed onto slides. Most bronchoscopy is performed with a fiberoptic bronchoscope, which is flexible. To remove foreign objects lodged in the larger airways, a rigid bronchoscope is usually used.

*Bronchoalveolar lavage (BAL)* is an additional technique, which can be performed with a fiber-optic bronchoscope. It is used to diagnose and manage interstitial lung disease. It is also being used in the diagnosis of lung cancer and pulmonary infections.

| | |
|---|---|
| **Purpose of the Test** | Bronchoscopy may be performed for therapeutic or diagnostic purposes. Bronchoscopy is used diagnostically to visualize possible tumors, obstructions, secretions, bleeding sites, or foreign objects in the tracheobronchial system. It permits the collection of secretions for cytologic and bacteriologic study as well as for assessing tumors for potential resection. Tissue for lung biopsy may be obtained through the bronchoscope.<br><br>Bronchoscopy is used therapeutically to remove foreign objects from the tracheobronchial tree and to remove secretions that are obstructing the air passages. A bronchoscope may be used to fulgurate (electrodesiccate) and excise lesions. |
| **Procedure** | A rigid (metal) or flexible fiberoptic bronchoscope may be used. The rigid bronchoscope employs a hollow metallic tube with a light at its distal end. It is useful in removing secretions, in evaluating future surgical interventions, and in dilating endobronchial strictures. The rigid bronchoscope has almost been replaced by the flexible fiberoptic bronchoscope. However, the physician may prefer the metal scope under certain circumstances, such as in the case of endobronchial tumor resection, massive hemorrhage, foreign body removal, and treatment of small children.<br><br>The bronchoscope is inserted through the nose (most common) or through the mouth. The tube is inserted as the physician observes the condition of the upper airways through the eyepiece and guides the tube to the area of the lung to be evaluated (Fig. 14–3).<br><br>If BAL is desired, the tip of the fiberoptic catheter is inserted until it wedges in the respiratory tract. Several boluses of 20 mL of normal saline at body temperature are injected distal to the wedge catheter. After each bolus, the BAL fluid is aspirated. Usually approximately 50% of the fluid is aspirated. Total bolus fluid should not exceed 300 mL or 3 mL/kg of patient's body weight. |
| **Findings** | Atelectasis<br>Bleeding<br>Bronchial adenomas<br>Foreign objects<br>Infection<br>Lung cancer<br>Sarcoidosis<br>Secretions<br>Tuberculosis<br>Tumors |
| **Interfering Factors** | • Patient distress (may require general anesthesia)<br>• For BAL: Less than 25 mL specimen volume |

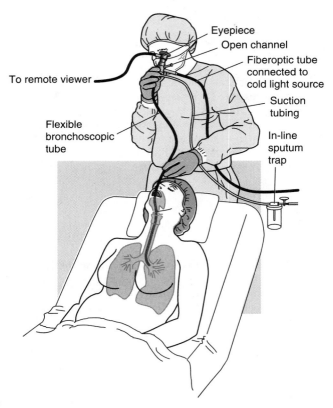

Eyepiece
Open channel
Fiberoptic tube
connected to
cold light source
To remote viewer
Suction
tubing
Flexible
bronchoscopic
tube
In-line
sputum
trap

**Figure 14–3**
Flexible fiberoptic bronchoscopy.

| **Nursing Implementation** | **Pretest** |
|---|---|

Ensure that a signed consent form has been obtained.

Assess for and report indications of hypoxia or history of asthma

Obtain a medication history to determine whether the patient is receiving anti-coagulant therapy or aspirin preparations.

If a prothrombin time (PT), a partial thromboplastin time (PTT), and a platelet count were ordered, check the results and report any clotting problems to the physician.

Instruct the patient not to eat or drink for 4 to 6 hours before the test.

Explain the purpose of and procedure for the test.

Warn the patient that the local anesthetic may taste bitter.

Inform the patient that as the tube is inserted it may feel like something is caught in the throat; provide reassurance that the airway is not blocked.

Record baseline vital signs.

Administer atropine as prescribed to reduce tracheobronchial secretions and inhibit vagal stimulation. A sedative, such as midazolam hydrochloride (Versed), may also be ordered and given. Codeine may be ordered and administered to decrease the cough reflex.

■

*Critical Thinking 14–8*
A bronchoscopy is planned for a patient who expresses anxiety about the procedure. How can you help the patient?

### During the Test

The patient is positioned in the semi-Fowler or Fowler's position.
Attach the pulse oximeter to the patient.
Provide the patient with emotional support.
To ensure patient comfort, a continuous infusion of diazepam is usually maintained.
A local anesthetic is sprayed onto the pharynx, and the solution is dropped onto the vocal cords, epiglottis, and trachea to abolish the gag reflex.
Encourage the patient to breathe through the nose or to pant.
Maintain supplemental $O_2$ for nonintubated patients.
Continuously monitor the patient's response, vital signs, and $Sao_2$.

### Posttest

■

*Critical Thinking 14–9*
Following a bronchoscopy, you note that the patient's larynx is shifting from the middle of the neck to the left side. Breath sounds are heard over the left lung fields, but sound is muted on the right side. What is your priority action at this time?

Assess vital signs.
Withhold food and fluids until the gag reflex returns.
Reassure the patient that hoarseness, sore throat, and blood-streaked sputum are common.
Provide throat lozenges or throat sprays as comfort measures.
Instruct the patient to expectorate rather than swallow saliva, because it may contain the local anesthetic.
If a biopsy or bronchoalveolar lavage has been performed, send the specimen to the histology laboratory and the microbiology laboratory.

| **Complications** | Complications are rare but include bleeding, drug reactions, hypotension, laryngospasm, bronchospasm, hypoxia, dysrhythmia, and cardiopulmonary arrest (Table 14–3). |

## Capnogram

Synonyms: Exhaled carbon dioxide, capnography, end-tidal carbon dioxide, $ETco_2$, $PETco_2$

| **Normal Values** | 35–45 mm Hg |

### Background Information

Capnography provides a $CO_2$ waveform, which visualizes a $CO_2$ elimination pattern during exhalation and a total percentage of $CO_2$ exhaled per breath.

$CO_2$ is measured at the end of exhalation, because at this point the exhaled $CO_2$ approximates arterial $CO_2$ levels. With normal perfusion of the lungs, arterial $CO_2$ will be a few millimeters higher (5 mm Hg) than end-tidal $CO_2$ ($ETco_2$). When perfusion is not adequate, this assumption cannot be made. Figure 14–4 shows a typical tracing of a capnogram.

The $ETco_2$ increases in hypermetabolic states, which increase the production of $CO_2$, and in hypoventilation, in which $CO_2$ is not excreted. The $ETco_2$ decreases when the metabolic rate is reduced, as production of $CO_2$ decreases, and when there is reduced perfusion, causing a decrease in pulmonary blood flow.

**Table 14–3   Complications of Bronchoscopy**

| Complication | Nursing Assessment |
| --- | --- |
| Bleeding | Hemoptysis |
| | Restlessness |
| | Hypotension |
| | Tachycardia |
| | Tension pneumothorax |
| Hypoxia | Low $Sao_2$ |
| | Restlessness |
| | Pallor, cyanosis |
| | Dyspnea |
| | Confusion |
| | Dysrhythmias |
| Bronchospasm | Wheeze |
| | Hypoxia |
| Laryngospasm | Stridor |
| Dysrhythmia | Abnormal electrocardiogram |
| Pneumothorax | Apprehension |
| (dependent on size | Feeling of tightness in chest |
| of pneumothorax) | Decreased or absent breath sounds over site |
| | Dyspnea |
| | Cough |
| | Depressed chest movement on affected side |
| | With a tension pneumothorax: mediastinal shift to unaffected side |

**Purpose of the Test**

Monitoring exhaled $CO_2$ permits continuous evaluation of alveolar ventilation, reducing the number of ABG determinations needed. $ETco_2$ may be used to evaluate ventilator changes and weaning parameters from mechanical ventilation. Although it is used for weaning patients from mechanical ventilators, capnography has not been shown to shorten the time of extubation or the number of ABG determinations done during the weaning process (Drew, 1998). It will confirm endotracheal intubation, because no capnographic waveform

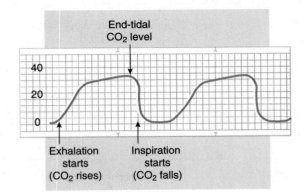

**Figure 14–4**

Capnographic tracing. On exhalation, the capnographic tracing shows a rapid rise in carbon dioxide followed by a plateau. At the end of exhalation, the end-tidal carbon dioxide level is obtained. As inspiration begins, there is a dramatic decrease in carbon dioxide.

will occur if the tube is in the esophagus. $ETco_2$ is also used to assess the adequacy of cardiopulmonary resuscitation.

Normally, $ETco_2$ closely approximates $Paco_2$; however, the nurse cannot assume that the patient has normal pulmonary function or physiology. To determine if a difference does exist, the nurse can calculate the gradient difference between the $Paco_2$ and the $ETco_2$, abbreviated $Pa\text{-}ETco_2$. The normal $Pa\text{-}ETco_2$ is 2 to 6 mm Hg. In critically ill patients, capnography can be used if the $Pa\text{-}ETco_2$ is abnormal but stable.

## Procedure

Exhaled $CO_2$ is measured with exhaled gas analyzers. These analyzers measure the $CO_2$ by mass spectrometry or infrared analysis. Mass spectrometry requires aspiration of exhaled gas, whereas the infrared gas analyzer is usually attached to the exhalation tubing on a ventilator. The recorded value refers to the amount of infrared light absorbed by the exhaled breath. The higher the $CO_2$ level, the more infrared light absorbed and the higher the reading.

## Findings

**Elevated Values**

| | | |
|---|---|---|
| Burns | Malignant hyper- | Multiple trauma |
| Hypermetabolic states | thermia | |
| Hypoventilation | | |

**Decreased Values**

| | | |
|---|---|---|
| Acute cardiac failure | Dislodgment of the | Hypovolemia |
| Anesthesia | endotracheal tube | Mucous plug |
| Bronchial spasms | Hypothermia | Pulmonary edema |
| Cardiac and pulmo- | Hypothyroidism | Pulmonary embolism |
| nary arrest | | |

## Interfering Factors

- Cardiopulmonary abnormalities
- Leak in system
- Metabolic disorders

## Nursing Implementation

■
*Critical Thinking 14–10*
The capnographic waveform disappears. What immediate nursing assessments would be appropriate?

**During the Test**

Check the capnographic waveform. It should return to zero baseline on inspiration. If it does not, check the seal of the expiratory demand valve on the ventilator and the fresh gas flow in the tube.

If the waveform disappears or drops to zero, it may indicate accidental extubation, obstruction, esophageal intubation, or cardiac arrest.

## Computed Tomography of the Chest

**(Tomography)**    Synonyms: Chest CT, CT scan of the chest

## Normal Values

No abnormalities noted

## Background Information

Computed tomographic (CT) scans are used to diagnose pulmonary lesions (benign or cancerous). They can detect primary and metastatic processes. With some bronchogenic cancers, CT scanning can be used to determine the invasive extent of the cancerous process into the chest wall, diaphragm, or mediastinum as well as extrathoracic metastasis. CT scans are used to plan radiation therapy for the patient with cancer of the lung.

CT scans can be performed with or without contrast dyes. Vascular problems such as arteriovenous malformations, central pulmonary emboli, and septic emboli may be identified with CT scanning when a contrast agent is used. With orally ingested dyes, esophageal lesions can be evaluated.

To obtain superior visualization of the bronchi, blood vessels, interstitial connective tissue, and air spaces, Novelline (1997) recommends high-resolution CT (HRCT).

CT scanning may be helpful in diagnosing silicosis, asbestosis, lung abscesses, and empyema. (See Chapter 12 for a complete discussion of CT scanning.)

## Lung Biopsy

(Pathology)     Synonym: Pulmonary biopsy

| **Normal Values** | Normal tissue |
|---|---|

## Background Information

A lung biopsy is performed to remove lung tissue so that the cells may be examined microscopically for pathologic features. A variety of methods are used to obtain these lung cells. Tissue samples may be obtained by bronchoscopy (see pp. 277–280), by fine needle biopsy (see pp. 289–291), or by open biopsy.

With an open biopsy, surgery is required, with its potential risks. It involves the resection of a small portion of tissue, which is sent to the laboratory for histologic examination.

| **Purpose of the Test** | A lung biopsy is performed to diagnose pulmonary disorders such as cancer and sarcoidosis. Lung biopsy can confirm the diagnosis of fibrosis and degenerative or inflammatory diseases of the lung. |
|---|---|
| **Procedure** | For an open biopsy of the lung, a thoracotomy is required, which is a surgical procedure. After a small incision is made in the chest wall, the lung is exposed and tissue is excised. A chest tube or tubes are inserted to restore negative pleural pressure. |
| **Findings** | Carcinomas<br>Granulomas<br>Infections<br>Sarcoidosis |
| **Interfering Factors** | • Noncompliance with dietary restrictions<br>• Smoking<br>• Obesity |

| | |
|---|---|
| **Nursing Implementation** | Follow hospital protocol for the preoperative and postoperative care of a patient requiring a thoracotomy. |
| **Complications** | Potential complications of an open lung biopsy are bleeding, pneumothorax, and empyema (Table 14–4). |

## Lung Scans

| | |
|---|---|
| **(Radiography)** | Synonyms: Ventilation scan, perfusion scan, ventilation-perfusion scan, V̇/Q̇ scan, ventilation-perfusion scintiphotography |
| **Normal Values** | Normal ventilation and perfusion<br>Ventilation-perfusion ratio of 0.85 or greater |

### Background Information

For adequate oxygenation, the lungs must receive adequate alveolar ventilation and blood flow to the ventilated alveoli. Thus, two types of lung scans exist: a *ventilation scan* and a *perfusion scan*. Ventilation scans are performed to evaluate the distribution of gas within the lungs. The patient inhales a radioactive gas, and a scanner records the distribution of the gas as it enters and leaves the lungs. Perfusion scans evaluate arterial pulmonary blood flow. A radioactive dye is given intravenously, and a scintillation camera records the distribution of the dye as it

passes through the right side of the heart to the pulmonary arterial bed.

Ventilation and perfusion scans (V̇/Q̇ scans) may be performed together so that they can be compared to identify mismatching of ventilation and perfusion. V̇/Q̇ scans are most often ordered to confirm the diagnosis of pulmonary emboli. The diagnosis of pulmonary emboli is difficult to confirm. Clinically, pulmonary emboli may be suspected because of chest pain, dyspnea, and hemoptysis, but pulmonary emboli are associated with other pulmo-

**Table 14–4  Complications of Open Lung Biopsy**

| Complication | Nursing Assessment |
|---|---|
| Bleeding | Tension pneumothorax |
| | Restlessness |
| | Tachycardia |
| | Hypotension |
| Pneumothorax | Dyspnea |
| | Tachypnea |
| | Decreased breath sounds |
| | Anxiety |
| | Restlessness |
| Empyema | Fever |
| | Tachycardia |
| | Malaise |
| | Elevated white blood cell count |

nary and cardiac disorders, which makes the diagnosis difficult to confirm. Although pulmonary angiography is the most specific diagnostic tool for pulmonary emboli, it is invasive. A V̇/Q̇ scan is less invasive and therefore less dangerous. It permits an evaluation of V̇/Q̇ mismatching. Figure 14–5 demonstrates how alveolar-capillary blood flow must interface for adequate oxygenation.

When the radioactively tagged albumin is given intravenously, it circulates through the pulmonary vasculature. If a pulmonary artery is occluded, the part of the lung served by that vessel does not "take up" the radioisotope, and the scan is positive. The scan can verify a pulmonary occlusion. It cannot verify that the tissue is necrotic (pulmonary infarction). With the ventilation scan, decreased areas of ventilation are lighter, indicating poorly ventilated lung tissue.

Various quantitative algorithms have been developed to improve interpretation of lung scans; however, clinical assessment (Henry, Gottschalk, & Leeper, 1996) and the experience of the observer of the scans (Klingensmith, 1996) provide the best reliability.

**Purpose of the Test**

Ventilation studies may be performed to evaluate patients with decreased pulmonary function. V̇/Q̇ scans are usually carried out to diagnose pulmonary emboli.

**Procedure**

With a ventilation scan, xenon 133, xenon 127, or krypton 81m is given via inhalation. Multiple scans are taken during (1) washin, as the radioactive gas builds up in the lung; (2) equilibrium, as the gas reaches its plateau within the lung; and (3) washout, as the radioactive gas is exhaled (Fig. 14–6).

For a perfusion scan, serum albumin is tagged with a radioisotope and given intravenously. As the tagged albumin passes through the right side of the heart into the pulmonary artery, a radiation detector scan of the lungs shows

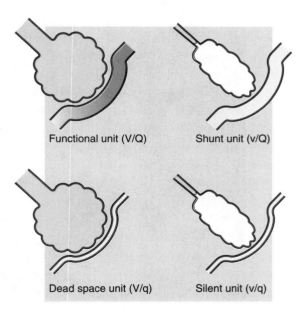

**Figure 14–5**
Alveolar-capillary interface. V = ventilated unit; Q = perfused unit; v = unventilated unit; q = unperfused unit.

Functional unit (V/Q)    Shunt unit (v/Q)

Dead space unit (V/q)    Silent unit (v/q)

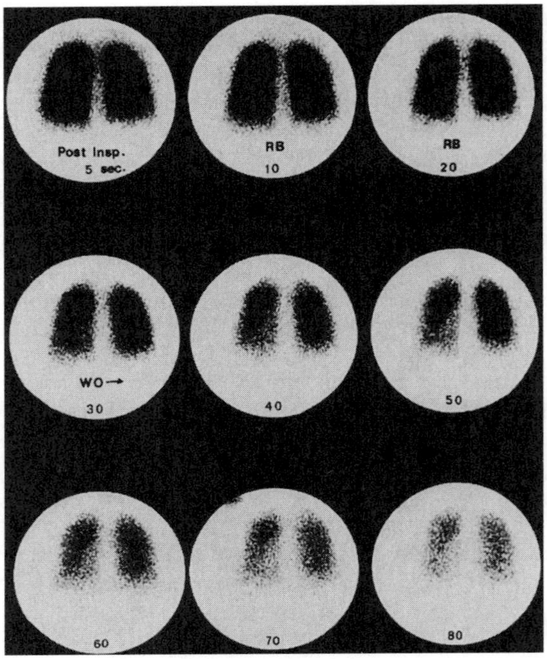

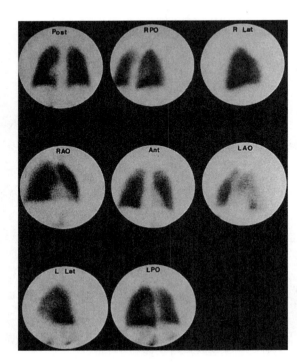

**Figure 14–6**
Normal ventilation lung scan. These are images of the lungs made from the patient's back. The patient inhales radioactive gas and rebreathes it for several seconds (RB), then additional images are made as the radioactive gas is allowed to wash out (WO) of the lungs for 30 to 80 seconds. (Reproduced with permission from Mettler, F. A., Jr. [1996]. *Essentials of radiology* [p. 137]. Philadelphia: W. B. Saunders.)

**Figure 14–7**
Normal perfusion lung scan. This nuclear medicine study is performed by intravenously injecting numerous very tiny particles that lodge in the pulmonary capillary bed, then obtaining perfusion images of the lungs in various projections. (Reproduced with permission from Mettler, F. A., Jr. [1996]. *Essentials of radiology* [p. 138]. Philadelphia: W. B. Saunders.)

the diffusion of the radioactive albumin throughout the pulmonary vessels (Fig. 14–7).

| | |
|---|---|
| **Findings** | Pulmonary vascular occlusion resulting from the following: |

Thrombus
Cysts
Abscesses
Carcinomas
Necrotizing pneumonia

Inadequate ventilation resulting from the following:

Atelectasis
Chronic obstructive pulmonary disease
Adult respiratory distress syndrome
Retained secretions
Pleural effusion
Pneumonia
Pneumothorax

| | |
|---|---|
| **Interfering Factors** | • Uncooperative patient |

**Nursing Implementation**

### Pretest

Inform the patient about the procedure and ensure patient cooperation.
Explain to the patient that the ventilation scan must be performed in the nuclear medicine department. Some hospitals have portable perfusion scanners.
Advise the patient that with the ventilation scan the inhaled gas should be held in the lungs for 20 seconds when the patient is instructed to do so.
Schedule other radionuclide tests for 24 to 48 hours after the perfusion scan.

### During the Test

Maintain the patient in an upright position for the ventilation scan. This position is maintained for at least 15 minutes.
If the patient is unable to maintain the upright position, a supine position may be used with the gamma camera underneath the patient.
After the radioactive gas is inhaled, encourage the patient to hold the breath for 20 seconds.
Radiolabeled albumin is given to the patient intravenously.
Six different views of the chest are obtained: anterior, posterior, right and left lateral, and right and left oblique.

## Magnetic Resonance Imaging of the Chest

**(Tomography)** Synonym: MRI of the chest

## Background Information

MRI of the chest is performed for cardiac, vascular, and neck imaging; however, its use for pulmonary evaluation is limited, as CT scanning is usually more precise. It has proved useful in imaging recurring tumors in the chest wall or pleural space after a pneumonectomy. MRI may also establish the diagnosis of arteriovenous malformation. (See Chapter 12 for a full discussion of MRI.)

Before MRI of the chest is performed, the patient is assessed for the presence of a permanent pacemaker. Cardiac pacemakers are considered a contraindication for MRI because they frequently contain ferromagnetic material and a magnetically activated relay switch. In addition, pacemaker leads may act as antennae, inducing electric current.

## Mediastinoscopy

**(Endoscopy)**          Synonyms: None

| **Normal Values** | No pathologic cells |
|---|---|

## Background Information

Mediastinoscopy is a surgical invasive procedure in which the mediastinum is entered to determine whether cancer has invaded the mediastinum or its lymph nodes. The procedure involves the insertion of an endoscope into the mediastinum, permitting visualization of the lymph nodes and biopsy of mediastinal nodes and tissue.

| **Purpose of the Test** | Mediastinoscopy is performed to determine invasion by lung cancer into the mediastinum; this determination can be used to "stage" lung cancer. Staging assists in determining appropriate treatment modalities. Mediastinoscopy may also be performed for diagnosing suspected granulomatous infections and other intrathoracic diseases, including sarcoidosis. |
|---|---|
| **Procedure** | With the patient under general anesthesia, a small incision is made over the suprasternal fossa, and a mediastinoscope is gently inserted. The mediastinum, with its lymph nodes, is visualized; it may be photographed and tissue samples removed. |
| **Findings** | Bronchogenic carcinoma<br>Esophageal cancer<br>Granulomatous infections<br>Lymphomas<br>Sarcoidosis |
| **Interfering Factors** | • Noncompliance with dietary restrictions<br>• Phenytoin hypersensitivity (may cause false-positive cytologic findings) |

**Nursing Implementation**

The nurse takes actions similar to those for thoracic surgery.

### Pretest

Reassure the patient, who is usually fearful of the outcome.
Explain the procedure to the patient.
Ensure that an informed consent form has been obtained.
Instruct the patient not to eat or drink after midnight.
Perform preoperative care according to hospital protocol.

### Posttest

Take vital signs every 15 minutes until they are stable and then every 4 hours for 24 hours.
Check the dressing to observe for bleeding or drainage.
Reassure the patient that chest discomfort is temporary.
Advise the patient to resume normal activities and diet when he or she has fully recovered from the anesthesia.

**Complications**

Complications are rare but include accidental puncture of the esophagus, the trachea, or a blood vessel.

## Percutaneous Needle Biopsy of the Lung

(Tomography)

Synonyms: PNB of the lung, fine needle biopsy of the lung, FNB of the lung, transthoracic needle biopsy

**Normal Values**

Normal tissue

### Background Information

Percutaneous needle biopsy of the lung has been made possible by the use of fluoroscopy and CT guidance. Intrathoracic lesions, especially of the lung parenchyma, can usually be visualized by bi-plane or C arm fluoroscopy technique. For small intrathoracic tumors or those located in the hilar or mediastinal area, a CT scan is used to guide the biopsy.

**Purpose of the Test**

A percutaneous needle biopsy of the lung is performed to determine the pathology of a lung lesion such as cancer, granuloma, infection, and sarcoidosis. It is used for staging of malignant tumors. Percutaneous needle biopsy is also indicated for diagnosis of mediastinal masses.

**Procedure**

Under the guidance of CT scanning or fluoroscopy, a biopsy needle is inserted into a lesion and a specimen is aspirated for histologic examination.

| | |
|---|---|
| **Findings** | Carcinomas |
| | Granulomas |
| | Infections |
| | Sarcoidosis |

**Nursing Implementation**

■

*Critical Thinking 14–11*
If your patient has a pulmonary artery catheter in place, what measurements would indicate pulmonary hypertension and therefore would be a contraindication to a percutaneous needle biopsy of the lung?

### Pretest

The patient is kept on nothing-by-mouth status for 4 hours before the procedure, but may take medications (except aspirin and anticoagulants).

Take and record baseline vital signs.

Assess the patient for bleeding disorders, because the needle path may be close to major vessels.

Instruct the patient about the procedure and the need to remain still and not cough when instructed not to move. Practice with the patient holding breath on command.

Assess the patient's history for contraindications to percutaneous needle biopsy: pulmonary hypertension, severe chronic obstructive lung disease, or arteriovenous malformation.

Warn the patient that minor discomfort may be experienced during the biopsy and that multiple biopsies may be necessary.

Ensure that an informed consent form is signed.

Transport the patient to the CT laboratory; if fluoroscopy is planned, bring the patient to the radiology department.

### During the Test

The patient is positioned according to the location of the lesion.

The skin is marked as a guide for needle insertion.

Apply pulse oximeter.

Check vital signs.

Have oxygen available in case a pneumothorax occurs.

Remind the patient not to cough or take deep breaths.

Skin preparation is carried out, and the area is draped.

A local anesthetic is given before the skin is nicked with a scalpel.

The biopsy needle is inserted, and samples are taken.

During insertion of the needle and any needle manipulation and biopsy, the patient is instructed to hold his or her breath and not move.

A pathologist may be present to prepare slides from the aspirated specimen. If a pathologist is not present, send the specimen in fixative to the laboratory.

Special techniques may be required depending on studies being done. Check with the physician for desired media.

### Posttest

Record vital signs every 15 minutes during the first hour.

Position the patient with the biopsy side down.

Observe the patient for a minimum of 2 hours.

Instruct the patient to avoid coughing and limit talking for 2 hours.

A chest x-ray study is usually ordered immediately after the procedure and again 2 hours later to identify any pneumothoraces.

Patients with small pneumothoraces (10% or less) are usually discharged (Mason & Templeton, 1996). If a significant pneumothorax occurs, the patient is admitted to the hospital.

Instruct the patient being discharged to rest at home, limit activities for the rest of the day, and return to the hospital if chest pain or discomfort or shortness of breath is experienced.

| Complications | The complications of percutaneous needle biopsy are pneumothorax, hemorrhage, bile leak, infection, and seeding of tumor cells (Table 14–5). |
|---|---|

## Pulmonary Angiography

(Radiology)

Synonym: Pulmonary arteriography

| Normal Values | Pulmonary vessels fill quickly and symmetrically, with no filling defects, narrowing, or obstruction. |
|---|---|

### Background Information

Pulmonary angiography is an invasive diagnostic procedure in which radiocontrast medium is injected into the pulmonary artery or its branches to visualize the pulmonary vascular bed. It is usually performed when a pulmonary embolism is suspected and other, less invasive procedures cannot exclude or confirm the diagnosis.

Risks are involved with pulmonary angiography; however, most of the problems are manageable, such as dysrhythmias, an allergic response to the contrast medium, and infection of the venous access site. Although there is no absolute contraindication for pulmonary angiography, certain conditions may require adaptations of the technique

**Table 14–5    Complications of Percutaneous Needle Biopsy of the Lung**

| Complication | Nursing Assessment |
|---|---|
| Pneumothorax | Dyspnea, shortness of breath |
| | Anxiety, restlessness |
| | Tachycardia, tachypnea |
| | Diminished breath sounds |
| | Pallor |
| Hemorrhage | Restlessness |
| | Cool, pale skin |
| | Tachycardia |
| | Hypotension |
| | Oliguria |
| Bile leak | Abdominal pain |
| | Nausea and vomiting |
| Infection | Tachycardia |
| | Fever, malaise |
| | Elevated white blood cell count |

used. These conditions include systemic anticoagulation, pregnancy, an uncooperative patient, severe hypoxia, pulmonary hypertension, right-sided endocarditis (risk of dislodging vegetation), left bundle branch block (risk of complete heart block), and amiodarone pulmonary toxicity.

## Purpose of the Test

Pulmonary angiography is used primarily to confirm the diagnosis of pulmonary embolism. It may be performed to diagnose congenital or acquired abnormalities of pulmonary vasculature.

## Procedure

The procedure is performed in an angiography laboratory in which cardiac monitoring equipment and emergency equipment are available. With the patient supine, a catheter is inserted via the antecubital or femoral vein into the right or left pulmonary artery, or both (the decision is based on previous testing). Multiple films are taken after the dye is administered through the catheter.

Additional imaging techniques are available in some laboratories and may be part of the angiography. These techniques include high-resolution cineangiography, balloon occlusion angiography, and *digital subtraction angiography*. Cineangiography has the advantage of delineating flow and motion and helping to distinguish questionable filling defects and overlapping structures. Balloon occlusion angiography involves occlusion of the pulmonary artery with a balloon catheter. A smaller amount of contrast dye is needed with balloon occlusion angiography, which permits excellent opacification. Digital subtraction angiography allows dye to be inserted into the superior vena cava or right atrium; thus, the procedure is less invasive.

## Findings

Pulmonary embolism
Pulmonary artery stenosis
Pulmonary arteriovenous fistula

## Interfering Factors

- Uncooperative patient
- Noncompliance with dietary restrictions

## Nursing Implementation

### Pretest

Perform and document baseline assessments.
Ensure that informed consent has been obtained.
Instruct the patient about the procedure.
Check blood test results for PT, PTT, and platelet determinations. If the patient is taking anticoagulants, the test is usually performed with the antecubital approach.
Check for a history of allergic reaction to contrast dyes or shellfish.
Maintain adequate hydration. A peripheral intravenous line is usually inserted.
Instruct the patient not to eat or drink, except for sips of water, for 4 to 6 hours before the procedure.
If a femoral vein is to be used as the access site, shave the area if necessary.

Ensure that a baseline electrocardiogram and electrolyte, blood urea nitrogen, creatinine, and ABG determinations are performed, that the results are in the patient's chart, and that abnormalities are reported.

Warn the patient that a warm, flushed, or nauseous feeling may ensue when the dye is injected but that this feeling passes quickly.

### During the Test

The patient is awake and will need reassurance and explanations during the procedure.

Place the patient on a cardiac monitor and observe cardiac rhythm during the procedure.

Position the patient in the supine position. The site of venous entry is exposed, and the patient is draped.

After a local anesthetic is given, right heart catheterization is performed under electrocardiographic monitoring and intermittent fluoroscopy.

As the catheter is inserted, record pressure readings and cardiac output.

Warm contrast dye to body temperature.

Reassure the patient that any discomfort felt when the dye is administered is temporary.

Monitor the patient for complications related to the dye (allergic reaction, anaphylaxis, bronchospasms) or to catheterization (dysrhythmias, cardiac perforation).

### Posttest

Maintain the patient on bedrest for 2 to 4 hours. Keep the patient warm.

Apply pressure to the site for a minimum of 5 minutes. Check the venous access site for hemostasis, and assess distal pulses.

Observe the patient for complications.

| | |
|---|---|
| **Complications** | Complications following pulmonary angiography are bleeding and arterial occlusion. In addition, observe for hypotension caused by osmotic diuresis and a delayed allergic reaction to the dye. |

## Pulmonary Function Studies

**(Spirometry)**                     Synonyms: None

| | |
|---|---|
| **Normal Values** | **ADULT (70-kg man; values are 20% to 25% lower in women)** |

**ADULT (70-kg man; values are 20% to 25% lower in women)**

| | |
|---|---|
| Tidal volume (Vt) | 500 mL |
| Inspiratory reserve volume (IRV) | 3,100 mL |
| Expiratory reserve volume (ERV) | 1,200 mL |
| Residual volume (RV) | 1,200 mL |
| Vital capacity (VC) | 4,800 mL |
| Inspiratory capacity (IC) | 3,600 mL |
| Functional residual capacity (FRC) | 2,400 mL |
| Total lung capacity (TLC) | 6,000 mL |
| $FEV_1$ | 84% |
| $FEV_2$ | 94% |
| $FEV_3$ | 97% |

## Background Information

Spirometry is a method of measuring the volume of gas that moves into and out of the lungs. The patient breathes through a tube connected to the spirograph, which records on a moving sheet of paper the volume of gas displaced in the spirometer. Two or more volumes form a pulmonary capacity (Fig. 14–8).

The pulmonary volumes consist of the tidal volume (Vt), inspiratory reserve volume (IRV), expiratory reserve volume (ERV), and residual volume (RV).

The Vt, the normal volume of air inhaled or exhaled during a single breath in a resting state, is normally 5 to 7 mL/kg body weight. *Minute volume (MV)* is obtained by multiplying the Vt by the respiratory rate.

The IRV is the amount of air that can be inspired over and above the inspired Vt. The ERV is the air remaining in the lungs, which can be expelled after a normal exhalation. The RV is the amount of air remaining in the lungs that cannot be forcibly expelled.

Pulmonary capacities consist of vital capacity (VC), inspiratory capacity (IC), functional residual capacity (FRC), and total lung capacity (TLC).

The VC is the amount of air that can be expelled from the lungs after a maximum inspiration: VC = Vt + IRV + ERV. A timed VC expresses the volume of air expelled forcibly over a certain amount of time. This *forced expiratory volume (FEV)* provides an index of pulmonary function. It is

the amount of gas exhaled over a given period. It is reported with a subscript to indicate time in seconds. The $FEV_1$ is the amount of air expelled in the first second of forced exhalation after a maximal inspiration. $FEV_2$ refers to the amount of air expelled in the first 2 seconds, and $FEV_3$ is the amount of air expelled in 3 seconds. FEV is reported as a percentage of the *forced vital capacity (FVC)*.

In cases of obstructive and restrictive lung disease, $FEV_1$ decreases. With obstructive lung disease, this decrease in $FEV_1$ is due to increased resistance to outflow. With restrictive lung disease, the decrease in $FEV_1$ is due to a decreased ability to inhale an adequate volume of air. Therefore, with restrictive lung disease, an $FEV_1$-to-FVC ratio is a more accurate parameter for evaluating patient status and treatment.

In addition to FEV, the average rate of flow for a specific segment of the FVC may be measured while the FVC is being assessed. The segment measured is usually between 25% and 75% of the FVC. Previously called the *maximum midexpiratory flow rate (MMEF)*, it is now called *forced expiratory flow* $(FEF_{25\%-75\%})$. The $FEF_{25\%-75\%}$ is the mean rate of expiratory air flow between 25% and 75% of the FVC.

The inspiratory capacity (IC) is the maximal amount of air that can be inspired: IC = Vt + IRV. The functional residual capacity (FRC) is the amount of air left in the lungs after a normal resting exhalation: FRC = ERV + RV. The total lung capacity

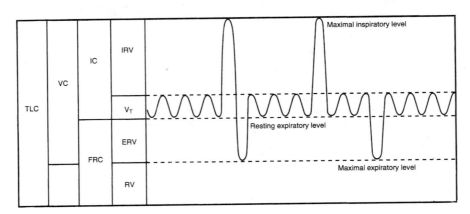

### Figure 14–8
Pulmonary volumes and capacities.

(TLC) is the amount of air in the lungs after a maximal inspiration: TLC = Vt + IRV + ERV + RV.

In addition to the volumes and capacities, a *maximum voluntary ventilation (MVV)* may or may not be determined. The MVV is the total amount of air that is moved into and out of the respiratory tract over 12 seconds with the patient's maximum effort to breathe quickly and deeply. The result is multiplied by 5 and expressed in liters per minute. It is sometimes called *maximum breathing capacity.*

An estimated volume of pulmonary function is called *dead space volume (Vds).* The Vds is that portion of inhaled air or gas that does not take part in gas exchange. It is made up of the anatomic dead space (Vd) (area from the nose and mouth to the terminal bronchioles) and alveolar Vd (areas of the lungs that are not perfused). Physiologic Vd consists of the anatomic Vd and the alveolar Vd. Normally, no measurable alveolar Vd exists. However, anatomic Vd usually is 1 mL of Vd per pound of body weight or 2 mL of Vd per kilogram of ideal body weight. The alveolar Vd increases with pathologic states that decrease blood flow to the lungs.

Pulmonary volumes may also be used to assess alveolar ventilation. *Alveolar ventilation* is estimated by taking the Vt and subtracting the Vds (Vt − Vds).

Varied measurements of the work of breathing can be obtained with pulmonary function studies, including the assessment of respiratory muscle strength. These measurements include the *Pimax test, Pdimax test, sniff test,* and *Pemax test.* The Pimax test involves measuring the intrathoracic pressure while the patient attempts to inspire as forcibly as possible against an occluded airway after a maximal exhalation. The Pdimax test measures transdiaphragmatic pressure (Pdi) while the patient tries to inspire as forcibly as possible against an occluded airway after a maximal exhalation. The sniff test is similar to the Pimax and Pdimax tests, only instead of attempting to inspire, the patient attempts a forceful maximal sniff. The Pemax test is measured while the patient attempts to forcibly exhale against an occluded airway after a maximal inspiration (Cherniack, 1992).

A challenge or provocation test is included as part of the pulmonary function studies in patients with suspected hypersensitivities of the airways. *Bronchial provocation tests* or *bronchial challenge tests* are performed as part of the pulmonary function studies for patients who have symptoms suggestive of asthma but who do not show evidence of air flow limitations. They may also be used to assess airway function over time and to evaluate various therapeutic interventions. The provocation tests are contraindicated for anyone whose baseline FEV is less than 1.5 L, who has a history of severe responses to identifiable antigens, or who has had a viral infection of the upper airway within 8 weeks before the test.

Various substances can be used in the provocation test. Inhalation challenges are performed with methacholine or histamine. The *methacholine challenge test* and the *histamine challenge test* use nonspecific agents, which are usually administered with a nebulizer. Specific agents may also be given by inhalation. These specific antigens are given in varying concentrations. When indicated, the patient may be exposed to occupational inhalants through inhalation.

Instead of inhalational stimulants, oral challenges may be given, but these take several hours or days. Substances ingested are acetylsalicylic acid (aspirin), tartrazine, sodium salicylate, metabisulfite, and monosodium glutamate.

An *exercise challenge* may be used to induce bronchospasms, which are characteristic of hyperresponsive airways when they occur after short-term exercise. Before the test is performed, a baseline $FEV_1$ is obtained. The exercise challenge is accomplished with either a treadmill or an exercise bike under controlled environmental temperature and humidity. With 5 to 10 minutes of exercise, the heart rate usually reaches at least 80% of the predicted maximum heart rate. The exercise is stopped, and the $FEV_1$ is measured.

The provocation tests are considered abnormal if there is a 20% or greater fall in $FEV_1$. At the end of the provocation test, a bronchodilator may be given by inhalation, and postbronchodilator pulmonary function may be evaluated.

---

**Purpose of the Test**    Pulmonary function studies are performed to evaluate the patient's respiratory status, especially in patients experiencing shortness of breath or other breathing difficulty. These studies may be used to evaluate the therapy for or progression of obstructive and restrictive lung disease. Portions of the test are used as parameters for weaning patients from mechanical ventilation and as part of preoperative evaluations.

A challenge or provocation test is included as part of the pulmonary function studies in patients with suspected hypersensitivity of the airways. *Bronchial provocation tests* or *bronchial challenge tests* are performed for patients who have symptoms suggestive of asthma but who do not show evidence of air flow limitations. They may be used to assess airway function over time and to evaluate various therapeutic interventions. The provocation tests are contraindicated for anyone whose FEV is less than 1.5 L, who has a history of severe responses to identifiable antigens, or who has had a viral infection of the upper airway within 8 weeks before the test.

| | |
|---|---|
| **Procedure** | Pulmonary function studies are usually performed in the respiratory therapy department or in a physician's office. To establish a closed system with the spirometer, a nose clip is placed over the patient's nose, and the spirometer's mouthpiece is held in the mouth with the patient's lips maintaining an airtight seal. The patient is then instructed when to breath normally, inhale maximally, and exhale maximally. This procedure is repeated several times. |

**Findings**

**Elevated Values**

FRC

Chronic obstructive
pulmonary disease

FEV

Chronic obstructive
pulmonary disease

**Decreased Values**

VT

| | | |
|---|---|---|
| Atelectasis | Pulmonary | Restrictive lung |
| Fatigue | congestion | disease |
| Pneumothorax | | Tumors |

IRV

| | |
|---|---|
| Asthma | Obstructive pulmo- |
| Exercise | nary disease |

ERV

| | | |
|---|---|---|
| Ascites | Pleural effusion | Pregnancy |
| Kyphosis | Pneumothorax | Scoliosis |
| Obesity | | |

RV

Advanced age
Obstructive pulmo-
nary disease

FEV

Restrictive pulmonary disease

FRC

Adult respiratory
distress syndrome

IC

Restrictive pulmonary
disease

VC

| Diaphragm restriction Drug overdose with hypoventilation | Neuromuscular diseases | Restrictive or depressed thoracic movement |

---

**Interfering Factors**

- Fatigue
- Lack of patient cooperation
- Smoking
- Abdominal distention or pregnancy
- Poor seal around mouthpiece (or tube)
- Medications
- Analgesics, bronchodilators, sedatives

---

**Nursing Implementation**

■

*Critical Thinking 14–12*
What would be the best time of day to schedule pulmonary function studies?

**Pretest**

Assess the patient's cardiac status. Hold the test and notify the physician if the patient has a history of angina or recent myocardial infarction.

Maximize patient cooperation by explaining the procedure and the need for full participation. Demonstrate the nose clip and mouthpiece. The patient should wear dentures if necessary for a proper mouth seal.

Instruct the patient not to smoke for 6 hours before the test.

Check with prescriber about administering bronchodilator and intermittent positive-pressure breathing therapy before the test.

Ensure that no constricting clothes are worn.

Ensure that oral intake is light to prevent stomach distention.

Instruct the patient to void immediately before the test.

Schedule the test before any other tests or procedures that may fatigue the patient.

**During the Test**

**Quality Control**

If an abnormal response to a specific substance occurs during a provocation test, a placebo substance should be given to ensure that the bronchospasms were not induced by the spirometry.

**Posttest**

Advise the patient to resume normal diet and activity. Advise the patient to resume taking medications or receiving therapy if the patient normally does.

## Pulse Oximetry

Synonym: $Spo_2$

| Normal Values | $Sao_2 > 95\%$ |
| --- | --- |

### Background Information

Pulse oximetry provides a continuous, noninvasive measurement of an individual's arterial oxygen saturation.

When the $Sao_2$ level is greater than 70%, pulse oximetry correlates accurately with $Sao_2$ measurements. When it is less than 70%, the reliability is questionable.

### Purpose of the Test

Pulse oximetry is frequently used as part of the ongoing pulmonary assessment of patients at risk for hypoxia. This test permits the nurse to assess the patient's response to varied nursing procedures, guiding adaptations in patient care and activity. Continuous $Sao_2$ measurements can assist in weaning the patient from mechanical ventilation and decrease the number of ABG measurements required.

### Procedure

The pulse oximeter is placed at the bedside and is attached to the patient by either a reusable or a disposable spectrophotometric probe (Fig. 14–9). The probe emits infrared and red light, which identify arterial pulsation. The probe then measures the amount of infrared and red light absorbed. Oxyhemoglobin absorbs infrared light, and reduced hemoglobin absorbs red light. The microprocessor in the oximeter then calculates the percentage of saturated hemoglobin. A digital readout of the patient's pulse rate and $Sao_2$ is continuous.

### Findings

Hypoxemia

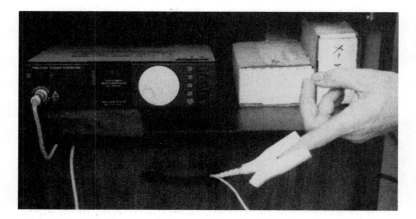

**Figure 14–9**
A pulse oximeter. (Reproduced with permission from Adler, A. M., & Carlton, R. R. [1994]. *Introduction to radiography and patient care* [p. 185]. Philadelphia: W. B. Saunders.)

| | |
|---|---|
| **Interfering Factors** | • Inadequate pulsation, as in hypotension, hypothermia, and vasoconstriction<br>• Severe anemia<br>• Carboxyhemoglobin<br>• Hyperbilirubinemia<br>• Radiopaque dyes<br>• Bright lights surrounding the probe<br>• Vasoconstricting drugs |

**Nursing Implementation**

### Pretest

Assess potential sites (finger, earlobe, nose, toe) for arterial pulsation. The fingers are the most common site in an adult. Remove nail polish if present. Apply warm packs if necessary to obtain adequate perfusion of the site.

**Quality Control**

Evaluate the patient, because the oximeter cannot distinguish between hemoglobin and carboxyhemoglobin. Was the patient at risk for smoke inhalation or carbon monoxide poisoning?

### During the Test

**Quality Control**

Ensure that the light-emitting diodes, which transmit the dual wavelengths, are aligned. The plastic reusable probes are designed to align. The disposable probes require proper application.

**Quality Control**

The use of the earlobe as a site for pulse oximetry has been controversial. If the earlobe is used, a specially designed ear clip should be used that reduces venous pooling. No ear sensor should be used on pierced sites (lobe or pinna), because the light from the diode will reach the sensor without going through an arterial vessel. Studies (Tittle & Flynn, 1997) have demonstrated that $Spo_2$ obtained by a finger probe correlates more closely with the patient's arterial oxygen saturation than an ear probe $Spo_2$.

■
*Critical Thinking 14–13*
Two patients have the same $Spo_2$ of 95%. Are both patients' oxygen needs being met?

Set the alarm limits on the oximeter.
Shield the probe from bright light.

**Critical Value**

**$Spo_2$ below 90%**

An $Spo_2$ below 90% correlates with a $Pao_2$ below 60%, which can lead quickly to a life-threatening situation. Notify the physician immediately, administer oxygen, assess vital signs, and prepare an order for ABGs.

## Roentgenogram of the Chest

**(Radiology)**        Synonyms: Chest x-ray, chest radiography

## Background Information

X-ray studies of the chest are an important diagnostic tool in assessing pulmonary and cardiac abnormalities as well as in evaluating therapies for these disorders. Chapter 9 discusses radiography in detail, including chest x-ray studies. Figure 14–10A presents a normal chest x-ray film. Compare this with a chest x-ray film showing emphysema (Fig. 14–10B) and one showing pneumonia (Fig. 14–10C).

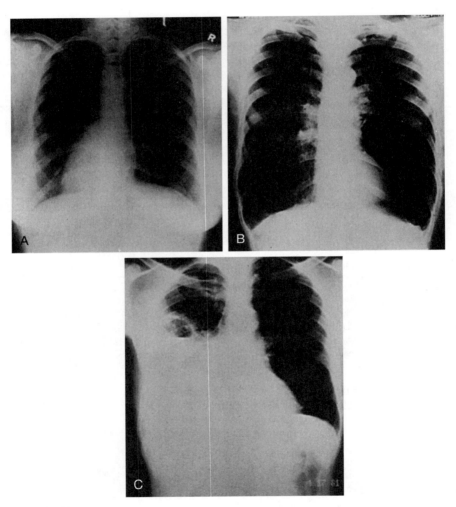

**Figure 14–10**

Chest roentgenogram. *A,* The normal chest x-ray film. *B,* Lung with emphysema. *C,* Lung with pneumonia. (Reproduced with permission from Thompson, M. A., Hall, J. D., Hattaway, M. P., & Dowd, S. B. [1994]. Principles of imaging science and protection [Vol. 2, Slides 207, 295, 296]. Philadelphia: W. B. Saunders.)

## Thoracentesis and Pleural Fluid Analysis

Synonym: Pleural tap

| Normal Values | Normal pleural fluid<br>No pathogens or malignant cells |
|---|---|

## Background Information

Thoracentesis is an invasive procedure used to remove fluid (effusion) from the pleural space. It may be performed for diagnostic or therapeutic reasons, or both. In addition to removing fluid, a percutaneous needle biopsy of the pleura may be performed to diagnose malignancy.

Pleural effusions (accumulation of fluid in the pleural space) may be a result of neoplastic or infectious processes or of leakage of fluid from the vascular system. If the effusion is due to neoplasms or infection, the fluid is usually called an *exudate*. If the fluid is due to leakage from the blood vessels, it is called a *transudate*. To distinguish between exudates and transudates, pleural fluid is evaluated for protein, specific gravity, and glucose, and a blood cell count with differential is performed.

Pleural fluid is also obtained for cultures to identify tuberculosis and fungal and various bacterial infections. Cytologic examination of the pleural fluid is performed to rule out malignancy.

## Purpose of the Test

Thoracentesis is performed to remove fluid from the pleural space for diagnostic or therapeutic reasons. An accumulation of fluid in the pleural space is abnormal. Examination of that fluid identifies or confirms diagnoses of cancer, infection, or severe fluid overload (congestive heart failure, liver failure, and systemic or pulmonary hypertension).

## Procedure

After the patient is positioned in a seated, upright position, the lower posterior chest is exposed and prepared, and a local anesthetic is given. A needle is inserted into the pleural space, and the fluid is aspirated. A pleural biopsy may be performed at this time.

If a *pleural biopsy* is planned, a special biopsy needle with a hooked biopsy trocar is used. Usually, three specimens are obtained from three pleural sites. Specimens are placed in fixative and sent to the laboratory immediately.

## Findings

Bacterial, viral, or fungal infection
Malignancy
Collagen disease
Lymphoma
Systemic lupus erythematosus
Liver failure
Nephrotic syndrome
Myxedema
Pancreatitis

| | |
|---|---|
| **Interfering Factors** | • Uncooperative patient |

**Nursing Implementation**

### Pretest

Explain the procedure and the purpose of the test to the patient.

Ensure that a signed consent form has been obtained.

Perform and document a baseline assessment. A blood pressure cuff is left in place to permit easy monitoring of the blood pressure during the procedure.

Check for allergy to local anesthetic.

Initiate supplemental $O_2$ if ordered.

Check the PT, PTT, and platelet count to identify potential bleeding problems.

Instruct the patient not to cough or move during the procedure.

Obtain a thoracentesis tray from the supply room.

### During the Test

Continuously monitor the patient's response to the procedure.

Observe the pulse oximeter, if in use, for changes in $Sao_2$.

Position the patient in an upright position, seated on the side of the bed with the legs resting on a footstool. The patient's arms should be supported on a padded overbed table (Fig. 14–11). If the patient is unable to sit up, he or she may lie on the unaffected side with the back flush with the edge of the bed. The head of the bed may be elevated 30 to 45 degrees.

Provide emotional support to the patient, because pressure pain may be experienced even though local anesthesia is given.

After the needle is inserted with a stopcock attached, fluid is drawn off for analysis. A catheter may be inserted at this point if a large amount of fluid is to be drained.

When a biopsy is performed, instruct the patient to exhale fully and perform Valsalva's maneuver to prevent air from entering the pleural space when the tissue sample is taken.

### Posttest

Check vital signs every 15 minutes until they are stable.

Assess for bilateral breath sounds.

Document amount, color, and character of the fluid obtained.

Obtain a chest radiograph as ordered to check for pneumothorax.

Encourage the patient to lie on the uninvolved side for 1 hour to improve oxygenation.

Check the small dressing over the site for bleeding or drainage.

Palpate around the site for subcutaneous emphysema.

**Complications**

The major complication following thoracentesis is pneumothorax. Another complication is reexpansion pulmonary edema. It occurs if large amounts of pleural fluid are removed, which causes an increase in negative intrapleural pressure. If the lungs do not reexpand to fill the space, edema can result. Bleeding is a rare complication. Because thoracentesis is an invasive procedure, infection is possible but extremely rare, because thoracentesis is performed with sterile technique (Table 14–6).

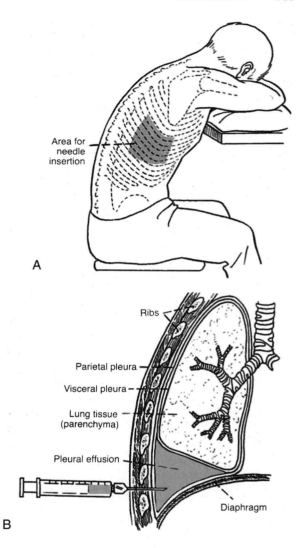

**Figure 14–11**

Thoracentesis. *A,* Thoracentesis position. Arms are raised and crossed. Head rests on folded arms. This position allows the chest wall to be pulled outward in an expanded position. If an overbed table is not available, the arms may be left down but positioned forward of the hips or crossed in front of the chest. *B,* The usual site for the insertion of a thoracentesis needle for a right-sided effusion. The actual site varies with each client, depending on the location and volume of the effusion. The physician tries to keep the needle as far away from the diaphragm as possible while at the same time inserting the needle close to the base of the effusion so that gravity can help with drainage.

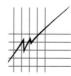

**Table 14–6   Complications of Thoracentesis**

| Complication | Nursing Assessment |
|---|---|
| Pneumothorax | Respiratory distress |
| | Diminished breath sounds |
| | Tracheal deviation to unaffected side (tension pneumothorax) |
| Pulmonary edema | Dyspnea, orthopnea |
| | Shortness of breath |
| | Crackles |

## Thoracoscopy

Synonyms: Videoscopic or video-assisted thoracic surgery, VATS

| Normal Values | No pleural fluid<br>No pathogens or malignant cells<br>Normal tissue |
|---|---|

### Background Information

A *thoracoscopy* is a surgical procedure that uses fiberoptic scopes inserted via small incisions on the chest wall. It may be performed for diagnostic or therapeutic reasons, or both. The procedure is used as an alternative to an open chest thoracotomy. Indications for a thoracoscopy and open thoracotomy are similar, but a thoracoscopy is less traumatic, with less blood loss, shorter hospital stay, more rapid wound healing, and less pain (Davidson & Colt, 1997).

A thoracoscopy has an advantage over a thoracentesis in that direct visualization of the pleura and pulmonary tissue is possible.

### Purpose of the Test

Thoracoscopy is used to identify causes of pleural thickening and recurrent effusions, to remove pleural fluid for diagnostic or therapeutic reasons (cultures, cytology), and to biopsy pleural or peripheral lung tissue.

Therapeutic uses of thoracoscopy include insertion of anti-infective or fibrinolytic agents, reinflation of the lungs by inserting chest tubes, removal of adhesions, and treatment of pleurodesis. It may also be used to remove blebs and bullae, to make pericardial windows, and to perform sympathectomy.

### Procedure

Thoracoscopy is an invasive procedure performed in the operating room under general anesthesia. Two or three 1- to 2-cm incisions are made between the ribs, and short hollow pleural trocars are inserted. For visualization through one trocar, a telescope is inserted with a side portal attached to a video camera. Through the other trocars, endoscopic instruments can be inserted depending on the tests to be performed (suction tubes, forceps, aspiration needles). At the completion of the procedure, a chest tube is attached for suction.

### Findings

Bacterial, viral, or fungal infection
Malignancy

### Interfering Factors

- Poor surgical risks

### Nursing Implementation

Follow hospital protocol for preoperative and postoperative care of a patient requiring open chest surgery. In addition, perform the following:

#### Pretest

Administer prophylactic antibiotics if ordered.
If blebs or bullae are suspected as the cause of pneumothoraces, instruct the

patient in the "huff" versus cough technique. With the huff technique, the person coughs with the epiglottis open.

### During the Test

Position the patient in the lateral decubitus position with the unaffected lung down.

### Posttest

Monitor chest tube drainage. Large amounts of straw-colored drainage are expected initially in patients with recurrent effusions.

■
*Critical Thinking 14–14*
Your patient, who is being mechanically ventilated, has a thoracoscopy done. Does mechanical ventilation influence the postprocedure critical pathway?

---

## Complications

Following a thoracoscopy, the nurse assesses for possible pulmonary complications of atelectasis, pneumothorax, and pneumonia. Atelectasis may result from positioning the unaffected lung down during the procedure.

---

## References

Askin, D. F. (1997). Interpretation of neonatal blood gases, part II: Disorders of acid-base balance. *Neonatal Network, 16,* 23–29.

Braun, M. A., Nemeck, A. A., & Vagelzang, R. L. (1997). *Interventional radiology procedure manual.* New York: Churchill Livingstone.

Carroll, P. (1997). Pulse oximetry—at your fingertips. *RN, 60,* 22–26.

Cherniack, R. M. (1992). *Pulmonary function testing* (2nd ed). Philadelphia: W. B. Saunders.

Colt, H. G. (1995). Thoracoscopy: A prospective study of safety and outcome. *Chest, 108,* 324–329.

Davidson, J. E., & Colt, H. G. (1997). Thoracoscopy: Nursing implications for optimal patient outcomes. *Dimensions of Critical Care Nursing, 16,* 20–27.

Drew, K., Brayton, M., Ambrose, A., & Bernard, G. (1998). End-tidal carbon dioxide monitoring for weaning patients: A pilot study. *Dimensions of Critical Care Nursing, 17,* 127–133.

Dubois, J. M., Bartter, T., & Pratter, M. R. (1995). Music improves patient comfort level during outpatient bronchoscopy. *Chest, 108,* 129–130.

Eisenberg, R. L. (1997). *Clinical imaging: An atlas of differential diagnosis* (3rd ed.). Philadelphia: Lippincott-Raven.

Emad, A. (1997). Bronchoalveolar lavage: A useful method for diagnosis of some pulmonary disorders. *Respiratory Care, 42,* 765–790.

Grap, M. J. (1998). Pulse oximetry. *Critical Care Nurse, 18,* 25–27.

Henry, J. W., Gottschalk, A., & Leeper, K. V. (1996). Scintigraphic lung scans and clinical assessment in critically ill patients with suspected acute pulmonary embolism. *Chest, 109,* 462–466.

Hudack, C. M., Gallo, B. M., & Morton, P. G. (1998). *Critical care nursing* (7th ed.). Philadelphia: J. B. Lippincott.

Khan, J., Akhtar, M., von Sinner, W. N., Bouchama, A., & Bazarbashi, M. (1994). CT-guided fine needle aspiration biopsy in the diagnosis of mediastinal tuberculosis. *Chest, 106,* 1329–1332.

Klingensmith, W. C. (1996). Lung scan interpretation: A user-friendly replacement for quantitative criteria. *Applied Radiology, 25,* 23–27.

LaValle, T. L., & Perry, A. G. (1995). Capnography: Assessing end-tidal $CO_2$ levels. *Dimensions of Critical Care Nursing, 14,* 70–77.

Marino, P. L. (1998). *The ICU book* (2nd ed.). Baltimore: Williams & Wilkins.

Mason, A. C., & Templeton, P. A. (1996). Transthoracic needle biopsy of the lung. *Applied Radiology, 25,* 7–12.

McConnell, E. A. (1997). Your role in thoracentesis. *Nursing 97, 27,* 76.

Novelline, R. A. (1997). *Squire's fundamentals of radiology* (5th ed.). Cambridge: Harvard University Press.

Ohmeda, Inc. (1996). *Accuracy of pulse oximeters.* Louisville, KY: Author.

Ovassapian, A., & Randel, G. I. (1995). The role of the fiberscope in the critically ill patient. *Critical Care Clinics, 11,* 29–50.

Regan, J. J., Mack, M. J., & Picetti, G. D. (1995). A technical report on videoassisted thoracoscopy in thoracic spinal surgery. *Spine, 20,* 831–837.

Roberts, W. L., & Johnson, R. D. (1997). The serum anion gap: Have the reference intervals really fallen? *Archives of Pathological Laboratory Medicine, 121,* 568–572.

Silver, M. R., & Balk, R. A. (1995). Bronchoscopic procedures in the intensive care unit. *Critical Care Clinics, 11,* 97–109.

Silverman, J. M., Julien, P. J., Herfkens, R. J., & Pele, N. J. (1994). Magnetic resonance imaging evaluation of pulmonary vascular malformations. *Chest, 106,* 1333–1337.

Sinclair, S. (1998). Dispelling myths of capnography. *Dimensions of Critical Care Nursing, 17,* 48–54.

Smatlak, P., & Knebel, A. R. (1998). Clinical evaluation of noninvasive monitoring of oxygen saturation in critically ill patients. *American Journal of Critical Care, 7,* 370–373.

Speicher, C. E. (1998). *The right test* (3rd ed.). Philadelphia: W. B. Saunders.

Stein, P. D., Goldhaber, S. Z., Henry, J. W., & Miller, A. C.

(1996). Arterial blood gas analysis in the assessment of suspected acute pulmonary embolism. *Chest, 109,* 78–81.

Szaflarski, N. L. (1996). Emerging technology in critical care: Continuous intra-arterial blood gas monitoring. *American Journal of Critical Care, 5,* 55–65.

Tietz, N. W. (1995). *Clinical guide to laboratory tests* (3rd ed.). Philadelphia: W. B. Saunders.

Tittle, M., & Flynn, M. B. (1997). Correlation of pulse oximetry and co-oximetry. *Dimensions of Critical Care Nursing, 16,* 88–94.

# Cardiac Function

The laboratory and diagnostic evaluation of cardiac function has evolved into many sophisticated techniques. The number of diagnostic procedures is proliferating. The number of tests and the various names and abbreviations for the same or similar tests can be confusing. This chapter emphasizes the knowledge required of the nurse for each of the studies presented and provides guidelines for assisting the patient in preparing for the procedure as well as for caring for the patient during and after the procedure.

The emotional needs of the patient and family during the diagnostic testing vary with the clinical condition of the patient, the purpose of the procedure, and the possible risks of the test.

Patients undergoing cardiac testing may or may not have experienced cardiac symptoms. The test may be a preamble to surgery or, because of the high incidence of cardiac disease, may be part of a routine physical examination.

Other tests not specific to the heart play an important role in identifying coronary problems. These tests include arterial blood gas and mixed venous gas determinations, a complete blood cell count, an erythrocyte sedimentation rate, a blood chemistry panel, and an electrolyte value. In addition, the importance of the patient's history and the clinical presentation cannot be overemphasized.

## Laboratory Tests

## Enzymes and Isoenzymes, Cardiac

**(Serum)**          Synonyms: None

| Normal Values | Creatine kinase (CK) | **Adult male:** 38–174 U/L *or* SI 0.65–29.6 µKat/L<br>**Adult female:** 26–140 U/L *or* SI 0.44–2.38 µKat/L<br>**Newborn:** 50–525 U/L *or* SI 0.85–8.93 µKat/L |
|---|---|---|

*Continued on following page*

*Continued*

| | |
|---|---|
| CK isoenzymes | |
| CK-BB, CK-1 (brain) | Trace or 0% of total CK *or* SI trace or 0.00 (fraction of total CK) |
| CK-MB, CK-2 (heart) | 0%–6% of total CK *or* SI 0.00%–0.06% (fraction of total CK) |
| CK-MM, CK-3 (skeletal muscles) | 90%–97% of total CK *or* SI 0.90–0.97 (fraction of total CK) |
| Aspartate aminotransferase (AST) or serum glutamic-oxaloacetic transaminase (SGOT) | **Adult:** 8–20 U/L *or* SI 0.14–0.34 µKat/L<br>**Older Adult**<br>Male: 11–26 U/L *or* SI 0.19–0.34 µKat/L<br>Female: 10–20 U/L *or* SI 0.17–0.34 µKat/L<br>**Child (<5 years):** 19–28 U/L *or* SI 0.32–0.47 µKat/L<br>**Infant:** 15–60 U/L *or* SI 0.25–1.02 µKat/L<br>**Newborn:** 16–72 U/L *or* SI 0.27–1.22 µKat/L |
| Lactate dehydrogenase (LDH) | **Adult:** 200–400 U/L |
| LDH isoenzymes | **Neonate:** 400–700 U/L |
| LDH₁<br>Heart, red blood cells | 14%–26% *or* SI 0.14–0.26 (fraction of total LDH) |
| LDH₂<br>Reticuloendothelial cells and kidneys | 29%–39% *or* SI 0.29–0.39 (fraction of total LDH) |
| LDH₃<br>Lungs, lymphatics, spleen, and others | 20%–26% *or* SI 0.20–0.26 (fraction of total LDH) |
| LDH₄<br>Kidney, placenta, and liver | 8%–16% *or* SI 0.08–0.16 (fraction of total LDH) |
| LDH₅<br>Kidney, liver, and skeletal muscle | 6%–16% *or* SI 0.06–0.16 (fraction of total LDH) |

## Background Information

Enzymes are complex compounds that are found in all tissues and that speed up the biochemical reactions of the body. Damage to body tissue causes release of the enzymes from the injured cells into the serum. Enzymes may be common to more than one type of tissue. Elevated serum levels of the enzymes reflect tissue damage, but because the enzymes are not specific, patterns of enzyme elevations are used to determine myocardial tissue damage.

Creatine kinase (CK) is an enzyme found in the heart, brain, and skeletal muscle. The individual with greater muscle mass has a higher CK level than does the average person. CK levels may be higher in African Americans. CK may be separated into three isoenzymes. Isoenzymes refer to the various forms of an enzyme, which can differ chemically, physically, or immunologically but catalyze the same reaction. The CK isoenzymes include CK-MM, CK-MB, and CK-BB. With myocardial damage, the elevated fraction is CK-MB.

Aspartate aminotransferase (AST), previously called serum glutamic-oxaloacetic transaminase (SGOT), is an enzyme found in the heart, kidneys, brain, red blood cells, liver, lungs, pancreas, and skeletal muscle. AST lacks specificity in diagnosing myocardial injury, because it is so widely distributed in the body.

Lactate dehydrogenase (LDH) is present in almost all metabolizing cells but is especially high in the heart, kidneys, brain, red blood cells, liver, and skeletal muscles. Because LDH is present in so many tissues of the body, the origin of its release cannot be determined without the use of electrophoresis, which separates out its five isoenzymes. $LDH_1$ and $LDH_2$ are used to assess myocardial damage.

Traditionally, the cardiac enzyme protocol consists of CK and its isoenzymes being collected three times, every 8 hours, after the onset of cardiac symptoms. CK, CK isoenzymes, LDH, LDH isoenzymes, and AST determinations are usually ordered at the onset of symptoms and thereafter every 24 hours for three additional times. Many institutions perform only serial CK and CK-MB determinations.

| | |
|---|---|
| **Purpose of the Test** | Cardiac enzyme and isoenzyme studies are used with clinical evaluation and electrocardiographic studies to diagnose myocardial injury. |

| | |
|---|---|
| **Procedure** | A venipuncture is necessary to obtain 5 to 10 mL of blood in a red-topped tube. Results of the enzyme levels will determine need for admission to the hospital and emergency treatment. Assays of CK-MB can be done in the emergency room, with results available within 20 minutes. |

**Findings**

■

*Critical Thinking 15–1*
What nursing actions ensure that the cardiac enzyme protocols are followed?

Multiple diagnoses cause changes in enzyme levels, because they are found in many body tissues. Because of this lack of specificity, enzymes alone do not establish diagnoses.

In diagnosing myocardial infarction, a pattern of enzyme changes *supports* the diagnosis. The first enzyme to rise is CK. CK levels begin to rise 6 hours after the infarction; they peak in 18 hours and return to normal in 2 to 3 days. CK-MB levels rise within 3 to 6 hours after an infarction, peak in 12 to 24 hours, and return to normal in 12 to 48 hours. An increase in CK-MB, expressed as a percentage of the total CK, supports the diagnosis of myocardial damage. The percentage accepted as diagnostic of an infarction varies from laboratory to laboratory. If the CK-MB level rises quickly and then drops quickly, myocardial contusion is suspected (Fig. 15–1).

AST levels will begin to rise 6 to 10 hours after an infarction, peak in 24 to 48 hours, and return to normal after 4 to 6 days.

LDH elevations do not occur until 24 to 48 hours after an infarction. They peak in 3 to 4 days and do not return to normal levels for 10 to 14 days after an infarction. $LDH_2$ levels are normally greater than $LDH_1$ levels. A "flipped" LDH, which occurs when $LDH_1$ levels become greater than those of $LDH_2$, is indicative of a myocardial infarction. The "flipped" LDH is especially helpful if the person delayed seeking help when chest pain occurred.

Because of their nonspecificity, other clinical problems may create changes in the enzyme levels. Common causes of these changes are as follows:

**Elevated Values**

CK

| | | |
|---|---|---|
| Amyotrophic lateral sclerosis | Burns | Central nervous system trauma, including cerebrovascular accident |
| Biliary atresia | Some cancers | |
| | Cardiomyopathy | |

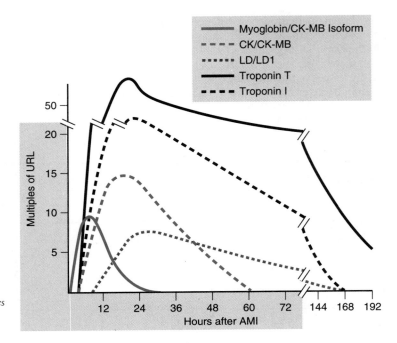

**Figure 15–1**
Cardiac enzyme pattern typical of patients with a myocardial infarction. (Reproduced with permission from Stepp, C. A., & Woods, M. A. [1998]. *Laboratory procedures for medical office personnel* [p. 224]. Philadelphia: W. B. Saunders.)

Hypokalemia, severe
Hypothermia
Hypothyroidism
Infarction: cerebral,
  bowel, myocardial

Intramuscular
  injections
Muscular dystrophy
Myocarditis
Organ rejection

Pulmonary edema
Pulmonary embolism
Renal insufficiency or
  failure
Surgery

**Decreased Values**

CK

Addison's disease
Anterior pituitary
  hyposecretion

Connective tissue
  disease
Cirrhosis, alcoholic

Metastatic cancer
Steroid administra-
  tion

**Elevated Values**

AST

Cirrhosis
Congestive heart
  failure

Hepatitis
Myocardial infarction
Pericarditis

Pulmonary infarction
Reye's syndrome

**Decreased Values**

AST

Severe liver failure

### Elevated Values

LDH

| | | |
|---|---|---|
| Alcoholism | Delirium tremens | Niacin |
| Anemia | Hepatitis | Pneumonia |
| Burns | Hypothyroidism | Pulmonary infarction |
| Cancer | Infectious mononu- | Procainamide |
| Cardiomyopathy | cleosis | Propranolol |
| Cerebrovascular | Codeine | Shock |
| accident | Lithium carbonate | Thyroid hormones |
| Cirrhosis | Meperidine | Ulcerative colitis |
| Convulsions | Morphine | |

### Decreased Values

LDH

Radiation therapy
Oxalates

**Interfering Factors**

- CPK: cardioversion, drugs (alcohol, aspirin, halothane, lithium, succinylcho-line), gross hemolysis of specimen, muscle trauma, recent vigorous exercise or massage, surgery
- AST: drugs (acetaminophen, antituberculosis agents, aspirin, chlorpropa-mide, dicumarol, erythromycin, methyldopa, sulfonamides, vitamin A), muscle trauma, not fasting, strenuous fasting
- LDH: pregnancy, prosthetic heart valves, recent surgery, hemolysis of specimen

**Nursing Implementation**

### Pretest

Reassure the patient, who is usually frightened and having chest pain and may also be in denial.

Do *not* give intramuscular injections or perform repeated venipunctures, if possible, until all the initial enzyme studies are completed.

Instruct the patient about the need to repeat blood sampling.

Determine if alcohol or drugs that affect results have been ingested.

### During the Test

If the tourniquet is in place too long, inaccurate results may occur.

### Posttest

Nursing actions are similar to those for any venipuncture.

## Lipids, Serum

**(Serum)**

Synonym: Lipoprotein-cholesterol fractionation

| Normal Values | Lipids, total | 400–800 mg/dL *or* SI 4.0–8.0 g/L |
|---|---|---|
| | Cholesterol, total | 120–200 mg/dL *or* SI 3.11–5.18 mmol/L |
| | Low-density lipoprotein (LDL) | <130 mg/dL *or* SI <3.37 mmol/L |
| | High-density lipoprotein (HDL) | **Male:** 44–45 mg/dL *or* SI 1.24–1.27 mmol/L |
| | | **Female:** 55 mg/dL *or* SI 1.425 mmol/L |
| | LDL:HDL ratio | <3 |
| | Triglycerides | **Male:** <40 years 46–316 mg/dL *or* SI 0.52–3.57 mmol/L |
| | | >50 years 75–313 mg/dL *or* SI 0.85–3.5 mmol/L |
| | | **Female:** <40 years 37–174 mg/dL *or* SI 0.42–1.97 mmol/L |
| | | >50 years 52–200 mg/dL *or* SI 0.59–2.26 mmol/L |

## Background Information

Most lipids are bound to protein in the blood and are called lipoproteins (Fig. 15–2). Lipoproteins are usually measured to identify persons at risk for coronary artery disease (CAD). In the laboratory, lipoproteins are separated by electrophoresis. Fractionation of the lipoproteins is then performed according to their density. The following groups have been identified:

Very low-density lipoproteins (VLDL), which are made up of 70% triglycerides

Low-density lipoproteins (LDL), which are made up of 45% cholesterol

High-density lipoproteins (HDL)

A high correlation exists between elevated VLDL and LDL levels and CAD. Research has shown that HDL may protect from CAD, because it seems to inhibit the uptake of LDL.

| Purpose of the Test | Lipid levels are used to identify individuals at risk for CAD and as an evaluation tool to determine the effectiveness of "heart healthy" changes in lifestyle. |
|---|---|
| Procedure | A venipuncture is necessary for a lipid profile. Two red-topped tubes of 7-mL capacity are required. If a cholesterol level determination is performed as a screening test, a drop or two of blood is obtained from a fingerstick using a sterile lancet, and the blood is collected in a capillary pipette (Fig. 15–3). |

### Findings

**Elevated Values**

CHOLESTEROL

| | | |
|---|---|---|
| Alcoholism | Diabetes mellitus | Myxedema |
| Arteriosclerosis | Hepatitis (early stage) | Obstructed bile duct |
| CAD | High-fat diet | Pancreatitis |

**Decreased Values**

CHOLESTEROL

| | | |
|---|---|---|
| Hyperalimentation | Liver disease | Malnutrition |
| Hyperthyroidism | Malabsorption | |

**A. Comparison of lipid content in lipoproteins**

| Lipoprotein in plasma | Lipid component — approximate % |
|---|---|
| Chylomicron | 90% triglyceride |
| VLDL | 25% cholesterol, 55% triglyceride |
| LDL | 65% cholesterol, 5% triglyceride |
| HDL | 20% cholesterol, 5% triglyceride |

**B. Comparison of HDL and LDL**

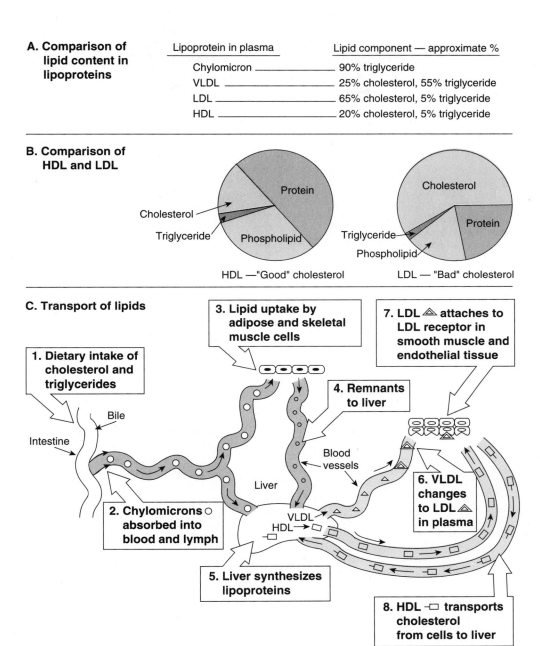

HDL —"Good" cholesterol          LDL — "Bad" cholesterol

**C. Transport of lipids**

**3. Lipid uptake by adipose and skeletal muscle cells**

**7. LDL ⬙ attaches to LDL receptor in smooth muscle and endothelial tissue**

**1. Dietary intake of cholesterol and triglycerides**

Bile

Intestine

**4. Remnants to liver**

Blood vessels

Liver

**6. VLDL changes to LDL ⬙ in plasma**

**2. Chylomicrons ○ absorbed into blood and lymph**

VLDL
HDL→

**5. Liver synthesizes lipoproteins**

**8. HDL ⬚ transports cholesterol from cells to liver**

**Figure 15–2**

Transport of lipids. (Reproduced with permission from Gould, B. E. [1997]. *Pathophysiology for health related professionals* [p. 182]. Philadelphia: W. B. Saunders.)

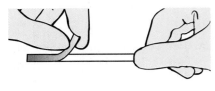

A

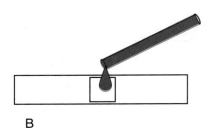

B

**Figure 15-3**
Cholesterol screening. *A*, Remove protective layer from strip.
*B*, Add blood to strip using capillary pipette.

**Elevated Values**

HDL

| | | |
|---|---|---|
| Alcoholism | Exercise | Nephrotic syndrome |
| Diabetes mellitus | Myxedema | Pancreatitis |

**Decreased Values**

HDL

| | | |
|---|---|---|
| Arteriosclerosis | Hypothyroidism | Malnutrition |
| Hyperalimentation | Malabsorption | |

**Elevated Values**

LDL

| | | |
|---|---|---|
| Alcoholism | Diabetes mellitus | Pancreatitis |
| CAD | Nephrotic syndrome | |

**Decreased Values**

LDL

| | | |
|---|---|---|
| Arteriosclerosis | Malabsorption | Malnutrition |
| Hyperalimentation | | |

**Elevated Values**

TRIGLYCERIDES

| | | |
|---|---|---|
| Alcoholism | Diabetes mellitus | Nephrotic syndrome |
| Arteriosclerosis | Myxedema | Pancreatitis |

**Decreased Values**

TRIGLYCERIDES

Hyperalimentation               Malabsorption               Malnutrition

---

**Interfering Factors**

- Diet affects the results of a lipid profile and fractionation outcome. Has the patient been dieting to lose weight? If the patient has had a recent traumatic event or infarction, results will also be affected. Smoking may affect results. Medications such as estrogen, steroids, birth control pills, and hypo-lipid agents cause an inaccurate lipid picture.
- For cholesterol screening, eating a diet high in saturated fats will affect the results.

**Nursing Implementation**

The nursing actions are similar to those of other venipunctures. In addition, review the following.

*Critical Thinking 15–2*
Does sex or age, or both, influence who would benefit from having a serum lipid determination done?

**Pretest**

Instruct the patient to fast for 10 to 12 hours before the blood sample is taken. If only a cholesterol screening is planned, instruct the patient to refrain from eating a high-fat diet for 12 hours before the blood is drawn.

Inquire if the patient has been on his or her normal diet for the last 2 to 3 weeks.

**Posttest**

Review results with the patient. If the patient is at risk for CAD, diet and exercise education may be necessary.

**Home Testing**

Home cholesterol screening is now possible. The use of such tests, however, is controversial. The controversy centers on the person's ability to interpret and act appropriately on the test results. Thompson (1994) reported that four out of five people using home cholesterol testing understand the relationship between cholesterol and CAD. Alger (1998) reported concerns by some persons about the accuracy of cholesterol testing at home. The reported accuracy for the home cholesterol test kits is 98%, which is consistent with tests done in physician offices. The accuracy of the home cholesterol test is dependent on the ability of the user to follow the manufacturer's guidelines.

Before home cholesterol testing is taught to a person, assess the medical history. The test is not recommended for anyone with a bleeding disorder or for anyone who is receiving anticoagulation therapy.

Instruct the person to avoid vitamin A, acetaminophen, and mesalamine for at least 4 hours before the test.

No dietary restrictions exist. Repeated tests should be done when the dietary intake is similar, for comparison purposes.

Warn the patient to check the packing of the kit for breaks and not to use the test if the foil package is not intact or if sterility of the lancet is questionable.

Home cholesterol testing requires capillary blood. Instruct the person to wash the hands before testing in warm soap and water. Warn the person not to use alcohol or hydrogen peroxide to clean the skin.

*Continued on following page*

*Continued*

> Instruct the patient to obtain the blood sample from the side of a fingertip, which has fewer pain sensors and a better blood supply than the center.
>
> Instruct the patient to follow the manufacturer's guidelines. Multiple steps are required, with different timings at different steps.
>
> Inform the person that cholesterol levels will be affected by diet. One test result is not adequate. Repeating the test is recommended.
>
> Instruct the person to notify his or her physician or nurse practitioner if results are greater than 200 mg/dL. Education about diet and exercise and possibly medication can be used to control high cholesterol levels.

## Myoglobin

(Serum)      Synonyms: Mb, S-Mgb

| Normal Values | <90 µg/L |
| --- | --- |

### Background Information

Myoglobin is an oxygen-binding protein found in striated muscle. It releases oxygen at very low tensions. Any injury to skeletal muscle will cause a release of myoglobin into the blood.

### Purpose of the Test

Myoglobin levels may be used with cardiac enzymes to diagnose myocardial infarction, evaluate muscle injury, or assess polymyositis. Myoglobin rises and falls within 2 to 6 hours of the onset of myocardial infarction; therefore, timing of the specimen is crucial. Myoglobin assays can be done in emergency rooms, with results available within 15 minutes.

### Procedure

A venipuncture is performed to obtain 5 mL of blood in a red-topped tube.

### Findings

**Elevated Values**

| | | |
| --- | --- | --- |
| Myocardial infarction | Polymyositis | Open heart surgery |
| Muscle injury or breakdown | Renal failure | Exhaustive exercise |

### Interfering Factors

- Myoglobin is nonspecific. Any trauma to skeletal muscle can cause an increase, which limits its usefulness in diagnosing a myocardial infarction.
- Recent administration of radioactive material, if radioimmunoassay (RIA) is used for analysis.

### Nursing Implementation

The nurse performs actions similar to those for other venipuncture procedures. No fasting is necessary.

# Troponin
**(Serum)**

Synonyms: Cardiac troponin T, $cT_nT$, cardiac troponin I, $cT_nI$

## Normal Values

| | |
|---|---|
| Cardiac troponin T: | <0.2 µg/L |
| Cardiac troponin I: | <0.35 µg/L |

## Background Information

Troponin is a protein found in skeletal and cardiac muscle fibers. Three forms of troponin exist, two of which are used in diagnosing cardiac disorders. Normally, cardiac troponin levels are very low, but the level increases rapidly with a myocardial infarction. Toponin I is found in the cardiac muscle complex; therefore, it is very specific to cardiac injury. This is especially important if the person being evaluated for a cardiac problem has renal disease or a musculoskeletal disorder, which would make interpretation of the CK-MB difficult. Troponin levels increase earlier than CK-MB levels; thus, their evaluation may be helpful in diagnosing myocardial infarction earlier than the traditional enzymes studies. Earlier diagnosis may lead to earlier treatment and salvaging more myocardium. Troponin assays can be done in the emergency room, with results available in less than 30 minutes.

## Purpose of the Test

Troponin levels are used to diagnose myocardial infarction and myocardial muscle damage.

## Procedure

A venipuncture is performed to obtain 5 mL of blood in a red-topped tube.

## Findings

**Elevated Values**

TROPONIN T & I

Acute myocardial infarction

TROPONIN T

| | | |
|---|---|---|
| Angina | Muscle trauma | Polymyositis |
| Renal failure | Rhabdomyolysis | Dermatomyositis |

## Interfering Factors

• Hemolysis of specimen

## Nursing Implementation

The nurse performs actions similar to those for other venipunctures.
Ensure that specimen is drawn on admission or on the occurrence of chest pain and then at 4, 8, 12, and 24 hours afterward.

## Diagnostic Procedures

## Catheterization, Cardiac

(Radiology)                    Synonyms: Angiocardiography, coronary arteriography

| Normal Values | Pressures | **Right atrium:** 2–6 mm Hg |
|---|---|---|
| | | **Neonate:** 0–3 mm Hg |
| | | **Child:** 1–5 mm Hg |
| | | **Right ventricle:** 20–30/2–8 mm Hg |
| | | **Neonate:** 30–60/2–5 mm Hg |
| | | **Child:** 15–30/2–5 mm Hg |
| | | **Pulmonary artery pressure:** 20–30/8–15 mm Hg |
| | | **Neonate:** 30–60/2–10 mm Hg |
| | | **Child:** 15–30/5–10 mm Hg |
| | | **Pulmonary artery wedge pressure:** 4–12 mm Hg |
| | | **Left atrium:** 4–12 mm Hg |
| | | **Neonate:** 1–4 mm Hg |
| | | **Child:** 5–10 mm Hg |
| | | **Left ventricle:** 90–140/4–12 mm Hg |
| | | **Neonate:** 60–100/5–10 mm Hg |
| | | **Child:** 80–130/10–20 mm Hg |
| | Cardiac output | 4–8 L/min |
| | Cardiac index | 2.5–4 L/min |
| | | **Neonate and child:** 3.5–4 L/min |
| | Stroke index | 30–60 mL/beat/min |
| | Ejection fraction | 55%–75% |
| | Oxygen saturation | 75% (right side of heart) |
| | | 95% (left side of heart) |
| | Oxygen content | 14–15 volume % (right side of heart) |
| | | 19 volume % (left side of heart) |
| | Oxygen consumption | 250 mL/min |
| | Volume | **Left ventricular end-diastolic:** 50–90 mL |
| | | **Left ventricular end-systolic:** 14–34 mL |
| | | **Right ventricular end-diastolic:** 70–90 mL |
| | | **Left atrium:** 57–79 mL |

| Mass | **Left Ventricular Thickness** |
|------|--------------------------------|
| | **Male:** 12 mm |
| | **Female:** 9 mm |
| | **Left Ventricular Wall Mass** |
| | **Male:** 99 g |
| | **Female:** 76 g |
| Wall motion | Normal |
| Valve gradient | None |
| Valve orifice areas | **Aortic valve:** 0.7 cm² |
| | **Mitral valve:** 1 cm² |

## Background Information

Cardiac catheterization is an invasive procedure that permits the assessment of anatomic abnormalities of the heart. Cardiac catheterization may assess (1) pressures, oxygen content, and oxygen saturation in the various heart chambers; (2) cardiac output and index; (3) patency of the coronary arteries; and (4) pressure gradients across the valves.

Cardiac catheterization may be a right-sided catheterization, a left-sided catheterization, or both. A right-sided catheterization is performed today in specialized units under the category of hemodynamic monitoring; therefore, this section will focus on left-sided catheterization.

The reader may wish to review the general principles of angiography in Chapter 11 before reading the specifics of cardiac angiography.

## Purpose of the Test

A cardiac catheterization is performed to (1) evaluate coronary artery disease with unstable, progressive, or new-onset angina or angina that is not responsive to medical therapy; (2) diagnose atypical chest pain; (3) diagnose complications of myocardial infarction such as septal rupture and refractory dysrhythmias; (4) diagnose aortic dissection; (5) evaluate the need for coronary artery surgery or angioplasty; (6) assess valvular function; and (7) determine the efficacy of a heart transplant. Rarely, a cardiac catheterization may be carried out to obtain a biopsy specimen.

## Procedure

A left-sided catheterization is performed in a cardiac catheterization laboratory. This laboratory is designed with fluoroscopy, electrocardiographic equipment, and emergency equipment and drugs (code cart). For a left-sided catheterization, a catheter must be threaded through an artery into the left side of the heart; therefore, arterial access is necessary. Pressure measurements are obtained in the aorta and left atrium and ventricle. Samples of blood are obtained for oxygen analysis. Cardiac output, stroke volume, and ejection fractions are measured.

When a *coronary angiogram* is included in the test, dye is instilled into the heart to visualize the size of the ventricles, wall motion, and contractility and to identify valvular dysfunction.

A *coronary arteriogram* may also be obtained. The catheter is withdrawn from the left ventricle and positioned at the coronary ostia, where small boluses of dye are injected into the coronary arteries while a series of x-ray films are taken.

| | |
|---|---|
| **Findings** | Cardiac catheterization provides a significant amount of data for analysis, which may support the following diagnoses:<br><br>CAD<br>Coronary occlusions and degree of blockage<br>Congenital abnormalities<br>Septal defects<br>Shunting<br>Aneurysms<br>Valvular defects |
| **Interfering Factors** | • Allergic reactions to contrast medium<br>• Uncontrolled congestive heart failure<br>• Dysrhythmias<br>• Renal insufficiency<br>• Electrolyte imbalances<br>• Infection<br>• Drug toxicity |

**Nursing Implementation**

**Pretest**

Verify that an informed consent has been obtained.

Instruct the patient about the purpose and procedure for the study. Explain to the patient that the table rotates and that the physician may ask the patient to change positions or cough. Explain to the patient that when the dye is given, a feeling of warmth, or flushing or a metallic taste may be sensed.

Assist with the precatheterization evaluation: blood tests, including a prothrombin time test and a partial thromboplastin time test; an electrocardiogram (ECG); and chest x-ray film if the procedure will be performed on an outpatient basis.

Obtain patient weight and height.

If contrast dye is going to be used, check for allergies. Report elevated blood urea nitrogen (BUN) or creatinine levels, because these patients are at risk for renal failure.

Assess the patient's fears. Correct any misperceptions and reassure the patient that the nurse, physician, and technicians to assist during the procedure will be continuously present.

The patient is to have nothing by mouth after midnight, except if the catheterization is planned for late in the afternoon. In that case, a clear liquid breakfast may be taken.

Cardiac drugs are usually held.

Prepare catheter site according to laboratory protocols. The femoral artery is commonly used for the percutaneous insertion of the catheter. Usually both sides of the groin are prepared.

Premedication is given as ordered to reduce the patient's anxiety. In some catheterization laboratories, the patient is premedicated to decrease the risk of allergic reaction to the contrast dye.

Encourage the patient to wear glasses, if required, to the catheterization laboratory.

The patient is instructed to void before going to the catheterization laboratory.

### During the Test

■
*Critical Thinking 15–3*
What can you do in the catheterization laboratory to reassure
the patient during the procedure?

The patient is awake. The nurse provides emotional support and reinforces
explanations given about the procedure.

Continuous cardiac monitoring is maintained.

A local anesthetic is used after the insertion site is prepared and draped.

The physician inserts the cardiac catheter under fluoroscopy.

The patient may be asked to change position or cough during the procedure.

Observe constantly for complications, especially dysrhythmia from catheter irritation or sensitivity to the contrast dye.

Heparin is usually given during the procedure to prevent emboli. At the end of
the procedure, protamine sulfate is given to reverse the heparin's effect.

### Posttest

Observe the insertion site for signs of bleeding. Palpate around the puncture
site to detect bleeding into tissue. If bleeding is present, exert pressure just
proximal to the puncture site with a gloved hand for a minimum of 15
minutes.

Monitor vital signs and cardiac monitor according to hospital protocol.

Check distal pulses for arterial patency.

Report any significant changes in vital signs, rhythm, and circulation or the
occurrence of chest pain.

Evaluate the patient's psychologic response to the procedure and its findings.

If cardiac catheterization is done as an outpatient procedure, instruct the
patient (1) not to drive or climb stairs for 24 hours; (2) to avoid heavy
lifting, sports, and strenuous housework for 3 days; and (3) to take no baths
until the wound is healed. Instruct outpatients that they may shower and
change the dressing after 24 hours.

| **Complications** | Table 15–1 summarizes the multiple complications that may occur with cardiac catheterization. Although many complications are possible, their incidence is infrequent. |
|---|---|

## Echocardiogram

**(Sonogram)** — Synonyms: ECHO, heart sonogram, transthoracic echocardiogram

| **Normal Values** | No anatomic or functional abnormalities |
|---|---|

## Background Information

An echocardiogram is a noninvasive test that uses
ultrasound techniques to detect enlargement of
the cardiac chambers or variations in chamber size
during the cardiac cycle. It also assesses valvular
function, septal defects, and pericardial effusion.
Echocardiography has been integrated into

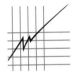

### Table 15–1    Complications of Cardiac Catheterization

| Complication | Nursing Assessment |
|---|---|
| Ventricular tachycardia, ventricular fibrillation | Observe monitor and patient |
| Supraventricular tachycardia | Observe monitor for paroxysmal supraventricular tachycardia, atrial fibrillation, and atrial flutter |
| Asystole | Observe monitor and patient, especially if patient had preexisting blocks |
| Vasovagal reaction | Observe monitor and pulse rate |
| Contrast medium reaction | See Chapter 11 |
| Retroperitoneal bleeding | Hypotension<br>Tachycardia<br>Low abdominal or flank pain<br>Drop in hematocrit |
| Air embolism | See Chapter 11 |
| Thrombus at catheter insertion site | Check distal pulses<br>Observe extremities for color and temperature change |
| Hematoma at catheter insertion site | As above |
| Cardiac tamponade | Decreased cardiac output<br>Muffled heart sounds<br>Increased right atrial pressure<br>Pulsus paradoxus |
| Myocardial infarction | Chest pain<br>Electrocardiographic changes<br>Elevated cardiac enzyme levels |
| Acute congestive heart failure, pulmonary edema | Crackles<br>Dyspnea<br>Pink, frothy sputum<br>Cyanosis<br>Cold, clammy skin |
| Cerebrovascular accident | Change in level of consciousness<br>Change in behavior<br>Hemiparesis<br>Aphasia |
| Infection | Fever<br>Tachycardia<br>Elevated white blood cell count |

stress testing. It is called *stress echocardiography* or *exercise echocardiography* (see Stress Testing, pp. 342–344). Stress echocardiography is similar to stress testing, but with an echocardiogram done at baseline and at each progressive level of exertion. It is especially helpful as a screening tool for women and for persons with a left bundle-branch block. If the patient is unable to use the treadmill or bicycle, stress can be induced with dobutamine or dipyridamole. Sometimes atropine is needed to reach the desired heart rate. *Dobutamine stress echocardiography (DSE)* is frequently used to assess "stunned" or "hibernating" myocardium.

## Purpose of the Test

An echocardiogram is performed for a variety of diagnostic reasons, such as to evaluate abnormal heart sounds; to evaluate heart size, chamber size, and valvular function; and to detect tumors, pericardial effusion, and wall motion abnormalities.

Figure 15–4 shows the diagnostic steps of the DSE protocol.

## Procedure

An echocardiogram may be carried out at the bedside, in a special laboratory, in a clinic, or in a doctor's office. A transducer is placed over the third and fourth intercostal spaces to the left of the sternum. The transducer emits ultrasonic beams of high-frequency sound waves that are inaudible to the human ear. The transducer then picks up the echos created by the deflection of the beams off the various heart structures. This creates a picture on the oscilloscope. The picture is created because the echo varies in intensity based on the differing densities of the structures.

## Findings

Abnormal heart valves
Aneurysm
Cardiomyopathy
Congenital heart disorders
Congestive heart failure
Idiopathic hypertrophic subaortic stenosis

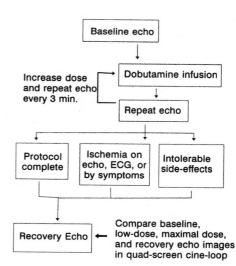

**Figure 15–4**

Protocol for dobutamine stress testing. (Reproduced with permission from Otto, C. M., & Pearlman, A. S. [1995]. *Textbook of clinical echocardiology* [p. 147]. Philadelphia: W. B. Saunders.)

Mural thrombi
Myocardial infarction
Pericardial effusion
Restrictive pericarditis
Tumor of the heart

| **Interfering Factors** | • Chest wall abnormalities<br>• Excessive movement<br>• Improper placement of transducer |
|---|---|

**Nursing Implementation**

**Pretest**

Instruct the patient that the test is noninvasive. The patient is awake during the test and is usually in a recumbent position.

Inform the patient that an electromechanical transducer will be positioned on the chest. The patient will sense only the conduction jelly and the movement of the transducer. No pain or risk is involved.

**During the Test**

The patient may be asked to breathe slowly or to hold the breath.

**Posttest**

Evaluate the patient's response to the procedure.
Cleanse the chest of conduction gel.

## Electrocardiogram

Synonyms: ECG, EKG, 12-lead ECG or EKG, 15-lead ECG or EKG, 18-lead ECG or EKG

**Normal Values**

Normal rate and rhythm with no abnormalities noted

### Background Information

The electrocardiogram (ECG) is an invaluable tool in the assessment of the heart. It records the heart's electric activity. Several lead systems are available for the measurement of the electric activity of the heart: 12-, 15-, and 18-lead ECG. The electrochemical physiology characteristics are the same for each of these systems; that is, each uses electrodes on the body surface, amplifies changes in electric potentials, and provides a graphic recording. This is made possible by the body's fluid system, which acts as a conductor of electric forces. A 12-lead ECG is the most common system used; it presents a graphic recording of 12 electric planes of the heart. By manipulating the skin electrodes, 12 various views of the heart's electric activity are seen.

In a 12-lead ECG, leads I, II, and III are limb leads. In lead I, the negative electrode of the electrocardiograph is connected to the right arm, and the positive electrode is attached to the left arm. In lead II, the negative electrode is placed on the right arm, and the positive electrode is placed on the left leg. In lead III, the negative electrode is placed on the left arm, and the positive electrode is placed on the left leg. Leads I, II, and III form a triangle, which is called Einthoven's triangle (Fig. 15–5).

The second three leads recorded by the electro-

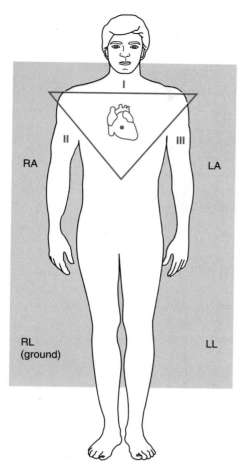

**Figure 15–5**
Einthoven's triangle.

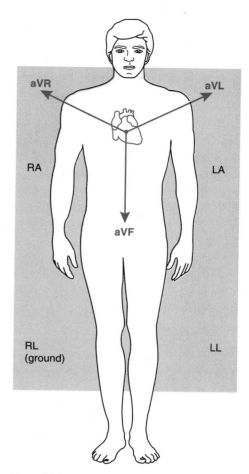

**Figure 15–6**
Augmented limb leads.

cardiograph machine are called augmented limb leads. In these leads, two limbs are attached to negative electrodes, and a third limb is attached to a positive electrode. If the positive electrode is placed on the right arm, the lead is called aVR (augmented voltage right arm). If the positive electrode is on the left arm, it is called aVL (augmented voltage left arm). When the positive electrode is on the left foot, it is called aVF (augmented voltage foot) (Fig. 15–6).

If one takes the three sides of Einthoven's triangle and moves them to the center, they form three intersecting lines of reference (Fig. 15–7A). If one superimposes the augmented limb leads, the lines of reference and the six limb leads form six

intersecting lines (one every 30 degrees). Each limb lead records a different angle and therefore a different view of the same electric activity (Fig. 15–7B).

For the precordial or chest leads, the positive electrodes are applied to the person's chest and the negative electrode is applied to the limbs. Usually, six chest leads are recorded. This is carried out by placing the positive electrodes at six different positions across the chest. The chest leads are identified as $V_1$ through $V_6$. The chest leads give various views of the horizontal plane of the left ventricle. The precordial leads can be visualized as spokes of a wheel, the center being the atrioventricular (AV) node (Fig. 15–8).

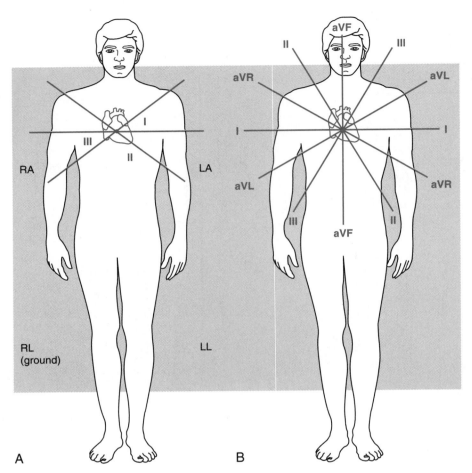

**Figure 15–7**
*A,* Intersecting limb leads. *B,* Intersecting limb and augmented leads.

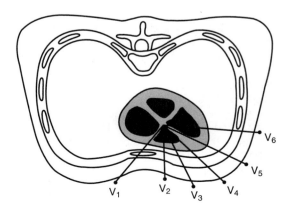

**Figure 15–8**
Precordial leads (V$_1$ to V$_6$).

## 15-Lead ECG

With growing recognition of right ventricular infarction, right-sided ECGs are increasing in frequency. Right ventricular infarctions present with ST elevations of at least 1 mm in the right precordial leads $V_{4r}$ and $V_{5r}$. Because the right coronary artery serves both the left ventricular inferior wall and the right ventricle, it is recommended that a right-sided or 15-lead ECG be done on any patient presenting with an inferior wall myocardial infarction.

## 18-Lead ECG

In the past, posterior wall infarctions were diagnosed by reciprocal changes seen on the 12-lead ECG. Now, when a posterior wall infarction is suspected (an inferior wall myocardial infarction has occurred), three additional leads are done with the 15-lead ECG. These are the posterior leads $V_7$, $V_8$, and $V_9$.

Understanding the lead system of the ECG is important for interpretation of its results. The morphologic features or shape of the varied waveforms is dependent on the lead. Whether the waveform is positive, negative, or biphasic depends on whether the mean electric axis is toward or away from the positive electrode of the lead.

Some newer monitor systems permit continuous 12-lead electrocardiographic monitoring.

| | |
|---|---|
| **Purpose of the Test** | The purpose of the 12-, 15-, and 18-lead ECG is to diagnose myocardial infarction, injury, and ischemia. It also assists in identifying hypertrophy, axis deviations, and electrolyte abnormalities and distinguishes between ventricular and supraventricular tachycardias. Left versus right hypertrophy can be distinguished by comparing the morphologic characteristics of the QRS complex in leads $V_1$ and $V_6$, by determining axis deviation, and by interpreting the P-wave. |
| **Procedure** | For a 12-lead ECG, the technician, the physician, or the nurse places the patient in a supine position. Conduction jelly is placed on the electrodes, and the electrodes are applied. The electrocardiograph's electrode wires are marked and color coded. It is essential that the chest leads be positioned correctly for accurate interpretation. |

The chest leads are applied as follows:

$V_1$: Fourth intercostal space at the right sternal border
$V_2$: Fourth intercostal space at the left sternal border
$V_3$: Midway between $V_2$ and $V_4$
$V_4$: Fifth intercostal space at the left midclavicular line
$V_5$: Fifth intercostal space at the anterior axillary line
$V_6$: Fifth intercostal space at the midaxillary line (Fig. 15–9)

Electrocardiographs vary. Older machines record one lead at a time. Newer machines simultaneously record the 12 leads and automatically mark them.

Leads for right ventricular assessment are placed at the right fifth intercostal space at the midclavicular line ($V_{4r}$), at the right intercostal space at the anterior axillary line ($V_{5r}$), and at the right fifth intercostal space at the midaxillary line ($V_{6r}$).

With the 18-lead ECG, a 15-lead ECG is taken, and then three chest electrodes are placed on the line level with the fifth intracostal space (ICS) at the posterior axillary line ($V_7$). The next electrode is placed at the fifth ICS at the posterior mid-clavicular line ($V_8$), and the last electrode is placed at the fifth ICS, left of the spinal column ($V_9$).

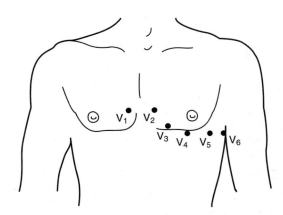

**Figure 15–9**
Chest lead placement.

---

**Findings**

Axis deviations (right or left)
Conduction disturbances
Dysrhythmias
Hypertrophy of the ventricles
Electrolyte imbalances
Pericarditis
Pulmonary infarctions
Therapeutic drug effects or toxicity, or both

As a myocardial infarction evolves, a sequence of electrocardiographic changes occurs. First, the ST segment changes. Elevation of an ST segment indicates myocardial injury. ST depression occurs as a reciprocal change in the ventricular wall opposite the infarction. The ST segment will return to normal within days or weeks after the infarction.

Within hours or days of the infarction, the T-wave inverts. It reflects ischemic changes in the heart. The T-wave will revert back to normal within weeks or months of the infarction.

Lastly, an abnormal Q-wave appears in the leads directly over the transmural myocardial infarction. An abnormal Q-wave is a Q-wave in a lead in which a Q-wave is not normally seen or one that is wider than 0.04 seconds or a third of the height of the QRS complex. A non–Q-wave infarction occurs when a subendocardial infarction occurs. A Q-wave indicates myocardial necrosis and may remain for years after the infarction.

Table 15–2 summarizes which leads reflect which walls of the left ventricle. Note that because leads are usually not placed over the posterior wall of the heart, posterior infarctions are diagnosed by reciprocal changes. Right ventricular infarctions are assessed by performing a right-sided 12-lead ECG.

---

**Interfering Factors**

- Patient movement, poor grounding, and poor skin contact can interfere with a clear recording of the ECG.

**Table 15–2    Electrocardiographic Changes with Acute Myocardial Infarction**

|  | Lead Changes | Reciprocal Changes |
|---|---|---|
| Inferior wall | II, III, aVF | I, aVL |
| Lateral wall | I, aVL, $V_5$, $V_6$ | $V_1$, $V_2$, $V_3$ |
| Anterior wall | $V_2$, $V_3$, $V_4$ | II, III, aVF |
| Anteroseptal | $V_1$, $V_2$, $V_3$, $V_4$ | II, III, aVF |
| Posterior wall | $V_7$, $V_8$, $V_9$ | $V_1$, $V_2$, $V_3$, $V_4$ |
| Right ventricular | $V_{4R}$, $V_{5R}$ | |

## Nursing Implementation

### Pretest

Explain to the patient the purpose and procedure for the ECG. No risk is involved.

No pretest restrictions are required.

Because electrodes are applied to the four extremities and the chest, clothing should permit easy access. If the male patient's chest is excessively hairy, the sites may need to be shaved.

### During the Test

Establish a relaxed environment.

Place the patient in a supine position.

Conduction jelly is placed on the electrodes, and the electrodes are applied.

The recording is made.

If a 15- or 18-lead ECG is done, clearly identify the lead placement on the ECG recording.

### Posttest

Remove the conduction jelly.

Help the patient to a comfortable position.

## Complications

Electrocardiography is a noninvasive procedure without complications.

# Electrophysiologic Studies

**(Radiology)**                    Synonym: EPS

## Normal Values

Normal cardiac rhythm; normal conduction, refractory, and interval times

## Background Information

Electrophysiologic studies are invasive procedures performed in special laboratories or in cardiac catheterization laboratories. These studies require the insertion of catheters into the right and some- times the left side of the heart. Several procedures are included: atrial stimulation, ventricular stimulation, His' bundle studies, and ventricular mapping.

| | |
|---|---|
| **Purpose of the Test** | Electrophysiologic studies are performed to diagnose dysrhythmias, to identify causes of ectopy and reentry phenomenon, and to determine a person's risk for lethal ventricular dysrhythmias. They are used to determine appropriate therapy for patients who have not obtained the desired effect from usual therapies and in whom noninvasive evaluation techniques have not provided the information necessary to determine which therapy or combination of therapies will be effective. |
| **Procedure** | Several procedures are included in the category of electrophysiologic studies. The patient may have one or all of the studies performed based on the clinical state. During the test, three or four multipolar pacing catheters are inserted percutaneously. One is positioned high in the atrium, one in the low-septal right atrium, one in the coronary sinus, and one in the right ventricle. Conduction intervals are measured to locate conduction delays by *programmed electrical stimulation (PES)*. Atrial pacing is carried out to assess sinoatrial node response, atrioventricular node response, and His' bundle and Purkinje conduction. If indicated, *atrial extrastimulus testing (AEST)* is performed. With this test, a premature atrial stimulus is initiated to assess atrial and atrioventricular node response. Atrial flutter or atrial fibrillation may be initiated. The focus or reentry pathway may then be identified. In some patients, *His' bundle electrographic studies* are performed to evaluate His' bundle conduction. |
| |     *Ventricular extrastimulus testing (VEST)* is performed to assess ventricular dysrhythmias. Ventricular tachycardia (VT) may be induced. If a right ventricular stimulus does not induce VT, a left-sided stimulation may be carried out. This requires the insertion of a multipolar pacing catheter through an artery. When VT is induced, its response to overdrive pacing or drugs, or both, can be evaluated. If the patient has recurrent VT, *ventricular endocardial mapping* may be performed to localize the origin of the dysrhythmia. If ventricular mapping is performed, VT is induced, and the ectopic focus is delineated by multiple intracardiac tracings. |
| |     If the electrophysiologic studies involve evaluation of drug responses, the test must be repeated, because only one drug or combination of drugs can be assessed at a time. If this is necessary, subclavian catheters are left in place between testings. |
| **Findings** | Electrophysiologic studies may identify dysrhythmias, conduction abnormalities, and appropriate treatment for these disturbances. |
| **Interfering Factors** | • See section on cardiac catheterization. |
| **Nursing Implementation** | The nursing actions are similar to those for cardiac catheterization, with the following additions. |

### Pretest

Reassure the patient that if dysrhythmias or blocks occur, resources are available to control and treat them.

Warn the patient that a "fluttering" sensation in the chest or hiccups may occur.

Antiarrhythmic drugs are usually discontinued for four half-lives (or four doses) before the test. In patients with potentially lethal dysrhythmias, cardiac monitoring is required.

The patient receives nothing by mouth for 6 hours before the procedure.

Premedication usually consists of diazepam (Valium), because it has no significant electrophysiologic effect. Avoid any medications with possible cardiac effect.

### During the Test

Actions are similar to those in cardiac catheterization except that only small doses of lidocaine are used as a local anesthetic to prevent systemic effects.

### Posttest

Assess site of catheter placement. If further studies are to be carried out, a catheter may have been left in place.

Check distal pulses if left-sided catheterization was performed.

Bedrest is maintained. For a right-sided study, bedrest is maintained for 2 hours; for a left-sided study, bedrest is maintained for 6 to 12 hours.

Encourage the patient to turn from side to side.

Avoid hip flexion if a femoral insertion was performed.

Evaluate the dressings for bleeding and infection. They should be kept dry and intact.

Anticoagulant therapy may be ordered if prolonged catheterization was required or if left ventricular stimulation or mapping was performed.

Patient and family teaching will depend on the findings of the studies and the indicated therapy.

---

**Complications**  See section on cardiac catheterization. In addition, if a subclavian insertion site was used, observe for pneumothorax.

---

## Endomyocardial Biopsy

**(Pathology)**  Synonyms: None

---

**Normal Values**  Normal cardiac tissue

---

### Background Information

Endomyocardial biopsy is an invasive procedure requiring cardiac catheterization. It permits sampling of right or left ventricular tissue.

---

**Purpose of the Test**  An endomyocardial biopsy is usually performed to determine if a transplanted heart is being rejected. Other purposes for the biopsy are to diagnose myocarditis or doxorubicin (Adriamycin)-induced cardiomyopathy and to determine the cause of restrictive heart disease.

| | |
|---|---|
| **Procedure** | The procedure involves a cardiac catheterization (see pp. 318–321). A catheter with a jawlike tip is inserted under fluoroscopy, and several small tissue samples are obtained. A right or left ventricular sample may be taken. For patients at high risk, such as those with a history of left ventricular thrombus or infarction, a right ventricular biopsy may be preferred. |
| **Findings** | Doxorubicin-induced cardiomyopathy<br>Cardiac amyloidosis<br>Cardiac fibrosis (especially radiation injury)<br>Chagas' cardiomyopathy<br>Myocarditis<br>Rejection of transplanted heart<br>Scleroderma<br>Toxoplasmosis<br>Tumor infiltrates<br>Vasculitis |
| **Interfering Factors** | • Bleeding disorders<br>• Severe thrombocytopenia<br>• Systemic anticoagulation<br>• Uncooperative patient |
| **Nursing Implementation** | See section on cardiac catheterization. |
| **Complications** | Although complications of endomyocardial biopsy are rare, they include accidental biopsy of papillary muscle or chordae tendineae, cardiac perforation, and hemopericardium. Other complications can occur but are related to the catheterization rather than to the biopsy itself. Table 15–3 provides assessments made by the nurse that indicate a complication. |

## Ergonovine Provocation Test

**(Radiology)**                    Synonyms: None

| | |
|---|---|
| **Normal Values** | No ST segment changes |

### Background Information

Ergonovine provocation testing is used to diagnose coronary artery spasm and vasospastic angina. Accurate diagnosis of coronary artery spasm is necessary, because treatment varies. Because of its risk, ergonovine provocation testing is limited to carefully selected patients.

### Table 15–3 Complications of Endomyocardial Biopsy*

| Complication | Nursing Assessment |
|---|---|
| Accidental biopsy of papillary muscle or chordae tendineae | New onset of a mitral or tricuspid murmur |
| Hemopericardium | Decreased cardiac output<br>Muffled heart sounds<br>Increased right atrial pressure<br>Pulsus paradoxus |
| Cardiac perforation | Same as hemopericardium<br>Shock |

*Complications other than those listed can occur, but they are related to cardiac catheterization.

## Purpose of the Test

Ergonovine provocation testing is indicated in patients with atypical angina in whom coronary artery spasm is *suspected*.

## Procedure

The ergonovine provocation test is usually performed as part of a cardiac catheterization. First, the cardiac catheterization must rule out severe coronary artery obstruction. A pacing wire is then inserted. Intravenous ergonovine maleate (Ergotrate Maleate) is given, which usually will stimulate a spasm within 3 to 6 minutes. Its effect lasts 10 to 15 minutes. If a positive response occurs, the spasm is reversed by administering nitroglycerin intravenously.

Bedside ergonovine provocation testing can be performed in the coronary care unit in patients who have had a cardiac catheterization to verify that the coronary arteries are not severely obstructed. Ergonovine is given intravenously every 5 minutes up to seven times. The ergonovine is stopped when ST segment changes are seen on the monitor, whether the patient has pain or not. Nitroglycerin is given to reverse the spasm.

## Findings

A positive response to ergonovine includes chest pain with ST segment abnormalities (rarely, chest pain does not occur), spasms visible on the arteriogram, serious dysrhythmias, or a combination of these responses.

## Interfering Factors

• Ergonovine provocation testing should not be performed if severe obstruction of a coronary artery or multivessel obstructive cardiac disease exists or in the presence of severe congestive heart failure, uncontrolled hypertension, pregnancy, acute myocardial infarction, or possible cerebral hemorrhage. It is contraindicated in anyone with a history of hypersensitivity to ergonovine.

## Nursing Implementation

See section on cardiac catheterization. In addition, review the following.

### Pretest

Warn the patient that chest pain is expected but will be treated immediately.
Discontinue vasoactive medications: nitrates for 4 hours before the test, calcium
channel blockers for 24 hours before the test, and beta-blockers for 48 hours
before the test.

### During the Test

Continuous cardiac and hemodynamic monitoring is performed. If major
adverse effects are noted, the ergonovine is stopped.

### Posttest

Assess the patient for chest pain with or without ST segment changes, as
spasms may recur after the nitroglycerin is stopped.
Maintain monitoring and bedrest for 1 to 2 hours if the procedure is performed
in the coronary care unit.

---

**Complications**

A variety of complications may occur with ergonovine provocation testing.
Close observation of the patient as well as assessment of subjective data
is essential. The complications range from nausea, vomiting, and headache to
atypical chest pain, myocardial infarction, dysrhythmias, bronchospasms,
and hyper- or hypotension. Table 15–4 summarizes the assessments with
each of these complications.

**Table 15–4    Complications of Ergonovine Provocation Testing**

| Complication | Nursing Assessment |
| --- | --- |
| Atypical chest pain | Patient report |
| Bronchospasms | Dyspnea<br>Wheeze |
| Dysrhythmias | Monitor for ventricular tachycardia, ventricular fibrillation, complete heart block, sinus arrest |
| Nausea, vomiting | Patient report<br>Emesis |
| Hypotension or hypertension | Monitor blood pressure<br>Hemodynamic monitoring |
| Headaches | Patient report |
| Myocardial infarction | Chest pain<br>Electrocardiographic changes<br>Elevated cardiac enzyme levels |

## Gated Blood Pool Studies

**(Radionuclide Imaging)**     Synonyms: Technetium 99 ventriculography, MUGA, multiple gated acquisition angiography

| Normal Values | Normal wall motion<br>Ejection fraction = 55%–75%<br>Response to exercise: Increase in ejection fraction greater than 5% |
|---|---|

### Background Information

A gated blood pool study is a noninvasive method of assessing myocardial function, particularly wall motion of the left ventricle. It also permits evaluation of left ventricular ejection without invasive catheterization.

**Purpose of the Test**     A gated blood pool study is performed to assess ventricular function by evaluating wall motion and determining ejection fractions.

**Procedure**     The procedure for the gated blood pool study is similar to that for myocardial imaging. The red blood cells are tagged with technetium 99m pyrophosphate, a gamma-emitting radionuclide. Because the bound technetium cannot diffuse through cell membranes, it remains in the blood. Its emissions are more concentrated in body cavities with large blood volumes, including the heart chambers.

During the procedure, the patient is monitored with a cardiac monitor, and the ECG is synchronized with the imaging equipment. Multiple images can be obtained. Results usually report the "first pass," which analyzes the radiotracing during the initial flow through the heart. In addition, a "gated" analysis is performed, which reports cardiac chamber responses of 200 to 300 cardiac cycles. Because left ventricular size can be measured at the end of diastole and systole, the ventricular ejection fraction can be measured. After a gated analysis, the patient may or may not be reassessed with exercise stress testing.

**Findings**     Hypokinesis (slightly diminished wall motion)
Akinesis (absence of wall motion)
Dyskinesia (paradoxical wall motion or bulging)
Decreased ejection fraction

**Nursing Implementation**     See sections on cardiac imaging and stress testing.

**Complications**     See section on stress testing.

## Holter Monitoring

Synonym: Ambulatory monitoring

| Normal Values | Normal rate and rhythm; no ectopy, reentry phenomenon, or changes in segments of the ECG with exercise or medication, or both |
| --- | --- |

## Background Information

Holter monitoring permits the recording of cardiac electric activity over time (usually 24 hours) on a cassette tape recorder. It allows the patient to perform normal daily activities so that cardiac responses to these activities can be determined.

## Purpose of the Test

The primary purpose of Holter monitoring is dysrhythmia detection. This procedure is helpful in identifying conduction defects and responses to therapeutic measures.

## Procedure

*Critical Thinking 15–4*
If the patient's ejection fraction is less than 20%, what adaptations in nursing care must be made?

With Holter monitoring, electrodes are applied to the patient's chest (placement varies with desired leads) and attached to a battery-operated cassette tape recorder. Most recorders permit simultaneous recording of two channels (frequently leads II and $V_5$ are chosen). Recorders are equipped with an event marker, which alerts the scanning technician that the patient experienced some symptom. A diary is kept by the patient, who records daily activities and the times at which they were performed, when and what medications were taken, and the presence and time at which symptoms occurred. The recordings are analyzed at 60 to 120 times real time by a microcomputer program. Any abnormalities are then recorded on the usual electrocardiograph paper.

## Findings

Conduction disturbances
Dysrrhythmias

## Interfering Factors

• Failure of patient to keep records of events and medications taken.

## Nursing Implementation

### Pretest

Inform patient regarding the purpose of the Holter monitoring and the vital role he or she plays in obtaining the needed information.
Check the Holter monitor's indicator light to determine if the battery is functioning.
The patient is instructed to keep a diary of activities and is taught how to trigger the event marker.

### During the Test

Apply electrodes to the chest. Shave the site if the chest is hairy.
Have the patient demonstrate triggering the event marker. The patient will push the marker whenever pain or other symptoms occur.
Give the patient a writing pad to record activities during the test time.

## Posttest

Remove electrodes and cleanse the site of gel.
Observe the skin for signs of irritation.

## Pericardiocentesis

**(Pathology)**             Synonym: Pericardial fluid analysis

| **Normal Values** | Fluid is sterile, clear, and colorless or straw-colored. |
| --- | --- |

## Background Information

Pericardiocentesis is a diagnostic and therapeutic procedure in which the pericardial space is accessed with a needle or cannula, and fluid is aspirated. For diagnostic purposes, the fluid is then analyzed. For therapeutic purposes, either fluid is drained on a one-time basis or a catheter is inserted and left in place for 1 to 48 hours (rarely, it may be kept in for 72 hours).

Normally, the pericardial space between the visceral and parietal pericardium contains approximately 20 to 50 mL of clear serous fluid. If the pericardium becomes inflamed or diseased or is disrupted, pericardial effusion may occur. As fluid builds up in the pericardial space, cardiac tamponade may result. Cardiac tamponade will eventually lead to a decrease in cardiac output, with an increase in right atrial pressure, pulsus paradoxus, and hypotension. If progressive and untreated, cardiac tamponade will result in death.

**Purpose of the Test**  Analysis of pericardial fluid is performed to determine the cause of and appropriate therapy for acute pericarditis, subacute effusive-constrictive pericarditis, neoplastic pericardial disease, and pericardial effusion of unknown cause.

**Procedure**  Pericardiocentesis for diagnostic purposes is not an emergency situation and can be performed in the controlled environment of an operating room or special procedure room. The procedure begins after skin preparation and infiltration of a local anesthetic, usually 1% lidocaine without epinephrine. A small incision is made in the skin, the site being determined by the desired approach.

The most common approach to the pericardial space is the left xiphocostal space. The needle is inserted through an incision made just under and to the left of the xiphoid process into the angle between the xiphoid process and the left costal margin. The physician points the needle toward the left shoulder and advances it until a "popping" or "giving" sensation is felt as the pericardium is entered. Traditionally, an electrocardiographic lead is attached to the pericardiocentesis needle. As the needle advances, a chest lead on the ECG is recorded. When the heart is punctured, a zone of injury pattern is noted, and the needle is withdrawn slightly. Some physicians do not recommend this technique, because poor electrocardiographic tracings prevent the zone of injury from being seen, which may lead to cardiac lacerations. Other approaches can be done, based on physician preferences. The sign of injury on the ECG also may not occur if the needle infiltrates an area of fibrosis, a tumor, or infiltrative cardiomyopathy tissue. A possibility of ventricular fibrillation exists if the electrocardiograph is not grounded properly, if electric leakage occurs, or if the individual performing the procedure accidentally touches the needle and electrocardiograph.

Once the needle is in position, approximately 20 mL of fluid is removed for analysis. If cytologic studies are performed, a heparinized container is necessary. The fluid is usually analyzed for color; hemoglobin concentration; hematocrit value; red blood cell, white blood cell, and differential counts; and protein and glucose determinations. In addition, Gram's stains and culture, fungal stains and culture, and cytologic studies are performed. Additional fluid is removed if viral and parasite studies, immunologic and serologic screens, or lipoelectrophoresis is planned.

If therapeutic pericarditis is desired after the specimens are obtained, a catheter is inserted and positioned to allow drainage.

| | |
|---|---|
| **Findings** | Bacterial, viral, or fungal infection <br> Malignancies |

| | |
|---|---|
| **Interfering Factors** | • Pericardiocentesis requires a patient who is cooperative and who will lie still during the procedure. Uncooperative patients may require sedation. Those receiving anticoagulant therapy, with bleeding disorders or thrombocytopenia, are not appropriate candidates. If cultures of the fluid are planned, administration of antibiotics will affect the results. |

**Nursing Implementation**

**Pretest**

Ensure that an informed consent form has been signed.
Explain the procedure to the patient.
Check laboratory work for bleeding problems.
Obtain a baseline ECG if ordered.
Document baseline vital signs and heart sounds.
Take medication history to check for anticoagulant use.
The patient maintains a nothing-by-mouth status for 4 to 6 hours before the test.
Administer sedation as prescribed.
Shave site as necessary.

**During the Test**

Position the patient. Usually a recumbent position is used, with the torso and head elevated 30 to 45 degrees.
Ensure that an intravenous infusion is present and patent.
Maintain telemetric or cardiac monitoring.
Frequent vital signs are taken.
Have a defibrillator and emergency drugs on hand.
Continue to reassure and support the patient, who will feel the local anesthetic being infiltrated and may experience a sharp pain when the pericardium is infiltrated.

**Posttest**

The patient may return to pretest activities gradually if vital signs are stable. Assess for recurrence of symptoms.

| Complications | Complications from pericardiocentesis include puncture or laceration of the cardiac chamber, laceration of a coronary artery, ventricular fibrillation, pneumothorax, and peritoneal puncture. Table 15–5 provides assessments of these complications. |
|---|---|

## Phonocardiogram

**(Sonogram)**    Synonyms: None

| Normal Values | No abnormalities |
|---|---|

### Background Information

A phonocardiogram is a graphic recording of cardiac sounds. It is a noninvasive test that amplifies cardiac sounds, which are recorded simultaneously with the electrocardiographic readings.

| Purpose of the Test | The phonocardiogram is performed to determine the exact timing of heart sounds; differentiate the varied sounds such as murmurs, splits, and clicks; and evaluate valvular function. |
|---|---|

| Procedure | A phonocardiogram may be carried out at the bedside, in the physician's office, in the clinic, or in a cardiac laboratory. Electrocardiographic equipment is necessary, and electrodes are applied. Microphones are placed over the heart in various positions. |
|---|---|

**Table 15–5   Complications of Pericardiocentesis**

| Complication | Nursing Assessment |
|---|---|
| Puncture or laceration of cardiac chamber | Bloody pericardial fluid<br>Acute cardiac tamponade |
| Laceration of coronary artery | Acute cardiac tamponade<br>Ventricular fibrillation |
| Ventricular fibrillation | Observed on monitor |
| Pneumothorax | Dyspnea<br>Absence of bilateral breath sounds |
| Peritoneal puncture | Straw-colored fluid if ascites is present |

| | |
|---|---|
| **Findings** | Valve disorders (stenosis or incompetence) |
| | Estimate of ventricular function |
| | Hypertrophic cardiomyopathies |

| | |
|---|---|
| **Interfering Factors** | • Improper placement of microphone |
| | • Muscle tremors |
| | • Obesity |
| | • Valsalva maneuver |

**Nursing Implementation**

### Pretest

Inform the patient as to the purpose and procedure of the study.
Explain to the patient that the test is painless and that no risk is involved.
Instruct the patient to remain quiet and still during the procedure.

### During the Test

Electrocardiograph electrodes are applied and attached to the electrocardiograph recorder.
Conduction jelly is applied to the chest wall.
As the phonocardiogram microphone is positioned at various sites over the chest wall, the patient may be asked to change position, perform muscle tightening, or change breathing patterns.

### Posttest

Remove conduction jelly from the chest and extremities.

## Roentgenogram, Cardiac

(Radiology)                    Synonym: Cardiac x-ray

| | |
|---|---|
| **Normal Values** | Normal size, shape, and positioning of the heart and great vessels |

### Background Information

A cardiac roentgenogram is a routine screening procedure in patients with suspected or known cardiac disorders. It provides information regarding the size of the heart, its shape, and the location of the cardiac structures and great vessels.

The x-ray study may also be used to evaluate pulmonary vasculature and determine the placement of evasive catheters and pacemaker wires.

See Chapter 9 for a full discussion of roentgenograms. The exception to the general preparation of the patient for a cardiac evaluation is that the electrodes used to monitor the patient are not usually removed when an x-ray film is taken.

| | |
|---|---|
| **Procedure** | Various views of the chest are usually obtained in a cardiac x-ray series. The four views commonly obtained are anteroposterior; posteroanterior; lateral, right anterior oblique; and left anterior oblique. During acute cardiac |

states, only portable chest x-ray studies are available to evaluate the client's progress. Because the plate is positioned under the client, an anteroposterior view is obtained.

## Signal-Averaged Electrocardiogram

**(Electrophysiology)**    Synonym: SAECG

| Normal Values | Normal cardiac rhythm and conduction times; normal Q-T interval |
|---|---|

### Background Information

Signal-averaged electrocardiography is a technique used to detect conduction defects that may precede ventricular tachycardia (VT). It is a noninvasive bedside test similar to a 12-lead ECG. With a signal-averaged ECG, the recording is obtained for 15 to 30 minutes, and the electric current from the heart is amplified 1,000 times. The machine then integrates all these signals and removes extraneous electric signals.

### Purpose of the Test

The cardiologist assesses the printout of the signal-averaged ECG for late potentials, which place the patient at risk for sustained VT. A late potential is seen as a QRS complex that extends 20 to 60 msec into the ST segment.

### Procedure

The procedure is similar to the 12-lead ECG, except that no limb electrodes are necessary and the six chest electrodes and ground lead are positioned differently on the chest.

### Interfering Factors

- Because the signal-averaged ECG averages the cardiac cycle of the patient, a relatively regular rhythm is needed during the test. *Frequent* premature atrial contractions or premature ventricular contractions will interfere with the results. Signal-averaged electrocardiography is also unable to detect late potentials in patients with right or left bundle branch block.

### Findings

Late potentials

### Nursing Implementation

The nursing actions are similar to those for electrocardiography. In addition, review the following.

#### Pretest

Check with the prescriber regarding discontinuing or administering the patient's antiarrhythmic medication.

#### During the Test

Keep the environment quiet.
Instruct others to stay out of the patient's room.

## Stress Testing, Cardiac

(Electrophysiology)

Synonyms: Graded exercise testing (GEX), graded exercise stress testing (GEST), exercise stress testing, exercise electrocardiography

| Normal Values | No unexpected changes in the ECG |
| --- | --- |

### Background Information

Stress testing is an important noninvasive procedure for evaluating the cardiovascular status of patients who are known to have cardiac disease or who are at risk for cardiac disease. The test increases the demand placed on the heart by increasing physical activity. Through electrocardiographic tracings, it can be determined whether the heart is able to meet the increased oxygen demand.

### Purpose of the Test

Stress testing is an invaluable technique for (1) assessing the at-risk population, (2) diagnosing chest pain syndromes and dysrhythmias associated with ischemia, (3) evaluating the effectiveness of therapy (surgical or pharmacologic), and (4) identifying the initial level of function in cardiac rehabilitation programs and evaluating the results.

### Procedure

Stress testing requires the use of a bicycle ergometer or a treadmill with continuous electrocardiac recording. The test is performed in a series of stages in which the patient exercises for 3 minutes. A variety of protocols are used in stress testing. The Bruce protocol involves gradual increase in speed and incline of the treadmill. The Ellestead protocol involves increasing speeds and intervals of shorter duration. At the end of each stage, a 12-lead ECG is recorded. After each stage, the workload or "graded load" is increased. This is accomplished by increasing the speed or resistance of the bicycle or treadmill. The stress testing continues until the patient reaches 85% of the maximum heart rate, becomes symptomatic, or displays electrocardiographic changes consistent with ischemia. The maximum heart rate is usually determined by normograms. A gross estimate of the maximum heart rate is 220 beats per minute minus the patient's age.

If a patient is physically unable to exercise to the point of 85% of the maximum heart rate, a *dipyridamole (Persantine) scan* may be performed. Dipyridamole may be given intravenously or by mouth. It causes coronary artery dilation similar to the response of the coronary arteries to exercise. After peak effect is reached (85% maximum heart rate), a thallium scan is performed (see pp. 344–345). A follow-up scan is performed 4 hours later.

Similar to dipyridamole stress testing is the use of adenosine. Adenosine also has a vasodilating effect but has a much shorter half-life then dipyridamole. It is also used with the thallium scan.

### Findings

A 1-mm depression of the ST segment is a positive stress test, indicating myocardial ischemia.

| | |
|---|---|
| **Interfering Factors** | • Severe anxiety may interfere with the patient's ability to participate fully in the stress testing. False-positive results may be due to bundle branch block, ventricular hypertrophy, or digitalization. False-negative results may be due to the use of beta-blockers. |

**Nursing Implementation**

**Pretest**

Inform the patient about the purpose and procedure of the test.

Instruct the patient to wear comfortable clothes and rubber-soled walking shoes.

Instruct the patient not to eat, smoke, or drink alcohol for 3 to 4 hours before the test.

If the adenosine stress test is being done, instruct the patient to avoid theophylline-based drugs, dipyridamole, over-the-counter drugs, and caffeine for 24 hours.

Routine cardiac medications are usually continued.

Assess for the following contraindications to stress testing: chest pain; hypertension; thrombophlebitis; second- or third-degree heart block; serious dysrhythmias; severe congestive heart failure; and neurologic, musculoskeletal, or vascular problems that would impede mobility on the bicycle or treadmill.

Warn the patient that he or she will feel his or her heart racing, and instruct the patient to report chest pain during the procedure.

**During the Test**

Have emergency equipment and drugs available (code cart).

The patient is attached to electrodes for recording a 12-lead ECG.

A blood pressure cuff is put in place for quick access. A baseline blood pressure reading is obtained.

As the graded exercises begin, a multichanneled ECG is recorded. A 12-lead ECG is recorded, and the blood pressure is checked as each workload ends (every 3-minute increment).

Observe for signs to stop the stress testing, for example, falling blood pressure, three consecutive premature ventricular contractions, chest pain, or exhaustion. The stressing may or may not be discontinued if ST depressions occur, blood pressure does not rise, or frequent or coupled premature ventricular contractions or bundle branch block occurs.

If dipyridamole or adenosine is used, assess for the following side effects: myocardial infarction, dysrhythmias, bronchospasms, chest pain, nausea, headache, flushing hypotension, and dizziness. Have aminophylline available to treat serious side effects.

**Posttest**

Cardiac monitoring is continued for 5 to 10 minutes after the testing to evaluate the patient's physiologic response.

Blood pressure is checked.

Remove conduction jelly and assist in robing the patient if necessary.

Evaluate the patient's physical and emotional response to the testing.

Instruct the patient to rest and not to take hot showers or baths for 2 to 4 hours.

| | |
|---|---|
| **Complications** | Stress testing is performed in a controlled environment; however, dysrhythmias and myocardial ischemia may occur (Table 15–6). |

## Thallium Testing

**(Radionuclide Imaging)**    Synonyms: Thallium scan, thallium exercise imaging, resting thallium scan

| | |
|---|---|
| **Normal Values** | Normal myocardial perfusion; no "cold" spots |

### Background Information

Thallium is a radioactive analog of potassium, which is rapidly taken up by myocardial cells. After thallium 201 is given, almost 90% of it is extracted by the myocardium within seconds. For this to occur, two factors are essential: (1) adequate perfusion and (2) cellular extraction efficiency. Since cellular ischemia does not seem to affect thallium uptake in the myocardium, its lack of uptake is an indication of an infarction.

Instead of thallium, technetium $T_c 99_m$ (sestamibi), a tracer agent, can be used. It has a shorter half-life than thallium. *Dual isotope studies* can also be performed using thallium and sestamibi. Uptake of sestamibi is similar to that of thallium, but it does not redistribute within the myocardium as quickly. This allows for poststress imaging to be done for up to 1 to 2 hours after the injection.

Traditionally, three main planes or projections are taken with thallium testing. An alternative is the use of single-photon emission computed tomography (SPECT). Thallium or sestamibi is given, and, with SPECT, the computer reconstructs tomographic images taken by the Anger camera.

| | |
|---|---|
| **Purpose of the Test** | Thallium imaging is used to assess coronary blood flow to determine areas of infarction and ischemia. It is used to diagnose CAD and assess revascularization following coronary artery bypass surgery. |

| | |
|---|---|
| **Procedure** | Thallium scanning is performed with an Anger gamma camera combined with a computer. Continuous counts of emitted photons are made during the cardiac cycle. The scan identifies "cold" spots, areas of decreased thallium uptake. Cold spots identify areas of ischemia and infarction. Thallium can be given under a state of no physical demand, which is known as a *resting thallium study,* or it can be part of a stress test, in which case it is called *exercise thallium imaging.* Exercise thallium imaging distinguishes ischemic sites from infarcted areas. Thallium scans are repeated, once during stress testing and then 3 to 4 hours after the thallium was given and the stress test was completed. |

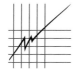

**Table 15–6    Complications of Cardiac Stress Testing**

| Complication | Nursing Assessment |
|---|---|
| Dysrhythmias | Monitor patient |
| Myocardial ischemia | Chest pain<br>ST depressions |

With the second imaging, if a cold spot remains, it is assumed to be an infarcted area. If the cold spot disappears, it is recognized as an ischemic area.

| | |
|---|---|
| **Findings** | Cold spots indicate and distinguish areas of infarction and ischemia. |

| | |
|---|---|
| **Interfering Factors** | • See section on stress testing. |

**Nursing Implementation**

Nursing care is similar to that in stress testing, except that an infusion of normal saline is started.

**Pretest**

Ensure that the patient is not pregnant.
Usually, long-acting nitrates are held for 8 to 12 hours before the test.
The patient fasts for 4 to 6 hours before the test but may drink water.
An infusion is started for intravenous access.
Inform the patient of the need to go to the nuclear medicine department twice.
If a SPECT scan is planned, check if the patient is claustrophobic.

**During the Test**

The thallium or adenosine is given intravenously about a minute before the completion of the stress test.
After the completion of the stress test, the patient is placed supine on the table, and multiple scintigraphic images are taken.
If a SPECT scan is done, the patient lies supine with arms over the head.
Between the two scans, the patient may drink clear, noncaffeinated fluids.

**Posttest**

Assess the patient's response.
Three to four hours later, the patient returns for repeat films.

## Transesophageal Echocardiography

**(Sonogram)**  Synonym: TEE

| **Normal Values** | No anatomic or functional abnormalities |
|---|---|

### Background Information

A transesophageal echocardiogram is an invasive procedure that uses ultrasound technique to detect enlargement of cardiac chambers and variations in chamber size during the cardiac cycle. It also assesses valvular function, septal defects, and pericardial effusion. Although these functions can be accomplished with a transthoracic echocardiogram, transesophageal echocardiography permits a better view of the posterior atrium and aorta. Transesophageal echocardiography is also indicated when a transthoracic approach is inadequate, such as when the patient is obese or has chest wall structure abnormalities.

**Purpose of the Test**

Indications for transesophageal echocardiography include diagnosis of (1) a thoracic aortic pathologic condition, including suspected aneurysms; (2) mitral valve disease; (3) suspected endocarditis; (4) congenital heart disease, for example, atrial septal defect; (5) left atrial intracardiac thrombi; and (6) cardiac tumors. It is also used to assess cardiac function during minimally invasive cardiac surgery (MICS) and to assess prosthetic valves.

**Procedure**

Transesophageal echocardiography is similar to transthoracic echocardiography except that the ultrasound probe is fitted into the end of a flexible gastroscopy tube and advanced down the esophagus behind the heart (Fig. 15–10).

**Findings**

See section on the echocardiogram.

**Interfering Factors**

- Transesophageal echocardiography should not be performed if the patient has a history of irradiation of the mediastinum, esophageal dysphagia, or structural abnormalities.

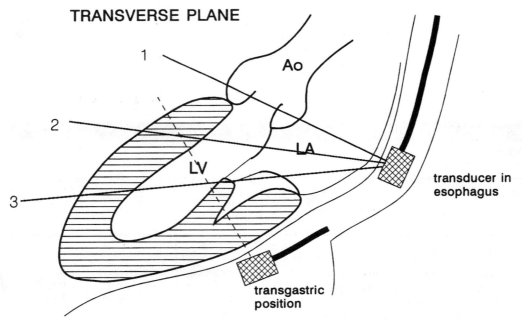

**Figure 15–10**

Transesophageal echocardiogram. (Reproduced with permission from Otto, C. M., & Pearlman, A. S. [1995]. *Textbook of clinical echocardiology* [p. 46]. Philadelphia: W. B. Saunders.)

**Nursing Implementation**

### Pretest

Ensure that a signed informed consent form has been obtained.

Question the patient about any disorder of the esophagus, stomach, throat, or vocal cords.

Inquire if the patient has dentures, bridges, or plates.

Report to the physician any history of arthritis of the neck, respiratory problems, or anticoagulation therapy.

Maintain the patient on a nothing-by-mouth status for 6 to 8 hours.

Describe the procedure to the patient, especially the need for a mouthguard, positioning, and the need to swallow when asked.

If the patient has prosthetic heart valves, prophylactic antibiotics may be prescribed.

Report any indications of infection in the mouth or throat.

Administer antianxiety medication as prescribed.

### During the Test

Administer medication to decrease secretions as ordered.

A topical anesthetic is sprayed into the throat.

Instruct the patient to gargle with viscous lidocaine and then to swallow it. Warn the patient that it will make the tongue and throat feel "swollen."

A mouthguard is placed to prevent the patient from biting down on the endoscope.

The patient is positioned on the left side in the chin-chest position. The head may be supported with a small pillow.

The probe is lubricated with lidocaine jelly and slowly inserted as the patient swallows.

Monitor the patient for a vasovagal response from the medication given to dry up secretions.

Check the patient for gagging.

Observe the oximeter for oxygen saturation readings.

### Posttest

Assess the patient for return of the gag reflex before resuming oral intake.

Instruct the patient to avoid hot liquids or foods for 2 hours.

If an outpatient, the patient must be accompanied home by another person.

Give lozenges for relief of throat discomfort.

**Complications**

Transesophageal echocardiography has several complications that are related to the placement of the probe in the esophagus, including esophageal perforation, transient hypoxia, dysrhythmias, and a vasovagal response. Table 15–7 provides a summary of assessments of each of these complications.

## Vectorcardiogram

**(Electrophysiology)**                Synonym: VCG

**Normal Values**        Normal cardiac axis

### Table 15–7   Complications of Transesophageal Echocardiography

| Complication | Nursing Assessment |
|---|---|
| Esophageal perforation | Bleeding<br>Pain |
| Transient dysrhythmias | Observe on monitor |
| Transient hypoxia | Observe pulse oximetry<br>Observe skin color and respiratory pattern |
| Vasovagal response | Observe monitor for bradycardia<br>Check pulse |

## Background Information

A vectorcardiogram is a graphic recording of electric forces of the heart. It is a noninvasive procedure that graphically records the direction and magnitude of the heart's electric forces by means of a continuous series of vector loops. Three planes of the heart are recorded (frontal, sagittal, and horizontal).

## Purpose of the Test

A vectorcardiogram is used to assess ischemia, conduction defects, and chamber enlargement (hypertrophy or dilation).

## Nursing Implementation

See section on electrocardiography for nursing care.

## References

Adams, J. E. (1997). Utility of cardiac troponins in patients with suspected cardiac trauma or after surgery. *Clinics of Laboratory Medicine, 17,* 613–623.

Adams, J. E., & Miracle, V. A. (1998). Cardiac biomarkers: Past, present, and future. *American Journal of Critical Care, 7,* 418–423.

Alger, A. (1998). Tests on demand. *Forbes, 161,* 208.

Arnold, S. E. (1997). What you should know about cardiac stress testing. *Nursing97, 27,* 58–61.

Beattie, S., & Staplton, A. (1997). Noninvasive evaluation of coronary artery disease and myocardial viability through stress echocardiography and myocardial perfusion imaging. *Nurse Practitioner, 22,* 32, 34, 39–40, 42, 45–46.

Beauregard, L. M., Volosin, K. J., Askenase, A. D., & Waxman, H. L. (1996). *Pace, 19,* 215–221.

Clochesy, J., Breu, C., Cardin, S., Whittaker, A., & Rudy, E. (1996). *Critical care nursing* (2nd ed.). Philadelphia: W. B. Saunders.

Fox, K. F. (1995). Cardiac enzymes. *Nursing Standard, 9,* 52–54.

Fraiti, A. F., Ineiestra, F., & Ariza, C. R. (1996). Acute effect of cigarette smoking on glucose tolerance and other cardiovascular risk factors. *Diabetes Care, 19,* 112–117.

Henderson, A. R. (1997). An overview and ranking of biochemical markers of ischemic cardiac disease: Strengths and limitations. *Clinics in Laboratory Medicine, 17,* 625–654.

Hudak, C. M., Gallo, B. M., & Morton, P. G. (1997). *Critical care nursing: A holistic approach* (7th ed.). Philadelphia: Lippincott.

Jaffe, A. S. (1997). Troponin, where do we go from here? *Clinics of Laboratory Medicine, 17,* 737–752.

Keffer, J. H. (1997). Why cardiospecificity is preeminent in myocardial markers of injury. *Clinics of Laboratory Medicine, 17,* 727–735.

Keteyian, S. J., Brawner, C. A., & Schairer, J. R. (1997). Exercise testing and training of patients with heart failure due to left ventricular systolic dysfunction. *Journal of Cardiopulmonary Rehabilitation, 17,* 19–28.

Kuczek, W. (1995). Understanding technique and applying the results—common cardiac tests. *Journal of the American Academy of Physician Assistants, 8,* 20–36.

Lane, P. (1997). Cardiac electrophysiology studies and ablation procedures: A literature review. *Intensive and Critical Care Nursing, 13,* 224–229.

Lehmann, C. A. (Ed.). (1998). *Saunders manual of clinical laboratory science.* Philadelphia: W. B. Saunders.

Littrell, K., Walker, D., & Worthy, C. (1995). Myocardial infarction and the nondiagnostic ECG: Strategies to meet the challenges. *Journal of Emergency Nursing, 21,* 287–295.

Mercer, D. W. (1996). A historical background in cardiac markers. *Medical Laboratory Observer, 28,* 45–51.

Montes, P. (1997). Managing outpatient cardiac catheterization. *American Journal of Nursing, 97,* 34–37.

National Heart Attack Alert Program. (1997). An evaluation of technologies for identifying acute cardiac ischemia in the emergency department: A report from a national heart attack alert program working group. *Annals of Emergency Medicine, 29,* 13–87.

Owen, A. (1995). Tracking the rise and fall of cardiac enzymes. *Nursing95, 25,* 35–38.

Parsa, M. B. (1995). Current body applications of MR angiography. *Applied Radiology,* (Suppl.), 34–40.

Pengue, S., Halm, M., Smith, M., Deutsch, J., van Roekel, M., McLaughlin, L., Dzubay, S., Doll, N., & Beahrs, M. (1998). Women and coronary disease: Relationship between descriptors of signs and symptoms and diagnostic and treatment course. *American Journal of Critical Care, 7,* 175–182.

Pitman, H., Umscheid, D., & Yablonsky, T.: Troponin T—cardiac marker of the future? *Laboratory Medicine, 27,* 499.

Sherman, D. L., & Balady, G. J. (1995). What's new in stress testing? 2. Cardiac imaging modalities. *Hospital Medicine, 31,* 37–43.

Sherman, D. L., & Balady, G. J. (1995). What's new in stress testing? 3. Pharmacologic approaches. *Hospital Medicine, 31,* 32–36.

Speicher, C. E. (1998). *The right test* (3rd ed.). Philadelphia: W. B. Saunders.

Steinberg, J. S., & Berbari, E. J. (1996). The signal-averaged electrocardiogram: Update on clinical applications. *Journal of Cardiovascular Electrophysiology, 7,* 972–988.

Straube, G. (1996). A safe way to take pictures of the heart. (1996). *RN, 59,* 61.

Thelan, L. A., Urden, L. D., Lough, M. E., & Stacy, K. M. (1998). *Critical care nursing diagnosis and management* (3rd ed.). St. Louis: Mosby.

Thompson, J. (1994). Cholesterol screening and heart disease. *Professional Care of Mother and Child, 4*(2), 32.

Travin, M. I., & Johnson, L. L. (1995). Current status and future directions in nuclear cardiology. *Journal of Nuclear Medical Technology, 23,* 27S–34S.

Turner, D. M., & Turner, L. A. (1995). Right ventricular myocardial infarction: Detection, treatment, and nursing implications. *Critical Care Nurse, 15,* 22–27.

Tymchak, W. J., & Armstrong, P. E. (1997). Spectrum of ischemic heart disease and the role of biochemical markers. *Clinics of Laboratory Medicine, 17,* 701–725.

VanRiper, S., & VanRiper, J. (1997). *Cardiac diagnostic tests.* Philadelphia: W. B. Saunders.

Vansant, J. (1995). Myocardial perfusion imaging: Clinical applications. *Applied Radiology, 24,* 11–14.

Verklan, M. T. (1997). Diagnostic techniques in cardiac disorders: Part I. *Neonatal Network, 16,* 9–15.

Verklan, M. T. (1997). Diagnostic techniques in cardiac disorders: Part II. *Neonatal Network, 16,* 7–13.

Waggoner, A. D., Harris, K. M., Braverman, A. C., Barzilai, B., & Geltman, E. M. (1996). The role of transthoracic echocardiography in the management of patients seen in an outpatient cardiology clinic. *Journal of the American Society of Echocardiography, 9,* 761–767.

Weiss, R. L., Brier, J. A., O'Connor, W., Ross, S., & Brathwaite, C. M. (1996). The usefulness of transesophageal echocardiography in diagnosing cardiac contusions. *Chest, 109,* 73–77.

Yager, M. (1996). Right ventricular infarction in the emergency department: A review of pathophysiology, assessment, diagnosis, treatment, and nursing care. *Journal of Emergency Nursing, 22,* 288–292.

# CHAPTER 16

# Peripheral Vascular Function

This chapter discusses the diagnostic procedures that identify abnormalities in the anatomic structure and the lumens of arteries and veins. Additionally, most of the procedures evaluate the alterations in blood flow that result from trauma or disease processes.

When the lumen of the artery is partially blocked, the descriptive term is *stenosis.* When the lumen of either the artery or the vein is completely blocked, the descriptive term is *occlusion.* In arterial peripheral vascular disease, the most common causes of stenosis and occlusion are atherosclerosis and thrombus, particularly affecting the aorta and the iliac and femoral arteries. In venous disease of the lower extremities, the most common cause of occlusion is thrombosis or thrombophlebitis, particularly affecting the deep femoral vein.

Many of the vascular diagnostic procedures are *invasive,* meaning that the blood vessel is penetrated by needle, catheter, or insertion of an instrument into the vascular lumen. Additionally, an iodine-based contrast agent is sometimes used to outline the lumen of the vessel and the abnormalities present. Arteriography, venography, and lymphangiography all use a contrast agent that is administered by needle or catheter insertion into the vascular lumen.

*Noninvasive* testing modalities also exist that offer minimal risk to the patient and provide excellent viewing of the blood vessels in the extremities. Ultrasound, plethysmography, computed tomography (CT), and magnetic resonance imaging (MRI) are used to assess the quality of the vascular system, quantify the amount of blood that can circulate through a partially occluded vessel, and identify tumors or other pathologic conditions that externally compress the blood vessel and impede circulation. Because they are safe and painless, these noninvasive procedures can be repeated as needed in the ongoing or long-term evaluation of the patient.

In recent years, many improvements, refinements, and modifications have been made in the design of catheters and guides and in the composition of contrast agents. These changes have resulted in greater safety for the patient. Also, major improvements have occurred in the quality of imaging because of the invention and use of x-ray image intensifiers, high-definition monitors, videotape or videodisc recorders, instant replay, and real-time subtraction techniques. These technologic developments have improved diagnostic accuracy because the images are much clearer.

The nurse can help the patient by preparing him or her for the procedure and explaining what to expect during the test. The advanced technology of the vascular laboratory can be intimidating. The results of the tests are a significant source of data for developing the patient's plan of care. The location, extent, and severity of peripheral vascular disease will require nursing modifications with regard for the patient's mobility, exercise, attainment of rest or comfort, and independence.

## Diagnostic Procedures

## Angiography

**(Radiography)**

Synonyms: Arteriography, digital subtraction angiography

Angiography uses an iodinated contrast agent, fluoroscopy, and x-ray studies to obtain images of the opacified artery and its target organ or organs. In peripheral arterial vascular disorders, angiography is used to investigate the origin, extent, and severity of arterial vascular disease. In peripheral vascular disease or arterial occlusive disease, the most common causes of stenosis or occlusion are atherosclerosis and thrombus, affecting the aorta and the femoral or iliac artery.

**Extremity Angiography.**   Following trauma to an arm or leg, such as from gunshot, stabbing, or automobile accident, extremity angiography may be required to investigate the status of the arterial circulation. An expanding hematoma or a bruit in the area of trauma or pulselessness, pallor, cold skin temperature, and neurologic abnormality in the distal part of the extremity are indicators of arterial damage.

A complete discussion of angiography is presented in Chapter 11.

## Cold Stimulation Test

**(Skin Temperature)**

Synonym: Cold sensitivity test

**Normal Values**

The temperature in the fingers returns to normal within 20 minutes.

## Background Information

In vasospastic disorders that affect the arterial circulation of the upper extremities, hypersensitivity to cold is a common complaint. In normal circulation, exposure of the hands and fingers to cold causes temporary vasoconstriction and a lowering of the temperature of the fingers. Once the cold temperature source is eliminated, the circulation improves and the temperature of the fingers returns to normal within 20 minutes. Patients with upper extremity vasospastic disorders require a much longer time to recover normal skin temperature (Fahey, 1994).

**Purpose of the Test**

The cold stimulation test assesses the symptom of upper extremity hypersensitivity to cold temperatures.

**Procedure**

The temperature of the fingers is recorded before and after the hands are immersed in ice water. The total time required for this test is 30 to 60 minutes.

| | |
|---|---|
| **Findings** | **Abnormal Values** |
| | Raynaud's syndrome    Systemic lupus |
| | Rheumatoid arthritis        erythematosus |
| | Scleroderma |

**Interfering Factors**

- Nicotine
- Caffeine
- Room temperature (excessively warm or cool)
- Gangrenous fingers
- Open wounds or infection in hands or fingers

**Nursing Implementation**

**Pretest**

Instruct the patient to refrain from smoking and ingesting caffeine (cola, cocoa, coffee, tea) for 24 hours before the test, because nicotine and caffeine are vasoconstrictive substances.

Remove any jewelry from the patient's fingers and wrists.

Inform the patient that the ice water can cause some temporary discomfort in the fingers but that it will disappear after the fingers are warm.

**During the Test**

Apply the thermistors to the distal part of the fingers of both hands. The thermistors record the skin temperature.

Record the baseline thermistor temperature.

Immerse the hands in ice water for 20 seconds.

Record the temperature immediately after removal of the hands from the water.

Record the temperature every 5 minutes until the temperature returns to the pretest baseline value.

**Posttest**

Remove the thermistors.

## Computed Tomography Angiography

**(Tomography Scan)**

Synonyms: CT scan, CT angiography

Computed tomography (CT) is a major diagnostic procedure in the assessment, diagnosis, and evaluation of vascular disease, particularly of the blood vessels of the torso. Often, the procedure uses an intravenous iodinated contrast medium to sharpen the view of the lumens of the arteries and surrounding organs.

CT provides visualization of the arterial wall and identifies other abnormalities, such as fluid or hematoma, that exist in the perivascular tissue. The cross-sectional views provide definition of the normal vascular anatomy and any significant, measurable abnormality (Fig. 16–1).

Preoperatively, it is the diagnostic procedure of choice to assess an abdominal aortic aneurysm, including its size, its location, and the extent of involvement of other arteries or organs.

**Figure 16–1**

Diagram of a cross-section of a diseased arterial wall. Computer-generated analysis of the average thickness of the aneurysmal wall and periaortic fibrosis calculated from computed tomographic (CT) scans of 12 patients with inflammatory abdominal aortic aneurysms. Note the increased thickness in the anterior wall. (Reproduced with permission from Fiorani, P., Faraglia, V., Speziale, F., Lauri, D., Massucci, M., & De Santis, F. [1991]. Extraperitoneal approach for the repair of inflammatory abdominal aortic aneurysm. *Journal of Vascular Surgery, 13,* 695.)

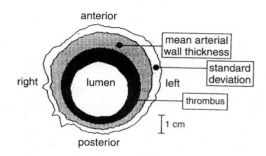

In arterial vascular disease, CT is used to diagnose an aneurysm of the thoracic or abdominal aorta or the iliac, femoral, or popliteal artery. It can also detect inflammation of the aneurysm, dissection, and any mural thrombus within the arterial defect. Postoperatively, it is used in the diagnosis of complications of a vascular graft and the evaluation of vascular stents and stent grafts.

In venous abnormalities, CT can identify the inferior vena cava and the presence of a thrombus, anatomic abnormality, or complication related to the placement of a vena cava filter. The presence of a deep vein thrombus can also be identified in the iliac–vena cava segment (Kim & Orron, 1992).

**Helical (Spiral) CT Scan.**   This scan is the newest type of CT and is of particular benefit in the diagnosis of aortoiliac aneurysmal or occlusive disease. With this technology, three-dimensional (3-D) longitudinal images of the entire aortoiliac system can be created from the data of the scan. The measurement of the exact size of an aortic aneurysm, the position of the branching arteries (celiac, superior mesenteric, renal, and iliac), and their patency are clearly visualized and documented. In addition, arterial stents and arterial grafts can be evaluated for patency, and arterial occlusive disease can be imaged and diagnosed (Rubin & Silverman, 1995).

A complete discussion of CT scanning is presented in Chapter 12.

## Doppler Ultrasound

**(Ultrasound)**          Synonyms: Doppler flow studies, Doppler testing

**Normal Values**

Arterial or venous examination: Normal frequency and volume of audio signal, normal waveform pattern, normal color for blood flow velocity, no evidence of vascular stenosis or obstruction

Ankle-brachial index (ABI): 0.9–1

Segmented pressures: <30 mm Hg difference in systolic pressure between the upper and lower segments of same extremity or between the right and left extremities

## Background Information

The Doppler ultrasound probe transmits low-intensity sound waves that are directed at a specific blood vessel. The transmitted sound waves strike moving red blood cells and bounce back to the transducer-receiver within the probe. The received impulses are translated into an audible signal or a waveform recording on graph paper. Additionally, the systolic pressure in the upper and lower extremities can be measured.

**Audible Signals.**   These signals are heard as the red blood cells circulate through the artery or vein and pass through the Doppler beam of sound waves. The instrument is sensitive and can detect even the most minimal blood flow. The frequency (pitch) of the sound is determined by the velocity of the blood flow. When erythrocytes circulate freely and rapidly in patent arteries or veins, the frequency is higher. Conversely, when blood flow is slowed because of stenosis, the pitch is lower.

The *loudness* of the sound is a measure of how many erythrocytes travel through the blood vessel and pass the Doppler beam. When the cells move rapidly and freely in a normal blood vessel, the sound is loud. Conversely, stenosis is indicated by softer, fainter sounds, and obstruction produces no sound at all.

*Waveform recordings* are Doppler signals that are transformed into a linear image. The waveforms are recorded on a graph-paper strip in a manner similar to the recording of an electrocardiogram (ECG).

The normal venous waveform is spontaneous and in phase with respirations. When the extremity and vein are compressed manually, signal augmentation occurs as seen by the upward spike in the waveform pattern. In abnormal venous flow, as in partial or total venous occlusion, the augmentation signal is absent. Reflux flow, such as that caused by incompetent venous valves, is also evident on the waveform.

The normal arterial waveform is characterized by three phases called the *systolic, diastolic,* and *wall rebound* phases (Fig. 16–2). When the artery is stenosed, the waveform pattern diminishes in height. In severe obstruction, the diastolic phase and wall rebound phase are absent.

The audio signal and waveform analysis are used to investigate peripheral vascular disease in the upper and lower extremities. In the diagnostic work-up for cerebrovascular disease, both components of the examination are used to assess the external carotid arteries in the neck.

**Ankle-Brachial Index and Segmented Pressures.**

These two measures assess systolic pressures within the arteries of the extremity. Both tests use blood pressure cuffs and the Doppler probe to obtain exact systolic readings at different levels of the extremities. They identify, locate, and quantify the drop in systolic blood pressure where it occurs. Stenosis or occlusion of the artery causes a drop in blood pressure distal to the site of the obstruction.

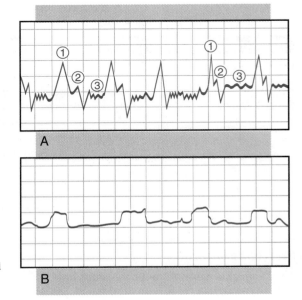

**Figure 16–2**

Normal versus abnormal Doppler arterial waveform patterns. *A,* Normal waveform with triphasic pattern of sharp upstroke and downstroke and good amplitude: *1,* systolic component; *2,* diastolic component; and *3,* elastic wall rebound. *B,* Abnormal waveform with monophasic pattern of low amplitude and flat waves. This pattern indicates severe arterial obstruction.

**Ankle-Brachial Index.**    The ABI compares the systolic pressure of the ankle with that of the arm. Normally, the systolic pressure of the ankle is equal or almost equal (90% to 100%) to that of the arm. The ABI is a comparison of the ankle pressure to the arm pressure and is expressed by one of the following mathematical formulas:

$$ABI = \frac{A \text{ (ankle pressure)}}{B \text{ (brachial pressure)}} \qquad ABI = A \div B$$

An ABI value of less than 0.9 is abnormal. It means that somewhere between the heart and the ankle a low systolic pressure has been caused by stenosis or occlusion of an artery. The numeric value of the ABI is inversely proportionate to the severity of the occlusion. An ABI of less than 0.5 indicates severe ischemia or gangrene.

**Segmented Pressures.**    These pressures are obtained when the ABI value is abnormal. The purpose is to locate the site of the diminished circulation in the extremity. Normal pressure differences should not exceed 30 mm Hg between the right and left limbs or segmentally between the upper and lower segments of the extremity.

**Quality Control**

The accuracy of the examination and the interpretation of the results depend on the expertise of the examiner. Additionally, some of the findings are subjective interpretations rather than measurable data (Fahey, 1994; Fleischer & Kepple, 1995).

## Purpose of the Test

Doppler ultrasound detects stenosis or occlusion in an artery or vein, assists with the diagnosis of peripheral vascular or cerebrovascular disease, evaluates the results of arterial reconstruction or vascular bypass surgery, and assesses for possible trauma to an artery.

## Procedure

■

*Critical Thinking 16–1*
The patient is scheduled for bone surgery on her foot. As you begin the Doppler ultrasound testing, the patient appears to be anxious. How do you respond?

**Venous and Arterial Doppler Tests.**    Acoustic gel and the Doppler probe are placed on the skin at the desired vascular sites. Audible signals are heard and interpreted. Three to five waveforms are recorded at each vascular site. The specific vascular sites and sides of the body (right or left) are identified to avoid confusion and error.

Venous sites of the lower extremities are the posterior tibial, greater saphenous, common femoral, superficial femoral, and popliteal veins. Venous sites of the upper extremities and neck are the brachial, axillary, subclavian, and jugular veins. Arterial pulse sites of the lower extremities are the common femoral, popliteal, dorsalis pedis, and posterior tibial pulses. Arterial pulse sites in the upper extremities and neck are the brachial, radial, ulnar, and carotid pulses.

**Segmented Pressures.**    Blood pressure cuffs are applied bilaterally to the upper thighs, above and below the knees, and above the ankles. Gel is applied to the skin. The pressure cuffs are inflated one at a time. On deflation of each, the Doppler probe identifies the systolic pressure by audio signal, and the numeric value is recorded. The ABI is calculated from the ankle and brachial pressures.

## Findings

**Abnormal Values**

Arterial stenosis or
    occlusion

Venous thrombosis

Venous valvular
    incompetency

| | |
|---|---|
| **Interfering Factors** | • Nicotine, alcohol, and caffeine<br>• Anxiety<br>• Uncooperative patient behavior |

| | |
|---|---|
| **Nursing Implementation** | **Pretest** |

Inform the patient about the test and obtain a written consent from the patient or the person legally designated to make health care decisions for the patient.

Instruct the patient to avoid nicotine, alcohol, caffeine, and other stimulants and depressants that will cause vasoconstriction.

Reduce the room lighting to promote relaxation.

Maintain a comfortable room temperature to prevent shivering and vasoconstriction.

Instruct the patient to remove all clothing and to wear a hospital gown.

For arterial tests, place the patient in the supine position. For venous tests of the lower extremities, place the patient in the supine position with two pillows under the legs to elevate them above the heart. The leg and hip are externally rotated, and the knee is flexed.

### During the Test

#### Venous Doppler Examination

Apply acoustic gel to the skin at the ankle, calf, thigh, and groin.

At each test point, use the probe and the audio mode to listen to the blowing sound that is in rhythm with the respirations.

Record three to five venous waveforms at each site, labeling each recording with the correct anatomic location.

#### Arterial Doppler Examination

Locate the pulse points on the upper or lower extremities and apply acoustic gel.

At each pulse point, apply the probe and the audio mode to listen to the blowing sounds.

Record three to five arterial waveforms at each site, labeling each recording with the correct anatomic location.

#### Ankle-Brachial Index

Place blood pressure cuffs on each arm and above each ankle.

Apply acoustic gel at the sites of the brachial, dorsalis pedis, and posterior tibial pulses.

Inflate each cuff (one at a time). Use the probe to identify the initial systolic beat as the cuff is deflated slowly.

Record the systolic pressures on the chart.

Calculate the ABI, using the arm with the higher pressure reading.

If the ABI value is less than 0.9, continue the examination with the segmented pressure examination.

#### Segmented Pressure Examination

Place additional cuffs at the top of the thighs and above and below the knees.

At the femoral and popliteal pulse sites, obtain the pressure readings by repeating the technique described previously. Waveforms may also be recorded at these sites.

Record all results on the chart.

### Posttest

Remove the blood pressure cuffs.
Remove the acoustic gel from the skin.

## Duplex Doppler Ultrasound

**(Ultrasound)**     Synonyms: Duplex scan, B-mode real-time imaging, duplex ultrasonography, vascular ultrasound

Duplex Doppler ultrasound combines the techniques of Doppler ultrasound and imaging to detect and identify abnormalities of arteries and veins. B-mode imaging locates and provides images of the affected vessel, and the Doppler component identifies the disturbance of blood flow caused by atherosclerotic plaque or thrombus. The two methods are complementary; their combination provides information that is clearer than the data obtained from a single modality.

**Color-Flow Doppler Ultrasound (CDU).**   The newest Doppler technology images and measures the blood flow velocity in color. In most systems, non-moving tissue (muscle or bone) is gray. Blood flow that moves toward the transducer is imaged as a shade of red. Blood flow that moves away from the transducer is imaged as a shade of blue. When blood flow within the artery or vein is normal, the color is intense, and the lumen of the blood vessel should be filled with color. With obstruction of the blood flow, such as with deep vein thrombosis, the color fades from red to orange or yellow or from blue to aqua or white. With turbulence of the blood flow, speckling is seen (Della Santina & Jolly, 1997; Hebdon & Letourneau, 1994).

Duplex Doppler ultrasound has been widely used to assess cranial neck vessels and is also used to assess the abdominal aorta and the peripheral vascular system. The technique can detect an embolus, stenosis, a thrombus, an aneurysm, and venous insufficiency.

Although venography remains the best imaging method for lower-extremity deep vein thrombosis in the femoral and popliteal veins, ultrasound is highly useful and accurate in detection of a thrombus. Additionally, ultrasound is advantageous because it is noninvasive and less painful and uses no contrast medium (Della Santina & Jolly, 1997).

Duplex Doppler ultrasound may also be used to assist with arteriography, angioplasty, placement of an inferior vena cava filter, thrombotic therapy, and the evaluation of bypass grafts and vascular access grafts.

A complete discussion of ultrasound is found in Chapter 8.

## Lymphangiography

**(Radiography)**     Synonyms: None

**Normal Values**     No evidence of obstruction, tumor, or enlarged nodes in the lymphatic system

## Background Information

The lymphatic system is an extensive network of capillaries, channels, and ducts that collect and transport lymphatic fluid. This system moves fluid from organs and tissues to the thoracic duct and then to the venous circulation. The lymph nodes are located at many sites within the system and serve as filters of the fluid. When the lymphatic system is obstructed, stasis and backflow of fluid will result. This causes lymphedema, which is the collection of lymphatic fluid in the interstitial spaces.

Several possible causes for blockage in the lymphatic system exist, including congenital abnormality, irradiation or other causes of fibrosis, surgical excision of lymphatic tissue, filariasis, and advanced malignancy. In the case of malignancy, usually metastatic involvement of the lymph nodes occurs in the pelvis, groin, and abdomen.

Lymphangiography is used infrequently today because of the effectiveness of CT scans, MRI, and ultrasound in the imaging of enlarged lymph nodes and the staging of malignancy. Additionally, lymphangiography is painful and carries a greater risk of complications than do the noninvasive imaging alternatives (Snopek, 1992).

| | |
|---|---|
| **Purpose of the Test** | Lymphangiography is used to diagnose the cause of lymphedema of the lower or upper extremities. It may also be used to investigate metastatic disease, lymphoma, and other cancers, including staging of the cancer and evaluation of cancer therapy. |
| **Procedure** | Under local anesthesia, methylene blue is injected subdurally into the webbing between the great toe and the second toe. The lymphatic system transports the dye upward along the dorsum of the foot until a larger lymphatic vessel is identified.<br><br>A 1-in incision is made over the dye-stained lymphatic vessel. After dissection, the vessel is cannulated with a fine needle that has tubing attached. Using a pump, iodized oil contrast material is instilled through the tubing and needle into the lymphatic vessel at a rate of 5 to 10 mL/hr. As the dye ascends through the lymphatic system, multiple x-ray films are taken to visualize the lymphatics and lymph glands of the lower extremities, groin, pelvis, and abdomen. The total time required for this test is 3 to 4 hours, with additional films taken after 12 to 24 hours. |

**Findings**

**Abnormal Values**

| | | |
|---|---|---|
| Hodgkin's lymphoma | Trauma | Primary lymphedema |
| Metastatic cancer | Inflammation | Filariasis |
| Retroperitoneal tumors | | |

**Interfering Factors**

- Allergy (iodine, shellfish, or contrast medium)
- Severe lung, heart, liver, or kidney disease

**Nursing Implementation**

**Pretest**

Identify any history of allergy to iodine or shellfish or any previous reaction to an x-ray study that used contrast material.

Provide instruction about the procedure and obtain informed consent from the patient or person who is legally responsible for making health care decisions for the patient.

Inform the patient of the following: the time required for the test and the need to return for additional films, the need to arrange for transportation home when the test is performed on an outpatient basis, the fact that the skin will have a blue streak and the stool will be blue for about 48 hours until the stain is cleared from the body, and the fact that a 1-in incision will be made on the back of the foot near the ankle.

Take baseline vital signs.

### During the Test

Instruct the patient to be still during the injections of the stain and the contrast medium and while x-ray films are taken.

Provide comfort and emotional support, because the test is distressing and painful. Pain is to be expected in the foot, back of the leg, and groin as the contrast medium reaches each area.

Monitor vital signs and observe for cardiopulmonary complications.

### Posttest

Monitor vital signs until they are stable.

Monitor the temperature every 4 hours for 48 hours. An infection or an inflammatory reaction may develop. Headache, sore throat, sore mouth, or swollen lymph glands often accompany the fever (Torres, 1993).

To reduce swelling, apply an ice pack to the incision.

Maintain a sterile dressing on the incision site for 2 days. Inform the patient that the incision may feel sore and that it is to be kept clean and dry. The sutures are removed in 7 to 10 days.

Instruct the patient to rest in bed for 24 hours with the foot elevated.

---

**Complications**

Lymphangiography can cause several complications. During the test, the patient can experience an allergic-type reaction to the iodine contrast medium, including cardiopulmonary distress. After the test, lymphangitis, cellulitis, or wound infection can occur. Although the methylene blue stain should disappear, it sometimes remains for a long time. A summary of the complications of lymphangiography appears in Table 16–1.

---

## Magnetic Resonance Angiography

**(Tomography)**

Synonym: MR angiography

Magnetic resonance angiography is a noninvasive procedure used to study blood flow and the structure and location of the major blood vessels. The blood acts as a physiologic contrast medium, so no pharmacologic contrast medium is needed. Generally, arterial blood flow appears dark and venous blood flow appears bright. The procedure can identify vascular stenosis, occlusion, thrombus, collateral vessels, tumor, aneurysm, and other abnormalities affecting an artery or vein. Additionally, the direction and rate of flow can be quantified (Muller & Edelman, 1995).

In vascular diagnostic procedures, magnetic resonance angiography of the

**Table 16–1   Complications of Lymphangiography**

| Complication | Nursing Assessment |
|---|---|
| Lymphangiitis | Generalized edema<br>Swelling of the extremity<br>Fever and chills<br>Enlarged nodes |
| Cellulitis and ascending infection | Redness<br>Swelling<br>Pain<br>Tenderness<br>Fever |
| Infection of suture line | Incisional redness, swelling<br>Tenderness<br>Purulence or serous drainage<br>Fever |
| Allergic-type reaction | Urticaria or itching<br>Erythema<br>Tachycardia<br>Respiratory distress or stridor<br>Cyanosis<br>Hypotension<br>Chest pain<br>Cardiac arrest |

abdominal vasculature can be used to identify abnormality of the inferior vena cava, renal veins, hepatic veins, portal vein, aorta, and renal arteries. In the study of the lower extremities, it provides a clear image of the circulation of the iliac arteries and veins and the femoral and popliteal veins. A complete discussion of magnetic resonance angiography is presented in Chapter 12.

## Plethysmography, Arterial

**(Manometry)**   Synonyms: Pulse cuff recording, PCR

| Normal Values | No evidence of arterial peripheral vascular disease; normal arterial waveform pattern |
|---|---|

### Background Information

Using blood pressure cuffs, plethysmography measures changes in the blood volume of the extremities. Normally, arterial flow is approximately equal to venous flow within an organ or extremity. If the

venous blood flow of an extremity is interrupted by using low pressure in the air cuffs, a subsequent increase occurs in the arterial blood volume of the extremity. This change in arterial volume can be detected by the plethysmograph. The machine records the linear waveform pattern on a strip of graph paper, much like the recording of an ECG (Blackburn & Peterson-Kennedy, 1994).

In normal arterial circulation, the waveform has a pulsatile pattern, with a characteristic rise, sharp peak, dicrotic notch, and down slope in each pulsation (Fig. 16–3). When the artery is stenosed or obstructed, a smaller volume of blood can pass through the arterial lumen. The abnormal waveform pattern is of low amplitude and reduced slope, with the loss of the dicrotic notch.

---

**Purpose of the Test**

Plethysmography is a noninvasive test that evaluates the arterial blood flow in the extremities. It detects the presence of peripheral arterial vascular disease.

---

**Procedure**

Plethysmographic cuffs are inflated at different levels on the extremities, and arterial waveforms are recorded. The test takes about 30 minutes to complete.

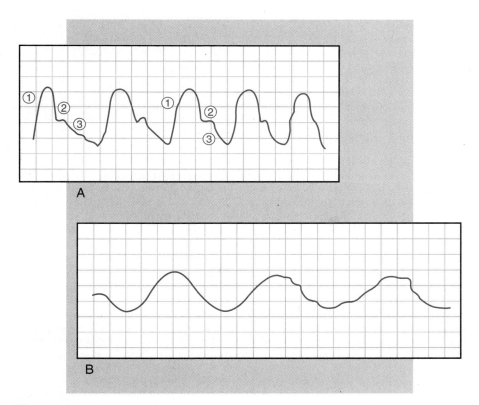

**Figure 16–3**

Normal versus abnormal arterial plethysmographic waveforms. *A,* The normal waveforms have characteristic *1,* sharp rise to peak; *2,* dicrotic notch; and *3,* downslope to baseline. *B,* Abnormal waveforms show a loss of the dicrotic notch, lower height, and rounding out of the peaks.

| **Findings** | **Abnormal Values** | | |
| --- | --- | --- | --- |
| | Peripheral vascular disease | Arterial occlusive disease | Arterial embolus Arterial trauma |

**Interfering Factors**

- Smoking
- Caffeine
- Alcohol
- Cold room temperature
- Anxiety

**Nursing Implementation**

### Pretest

Explain the procedure to the patient and obtain written consent from the patient or person responsible for the patient's health care decisions.

Instruct the patient to refrain from smoking and ingesting alcohol and caffeine before the test, because stimulants, depressants, and vasoconstrictive substances will alter the results.

Assist the patient in removing all clothing and putting on a hospital gown. Restrictive clothing can alter the circulatory flow to the extremities.

Place the patient in a supine position with a pillow under the head.

Maintain a comfortable room temperature and dim the room lighting. Cool temperatures, anxiety, and muscle tension will alter the results.

Instruct the patient to refrain from talking and moving during the test.

### During the Test

The pressure cuffs are applied to both legs at the level of the upper thighs, above and below the knees, and above the ankles.

At the first cuff site, inflate the cuff to 75 mm Hg for 2 to 3 seconds and then lower the pressure to 65 mm Hg.

Record four to five waveforms. Label the recording with the correct identification of the cuff level and right or left side. Repeat this procedure at each cuff site.

### Posttest

Deflate and remove the cuffs.

## Plethysmography, Venous

**(Manometry)**   Synonym: Impedance plethysmography, venous

| **Normal Values** | Normal waveform patterns with adequate venous capacity and maximum venous outflow; no evidence of deep vein thrombosis |
| --- | --- |

## Background Information

Using blood pressure cuffs and electrodes, venous plethysmography measures the change in blood volume of the extremities. The electrodes and the recorder produce a linear waveform pattern that is recorded on a graph-paper strip, as in the recording of an ECG.

In normal venous circulation, the blood moves toward the heart from the distal extremities. If a vein is compressed temporarily by a blood pressure cuff, the venous flow is interrupted. Distal to that compression point, the veins become engorged. On deflation of the cuff and release of the compression, the vein quickly empties of its excess blood and resumes normal venous outflow (Katz & McCulla, 1995).

When a deep vein is obstructed by a thrombus,

back-up of the venous blood and engorgement of the distal vessel also occur. Once the vein is compressed temporarily by the blood pressure cuff, the blood flow is further interrupted. Increased engorgement of the distal vein cannot occur, because the vein has already filled to capacity. On deflation of the cuff and release of the compression, only minimal venous blood flow resumes, because the thrombus continues to obstruct the lumen.

As the compression is applied to a normal vein, the venous plethysmographic waveform pattern shows a gradual rise in height from the baseline. This phase is called *venous capacitance* and represents the filling of the distal vein to its fullest capacity. On release of the compression, the waveform drops rapidly and returns to baseline (Fig. 16–4). In

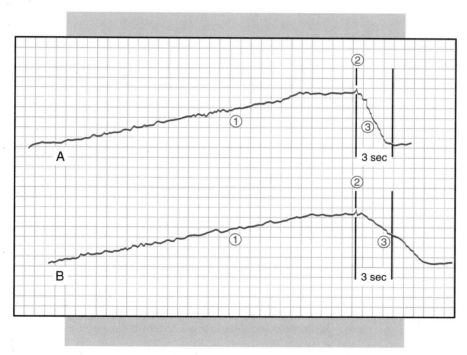

**Figure 16–4**

Normal versus abnormal venous plethysmographic waveforms. *A,* The normal waveform demonstrates *1,* venous capacitance; *2,* release of the thigh cuff; and *3,* rapid venous outflow that completes in 3 seconds. *B,* The abnormal waveform demonstrates *1,* venous capacitance; *2,* release of the thigh cuff; and *3,* slow venous outflow. It takes longer than the normal 3 seconds for the waveform to return to the baseline level.

an obstructed vein, the release of the pressure cuff relieves the venous compression, but limited venous outflow and slow emptying of the engorged vein occur. Correspondingly, the waveform demonstrates a limited, slow return to baseline.

| | |
|---|---|
| **Purpose of the Test** | Venous plethysmography is used to help detect deep vein thrombosis and to screen patients who are at high risk for the development of venous thrombosis. |

| | |
|---|---|
| **Procedure** | Plethysmographic cuffs and electrodes are applied to the thigh and calf to control and monitor venous blood flow. The cuffs are inflated, and the recorded waveforms demonstrate the filling of the vein to maximal capacity. On rapid release of the cuffs, the waveform demonstrates the venous outflow of the distal vein. The total time required to complete the test is 30 to 45 minutes. |

**Findings**

**Abnormal Values**

Venous thrombosis
Thrombophlebitis

Venous obstruction
(partial or complete)

**Interfering Factors**

- Nicotine, alcohol, and caffeine
- Anxiety and muscle tension
- Uncooperative patient behavior
- Compression of pelvic veins (caused by a tumor or tight bandages)
- Low cardiac output
- Shock
- Arterial occlusive disease

**Nursing Implementation**

**Pretest**

Inform the patient about the procedure and obtain written consent from the patient or person legally designated to make the patient's health care decisions.

Instruct the patient to refrain from smoking and ingesting alcohol and caffeine before the test, because stimulants and depressants alter the test results.

Help the patient remove all clothing and put on a hospital gown. Any compression from restrictive clothing alters the venous circulation from the extremities. Maintain a comfortable room temperature and dim the lights, because anxiety and muscle tension alter the results.

Place the patient in the supine position with the legs elevated above the heart and supported by pillows. The affected leg and hip are externally rotated, and the knee is flexed.

Instruct the patient to refrain from movement and talking during the test.

**During the Test**

Place blood pressure cuffs on the thigh and calf of the affected leg (Fig. 16–5). Apply the conductive gel and electrodes to the skin.

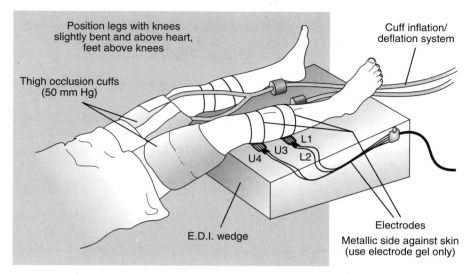

Position legs with knees slightly bent and above heart, feet above knees

Cuff inflation/ deflation system

Thigh occlusion cuffs (50 mm Hg)

L1
U3
L2
U4

E.D.I. wedge

Electrodes
Metallic side against skin
(use electrode gel only)

**Figure 16–5**

Impedance plethysmography. Setup for a patient undergoing impedance plethysmography in both lower extremities. Inflatable cuffs are placed around the thighs for venous compression. A cuff with electrodes is applied around each calf for recording the results. (Reproduced with permission from Katz, R. T., & McCulla, M. M. [1995]. Impedance plethysmography as a screening procedure for asymptomatic deep vein thrombosis in a rehabilitation hospital. *Archives of Physical Medicine and Rehabilitation, 76*[9], 834.)

Inflate the cuff on the calf to 15 mm Hg of pressure. The cuff and electrode monitor the inflow of the venous system.

Inflate the cuff on the thigh to 50 mm Hg of pressure. This pressure level obstructs the venous outflow but allows the arterial flow to fill and engorge the distal vein segment.

Start the recorder to trace the waveform. Once the tracing has risen to its maximum level and formed a plateau, the venous filling is completed.

Quickly release the pressure on the thigh cuff to open the venous outflow of the vein. The waveform pattern will continue and provide the linear recording of the return to the baseline reading.

Repeat the procedure until three to five waveforms are recorded. Label the paper, correctly identifying the extremity.

Repeat the entire procedure on the opposite extremity to provide comparison data.

### Posttest

Remove the deflated cuffs and electrodes.
Wipe the conductive gel off the skin.

## Venography

**(Radiography)**                        Synonym: Phlebography

| **Normal Values** | No evidence of intraluminal filling defects, obstruction, incompetent venous valves, calcifications, or dilations of collateral veins |
|---|---|

## Background Information

Venography is an invasive technique that provides radiographic visualization of the venous system, particularly in the lower extremities. In this location, the venous system consists of the superficial veins, the deep veins, and the perforating veins. The lower leg veins provide a passive conduit for the return of the blood to the heart and also serve as a reservoir for the large volume of circulating blood.

The valves within the veins are the most important functional feature. Each valve has a pair of fibrous leaflets that control the direction of the blood flow upward toward the heart and from the superficial to the deep veins. When valves are competent, no reflux or backflow occurs. Incompetent valves cause a reflux of blood into the superficial vein system and the ultimate formation of varicosities. Incompetence of the perforating veins usually is caused by deep vein thrombosis or other sources of obstruction.

Deep vein thrombosis and thromboembolism are caused by three general pathologic conditions: damage to the blood vessel, venous stasis, and decreased fibrinolytic activity. Thrombosis is the most common venous pathologic condition. As the thrombus enlarges, it occludes the lumen of the vein and ultimately destroys the venous valve or valves. In the early stage of formation, the thrombus is soft and friable. When located in the leg, a piece of the thrombus can break off, travel, and lodge in the lung as a pulmonary embolus. A thrombus that is 24 to 48 hours old becomes firm and adheres to the vein wall. Eventually, the thrombus will partially or completely resolve by fibrinolysis.

Examination of the veins by venography is carried out by several methods. *Ascending venography* is used to identify the presence and location of deep vein thrombosis and to assess the patency of the deep venous system. *Descending venography* is used to assess valve competency (Vogelzang & Methe, 1994). *Venography of the upper extremities* evaluates occlusion, lesions, or thrombosis in the subclavian or axillary veins. *Venacavography* evaluates the inferior vena cava for obstruction, malformation, traumatic injury, and placement of the inferior vena cava filter.

Noninvasive technologies such as ultrasound, plethysmography, and compression sonography are used to identify deep vein thrombosis of the lower extremities. CT and MRI are the preferred methods to image the vena cava. When these procedures are inconclusive, however, the venogram is used to clarify the data. Venography is the best method to identify a deep vein thrombosis below the knee (Della Santina & Jolly, 1997).

| **Purpose of the Test** | Venography is used to investigate venous function, suspected obstruction, venous insufficiency, postphlebotic syndrome, and the source of pulmonary embolism. It also evaluates veins before and after bypass surgery, reconstructive surgery, or thrombolytic therapy to determine the effectiveness of treatment. |
|---|---|

| **Procedure** | Contrast medium is injected into the vein via a butterfly needle or an intravenous catheter. With use of a tilt table, fluoroscopy, and x-ray studies, the contrast medium illustrates the flow patterns of the venous circulation and identifies the site of occlusion in the vein. |
|---|---|
| | In venography of the lower extremities, either ascending or descending venography may be used. Ascending venography uses a butterfly needle placed in a small vein on the dorsum of the foot (Fig. 16–6). In descending venog- |

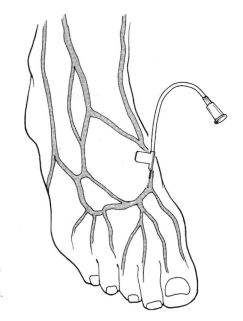

**Figure 16–6**
Technique of ascending venography. Diagrammatic
representation of the ideal needle position to instill the contrast
medium. (Reproduced with permission from Kim, D., &
Orron, D. E. [1992]. *Peripheral vascular imaging and intervention.*
St. Louis: Mosby–Year Book.)

raphy, a catheter is placed in the common femoral vein via a
percutaneous femoral approach.

| **Findings** | **Abnormal Values** | | |
|---|---|---|---|
| | Deep vein thrombosis | Venous compression | Congenital malforma- |
| | Tumor (extrinsic | syndrome | tion |
| | compression) | Venous insufficiency | Traumatic injury to |
| | Vascular tumor | Varicose veins | the vein |
| | (intrinsic blockage) | | |

| **Interfering Factors** | • Allergy to iodine or contrast medium |
|---|---|
| | • Renal failure |
| | • Congestive heart failure |
| | • Severe pulmonary hypertension |

**Nursing Implementation**

*Critical Thinking 16–2*
Following a venography, what
should you instruct the aide
to report about the patient?

**Pretest**

Identify any allergy to iodine or shellfish or any allergic reaction to a previous
x-ray study that used contrast medium.
Instruct the patient regarding the procedure and pretest preparation. Obtain
written consent from the patient or person legally designated to make
health care decisions for the patient.
Ensure that the pretest blood urea nitrogen and creatinine determinations are
performed and that the results are posted in the patient's chart. This is

carried out to ensure that renal function is adequate, because the kidneys must clear the contrast material from the body.

Solid foods are omitted for 4 hours before the test, but water and clear liquids are permitted.

Record baseline vital signs.

### During the Test

The patient is positioned according to the views that are required. In general, most lower extremity views are done with the patient in a supine position or tilted upward by 45 to 60 degrees to a semi-erect position (Snopek, 1992).

Provide emotional support during the period of discomfort. The injection of contrast material is painful.

On completion of the test, an intravenous solution of 200 to 300 mL of heparinized saline is administered. This flushes the contrast medium from the veins.

### Posttest

Obtain vital signs and record the results.

Assess the puncture site for signs of swelling, pain, redness, or hematoma.

Keep the patient on bedrest for 2 hours.

Resume the previous dietary status. Instruct the patient to drink extra fluids for 24 hours to help flush the remaining contrast medium from the veins and kidneys. Frequent urination is expected until the diuresis is complete.

**Complications**

If more than 5 to 10 mL of contrast material infiltrates the tissue, chemical cellulitis will result. The contrast medium also can cause postvenographic thrombosis or phlebitis. The onset of these posttest complications can begin in

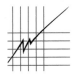

**Table 16–2   Complications of Venography**

| Complication | Nursing Assessment |
| --- | --- |
| Cellulitis | Redness<br>Swelling<br>Pain or tenderness |
| Thrombophlebitis | Pain<br>Redness<br>Swelling |
| Allergic-type reaction | Urticaria or itching<br>Erythema<br>Respiratory distress or stridor<br>Cyanosis<br>Hypotension<br>Tachycardia<br>Chest pain<br>Cardiac arrest |

2 to 12 hours, peak in 12 to 24 hours, and gradually subside in a few days. During the test, an allergic-type reaction to the contrast medium can occur. A summary of the complications of venography is presented in Table 16–2.

## References

Alving, B. M., & Griffin, J. H. (1995). Venous thrombosis: How to make the best use of the laboratory to guide therapy. *Consultant, 35*(1), 64–66.

Blackburn, D. R., & Peterson-Kennedy, L. (1994). Noninvasive vascular testing. In V. A. Fahey, *Vascular nursing* (2nd ed.). Philadelphia: W. B. Saunders.

Borrelo, J. A. (1993). MR angiography versus conventional x-ray in the lower extremities: Everyone wins. *Radiology, 187*(3), 615–617.

Carpenter, J. P., Owen, R. S., Holland, G. A., Baum, R. A., Barker, C. F., Perloff, L. J., Golden, M. A., & Cope, C. (1994). Magnetic resonance angiography of the aorta, ilial and femoral arteries. *Surgery, 116*(1), 17–23.

Della Santina, P. J., & Jolly, B. T. (1997). Vascular ultrasonography. *Emergency Medicine Clinics of North America, 15*(4), 849–873.

Dowd, S. B., Wilson, B. G., Hall, J. D., Steves, A., & Benson, T. (1996). Review of techniques used to image aortic dissection. *Radiologic Technology, 67*(3), 223–232.

Eftychiou, V. (1996). Clinical diagnosis and management of the patient with deep vein thromboembolism and acute pulmonary embolism. *Nurse Practitioner: American Journal of Primary Health Care, 21* 3, 52, 52, 58.

Fahey, V. A. (Ed.). (1994). *Vascular nursing* (2nd ed.). Philadelphia: W. B. Saunders.

Fleischer, A. C., & Kepple, D. M. (1995). *Diagnostic sonography. Principles and clinical applications* (2nd ed.). Philadelphia: W. B. Saunders.

Hebdon, B., & Letourneau, J. G. (1994). Duplex sonography of extremity arteries and veins, part 2. *Applied Radiology, 23*(4), 39–48.

Hertz, S. M., Baum, R. A., Owen, R. S., Holland, G. A., Logan, D. R., & Carpenter, J. P. (1993). Comparison of magnetic resonance angiography and contrast angiography in peripheral artery stenosis. *American Journal of Surgery, 166*(8), 112–116.

Kandarpa, K., & Aruny, J. E. (1996). *Handbook of interventional radiologic procedures* (2nd ed.). Boston: Little, Brown.

Katz, R. T., & McCulla, M. M. (1995). Impedance plethysmography as a screening procedure for asymptomatic deep vein thrombosis in a rehabilitation hospital. *Archives of Physical Medicine and Rehabilitation, 76*(9), 833–839.

Kim, D., & Orron, D. E. (1992). *Peripheral vascular imaging and intervention.* St. Louis: Mosby–Year Book.

McConnell, E. A. (1995). Monitoring peripheral pulses with a Doppler ultrasound device. *Nursing95, 25*(3), 18.

Mettler, F. A. (1996). *Essentials of radiology.* Philadelphia: W. B. Saunders.

Muller, M. F., & Edelman, R. R. (1995). Magnetic resonance angiography of the abdomen. *Gastroenterology Clinics of North America, 24,* 2, 435–453.

Rice, K. L., & Walsh, M. E. (1998). Peripheral arterial occlusive disease, part 1: Navigating a bottleneck. *Nursing98, 28*(2), 33–38.

Rubin, G. D., & Silverman, S. G. (1995). Helical (spiral) CT of the retroperitoneum. *Radiologic Clinics of North America, 33*(5), 903–932.

Snopek, A. M. (1992). *Fundamentals of special radiographic procedures* (3rd ed.). Philadelphia: W. B. Saunders.

Torres, L. S. (1993). *Basic medical techniques and patient care for radiologic technologists.* Philadelphia: J. B. Lippincott.

Vogelzang, R. L., & Methe, D. M. (1994). Percutaneous vascular intervention and imaging techniques (pp. 104–134). In V. A. Fahey (Ed.), *Vascular nursing* (2nd ed.). Philadelphia: W.B. Saunders.

# CHAPTER 17

# Hematologic Function

In hematologic testing, the laboratory tests provide information regarding the number, concentration, structure, and characteristics of the cells in the blood. The diagnostic procedures of bone marrow aspiration, biopsy, and nuclear scanning provide information about the marrow tissue that forms the blood cells.

Many blood cell alterations have their origin in abnormal bone marrow function. The marrow can be altered by malignancy, inadequate nutrition, infection, genetics, radiation, chemical toxins, or an adverse reaction to medication. The abnormal changes can include excess production of cells, diminished production or lack of production of cells, errors in the maturation of cells, and production of defective cells.

Some diseases, such as leukemia, directly affect the bone marrow and its ability to produce blood cells. Other diseases, such as renal failure, cause changes in hematopoietic function even though the bone marrow cells are healthy. Additionally, some diseases or conditions of the body directly alter the blood cells. Examples include some parasitic infections and antigen-antibody reactions.

The cells of the blood consist of erythrocytes, leukocytes, and platelets (Table 17–1). The plasma also contains clotting factors, antibodies, and other plasma proteins, including albumin. In hematologic testing, the number and concentration of each type of cell provide important estimates about bone marrow function. The marrow responds to the signals of the microenvironment and to the presence of colony-stimulating factors for the regulation of its activity in formation, differentiation, and maturation of blood cells (Rodak, 1995).

The study of the structure and characteristics of the blood cells provides important data for accuracy in diagnosis of hematologic disorders. In the investigation of anemia, studies of blood cells and bone marrow help differentiate among the types of anemia, identify abnormal erythrocytes and cell membrane characteristics, and identify the source of the problem. Broadly defined, anemias are caused by acute or chronic blood loss, by abnormal formation of erythrocytes or their hemoglobin content, or by hemolysis or the early destruction of erythrocytes.

Diseases of the phagocytic and immune systems are defined through the study of leukocytes. Excessive or diminished numbers of one or more types of leukocyte may exist. Immature or abnormal forms of these cells may also exist in the blood.

For more information on other tests related to cells of the blood, the quantitative tests, including the complete blood count, are presented in Chapter 4. The laboratory tests for clotting are presented in Chapter 6.

## Table 17–1   Formed Elements of the Blood

| | |
|---|---|
| Erythrocytes | Agranular leukocytes |
| Reticulocytes | Lymphocytes |
| Leukocytes | Plasma cells |
| Granular leukocytes | T cells |
| Neutrophils | Monocytes |
| Eosinophils | Thrombocytes |
| Basophils | Platelets |

## Laboratory Tests

## Antiglobulin Tests

**(Blood)**    Synonyms: Antiglobulin test, direct; AGT; direct Coombs' test; antiglobulin test, indirect; indirect Coombs' test

**Normal Values**    Negative

### Background Information

The antiglobulin tests consist of direct and indirect tests. They are used to detect the presence of antibodies in the serum and antigens on erythrocytes (Fig. 17–1). When an antigen-antibody reaction has occurred in the blood, the erythrocytes become coated with antibody globin, and the erythrocytes agglutinate. In severe conditions, phagocytosis of the cell membranes and lysis of the coated erythrocytes occur. The lysis of many erythrocytes results in hemolytic anemia.

**Direct Antiglobulin Test.**   The direct antiglobulin test, or direct Coombs' test, looks for antibodies attached to red blood cells. In this antigen-antibody reaction, the immunoproteins, immunoglobulin

G (IgG), and complement cling to the erythrocytes and coat the red blood cells with globin. The coated cells are "sensitized" and then clump together in the process called *agglutination*. The severity of the reaction depends on the number of antibodies produced and the number of erythrocytes affected.

In transfusion of incompatible blood, the recipient's anti-Rh$_0$ IgG antibodies detect the foreign antigens on the cells of the donor blood. The antibodies move to attack and destroy the foreign cells in a massive antigen-antibody response. During the pregnancy of an Rh$_0$-negative mother who carries an Rh$_0$-positive baby, the maternal Rh$_0$ anti-

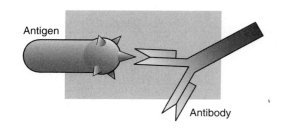

**Figure 17–1**
Antigen and antibody. A specific antibody matches the antigen based on the characteristic shape that protrudes from the antigen surface. Once the antibody locks onto the antigen, the antigen is destroyed by phagocytosis, an enzyme toxin from complement, or other biochemical response of the immune system.

bodies and complement pass through the placenta and into the fetus's circulation. Because the blood types of the mother and fetus are incompatible, the maternal antibodies attack the erythrocytes of the fetus. As the erythrocytes of the fetus become coated, agglutinate, and undergo hemolysis, erythroblastosis fetalis or hemolytic anemia of the newborn develops.

Some medications also cause elevation of the direct antiglobulin test. Methyldopa (Aldomet), acetaminophen, and quinidine are the medications often involved, but others are penicillin, cephalosporin, tetracycline, sulfonamides, levodopa, and insulin. Protein in the medication is the antigenic substance, and IgG or complement causes the erythrocytes to become coated. In most of these cases, the direct antiglobulin test result is elevated, but in a few cases, hemolytic anemia results (Jacobs et al., 1996; Tietz, 1995; Waterbury, 1996).

The direct antiglobulin test examines the patient's erythrocytes for antibodies. The red blood cells of the specimen are immersed in laboratory antiglobulin serum. After the erythrocytes are washed to remove other serum proteins, the antibodies remain attached to the antigens on the cellular surfaces of erythrocytes.

**Indirect Antiglobulin Test.**　The indirect antiglobulin test, or indirect Coombs' test, looks for the presence of antibodies in the patient's serum. In the laboratory analysis, the patient's serum is mixed with known reagents of red blood cells, and the result is observed for an antigen-antibody reaction. If circulating antibodies are present in the patient's serum, they adhere to and coat the reagent red blood cells. Agglutination of the erythrocytes occurs when the level of antibodies is high.

In the first trimester of pregnancy, this test is used to screen $Rh_0$-positive and $Rh_0$-negative expectant mothers. When the test results are negative, the test is repeated in the 28th week of pregnancy and at delivery. Whenever the test becomes positive for the presence of antibodies, it is followed up with antibody identification, a titer reading, and possible amniocentesis. The development of maternal antibodies occurs in the Rh-negative mother who carries an Rh-positive fetus. The antibodies cross the placental barrier, enter the fetal circulation, and result in the coating and agglutination of fetal erythrocytes.

Methyldopa is a common drug cause of elevated indirect antiglobulin test results (Jacobs et al., 1996).

---

**Purpose of the Test**　The *direct antiglobulin test* detects antibodies on the erythrocytes. It is part of the posttransfusion work-up to detect red blood cell incompatibility between donor and recipient blood. It is also used to help diagnose erythroblastosis fetalis, or hemolytic disease of the newborn, and helps confirm the diagnosis of hemolytic anemia.

The *indirect antiglobulin test* detects unknown antibodies in the serum. It is used as an antibody screen in type and crossmatch testing in preparation for blood transfusion. It detects maternal-fetal blood incompatibility and predicts the hematologic risk to the fetus. It is used to evaluate the need for $Rh_0$(D) immune globulin administration and helps confirm the diagnosis of hemolytic anemia.

**Procedure**

**Direct Antiglobulin Test.** One red-topped tube and one lavender-topped tube are used to collect 10 mL and 7 mL, respectively, of venous blood. In the newborn, venous cord blood may be collected.

**Indirect Antiglobulin Test.** A red-topped tube is used to collect 10 mL of venous blood.

**Quality Control**

> The tourniquet must not be applied tightly or for a prolonged time. Venipuncture technique must be smooth, with a blood flow that fills the tube readily. If the blood flow has excessive turbulence because of flawed venipuncture technique, hemolysis of the erythrocytes will alter the test results.

**Findings**

**Positive Values**

DIRECT ANTIGLOBULIN TEST

Autoimmune hemo-
lytic anemia
Hemolytic transfu-
sion reaction
Hemolytic disease of
the newborn

Lymphoma
Systemic lupus
erythematosus
Mycoplasmal
infection

Infectious mono-
nucleosis
Sensitivity to particu-
lar medications

INDIRECT ANTIGLOBULIN TEST

Maternal-fetal blood
incompatibility

Autoimmune hemo-
lytic anemia

Sensitivity to particu-
lar medications

**Interfering Factors**

- Hemolysis
- Inadequate identification of the specimen

**Nursing Implementation**

**Pretest**

Include the following information on the requisition form: recent history of blood transfusion or plasma expanders and the pertinent medications taken.

**Posttest**

Ensure that the specimen label and requisition slip include the patient's name and identification number and the source of the blood (venous, cord).
Arrange for prompt transport of the specimen to the laboratory.

**Quality Control**

> For accurate results, the serum must be separated from the cells without delay.

## Complement, Total

(Serum)                    Synonyms: $CH_{50}$, complement assay

| Normal Values | 75–160 $CH_{50}$ U/mL or SI 75–160 $CH_{50}$ kU/L |
| --- | --- |

### Background Information

Complement is a system of 25 plasma proteins and cell-membrane–associated proteins that circulate as inactive precursors in the blood. When activated, they serve to mediate the defense system and protect against infection. In supporting the work of antibodies, the complement cells facilitate phagocytosis, eliminate antigen-antibody complexes, and puncture the cell membranes of bacteria. In an active form, complement induces an inflammatory response.

When complement is activated, it follows the *classic component pathway* (Fig. 17–2) or an *alternative pathway*. The activation of the classic component pathway usually occurs when an antibody locks onto an antigen. In the alternative pathway, the process usually starts when complement C3 interacts with other factors. Ultimately, both pathways finalize with the formation of a membrane attack complex. This complex penetrates the wall of the molecule and causes lysis of the cell.

Complement proteins increase in an acute response to inflammation or infection and are decreased or absent in hypercatabolism (autoimmune disease), hereditary deficiency, and overexpenditure of the complexes.

### Purpose of the Test

Total complement is used to evaluate or monitor systemic lupus erythematosus and its response to therapy. The test is also used to diagnose complement deficiency and to detect disease caused by the immune complex.

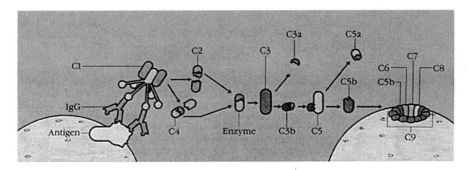

**Figure 17–2**

The complement cascade. The classic complement pathway becomes activated when the first complement molecule, C1, recognizes an antigen-antibody complex. Each of the remaining complement proteins, in turn, performs its specialized job, cleaving or binding to the complement molecule next in line. The end product is the cylindrical membrane attack complex. (Reproduced with permission from Schlindler, L. W. [1988]. *Understanding the immune system* [NIH Publication No. 88-529, p. 10]. Washington, DC: U. S. Department of Health, Public Health Service, National Institutes of Health.)

| | |
|---|---|
| **Procedure** | A red-topped tube is used to collect 10 mL of venous blood. |

**Findings**

**Elevated Values**

Chronic infection
Rheumatoid arthritis
Acute rheumatic fever

Ulcerative colitis
Diabetes mellitus
Thyroiditis

Congestive heart
  failure
Osteoarthritis

**Decreased Values**

Systemic lupus
  erythematosus
Multiple myeloma
Acute post-
  streptococcal
  glomerulonephritis

Hypogammaglob-
  ulinemia
Trauma

Advanced cirrhosis of
  the liver
Acute vasculitis

**Interfering Factors**

• None

**Nursing Implementation**

Nursing care includes care of the venipuncture site.
No other specific patient instruction or intervention is needed.

## Fetal Hemoglobin

**(Whole Blood)**     Synonyms: HbF, hemoglobin F

**Normal Values**

6 months–adult: <2% HbF *or* SI <0.02 mass fraction HbF
Infant (0–6 months): <75% HbF *or* SI 0.75 mass fraction HbF
**Kleihauer Betke Method**
Adult: <0.01% HbF *or* SI 0.0001 mass fraction HbF
Newborn, full term: >90% HbF *or* SI >0.9 mass fraction HbF

### Background Information

Hemoglobin F (HbF) is one of three distinct types of hemoglobin and is the major hemoglobin in the fetus and newborn infant. During the first year of life, the production of HbF gradually decreases and the production of hemoglobins A and $A_2$ (HbA and $HbA_2$), the predominant hemoglobins of childhood and adulthood, gradually increases. By age 1 year, very little HbF should exist in the erythrocyte pool. When HbF remains at an elevated level, it can be caused by a hereditary disorder or by an acquired disorder.

**Hereditary Persistence of Fetal Hemoglobin.** This is a group of conditions that persist after infancy but cause little hematologic abnormality. The HbF content varies from 20% to 30% of total hemoglobin in those who have the heterozygous type of hereditary persistence of fetal hemoglobin. In those who have the homozygous type of condition, the hemoglobin is 100% HbF, with no HbA or $HbA_2$. These individuals demonstrate slightly macrocytic, microchromic erythrocytes, but no anemia exists. The HbF is distributed uniformly throughout each erythrocyte.

**Hemoglobinopathy.** This is an alteration of the structure of hemoglobin that may or may not result in significant hematologic disease. Elevated levels of HbF are found to coexist in some of these hemoglobin disorders. In beta-thalassemia disorders, HbF is unevenly distributed among the erythrocytes. This means that some of the erythrocytes have HbF present and others do not.

**Fetal-Maternal Hemorrhage.** The Kleihauer Betke method of analysis is used after fetal-maternal hemorrhage. It detects the amount of fetal cells and HbF in the maternal and newborn circulation. Based on the calculation of fetal blood contamination in the mother, she is given the proper dose of $Rh_0(D)$ immune globulin to prevent the formation of anti-D antibodies and the development of erythroblastosis fetalis in a subsequent pregnancy. Maternal erythrocytes may have entered the blood of the newborn. The quantity of HbF is measured before blood transfusions are given.

---

**Purpose of the Test**

HbF is measured to help diagnose some forms of anemia, evaluate hemoglobinopathies, assess the severity of fetal-maternal hemorrhage in the newborn and mother, and diagnose hereditary persistence of fetal hemoglobin.

---

**Procedure**

A lavender-topped tube is used to collect 7 mL of venous blood. In cases of fetal-maternal hemorrhage, three separate lavender-topped tubes are used to obtain 7 mL of blood from the mother and from the cord blood and 0.6 mL to 2 mL from the newborn. The cord blood serves as a control specimen.

---

**Findings**

**Elevated Values**

HEREDITARY DISORDERS

| | |
|---|---|
| Beta-thalassemia anemia | Sickle cell anemia |
| Hereditary persistence of fetal hemoglobin | Trisomy 21 (Down syndrome) |

ACQUIRED DISORDERS

| | | |
|---|---|---|
| Pernicious anemia | Acute leukemia | Chronic renal disease |
| Refractory normoblastic anemia | Erythroleukemia | Hyperthyroidism |
| Sideroblastic anemia | Benign monoclonal gammopathy | Pregnancy |
| Aplastic anemia | Metastatic cancer of bone marrow | Molar pregnancy |
| Juvenile chronic myeloid leukemia | | Fetal-maternal hemorrhage |

---

**Interfering Factors**

- Hemolysis
- Improper labeling of specimens

---

**Nursing Implementation**

Nursing care includes care of the venipuncture site.

**Pretest**

Ensure that all specimens and laboratory requisition slips are identified with the patients' names and sources of blood (i.e., mother, newborn, cord blood).

**Posttest**

Arrange for prompt transportation of the blood to the laboratory.

**Quality Control**

The analysis is performed on fresh blood within 6 hours. Once slides are prepared, a fixative must be applied within the hour to prevent deterioration of the specimen.

## Glucose-6-Phosphate Dehydrogenase Screen

**(Blood)**                    Synonym: G-6-PD screen, blood

| **Normal Values** | G-6-PD enzyme activity is present. |
|---|---|

### Background Information

Genetic defects in erythrocyte metabolism are responsible for many forms of hemolytic anemia. With deficient or diminished enzyme activity, the erythrocytes have a shorter life span. The deficiency of the glucose-6-phosphate dehydrogenase (G-6-PD) enzyme in the erythrocyte is the most frequent and important of this type of chronic hemolytic anemia. The deficiency of this enzyme is hereditary and linked to the X chromosome (Brown, 1996b).

This type of hemolytic anemia is seen most frequently in African Americans, and it is usually a mild condition. A more severe, but rare, form of the disorder affects individuals from Asia and the countries of the Mediterranean. It can cause hemolytic disease of the newborn (Mehta, 1994).

A sudden, acute episode of severe hemolytic anemia is usually triggered by the administration of particular drugs, an infection, or an illness. The medications include sulfonamides, antimalarial drugs, and a variety of other medications. The illnesses that can trigger hemolytic episodes are usually acute bacterial or viral infections or metabolic disorders, including acidosis. In severe infection, the anemia can be life-threatening.

When the screening test result is positive, a quantitative blood test is performed to evaluate the severity of the defect. The screening test cannot detect the deficiency of the G-6-PD enzyme after the hemolytic episode is over because the defective erythrocytes are destroyed by hemolysis.

| **Purpose of the Test** | This screening test is used to detect a G-6-PD enzyme defect in erythrocytes and determine that it is the cause of hemolytic anemia. |
|---|---|

| **Procedure** | A lavender-topped tube is used to collect 7 mL of venous blood. |
|---|---|

| **Findings** | **Decreased Values** |
|---|---|
| | G-6-PD anemia, mild to moderate    G-6-PD anemia, severe |

| **Interfering Factors** | • Sudden, severe hemolysis |
|---|---|

| **Nursing Implementation** | Nursing care includes care of the venipuncture site. No other specific patient instruction or intervention is needed. |
| --- | --- |

## Haptoglobin

| (Serum) | Synonyms: HAP, HP, Hp |
| --- | --- |

| **Normal Values** | Adult: 40–180 mg/dL *or* SI 0.4–1.8 g/L<br>Newborn–4 months: 5–48 mg/dL *or* SI 0.05–0.48 g/dL |
| --- | --- |

### Background Information

Haptoglobins are small plasma proteins that are manufactured by the liver and released into the blood. When erythrocytes undergo hemolysis by normal or abnormal processes, the circulating haptoglobins bind to the free hemoglobin, forming hemoglobin-haptoglobin complexes. Because the hemoglobin-haptoglobin complexes cannot be filtered through the renal glomeruli, hemoglobin is protected from excretion in the urine. These complexes are carried to the reticuloendothelial system for physiologic breakdown and conservation of the iron that was in the hemoglobin.

**Increased Values.** Inflammation is a powerful stimulant for the increased manufacture of haptoglobin. The haptoglobin level usually rises as a result of inflammation, infection, conditions of stress, and conditions of tissue destruction. These conditions, however, do not consistently cause an increase in haptoglobin. Because of other physiologic variables, the haptoglobin level may increase, remain steady, or even decrease.

**Decreased Values.** A decreased haptoglobin value may occur gradually, chronically, or suddenly, depending on the cause of hemolysis. As the red blood cells are destroyed, available haptoglobin is rapidly consumed as it binds to hemoglobin.

A moderately or chronically decreased value may be caused by ineffective erythropoiesis by the bone marrow, as in hemolytic anemia. Abnormal erythrocytes have a shorter life span and undergo hemolysis at a more frequent rate. Additional causes of lower haptoglobin levels include impairment of the liver's ability to manufacture haptoglobin and trauma to the erythrocytes as from mechanical heart valves or sports activities such as running or aerobic dancing (Burtis & Ashwood, 1999).

Because the results vary from one test to another, serial testing is more accurate than a single value in the monitoring of nonacute conditions. In a first-time evaluation of haptoglobin, a severely decreased value is an indicator of acute hemolysis.

| **Purpose of the Test** | Haptoglobin measurement is useful in the work-up for hemolytic conditions. It is also used for monitoring or detection of acute-phase reactions that involve hemolysis of erythrocytes. |
| --- | --- |

| **Procedure** | A red-topped tube is used to collect 7 mL of venous blood. |
| --- | --- |

**Quality Control**

The tourniquet must not be applied too tightly or for very long. Venipuncture technique must be smooth, with a blood flow that fills the vacuum tube readily. If the blood has excessive turbulence because of flawed venipuncture technique, the hemolysis of the erythrocytes alters the test results.

| Findings | **Elevated Values** | | |
|---|---|---|---|
| | Collagen diseases | Acute rheumatoid | Infection |
| | Corticosteroid | arthritis | Biliary obstruction |
| | therapy | Nephrotic syndrome | Advanced malignancy |

**Decreased Values**

| | | |
|---|---|---|
| Hemolytic transfu- | Folate deficiency | Infectious mono- |
| sion reaction | G-6-PD deficiency | nucleosis |
| Advanced liver | Hereditary sphero- | Acute thermal injury |
| disease (cirrhosis) | cytosis | Malaria |
| Nephrotic syndrome | Oral contraceptives | |
| Sickle cell anemia | (estrogen) | |
| Thalassemia | | |

| | |
|---|---|
| **Interfering Factors** | • Hemolysis from a traumatic venipuncture |

| | |
|---|---|
| **Nursing Implementation** | Nursing care includes the care of the venipuncture site. |

**Pretest**

This test may be used to monitor for a blood transfusion reaction. If prescribed, ensure that the haptoglobin specimen is drawn before starting the transfusion.

**Posttest**

Compare the current results with the patient's baseline value to monitor for the level and direction of change.

| | |
|---|---|
| **Critical Value** | **<40–50 mg/dL (SI <0.4–0.5 mg/dL)** |

The sudden and severe decrease of haptoglobin is an indicator of acute hemolysis of erythrocytes. If the test result is below the critical value, the physician must be notified immediately. The cause of the hemolysis and the acuity of the illness will determine the interventions that are needed. Assess any fresh sample of urine for change in color, and review any subsequent urinalysis reports. With little haptoglobin remaining, the excess free hemoglobin is filtered out of the blood into the urine. Hemoglobin changes the color of the urine to dark red or brown.

## Heinz Bodies

(Blood)          Synonyms: Heinz body stain, methyl violet stain for Heinz bodies

| | |
|---|---|
| **Normal Values** | No Heinz bodies are identified. |

## Background Information

Heinz bodies are precipitates or particles present in abnormal hemoglobin and are visible in the presence of methyl violet stain. The Heinz bodies represent the end product of denatured hemoglobin and are associated with some form of hemolytic anemia.

The life span of the normal erythrocyte is 120 days. This time is shortened by intrinsic or extrinsic factors that alter the erythrocytes and result in their premature destruction and removal. Five types of change cause premature destruction of red blood cells and hemolytic anemia: (1) osmotic lysis, (2) phagocytosis of the erythrocytes, (3) complement-induced cytolysis, (4) fragmentation of the erythrocytes and denaturation, and (5) the alteration of the chemical or biologic properties of the erythrocytes. The premature destruction of red blood cells is observed in some hemolytic anemias, but the causes and importance of these five mechanisms are not fully understood.

In normal physiology, the iron in hemoglobin must remain in a reduced state so that oxygen molecules can be transported. The erythrocytes protect the hemoglobin from internal and external agents and prevent excess oxidation of iron. If these mechanisms fail, the hemoglobin becomes nonfunctional.

Abnormalities in the erythrocytes occur because of exposure to oxidant drugs or toxins, defects in the intrinsic protective mechanisms of the erythrocytes, and genetic abnormalities of hemoglobin. Once the hemoglobin is oxidized, the end product of the change produces precipitates, called Heinz bodies.

The Heinz bodies exist within the damaged erythrocytes and may be attached to the cell membrane. With methyl violet staining of the erythrocytes, the microscopic examination of the slides reveals deep purple, small, irregular forms. Their presence reflects either metabolic derangement or altered hemoglobin. The formation of the Heinz bodies is usually followed by the destruction of the erythrocyte.

| Purpose of the Test | The test is used to identify hemolytic disorders associated with Heinz body formation. |
| --- | --- |

## Procedure

A lavender-topped tube is used to collect 7 mL of venous blood.

### Quality Control

The tourniquet must not be applied too tightly or for very long. Venipuncture technique must be smooth, with a blood flow that fills the vacuum tube readily. If the blood has excessive turbulence because of flawed venipuncture technique, the hemolysis of the erythrocytes alters the test results.

## Findings

### Abnormal Values

G-6-PD deficiency
Congenital Heinz
   body hemolytic
   anemia

Drug-sensitive
   hemolytic anemia
Postsplenectomy

## Interfering Factors

• Hemolysis
• Coagulation of the specimen

**Nursing Implementation**   Nursing care includes care of the venipuncture site.

### Pretest

No specific patient instruction or intervention is needed.

### Posttest

Arrange for prompt transport of the specimen to the laboratory to prevent clotting of the specimen.

## Hemoglobin Electrophoresis

(Blood)                              Synonyms: None

**Normal Values**

HbA: 95%–98%
$HbA_2$: 1.5%–3.5%
HbF: 0%–2%
HbC: Absent
HbS: Absent

## Background Information

In the normal adult, the three types of hemoglobin found in erythrocytes are HbA, $HbA_2$, and HbF. Abnormal hemoglobins are produced by a single amino acid substitution in one of the polypeptide chains in the globin part of the molecule.

More than 400 variants of hemoglobin are identified by letters other than A, $A_2$, and F. To further subclassify the variants, the name may include a geographic region, city, or place of discovery, such as $HbM_{Boston}$. Of all the abnormal variants, HbS, or sickle cell hemoglobin, is the most predominant. Other relatively common variants are HbC, $HbD_{Punjab}$, and HbE.

*Hemoglobinopathy* is the general term used to describe altered hemoglobin and some forms of hemolytic anemia. A range of intensity of anemia can exist in individuals with a hemoglobin defect. The differences include a general alteration of the globin molecule, a homozygous (pure) state that produces disease, and a heterozygous (mixed) state that produces the trait but not the disease.

**Hemoglobin $A_2$.** Although this is a normal hemoglobin, little of it should be present. Hemoglobin electrophoresis evaluates the amount of $HbA_2$ in the investigation of beta-thalassemia trait and differentiates beta-thalassemia diseases from iron deficiency anemia. The beta-thalassemia diseases are a group of disorders that produce a range of conditions varying from no clinical change to severe hypochromic, microcytic anemia. The amount of $HbA_2$ is increased in the beta-thalassemia trait. Abnormal elevations of $HbA_2$ may include up to 7% of the total hemoglobin content.

**Hemoglobin F.** HbF is the hemoglobin present in fetal life; it is gradually replaced by HbA and $HbA_2$ during infancy. Adults can have abnormal quantities of HbF in hereditary persistence of fetal hemoglobin. The homozygous state produces mildly microcytic, hypochromic erythrocytes without anemia. The hemoglobin electrophoresis test reveals 100% HbF. The heterozygous state produces no hematologic abnormality, but hemoglobin electrophoresis reveals 30% to 40% HbF.

**Hemoglobin S.** In the homozygous state, HbS (HbSS) produces sickle cell anemia, a type of severe hemolytic anemia. Hemoglobin electrophoresis demonstrates no HbA, with a large percentage of HbS and elevated amounts of HbF and $HbA_2$. In the heterozygous form, or sickle cell trait, hemoglobin electrophoresis demonstrates 30% to 35% HbS mixed with HbA and $HbA_2$ and a normal percentage of HbF. Sickle cell trait (HbAS) produces no disease or hematologic abnormality unless the person experiences hypoxia, acidosis, or thrombotic phenomena. One of the thalassemia disorders may coexist with the sickle cell trait.

**Hemoglobin C.**   In the homozygous state of HbC disease (HCC), a mild hemolytic anemia often exists that is usually asymptomatic. On electrophoresis, no HbA is present. Most of the hemoglobin is HbC, with smaller quantities of other forms of hemoglobin. In the heterozygous state (HbAC), 30% to 40% is HbC, with about 50% to 60% HbA pre-

sent. One of the thalassemia disorders may coexist with the HbC trait.

Hemoglobin electrophoresis separates the normal from the abnormal hemoglobin in the blood sample. Hemoglobin molecules in alkaline solution have a net negative charge. The different types of hemoglobin molecules move at different rates toward the anode of the electrophoresis test. For screening purposes, different media and buffers separate the distinct types of hemoglobin.

## Purpose of the Test

Hemoglobin electrophoresis is used to detect hemoglobinopathy, help confirm the diagnosis of thalassemia, evaluate hemolytic anemia, identify the presence of HbC, identify sickle cell hemoglobin, and differentiate between sickle cell disease and sickle cell trait.

## Procedure

A lavender-topped tube is used to collect 7 mL of venous blood. A fingerstick or earlobe puncture is used to obtain two lavender-topped capillary tubes of blood.

### Quality Control

The tourniquet should not be tied tightly and should not remain tied for a prolonged period. Venipuncture technique must be smooth, with a blood flow that fills the vacuum tube readily. If the blood has excessive turbulence because of flawed venipuncture technique, hemolysis of the erythrocytes will alter the results.

## Findings

### Elevated Values

| | | |
|---|---|---|
| Beta-thalassemia minor or major | Sickle cell disease | HbC trait |
| | Sickle cell trait | HbH disease |
| Hereditary persistence of fetal hemoglobin | HbC disease | Megaloblastic anemia |

### Decreased Values

DEFICIENCY OF HbA$_2$

| | |
|---|---|
| Sideroblastic anemia | Erythroleukemia |
| Untreated iron deficiency anemia | Hereditary persistence of fetal hemoglobin |
| HbH disease | |

## Interfering Factors

- Blood transfusion in the preceding 4 months
- Hemolysis
- Coagulation of the specimen

| **Nursing Implementation** | **Pretest** |
|---|---|

Ask the patient about any transfusion of blood within the preceding 3 to 4 months. A recent transfusion would make the findings of the test inconsistent.

**Posttest**

Gently rotate the tube several times to mix the anticoagulant with the blood. This prevents clotting of the specimen.

Arrange for prompt transport of the blood to the laboratory.

**Quality Control**

> The specimen must be fresh or refrigerated.

Provide support to the parent as the infant is tested. Once a sickle cell screening test is positive, this test is done to verify a condition of trait or disease. Other inherited hemoglobinopathies may be identified, many of which cause a form of chronic anemia. The parent may express feelings of concern, guilt, fear, and worry about the well-being of the infant.

Encourage the parent (or the adult patient) to return to the primary physician for the test results and guidance that includes genetic counseling and education about any specific health care needs (Waterbury, 1996).

## Hemosiderin, Urinary

**(Urine)**                                  Synonyms: None

| **Normal Values** | Negative |
|---|---|

## Background Information

Hemosiderin granules are indicators of hemoglobin in the urine resulting from significant acute or chronic intravascular hemolysis. With the lysis of many erythrocytes, hemoglobin is released into the blood and is metabolized in the renal tubules to form ferritin and hemosiderin. The hemosiderin granules are present in the cells or casts in urinary sediment. They appear in the urine on the second or third day after the hemolytic episode. The source of the urinary hemosiderin may also be diseases that cause siderosis of the renal parenchyma, such as hematochromatosis.

The presence of hemoglobin in the urine may not be detected by a reagent strip. When the urinary sediment is stained with Prussian blue stain, however, the iron in hemosiderin appears as blue-stained granules. The results are seen by microscopic examination of the slides, which contain urinary cells and casts.

| **Purpose of the Test** | Urinary hemosiderin is used to identify hemolytic anemia that is associated with intravascular hemolysis. |
|---|---|

| **Procedure** | A random sample of 30 to 60 mL of urine is collected in a clean glass container. |

**Quality Control**

> To avoid the introduction of iron from extraneous sources, the container, slides, and covers must be free of iron.

**Findings**    **Elevated Values**

| | | |
|---|---|---|
| Blood transfusion reaction | G-6-PD deficiency | Paroxysmal cold hemoglobinuria |
| Microangiopathic hemolytic anemia | Thalassemia major | Severe infectious organisms (malaria, *Clostridium perfringens*) |
| Mechanical trauma to erythrocytes | Severe megaloblastic anemia | |
| Exposure to oxidant drugs or chemicals | Sickle cell anemia | |
| | Hematochromatosis | |

**Interfering Factors**    • None

**Nursing Implementation**    No special patient instruction or intervention is needed.

## Human Leukocyte Antigen

**(Blood)**    Synonyms: HLA typing; tissue typing, crossmatch; crossmatch lymphocyte; transplant tissue typing

**Normal Values**    No destruction of lymphocytes

## Background Information

Human leukocyte antigens (HLAs) are genetic products that are major determinants of histocompatibility. These antigens exist in an exact sequence or pattern that is specific and different for each individual. The only exception is in identical twins, who have the same HLA antigens. The unique protein sequence is found on every cell of the body, including on leukocytes.

HLA antigens are produced by chromosome 6. The chromosome loci are identified as HLA-A, HLA-B, and HLA-C (class I) and HLA-DR, HLA-DQ, HLA-DP, and HLA-DW (class II). Class I antigens are derived from T lymphocytes, and class II antigens are derived from B lymphocytes. The HLA-A, HLA-B, and HLA-C antigens are present on almost all nucleated cells. HLA-D antigens are present on B lymphocytes, monocytes, and possibly endothelial cells.

Circulating leukocytes are in contact with other cells. During the moment of contact, the leukocytes compare the HLA sequence on the cell surface with their own HLA sequence. When the HLA sequence is the same, the leukocyte does not react. When the HLA sequence is different, the leukocyte recognizes the cell as a foreign substance and initiates an inflammatory reaction to inactivate and destroy the cell with a different HLA sequence (Myhre, 1996).

In organ transplantation, HLA matching of the organ donor and transplant recipient is essential.

Tissue matching improves the chance of acceptance of the tissue graft and increases the long-term survival of the transplanted tissue. When HLA matching is less than optimal, the recipient's immune system is activated with the recognition of a foreign HLA antigen. Mismatching results in graft-versus-host disease, graft failure, and possible increased sensitization of the recipient when retransplantation is needed.

A number of disease syndromes are associated with a single leukocyte antigen (Table 17–2), although the clinical significance of the tissue marker is not yet understood. The specific HLA antigens are statistically correlated with illnesses that are thought to have autoimmune characteristics. A discussion of HLA-B27 is presented in Chapter 24.

In the past, HLA typing was used to help exclude paternity. That is still true, but the test is used less often for this purpose. DNA testing is preferred because it provides more definite information that establishes or excludes paternity (Jacobs et al., 1996; Myhre, 1996).

**Purpose of the Test**

In organ transplantation, HLA tissue typing is used to determine tissue compatibility between the donor and the recipient. HLA testing may also be performed to exclude paternity, and it may be used as a source of data in genetic counseling.

**Procedure**

**Donor Specimen.** Two green-topped tubes are each filled with 7 mL to 10 mL of venous blood.

**Recipient's Blood.** A red-topped tube is used to obtain 7 mL to 10 mL of venous blood.

**HLA Typing.** A green-topped, heparinized tube is filled with 7 mL to 10 mL of venous blood.

**Table 17–2    HLA Antigen Associated Diseases**

| Specific HLA Antigens | Diseases |
| --- | --- |
| B27 | Ankylosing spondylitis<br>Reiter's syndrome<br>Anterior uveitis |
| B47 | Congenital adrenal hyperplasia |
| B35 | Subacute thyroiditis |
| B8 | Chronic autoimmune hepatitis |
| Cw6 | Psoriasis |
| D/DR3 | Myasthenia gravis<br>Systemic lupus erythematosus<br>Celiac disease<br>Graves' disease<br>Idiopathic Addison's disease |
| D/DR4 | Pemphigus<br>Rheumatoid arthritis |

| Findings | Abnormal Values | |
|---|---|---|
| | HLA-A, HLA-B, or HLA-DR mismatch | Incompatibility of donor and recipient tissues |

| Interfering Factors | • Recent blood transfusion<br>• Inadequate lymphocytes in the specimen |
|---|---|

**Nursing Implementation**

Nursing care includes care of the venipuncture site.

**Pretest**

Schedule this test before or 72 hours after any blood transfusion.

**Posttest**

Arrange for prompt transport of the specimen to the laboratory. The analysis must be performed immediately on a fresh blood sample.

**Quality Control**

A prolonged delay or refrigeration of the specimen will yield an insufficient number of lymphocytes for the test.

## Intrinsic Factor Antibodies

(Serum)                          Synonym: Anti-IF antibodies

| Normal Values | Negative; no intrinsic factor antibodies are present. |
|---|---|

## Background Information

Intrinsic factor is a glycoprotein manufactured by the parietal cells of the gastric mucosa. The function of intrinsic factor is to bond with ingested cobalamin (vitamin $B_{12}$) and then adhere to receptor sites in the distal ilium. At these receptor sites, the cobalamin is absorbed into the blood. Most of it is transported to the liver for storage, and some goes to the bone marrow for hematopoiesis. Pernicious anemia is a megaloblastic anemia that results from inadequate manufacture of intrinsic factor, interference with the bonding of intrinsic factor-cobalamin, or interference with the bonding of the intrinsic factor-cobalamin complex at the ileal receptor sites.

Interference with the function of intrinsic factor is caused by intrinsic factor antibodies. These antibodies are autoimmune complexes that are present in many cases of pernicious anemia. Two types of intrinsic factor antibody exist. Type 1, the "blocking" antibody, interferes with the bonding of intrinsic factor to cobalamin. Type 2, the "binding" antibody, interferes with the attachment of the intrinsic factor-cobalamin complex to the ileal receptor sites.

It is unclear whether the antibodies cause the pernicious anemia or develop as a result of it. Adult pernicious anemia may be an autoimmune gastritis of genetic origin, but the relationship of the autoantibodies to the gastritis is unclear (Henry, 1996). Intrinsic factor antibodies are also present in a small percentage of patients who have hyperthyroidism or insulin-dependent diabetes without pernicious anemia.

When pernicious anemia is diagnosed by the triad of megaloblastic anemia, decreased serum cobalamin, and the presence of intrinsic factor antibodies, it is not necessary to perform a Schilling test or gastric analysis.

| **Purpose of the Test** | This test is performed to differentiate pernicious anemia from other causes of megaloblastic anemia. |

| **Procedure** | A red-topped tube is used to obtain 10 mL of venous blood. |

**Findings**

**Positive Values**

Pernicious anemia
Hyperthyroidism
(Graves' disease)

Diabetes mellitus
(insulin depen-
dent)

**Interfering Factors**

- Recent radioisotope scan
- Recent vitamin $B_{12}$ injection

**Nursing Implementation**

**Pretest**

Schedule this test before any radioisotope scan. The radioisotopes of the nuclear scan interfere with the radioimmunoassay method of analysis used in this test.

Instruct the patient to withhold any injection of vitamin $B_{12}$ for 48 hours before the test. Recent injection of this vitamin could cause a false-positive result.

**Posttest**

Arrange for prompt transport of the specimen to the laboratory.

## Iron Studies

**(Serum)**

Synonyms: Serum iron, Fe; transferrin, Tf; siderophilin; total iron-binding capacity, TIBC; transferrin saturation, iron saturation

**Normal Values**

**Serum Iron**
Adult male: 65–175 µg/dL *or* SI 11.6–31.3 µmol/L
Adult female: 50–170 µg/dL *or* SI 9–30.4 µmol/L
Child: 50–120 µg/dL *or* SI 9–21.5 µmol/L
Infant: 40–100 µg/dL *or* SI 7.2–17.9 µmol/L
Newborn: 100–250 µg/dL *or* SI 17.9–44.8 µmol/L
**Transferrin**
Adult >60 years: 190–375 mg/dL *or* SI 1.9–3.75 g/L
Adult 16–60 years (male): 215–365 mg/dL *or* SI 2.15–3.65 g/L
(female): 250–380 mg/dL *or* SI 2.50–3.80 g/L

*Continued on following page*

*Continued*

Child 3 months–16 years: 203–360 mg/dL *or* SI 2.03–3.6 g/L
Newborn: 130–275 mg/dL *or* SI 1.3–2.75 g/L
**Total iron-binding capacity:** 250–425 µg/dL *or* SI 44.8–76.1 µmol/L
**Transferrin saturation:** 20%–50% *or* SI 0.20–0.50 fraction saturation
**Ferritin**
Adult male: 20–250 ng/mL *or* SI 20–250 µg/L
Adult female: 10–120 ng/mL *or* SI 10–120 µg/L
Child 6 months–15 years: 7–140 ng/mL *or* SI 7–140 µg/L
Infant 2–5 months: 50–200 ng/mL *or* SI 50–200 µg/L
Newborn: 25–200 ng/mL *or* SI 25–200 µg/L

## Background Information

Iron is an inorganic ion that is essential to many vital body processes, including erythropoiesis, the transport of oxygen to tissues, and cellular oxidation mechanisms. In normal physiology, the total iron content remains relatively constant throughout life. The body has an efficient method to conserve the iron from senescent erythrocytes and reuse it in erythropoiesis and hemoglobin synthesis (Fig. 17–3).

**Absorption.** Iron homeostasis is regulated by the function of intestinal absorption of the iron in foods. Because the body has a limited ability to excrete iron, the intestine absorbs only 5% to 10% of the daily iron intake. This prevents the retention of an excessive or toxic amount. Most of the iron is absorbed from the duodenum and jejunum, with enhanced absorption in the presence of gastric acids. In times of greater demand, as in pregnancy or after blood loss, the intestinal tract absorbs a greater quantity of iron to meet the body's need.

**Transport.** Once absorbed, iron enters the blood and the unbound iron attaches to transferrin, a plasma protein. At the bone marrow, iron is passed into developing erythrocytes to become heme molecules and part of hemoglobin.

**Storage.** Some of the absorbed iron combines with apoferritin to form ferritin, and the remainder is deposited into tissues in the form of hemosiderin. Both ferritin and hemosiderin are used to store the iron reserves, and the stored iron can be released when needed. The stored iron reserves are located in the tissues of the liver and in the reticuloendothelial cells of the bone marrow, spleen, and liver.

**Circulation.** Iron is present in the hemoglobin content of erythrocytes. Each hemoglobin molecule has iron-containing pigment called *heme*. As the erythrocytes are damaged or become senescent, they are removed from the circulation by hemolysis. During this process, the reticuloendothelial tissues extract the iron. The iron is either bound to transferrin for transport or stored as hemosiderin in the reticuloendothelial tissues and the liver.

**Elevated Values.** Iron overload occurs in some types of anemia, in liver disease, in excessive iron replacement therapy, and after multiple transfusions.

**Decreased Values.** Iron deficiency occurs when the supply of iron is insufficient to meet the body's demand and the iron reserves are also depleted. The source of the problem can be insufficient intake, impaired absorption, blood loss, or increased demand because of pregnancy or lactation (Table 17–3).

**Laboratory Testing.** No one test fully measures iron deficiency, iron overload, and iron storage. A battery of several tests is used to provide a complete assessment, including the complete blood count. The laboratory assessment of iron stores includes serum iron, transferrin, total iron-binding capacity, transferrin saturation, and ferritin.

**Serum Iron.** This is the amount of iron bound to transferrin. In the laboratory analysis, the iron must first be separated from the transferrin so that the measurement is accurate. As a single laboratory test, a serum iron determination is used to evaluate iron toxicity. The value is decreased in iron deficiency anemia and in the anemia associated with chronic disease. The test is useful when serum iron is measured along with transferrin and transferrin saturation.

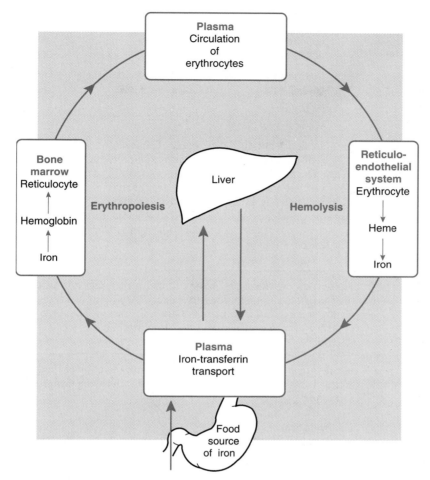

**Figure 17–3**

The use and conservation of iron. Some iron is readily available in the plasma and bone marrow for the synthesis of hemoglobin and erythropoiesis. After the hemolysis of old or damaged erythrocytes, the body is very efficient in the conservation and storage of iron in the liver and bone marrow. Whenever the immediate supply of iron is low, the liver releases the stored iron for erythropoiesis.

**Transferrin.** This is the major protein that binds serum iron and transports it in the blood. In normal physiology, about one third of the transferrin is bound with iron, and the remainder is available in reserve. Transferrin is elevated in iron deficiency anemia and is decreased with iron overload. It is a useful index of nutritional status because it is elevated in uncomplicated iron deficiency but is in the normal to low-normal range in other types of anemia.

**Total Iron-Binding Capacity.** This is the maximum iron-binding capacity of transferrin and other iron-binding globulins. The serum value also provides data regarding the nutritional status of the individual. The results of the total iron-binding capacity determination correlate with the transferrin value, meaning that the total iron-binding capacity rises in iron deficiency anemia and decreases in the presence of iron overload.

**Table 17–3  Factors That Contribute to Iron Deficiency**

| Insufficient Intake | Impaired Absorption | Blood Loss | Increased Demand |
|---|---|---|---|
| Fad diets | Gastric surgery | Gastrointestinal bleeding | Pregnancy |
| Pica | Celiac disease | Excessive menstruation | Lactation |
| Poverty | Achlorhydria | | |

**Transferrin Saturation.** This is a calculation of the iron storage, expressed as the ratio of serum iron to total iron-binding capacity. The result is the percentage of transferrin that is saturated with iron. The value is decreased in iron deficiency, but a value of less than 15% indicates iron deficiency erythropoiesis.

**Ferritin.** This is a reliable indicator of total iron storage. The level is decreased in iron deficiency anemia and elevated in iron overload. When a ferritin determination is combined with other iron studies, the results differentiate among the different types of microcytic, hypochromic anemias. Iron deficiency anemia is indicated by a serum ferritin value of less than 10 ng/mL (SI <10 µg/L).

---

**Purpose of the Tests**

These tests provide an estimate of total iron storage and information regarding the nutritional status of the individual. They help distinguish between iron deficiency anemia and the anemia of chronic disease. They also confirm the presence of iron overload and hematochromatosis.

---

**Procedure**

A red-topped tube is used to collect 10 mL of venous blood. This blood sample is drawn before other blood samples that require vacuum tubes with anticoagulant.

**Quality Control**

The tourniquet is applied loosely and is not kept in place for long. The venipuncture must be smooth, with a blood flow that fills the vacuum tube readily. If the blood has excessive turbulence because of flawed venipuncture technique, the hemolysis of the erythrocytes will alter the results.

---

**Findings**

**Elevated Values**

SERUM IRON

| | | |
|---|---|---|
| Anemias (pernicious, aplastic, hemolytic) | Excess iron replacement | Lead poisoning |
| Hematochromatosis | Multiple transfusions | Vitamin B$_6$ deficiency |
| Thalassemia | Iron poisoning | Acute leukemia |

TRANSFERRIN

| | | |
|---|---|---|
| Iron deficiency anemia | Elevated estrogen levels | Pregnancy |

TOTAL IRON-BINDING CAPACITY

| | | |
|---|---|---|
| Hypochromic anemias | Iron deficiency anemia | Acute hepatitis |
| | | Pregnancy |

FERRITIN

| | | |
|---|---|---|
| Thalassemia | Hemochromatosis | Nephrosis |
| Iron toxicity | Viral hepatitis | |

TRANSFERRIN SATURATION

| | | |
|---|---|---|
| Hemochromatosis | Acute leukemias | Infectious diseases |
| Liver disease | Inflammatory | |
| Iron overload | diseases | |

### Decreased Values

SERUM IRON

| | | |
|---|---|---|
| Iron deficiency anemia | Nephrosis | Malignancy |
| Pernicious anemia (in remission) | Hypothyroidism | Starvation |
| | Acute or chronic infection | |

TRANSFERRIN

| | |
|---|---|
| Inflammation or necrosis | Multiple myeloma |
| Malignancy | Hepatocellular diseases |
| Malnutrition | Nephrotic syndrome |

TRANSFERRIN SATURATION

| | | |
|---|---|---|
| Iron deficiency anemia | Anemia of chronic infection | Malignancy |

TOTAL IRON-BINDING CAPACITY

| | | |
|---|---|---|
| Anemias (non–iron-deficient) | Hemochromatosis | Renal disease |
| | Malignancy | Thalassemia |

FERRITIN

Iron deficiency
   anemia

---

**Interfering Factors**

- Recent administration of radioisotopes (ferritin)
- Hemolysis (serum iron, iron saturation)
- Lipemia (transferrin)
- Recent blood transfusion (serum iron)

---

**Nursing Implementation**

Nursing care includes care of the venipuncture site.

### Pretest

Schedule these laboratory tests before or a few days after a blood transfusion to obtain the most accurate results.

Schedule these laboratory tests before any nuclear scans, because the radioactive isotopes of the scan interfere with the radioimmunoassay method for testing of ferritin.

Schedule these tests to be performed in the morning. Serum iron has a diurnal rhythm, with the highest value in the early morning. The serum iron values fluctuate widely between day and night and also on different days.

Instruct the patient to fast from food and fluids for 8 hours before the test for transferrin levels. Lipemia interferes with the transferrin values.

If the patient takes an iron supplement, include this information on the requisition slip.

### Posttest

Arrange for prompt transport of the specimen to the laboratory.

**Quality Control**

The cells must be separated from the serum without delay. This avoids false elevation due to hemolysis.

## Neutrophil Alkaline Phosphatase

**(Peripheral Blood)**        Synonyms: NAP, leukocyte alkaline phosphatase (LAP)

| Normal Values | Rating score of 40–130 (Tietz, 1995) |
|---|---|

### Background Information

Chronic myeloproliferative diseases are hematologic malignancies that produce rapid, excessive cloning of a multipotential cell of the bone marrow. The cloning can proceed along different granulocytic, erythroid, or megakaryocytic lines, producing excessive neutrophils, erythrocytes, platelets, or other related cells derived from progenitors. The four chronic myeloproliferative diseases are chronic myelogenous leukemia, polycythemia vera, myelofibrosis, and essential thrombocytopenia.

The neutrophil alkaline phosphatase test produces a characteristic chemical reaction that helps to differentiate among these myeloproliferative disorders. Neutrophil alkaline phosphatase is an enzyme located in neutrophils. The enzyme is detected in an alkaline medium and in the presence of dye.

In the test method, 100 stained neutrophils are given a rating score of 0 to 4, based on the intensity of the color of the reaction. Thus, the range is 0 to 400, and the reference range or normal range is 40 to 130. The scoring is somewhat subject to color interpretation, and the reference range varies among laboratories.

Among the myeloproliferative disorders, chronic myelogenous leukemia tends to produce low scores regardless of the total white cell count. The other myeloproliferative disorders have higher scores.

### Purpose of the Test

This test helps differentiate chronic myelogenous leukemia from leukemoid reaction and other myeloproliferative diseases. It is also useful in the evaluation of Hodgkin's disease and its response to therapy.

| | |
|---|---|
| **Procedure** | Fingerstick puncture is used to make six slides with smears of the peripheral blood. As an alternative, a green-topped tube with heparin or oxalate anticoagulant is used to collect 10 mL of venous blood. |

**Findings**

**Elevated Values**

| | | |
|---|---|---|
| Polycythemia vera | Leukemoid reactions | Neutrophilia secondary to infection |
| Hairy cell leukemia | Hodgkin's disease | |
| Myelofibrosis | Acute lymphoblastic | |
| Down syndrome | leukemia | |

**Decreased Values**

| | | |
|---|---|---|
| Chronic myelogenous leukemia | Sideroblastic anemia | Acute monocytic leukemia |
| Cirrhosis of the liver | Gout | Hereditary hypophosphatemia |
| Acute myeloid leukemia | Thrombocytopenic purpura | Collagen disease |
| Congestive heart failure | Diabetes mellitus | |

**Interfering Factors**

- Pregnancy
- Acute stress
- Neutropenia
- Delay in the final preparation of slides

**Nursing Implementation**

Nursing care includes care of the site of the venipuncture or fingerstick puncture.

**Pretest**

To ensure a valid test, verify that the recent peripheral blood neutrophil count is greater than 1,000/mm³.

**Posttest**

Arrange for immediate transport of the slides or blood specimen to the laboratory.

**Quality Control**

To avoid rejection of the specimen, the slides must be fixed in preservative within 30 minutes.

## Osmotic Fragility

**(Whole Blood)**     Synonyms: OF, erythrocyte fragility, RBC fragility

| **Normal Values** | Initial hemolysis of erythrocytes: 0.45% sodium chloride (NaCl) *or* SI 4.5 g/L NaCl |
|---|---|
| | Complete hemolysis of erythrocytes: 0.35% NaCl *or* SI 3.5 g/L NaCl |

## Background Information

Osmotic fragility refers to the ability of erythrocytes to absorb water without lysis of the cell membrane. The variation of time in the results is based on the surface area and cell volume. Abnormal erythrocytes, such as spherocytes, have greater than normal volume. They demonstrate lysis in the presence of a hypotonic saline solution because of increased osmotic fragility. Abnormal erythrocytes, such as hypochromic cells, have a greater than normal surface area. They resist lysis in the presence of a hypotonic saline solution because of decreased osmotic fragility.

## Purpose of the Test

Osmotic fragility is used in the evaluation of immunohemolytic conditions, including hemolytic anemia and hereditary spherocytosis.

## Procedure

A lavender-topped tube with EDTA or a green-topped tube with heparin is used to collect 7 or 10 mL of venous blood.

### Quality Control

The tourniquet must not be applied tightly or kept in place long. Venipuncture technique must be smooth, with a blood flow that fills the vacuum tube readily. If the blood has excessive turbulence because of flawed venipuncture technique, the hemolysis of the erythrocytes alters the test results.

## Findings

### Elevated Values

Hereditary sphero-
  cytosis
Acquired immune
  hemolytic anemia
  with spherocytosis

Hereditary stomato-
  cytosis

### Decreased Values

Iron deficiency
  anemia
Microcytic anemia

Hemoglobinopathy
Thalassemia

Leptocytosis

## Interfering Factors

- Hemolysis
- Clotting of the blood sample
- Delay in analysis of the blood

| | |
|---|---|
| **Nursing Implementation** | **Pretest** |

Nursing care includes care of the venipuncture site.
No special teaching or intervention with the patient is needed.

**Posttest**

Arrange for prompt transport of the specimen to the laboratory.

**Quality Control**

The results are most accurate when the test is performed on fresh cells. A delay of more than 6 hours before analysis or the clotting of the specimen results in an invalid test.

## Parietal Cell Antibody

**(Serum)**          Synonym: PCA

| | |
|---|---|
| **Normal Values** | Negative; no parietal cell antibodies are present. |

### Background Information

The parietal cells of the gastric mucosa manufacture intrinsic factor, the glycoprotein that promotes intestinal absorption of cobalamin (vitamin $B_{12}$). When the parietal cells are destroyed, cobalamin deficiency and pernicious anemia develop. Parietal cell antibodies can be detected in most cases of pernicious anemia and atrophic gastritis. The two conditions often coexist and are characterized by the absence of parietal and chief cells in the gastric mucosa.

The presence of parietal cell antibodies and intrinsic factor antibodies suggests that pernicious anemia and some cases of atrophic gastritis are autoimmune disorders.

| | |
|---|---|
| **Purpose of the Test** | The parietal cell antibody test is useful in the diagnosis of pernicious anemia and some cases of atrophic gastritis. |

| | |
|---|---|
| **Procedure** | A red-topped tube is used to collect 10 mL of venous blood. |

| | |
|---|---|
| **Findings** | **Elevated Values** |

| | | |
|---|---|---|
| Pernicious anemia | Addison's disease | Iron deficiency |
| Atrophic gastritis | Myasthenia gravis | anemia |
| Hashimoto's thy- | Juvenile diabetes | Sjögren's syndrome |
| roiditis | Gastric ulcer | |

| | |
|---|---|
| **Interfering Factors** | • None |

**Nursing Implementation**    **Pretest**

No specific patient instruction or intervention is needed.
Nursing care includes care of the venipuncture site.

**Posttest**

Arrange for prompt transport of the specimen to the laboratory.

**Quality Control**

The cells must be separated from the serum without delay.

## Schilling Test

**(Urine)**

Synonyms: Vitamin $B_{12}$ absorption test, radioactive vitamin $B_{12}$ absorption test with (without) intrinsic factor

**Normal Values**

> **Stage 1:** >10% cobalt 58–labeled vitamin $B_{12}$ excretion/24-hour urine collection *or* SI >0.10 (fraction of dose excreted)
> **Stage 2:** 0%–42% cobalt 57–labeled vitamin $B_{12}$ plus intrinsic factor excretion per 24-hour urine collection *or* SI 0.000.42 (fraction of dose excreted)
> **Cobalt 57–to–cobalt 58 ratio:** 0.7–1.3

## Background Information

When vitamin $B_{12}$ is poorly absorbed from the small intestine, pernicious anemia, a form of megaloblastic anemia, develops gradually. The poor absorption of vitamin $B_{12}$ can be caused by malabsorption in the small intestine or by a defect of intrinsic factor. The Schilling test measures the ability of the small intestine to absorb vitamin $B_{12}$ and also identifies the source of the problem.

In normal physiology, vitamin $B_{12}$ is absorbed in the terminal segment of the small intestine in the presence of intrinsic factor. Once vitamin $B_{12}$ enters the bloodstream, it is bound to plasma proteins or is stored by the liver. It is an essential ingredient for normal hematopoiesis.

In stage 1 of the test, a measured oral dose of cobalt 58–labeled vitamin $B_{12}$ is absorbed. It has been blocked from the liver and plasma proteins, so it must be excreted in the urine. In the 24-hour urine collection, the normal excretion is >10% of the oral dose of cobalt 58–labeled vitamin $B_{12}$. The normal value indicates that intrinsic factor is sufficient and that the intestine is functional for the ab-

sorption of vitamin $B_{12}$. When the stage 1 urine value is less than 7%, the results indicate that pernicious anemia or malabsorption exists. Stage 2 of the test is used to distinguish between these two causes.

In stage 2, the process is repeated, but the radiolabeled vitamin $B_{12}$ contains intrinsic factor (cobalt 57–labeled vitamin $B_{12}$ plus intrinsic factor). In the 24-hour urine collection, the normal excretion is 10% to 42% of the oral dose of cobalt 57–labeled vitamin $B_{12}$ plus intrinsic factor. When the result remains lower than normal, the problem is malabsorption. Low values in the presence of intrinsic factor imply that the problem concerns the structure and integrity of the intestinal mucosa.

It is also possible to perform both stages of this test at the same time. The radionuclides in the urine can be measured separately because of the different energies of cobalt 57 and cobalt 58. The results are expressed as the ratio of cobalt 57 to cobalt 58. In normal function, they are absorbed and excreted in almost equal amounts. When the value of cobalt 57–labeled vitamin $B_{12}$ plus intrinsic factor is normal, but the value of cobalt 58–labeled vitamin $B_{12}$ without intrinsic factor is low, the cause is pernicious anemia. In this case, the cobalt 57–to–cobalt 58 ratio is greater than 1.7.

This alternative method requires only one test period and minimizes the opportunity for error that results from incomplete collection of urine.

---

**Purpose of the Test**

The 24-hour urine test measures vitamin $B_{12}$ absorption before and after the administration of intrinsic factor to differentiate between pernicious anemia and malabsorption of the small intestine.

---

**Procedure**

**Traditional Method, Stage 1.** After administration of an oral dose of cobalt 58–labeled vitamin $B_{12}$ and an intramuscular dose of unlabeled vitamin $B_{12}$, urine is collected for 24 hours.

**Traditional Method, Stage 2.** Five days later, after administration of an oral dose of cobalt 57–labeled vitamin $B_{12}$ plus intrinsic factor and an intramuscular dose of unlabeled vitamin $B_{12}$, urine is collected for 24 hours.

**Combined Method.** After oral administration of cobalt 58–labeled and cobalt 57–labeled vitamin $B_{12}$ plus intrinsic factor, urine is collected for 24 hours.

---

**Findings**

**Decreased Values**

| | | |
|---|---|---|
| Pernicious anemia | Chronic pancreatitis | Total gastrectomy |
| Abnormality of the small intestine | Crohn's disease | Radiotherapy |
| Severe ileal disease | Giardiasis | Celiac disease |

---

**Interfering Factors**

- Failure to maintain pretest nothing-by-mouth status
- Failure to administer vitamin $B_{12}$ intramuscularly
- Incomplete urine collection
- Renal dysfunction
- Recent vitamin $B_{12}$ injection
- Recent radioisotope scan
- Fecal contamination of urine specimen
- Pregnancy or lactation

---

**Nursing Implementation**

**Pretest**

Schedule the bone marrow examination, serum folate determination, and serum vitamin $B_{12}$ determination before the Schilling test, because the administered vitamin $B_{12}$ will alter the bone marrow and serum levels of these other tests.

Schedule the Schilling test before any radioactive scans, because the radioactive materials of the scans will alter the count of the radiolabeled vitamin $B_{12}$. Instruct the patient to discontinue food intake at midnight before the test (Jacobs et al., 1996). Water is permitted.

Explain the procedure to the patient, including the need to save all urine for each 24-hour collection period.

### Quality Control

No fecal material can be mixed in with the urine. The unabsorbed radiolabeled vitamin $B_{12}$ is excreted in the feces. If fecal contamination occurs, the urine will have a falsely elevated result.

## During the Test

### Stage 1

Before the vitamin $B_{12}$ is given to start the test, have the patient void to empty the bladder in preparation for the 24-hour urine collection.

Administer the oral dose of cobalt 58–labeled vitamin $B_{12}$.

At the same time or within 2 hours, administer the "flushing dose" of vitamin $B_{12}$, 1,000 µg intramuscularly.

Instruct the patient to resume food and beverage intake 1 to 2 hours after the oral dose of radiolabeled vitamin $B_{12}$ is given. Encourage extra water and fluids throughout the test to ensure the production of at least 1 L of urine in the 24-hour period.

Collect all urine for 24 hours, starting with the time of the oral dose of radiolabeled vitamin $B_{12}$.

### Stage 2

Five days later, begin the second stage of the test.

Instruct the patient to void and empty the bladder in preparation for the 24-hour collection of urine.

Administer the oral dose of cobalt-57–labeled vitamin $B_{12}$ with 60 mg of active hog intrinsic factor to the fasting patient.

At the same time or within 2 hours, administer the flushing dose of unlabeled vitamin $B_{12}$, 1,000 µg intramuscularly.

Instruct the patient to collect all urine for 24 hours, starting at the time of the oral dose of radiolabeled vitamin $B_{12}$ and intrinsic factor.

Instruct the patient to resume food and beverage intake 1 to 2 hours after the oral dose of radiolabeled vitamin $B_{12}$ and intrinsic factor is given. Encourage sufficient extra fluids to produce at least 1 L of urine in the collection period.

### Combined Method

Instruct the patient to void and empty the bladder in preparation for the 24-hour collection of urine.

Administer the capsule of cobalt-58–labeled vitamin $B_{12}$ simultaneously with the cobalt-57–labeled vitamin $B_{12}$ plus intrinsic factor to the fasting patient. At the same time or within 2 hours, administer the flushing dose of unlabeled vitamin $B_{12}$, 1,000 µg intramuscularly.

Instruct the patient to collect all urine for 24 hours, resume food and fluid intake, and drink extra fluids, as described previously.

## Posttest

Ensure that the urine container and requisition slip have the patient's name and the dates and times of the start and finish of the collection period.

Arrange for prompt transport of the urine specimen to the laboratory.

■
*Critical Thinking 17–1*
The patient had an abnormal Schilling test result and was diagnosed with pernicious anemia. If vitamin $B_{12}$ treatment is effective, which laboratory tests provide pertinent evaluation data?

# Sickle Cell Tests

(Blood)                    Synonyms: Dithionite test, metabisulfate test, sickle cell solubility test, Sickledex

| Normal Values | Negative |
|---|---|

## Background Information

The normal adult forms of hemoglobin are identified as HbA, HbA$_2$, and HbF. Common variant hemoglobins are identified as HbS, HbC, HbD, and HbE, but sickle cell hemoglobin (HbS) is the most common of the abnormal hemoglobins. The term *sickled* is used because in deoxygenated states, HbS converts the erythrocytes into sickle or crescent shapes (Fig. 17–4).

The homozygous (pure) form of HbS produces sickle cell anemia. The infant inherits the HbS from both parents, and the erythrocytes have only HbS, with no HbA or HbA$_2$ present. Other forms of sickle cell anemia are inherited when one parent has HbS and the other parent has beta-thalassemia or abnormal hemoglobin (Table 17–4). The heterozygous (mixed) form of HbS produces sickle cell trait, and each erythrocyte has some HbA and some HbS. In the trait condition, the proportion of

normal hemoglobin is always greater than that of HbS, usually in the 55% to 65% range.

Because all infants are born with 100% HbF, sickle cell anemia may not be detected by these test methods until the baby is 3 to 6 months old. By this time, affected infants have replaced the HbF with HbS, and the test result is positive (Jacobs et al., 1996).

These tests have a number of limitations. Polycythemia or hyperglobulinemia may produce a false-positive result. Patients who have severe anemia will have a false-negative result. When the test result is positive, no differentiation exists between sickle cell anemia and sickle cell trait. With suspicious findings, the test should be repeated. Hemoglobin electrophoresis is the preferred method to confirm the diagnosis and differentiate between sickle cell disease and sickle cell trait.

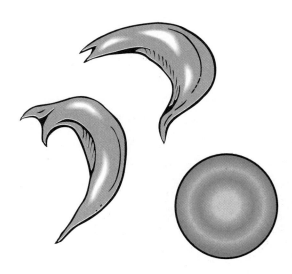

**Figure 17–4**
Sickled cells differ markedly from normal cells. (Reproduced with permission from Stepp, C. A., & Woods, M. A. [1998]. *Laboratory procedures for medical office personnel* [Figure 12–24, p. 164]. Philadelphia: W. B. Saunders.)

### Table 17–4   Sickle Cell Diseases with Abnormal Variant Hemoglobins

Sickle cell anemia
HbSC disease
Sickle beta-thalassemia
HbSD$_{Punjab}$
HbSE disease
HbSO$_{Arab}$
HbS$_{Lepore}$

## Purpose of the Test

The sickle cell test is a screening test that is used to detect HbS, the sickling hemoglobin; to evaluate hemolytic anemia; and to help identify the cause of hereditary anemia.

## Procedure

A lavender-topped or green-topped tube is used to collect 7 to 10 mL of venous blood. As an alternative method, a fingerstick or earlobe puncture can be performed to obtain a capillary specimen.

### Quality Control

With venipuncture, the tourniquet must not be applied tightly or for a prolonged time. The venipuncture should be smooth, with a blood flow that fills the tube readily. If the blood has excessive turbulence because of flawed venipuncture technique, the hemolysis of the erythrocytes will alter the test results.

## Findings

**Positive Values**

Sickle cell anemia
Sickle cell trait

Other sickling
disorders

## Interfering Factors

- Hemolysis
- Coagulation of the specimen
- Blood transfusion within the past 3 to 4 months

## Nursing Implementation

Nursing care includes care of the venipuncture or capillary puncture site.

### Pretest

No specific patient instruction or intervention is needed.

### Posttest

Provide support to parents who become upset when they learn of the abnormal findings. Additional testing must be performed before any diagnosis is confirmed. With a positive screening test result, assist with the scheduling of a repeat test or hemoglobin electrophoresis that determines the exact diagnosis (trait versus disease).

## Total Blood Volume

**(Blood)**                    Synonyms: Plasma blood volume; blood volume, total

| Normal Values | **Red Blood Cell Volume** |
| --- | --- |
| | Male: 25–35 mL/kg |
| | Female: 20–30 mL/kg |
| | **Plasma cell volume:** 40–50 mL/kg |
| | **Total blood volume:** 60–80 mL/kg |

### Background Information

The total blood volume test consists of the red blood cell volume test and the plasma volume test. The normal amounts of red blood cells and plasma fluid vary with the individual's body surface, weight, height, sex, and age. Many pathophysiologic conditions exist that also alter the number of red blood cells or the fluid volume of the plasma, or both.

Polycythemia vera is caused by an increase in red blood cell volume or red blood cell mass. It is indicated by laboratory test results showing elevated hemoglobin, hematocrit, and red blood cell count. An elevation of the red blood cell volume can be caused by polycythemia vera or relative polycythemia. In severe, absolute polycythemia, the red blood cell volume, plasma volume, and total blood volume increase. In relative polycythemia, the plasma volume and total blood volume decrease. Although a relative increase in the red blood cell volume occurs, it is a result of hemoconcentration and not of an increase in the number of erythrocytes.

The red blood cell volume test may also be used in the assessment of anemia. In moderate to severe anemia, the red blood cell volume decreases, with normal to decreased total blood volume. The decrease of the red blood cell volume is a result of smaller, thinner, or fewer erythrocytes, or a combination of these factors, in a stable plasma volume.

Red blood cell volume or red blood cell mass is measured by radioactive sodium chromate (chromium 51) bound to erythrocytes. The plasma volume is measured by radioactive iodine (iodine 125 or iodine 131) bound to albumin. In both tests, the radiolabeled tracers are injected intravenously and blood is drawn at timed intervals. A scintillation counter is used to measure the test values.

### Purpose of the Test

The three tests of red blood cell volume, plasma cell volume, and total blood volume are used to distinguish between absolute polycythemia vera and relative polycythemia vera. Red blood cell volume is used to help assess anemia and the effect of cancer chemotherapy or radiation. The plasma volume or total blood volume, or both, can be used to help evaluate complicated fluid and electrolyte problems.

### Procedure

**Red Blood Cell Volume.**   Two green-topped, heparinized tubes are used to obtain 10 mL of venous blood. Chromium 51 radioisotope is added to the erythrocytes, and the cells are diluted in saline. The radioisotope-tagged erythrocytes are injected intravenously into the patient. After 10 minutes, a green-topped, heparinized tube is used to obtain 10 mL of venous blood from the opposite arm. A scintillation counter measures the radioactive erythrocyte count, and the red blood cell volume is calculated.

■

*Critical Thinking 17–2*
When genetic screening for sickle cell carriers is performed, what additional health care services should be provided to the patients and families who have positive results?

**Plasma Volume.**   Two green-topped, heparinized tubes are used to obtain 10 mL of venous blood. In the laboratory, radiolabeled albumin is added to the patient's plasma. This plasma preparation is injected intravenously into the patient. Using two green-topped, heparinized tubes, blood samples are drawn 10, 20, and 30 minutes later. In some laboratory methods, only one posttest sample is drawn after 10 minutes. A scintillation counter performs the radioactive albumin count, and the plasma volume is calculated.

**Total Blood Volume.**   The total volume of the blood is calculated by adding the test values for the red blood cell volume and the plasma volume.

---

**Findings**

**Elevated Values**

TOTAL BLOOD VOLUME

| | | |
|---|---|---|
| Absolute polycythemia vera | Overhydration | Pregnancy |
| Cardiac failure | Starvation | Renal insufficiency |
| Pulmonary diseases | Thyrotoxicosis | Congenital cardiac abnormality |
| | Acidosis | |

RED BLOOD CELL VOLUME

| | | |
|---|---|---|
| Absolute polycythemia vera | Relative polycythemia vera | Hemoglobinopathy |
| Pulmonary diseases | Neoplasm | Congenital cardiac abnormality |

PLASMA VOLUME

| | | |
|---|---|---|
| Anemia | Macroglobulinemia | Cirrhosis |
| Absolute polycythemia vera | Vasodilation | Acidosis |
| Splenomegaly | Overhydration | Renal insufficiency |
| | Cardiac failure | Pregnancy |

**Decreased Values**

TOTAL BLOOD VOLUME

| | | |
|---|---|---|
| Severe anemia | Diabetes mellitus | Chronic renal failure |
| Vomiting, diarrhea | Burns | Starvation |
| Hemorrhage | Dehydration | |

RED BLOOD CELL VOLUME

| | | |
|---|---|---|
| Anemia | Starvation | Chronic renal failure |
| Chronic infection | Pheochromocytosis | |
| Acute and chronic blood loss | | |

PLASMA VOLUME

| | | |
|---|---|---|
| Dehydration | Vomiting, diarrhea | Radiation |
| Chronic infection | Acute hemorrhage | Tissue hypoxia |
| Preeclampsia | | |

---

**Interfering Factors**

- Recent radioactive isotope scan
- Bleeding or edematous tissue
- Time delay in obtaining second blood specimens

| **Nursing Implementation** | **Pretest** |
|---|---|

Schedule this test before any other radioisotope tests.

Obtain the patient's accurate weight and height and record them in the chart.

Because of the administration of radioisotopes, a written consent may be needed.

Explain to the patient that several sets of blood samples will be drawn before and after the administration of the radioisotopes.

### During the Test

Ensure that the patient is present and available for the second set of blood tests, which are carried out on a timed basis.

### Posttest

Write the patient's height, weight, and age on the requisition slip.

If the health condition permits it, encourage the patient to drink extra fluids and to void. The half-life of the radioisotopes is only a few hours, so exposure to low-dose radiation is minimal. The radioisotopes are excreted in the urine.

## Type and Crossmatch

**(Blood)**      Synonyms: Blood compatibility testing, crossmatch

| **Normal Values** | Not applicable |
|---|---|

### Background Information

Human blood is typed by group, based on the presence or absence of A, B, AB, O, and Rh antigens. Blood group A has A antigens on the erythrocytes and anti-B antibodies in the serum. Blood group B has B antigens on the erythrocytes and anti-A antibodies in the serum. Blood group AB (universal receiver) has a double set of antigens on the erythrocytes and no antibodies in the serum, whereas blood group O (universal donor) has no antigens on the erythrocytes and a double set of antibodies in the serum (Table 17–5). When Rh antigens are also present on the erythrocytes, the person is classified as Rh positive. With no Rh antigens on the erythrocytes, the person is classified as Rh negative.

In preparation for blood transfusion, the intended recipient's blood is tested for ABO/$Rh_0$(D) type and antibody screening. In the crossmatch part of the test, the donor's blood type is determined and the blood is screened to identify antibodies. In se-

**Table 17–5    Erythrocyte Antigens and Antibodies: ABO System**

| Blood Group | Erythrocyte Antigens | Serum Antibodies |
|---|---|---|
| A | A | Anti-B |
| B | B | Anti-A |
| AB | AB | None |
| O | None | Anti-A, anti-B |

lecting a donor's blood that matches that of the recipient, a compatibility of antigens and antibodies must exist so that the transfusion is safe for the recipient. Incompatibility results in agglutination and hemolysis of the erythrocytes. Incompatible blood must not be administered to the patient.

The process of typing and crossmatching the blood determines a probable compatibility between the blood of the donor and that of the recipient. Despite careful work, some incidence of transfusion reaction occurs. The process of typing and crossmatch cannot detect all possible antibodies, and it cannot detect reactions to components other than erythrocytes. Most cases of severe transfusion reaction are a result of clerical error, including administration of the wrong unit of blood to the patient or identification of the wrong patient. Complications of a severe transfusion reaction include a shortened life span or hemolysis of the erythrocytes, anaphylaxis, or sudden death.

---

**Purpose of the Test**

In preparation for transfusion, these tests are performed to determine the major blood groups, to screen for antibodies, and to determine the compatibility of the blood of the recipient and that of the potential donor.

---

**Procedure**

**Intended Recipient's Blood.**   Two red-topped tubes and one lavender-topped tube are used to collect 7 mL of venous blood in each tube.

**Quality Control**

To prevent hemolysis of the erythrocytes, the tourniquet must be tied lightly and for a brief time only. Venipuncture technique must be smooth, with a blood flow that fills the vacuum tube readily. If the blood has excessive turbulence because of flawed venipuncture technique, hemolysis will alter the test results.

---

**Findings**

**Positive Crossmatch**

Incompatibility between the donor's blood and the recipient's blood

**Negative Crossmatch**

Probable compatibility between the donor's blood and the recipient's blood. The donor unit of blood is considered safe for transfusion to the recipient.

---

**Interfering Factors**

- Hemolysis
- Inadequate identification procedure

## Nursing Implementation

■
*Critical Thinking 17–3*
The patient calls you over and shows you a transfusion identification wristband that is taped to the bed. It has the wrong name on it. What are the potential complications of this error? How can you intervene so that this error is not repeated?

### Pretest

Ask the intended recipient about a history of blood transfusion in the past 3 months. Antibodies from a previous transfusion may be present. Additional testing is needed when the antibody screen is positive.

### During the Test

When blood is to be drawn, the intended recipient must be identified with absolute certainty by the person who draws the blood using the following steps: the intended recipient states his or her name, and the hospital wristband is compared with the verbal identification.

A transfusion wristband is also applied to the recipient's wrist. This wristband contains the recipient's name and hospital identification number and the date and initials of the phlebotomist. In some institutions, additional information includes the patient's birth date and sex, the physician's name, and the room and bed numbers.

The specimen tubes and the requisition form are also labeled with the same identification information.

The requisition form is signed by the phlebotomist, indicating that all identification information has been verified on the two wristbands and by the intended recipient.

### Posttest

Once the type and crossmatch is completed, the donor blood units are available for the recipient. Donor crossmatched blood is usually held for no more than 24 hours.

Use the same careful identification procedure when the blood is to be administered (Craig & Bower, 1997). The consequences of an error in identification are profound and can result in the death of the patient.

## Vitamin B₁₂ Assay

(Serum)                     Synonyms: None

| Normal Values | Adult: 200–835 pg/mL *or* SI 148–616 pmol/L<br>Adult (60–90 years): 110–770 pg/mL *or* SI 81–568 pmol/L<br>Newborn: 160–1,300 pg/mL *or* 118–959 pmol/L |
| --- | --- |

## Background Information

Vitamin B₁₂, also known as cobalamin, is an essential vitamin and coenzyme needed for the formation of normal erythrocytes and other bone marrow functions. In terms of dietary intake, this vitamin is present in meat, dairy products (milk, butter, cheese), fish, and eggs. The absorption of the vitamin occurs in stages. Initially, it is bound to intrinsic factor, manufactured by the gastric parietal cells. In the ileum, it is absorbed into the portal vein system, aided by intrinsic factor and pancreatic enzymes. Once it is in the circulation, some of the vitamin is stored in the liver, and the remainder is used by the bone marrow in hematopoiesis (Rodak, 1995).

**Elevated Level.** The vitamin B₁₂ level is elevated in the blood when a disorder exists that increases the manufacture of transport substances or increases hematopoiesis. The organs involved include the liver, stomach, and bone marrow.

**Decreased Level.** Several possible causes exist for a decreased amount of vitamin $B_{12}$ in the blood. The most common cause is a problem with the production and function of intrinsic factor. Without intrinsic factor, the available vitamin $B_{12}$ cannot enter the circulation from the intestinal tract. Defective absorption may also be the cause. Disorders that impair the absorption in the ileum also prevent the absorption of the vitamin. A lack of dietary intake of the vitamin may be the cause, but it is not a very common occurrence. Persons who are strict vegetarians are the most vulnerable (Henry, 1996).

With an absence of sufficient vitamin $B_{12}$ in the blood and a depletion of the vitamin reserves that were stored in the liver, the patient develops megaloblastic anemia, with erythrocytes that are too large. Because of their size, the erythrocytes have difficulty passing through the microcirculation, and they become damaged. The life span of these erythrocytes is only 27 to 35 days before hemolysis occurs. Because of hemolysis, the patient's indirect bilirubin rises. In addition, the lack of this vitamin impairs the bone marrow function of white blood cells and platelets, causing thrombocytopenia and leukopenia.

The normal values vary according to laboratory methodology. The nurse should refer to the reference value provided by the laboratory that performs the test.

| | |
|---|---|
| **Purpose of the Test** | This test is used to identify vitamin $B_{12}$ deficiency or to investigate the cause of hematologic and neurologic symptoms that suggest a vitamin $B_{12}$ deficiency. |

| | |
|---|---|
| **Procedure** | A red-topped tube is used to collect 10 mL of venous blood. |

**Findings**

**Elevated Values**

| | | |
|---|---|---|
| Chronic leukemia | Polycythemia vera | Liver metastases |
| Chronic renal failure | Liver disease | |

**Decreased Values**

| | | |
|---|---|---|
| Pernicious anemia | Malabsorption in the ileum | Fish tapeworm |
| Intrinsic factor antibodies | Atrophic gastritis | Pancreatic insufficiency |
| Postgastrectomy | Chronic pancreatitis | Giardiasis |

**Interfering Factors**

- Failure to maintain nothing-by-mouth status
- Radioactive isotopes
- Hemolysis
- Exposure of the specimen to sunlight

**Nursing Implementation** Nursing care includes care of the venipuncture site.

**Pretest**

Schedule this test before a Schilling test or radioisotope scan, because the radioisotopes of these procedures interfere with the radioimmunoassay method of analysis for this test.

Schedule this test before a blood transfusion is administered or a trial of vitamin $B_{12}$ treatment is started.

Instruct the patient to fast from food for 8 hours before the test (Tietz, 1995).

### Posttest

Send the specimen to the laboratory without delay. If a delay in analysis occurs, the specimen must be protected from exposure to sunlight.

## Diagnostic Procedures

## Bone Marrow Examination

**(Microscopy)**                    Synonym: Bone marrow aspiration and biopsy

**Normal Values**          Normal bone marrow

## Background Information

The bone marrow is responsible for *hematopoiesis*—the formation of blood cells. Shortly after birth, the entire medullary cavity is occupied by hematopoietic red marrow. With physical growth, the bones and the medullary spaces also increase in size, and the excess space in the medullary cavities fills with fat cells or yellow marrow. By later childhood and throughout adulthood, the only bones that have red marrow are the flat bones of the skull, vertebrae, shoulder, pelvis, sternum, and rib cage and the proximal ends of long bones.

In the marrow, it is believed that a pluripotential cell is capable of producing more differentiated stem cells for hematopoiesis (Fig. 17–5). The lymphoid stem cells and hematopoietic stem cells evolve into a variety of committed precursor cells, based on microenvironmental factors and the presence of colony-stimulating factors. Once the precursor cells are committed, blood cells proliferate and mature along specific lines. In their mature forms, cells are released from the marrow and enter the blood.

Most of the formed cells of the blood originate from hematopoietic stem cells. The hematopoietic line further differentiates into particular groups of cells of a particular line, including the granulocyte, erythroid, monocyte, and megakaryocyte lines. The mature forms of blood cells include the erythrocytes, leukocytes, and platelets.

The lymphoid stem cell and its lymphoid precursor cells produce the B lymphocytes and plasma cells (Post-White, 1996). The lymphocytes are small white blood cells that carry out the activities of the immune system. In the blood, other cells of the immune system exist, but they are produced by the thymus and secondary lymphoid tissue rather than by the bone marrow.

**Examination of the Marrow.**    The aspirated cells of the bone marrow are used to investigate hematologic disorders. A small sample of the cells is often representative of the whole marrow. Microscopic examination of the cells provides information about the cause, type, and extent of the abnormality. A peripheral blood smear is performed on the same day to compare and incorporate pertinent findings.

The marrow cells are examined for characteristics of the tissue. *Cellularity* indicates the proportion of aspirate that is hematopoietic cells rather than fat cells. *Distribution* provides an estimate or count of the number of each type of cell found in the marrow specimen. The marrow cells should be in proper proportion to each other, without excessive or diminished cells of a particular type. The *maturation* of the cells is also observed. Nuclear and cytoplasmic development should be in balance, without deficiency or impairment in either stage. Bizarre maturation can be caused by some leukemias and by toxicity from some medications. Some forms of anemia cause impairment of nuclear or cytoplasmic development. The term *abnormal cells* refers to the presence of irregular or

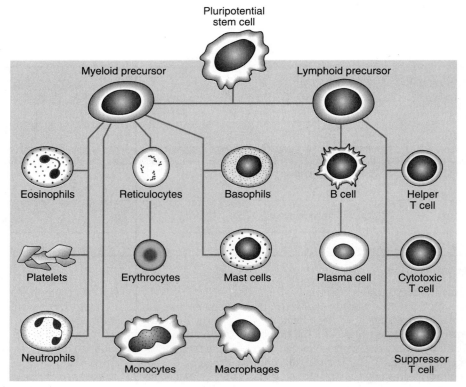

**Figure 17–5**
Cells of the bone marrow and blood.

abnormal cells in the marrow. These include mast cells, osteoblasts, osteoclasts, and metastatic neoplastic cells (Henry, 1996).

**Iron Staining of the Marrow.**   In microcytic anemia, the bone marrow examination evaluates the iron stores and sideroblasts that are present. Sideroblasts are early forms of marrow cells that contain iron pigment. As the slides of the marrow are prepared, iron stain is applied. When iron is present in the cytoplasm, Prussian blue, a dark blue precipitate, emerges. About one third of the rubricytes should be iron-positive sideroblasts.

When the amount of iron stain in the cells is abnormally high, it is caused by excess iron storage or excess formation of sideroblasts. The underlying diseases include hemolytic or sideroblastic anemia, the anemia associated with decreased erythropoiesis, ineffective erythropoiesis, or chronic inflamma-

tory disease. When the iron stores or number of sideroblasts is decreased, it may be due to iron deficiency anemia or to the anemia of chronic disease.

**Anemias.**   In addition to microcytic anemia, the examination of the marrow can demonstrate a megaloblastic process that is associated with macrocytic anemia. In macrocytic anemia, the erythrocytes are enlarged in diameter or cell volume, or both. In normocytic anemia, without an increase in the reticulocytes in the peripheral blood, the marrow is assessed for abnormal or deficient erythropoiesis.

**Cytopenia.**   When the peripheral blood demonstrates deficiencies of cells, the examination of the marrow is performed to identify the presence and quality of precursor cells. In the blood, neutropenia is the deficiency of neutrophils, thrombocytopenia is the deficiency of platelets, and pancytopenia is the overall lack of blood cells. The possible causes include decreased production, impaired maturation, or increased destruction of one or more types of precursor cell. The examination of the marrow sometimes identifies leukemia or another hematologic malignancy as the cause.

**Immunoglobulins.** The infiltration of abnormal plasma cells or lymphocytes in the marrow can cause immunoglobulin abnormality. These abnormal changes in the marrow are the cause of plasma cell myeloma or macroglobinemia.

**Purpose of the Test**

The bone marrow aspiration and biopsy, with microscopic examination of the tissue, is used to evaluate hematopoiesis, including erythroid, myeloid, megakaryocyte, and lymphoid processes. It diagnoses malignancy of primary and metastatic origin and determines the cause of infection. The examination of the marrow also is used to evaluate the progression of some hematologic diseases or the response of the marrow to chemotherapy treatment, such as in Hodgkin's disease and acute myelogenous leukemia (Larson & McCurley, 1996).

**Procedure**

A local anesthetic is used for the procedure. In bone marrow aspiration, a bone marrow needle is inserted into the medullary cavity of a bone. Fluid and marrow cells are aspirated into several syringes. When a bone marrow biopsy is required, the biopsy needle removes a core of marrow tissue. Slides are prepared, and tissue specimens are collected. When indicated, culture specimens are obtained (Hodges & Koury, 1996).

The aspiration sites include the sternum, iliac crest, spinous process of the vertebrae, and proximal tibia (Fig. 17–6). In adults, the posterior iliac crest is the most common site. In infants and young children, the proximal tibia is used.

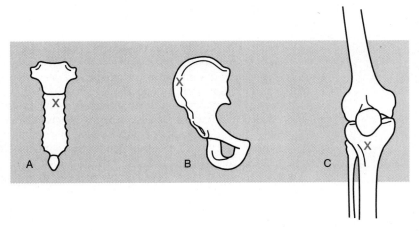

**Figure 17–6**

Anatomic sites (X) for bone marrow aspiration. *A,* The sternum between the second and third intercostal spaces. *B,* The iliac crest on the rim or upper posterior surface. *C,* The proximal tibia about 1 to 2 inches below the patella of the infant or small child.

| Findings | **Abnormal Values** | | |
|---|---|---|---|
| | Iron deficiency anemia | Megaloblastic anemia | Parasitic disease: malaria, leishmaniasis |
| | Infection: histoplasmosis, miliary tuberculosis, infectious mononucleosis | Macroglobulinemia | Hodgkin's disease |
| | | Agammaglobulinemia | Lymphoma |
| | | Myelofibrosis | Metastatic bone cancer |
| | | Aplastic anemia | |
| | Sideroblastic anemia | Leukemia | |
| | Anemia of chronic disease | Collagen disease | |
| | | Multiple myeloma | |

| **Interfering Factors** | • Failure to obtain an adequate specimen |
|---|---|

**Nursing Implementation**

### Pretest

The physician explains to the patient the reason for the bone marrow examination and how the procedure will be done.

Assess the patient for anxiety or the need for additional information. Common sources of anxiety are fear of the procedure and fear of the possible diagnosis.

Obtain a signed consent form from the patient or the person who is legally responsible for the patient's health care decisions.

### During the Test

Position the patient according to the site that will be biopsied. For a sternal or tibial biopsy, the supine position is used. Biopsy of the iliac crest requires a lateral recumbent or prone position. Vertebral biopsy is performed with the patient in a seated position.

Prepare the skin by cleansing it with an antiseptic solution.

Provide support and reassurance as the local anesthetic is instilled. The patient feels brief discomfort as the needle and anesthetic solution penetrate the skin and infiltrate the periosteum.

Caution the patient to remain immobile as the biopsy needle is inserted into the marrow. Some pain is felt as the marrow is aspirated.

Assist with the preparation and labeling of the slides. The clot and biopsy tissue are placed in a sterile specimen jar that contains fixative (formalin or Zenker's solution).

Once the needle is removed, apply pressure to the site, using a small sterile gauze. After bleeding has stopped, apply a small sterile dressing. The patient with a low platelet count is prone to prolonged bleeding.

### Posttest

Arrange for prompt transport of the specimens and slides to the laboratory.

Reassure the patient that for a few days, mild discomfort at the biopsy site is expected. Any signs of persistent bleeding or infection should be reported to the physician.

# Bone Marrow Scan

**(Nuclear Scan)** | Synonyms: None

The bone marrow scan uses technetium sulfur colloid (technetium 99m) to image the reticuloendothelial system of the bone marrow. Once the radio-isotope is injected intravenously, it moves to the marrow, because the colloid particles undergo phagocytosis by the reticuloendothelial system. In a whole body scan, the images demonstrate the presence of hematologic malignancy, bone marrow infarct, aplastic anemia, myelofibrosis, or abnormal distribution of the marrow. The scan also locates active sites of marrow tissue for biopsy purposes and identifies extramedullary sites of hematopoiesis such as the liver or spleen. The scanning process is performed in 24 to 48 hours, after active marrow cells absorb the tracers.

A complete discussion of nuclear scans is presented in Chapter 10.

## References

Anderson, C. (1995). Drawing serum haptoglobin levels to determine hemolysis due to use of an incorrect reprocessed dialyzer. *ANNA Journal, 22*(4), 418, 426.

Baer, D. M. (1994). Schilling test. *Medical Laboratory Observer, 26*(1), 10.

Baer, D. M. (1995). Hematology testing at the bedside. *Laboratory Medicine, 26*(1), 48–53.

Baird, M. L. (1996). Use of DNA identification for forensic and paternity analysis. *Journal of Clinical Laboratory Analysis, 10*(4), 350–358.

Brown, K. A. (1996a). Hematology I. Erythrocyte metabolism and enzyme defects. *Laboratory Medicine, 27*(5), 229–233.

Brown, K. A. (1996b). Hematology II. Glucose-6-dehydrogenase deficiency and other enzyme defects. *Laboratory Medicine, 27*(6), 390–395.

Burtis, C. A., & Ashwood, E. R. (Eds.) (1999). *Tietz textbook of clinical chemistry* (3rd ed.). Philadelphia: W. B. Saunders.

Cassetta, R. A. (1993). Sickle cell guidelines stress screening. *American Nurse, 25*(6), 9.

Chatta, G. S., Price, T. H., Stratton, J. R., & Dale, D. C. (1994). Aging and marrow neutrophil reserves. *Journal of the American Geriatric Society, 42*(1), 77–81.

Cook, L. S. (1997). Nonimmune transfusion reactions: When type-and-cross match aren't enough. *Journal of Intravenous Nursing, 20*(1), 15–22.

Craig, V., & Bower, J. O. (1997). Perioperative pharmacology. Blood transfusion in perioperative settings. *AORN Journal, 66*, 133–136, 138, 140–143.

Erickson, J. M. (1996). Anemia. *Seminars in Oncology Nursing, 12*(1), 2–14.

Fitzpatrick, L., & Fitzpatrick, T. (1997). Blood. Keeping your patient safe. *Nursing97, 27*(8), 34–41.

Gore, M. J. (1996). What's new in blood banking? Plenty. *Clinical Laboratory Science, 9*(1), 5–9.

Henry, J. B. (Ed.). (1996). *Clinical diagnosis and management by laboratory methods* (19th ed.). Philadelphia: W. B. Saunders.

Hodges, A., & Koury, M. J. (1996). Bone marrow. Needle aspiration and biopsy in the diagnosis and monitoring of bone marrow diseases. *Clinical Laboratory Science, 9*(6), 349–353.

Jacobs, D. S., Dermott, W. R., Grady, H. J., Horvat, R. T., Huestis, D. W., & Kasten, B. L. (Eds.). (1996). *Laboratory test handbook* (4th ed.). Baltimore: Williams & Wilkins.

Larson, R. S., & McCurley, T. L. (1996). Cutting edge technologies in the evaluation of bone marrow samples. *Clinical Laboratory Science, 9*(6), 354–357.

Lehmann, C. A. (1998). *Saunders manual of clinical laboratory science*. Philadelphia: W. B. Saunders.

McCurley, T. L., & Larson, R. (1996). Clinical applications of flow cytometry in hematology and immunology. *Clinical Laboratory Science, 9*(6), 358–362.

Mehta, A. B. (1994). Glucose-6-phosphate dehydrogenase deficiency. *Postgraduate Medicine, 70*(12), 871–877.

Myhre, B. A. (1996). HLA typing . . . human leukocyte antigen. *Medical Laboratory Observer, 28*(6), 14.

Pelehach, L. (1996). The story of the stem cell. *Laboratory Medicine, 27*(9), 588–599.

Post-White, J. (1996). The immune system. *Seminars in Oncology Nursing, 12*(2), 89–96.

Rodak, B. F. (1995). *Diagnostic hematology*. Philadelphia: W. B. Saunders.

Stepp, C. A., & Wood, M. A. (1998). *Laboratory procedures for medical office personnel*. Philadelphia: W. B. Saunders.

Tietz, N. W. (Ed.) (1995). *Clinical guide to laboratory tests* (3rd ed.). Philadelphia: W. B. Saunders.

U. S. Public Health Service, Agency for Health Care Policy and Research. (1993). Sickle cell disease: Screening, diagnosis, management, and counseling in newborns and infants. Clinical practice guideline number 6 (AHCPR Publication No. 93-0562). Washington, DC: U. S. Department of Health and Human Services.

Waterbury, L. (1996). *Hematology* (4th ed.). Baltimore: Williams & Wilkins.

# CHAPTER 18

# Gastrointestinal Function

This chapter discusses the laboratory tests and diagnostic procedures that identify abnormalities in the structure and function of the alimentary canal. The organs include the esophagus, stomach, small bowel, and large bowel. Additionally, this chapter includes discussion of the tests that assess the peritoneum and peritoneal cavity.

The laboratory tests measure the specific aspects of secretion, digestion, absorption, and elimination as functions performed by the gastrointestinal tract. Additionally, tissue biopsy, culture, and microscopic examination of the secretions and fecal matter provide data about the disease process and cause of tissue damage.

Many of the diagnostic procedures use an endoscope or x-ray studies with barium to visualize the intestinal lumen and its mucosal lining. Nuclear scans also provide visualization of the function of specific parts of the alimentary tract. Because these diagnostic procedures visualize segments of the intestinal tract, more than one test may be required for a complete assessment of the intestinal problem.

In addition to a diagnosis, the examiner provides descriptive data about the pathologic condition, including specific information about the length, depth, and location of the abnormality, as well as any alteration of function that is observed.

The extent of involvement is described by a specific vocabulary. A *diffuse process* involves the entire alimentary canal or an entire organ, such as the colon. A *regional process* concerns a complete portion of an organ, such as the ileum of the small bowel. A *focal process* involves a small area, such as a single lesion in the cecum.

The *depth* of the pathologic condition refers to the penetration of the disease process into the various layers of intestinal tissue. The alimentary tract consists of four layers of tissue. From the lumen outward, the layers are the mucosa, submucosa, muscularis, and adventitia or serosa. A lesion, therefore, may involve only the mucosal layer or may penetrate more deeply into the submucosal or muscularis layers. A *transmural lesion* involves all four layers of the tissue wall.

The diameter of the lumen of the alimentary tract can be altered by a pathologic condition. Narrowing or obstruction of the lumen may be caused by inflammation, edema, strictures, stenosis, adhesions, or twisting (volvulus) of the intestinal tissue. Altered neuromuscular function can dilate or relax tissue walls, with a resultant widening of a portion of the bowel and loss of peristaltic activity. Depending on the extent of the disease process, alteration of the size of the lumen affects the passage of food, fluid, gas, and fecal matter through the intestinal tract.

Malignant growths in the intestinal tract incorporate all these dimensions. Cancerous tumors tend to grow inward, narrowing the lumen. As they grow, they also extend in length. Additionally, the depth of tissue involvement increases, and the tumor may become a transmural lesion or even break out beyond the tissue border to spill into the peritoneal cavity or extend into a contiguous organ.

## Laboratory Tests

## Carcinoembryonic Antigen

**(Serum, Effusion Fluid)**         Synonym: CEA

**Normal Values**

> Adult nonsmoker: <2.5 ng/mL *or* SI 2.5 µg/L
> Adult smoker: Up to 5 ng/mL *or* SI 5 µg/L

### Background Information

As a tumor marker, carcinoembryonic antigen (CEA) is the best test to estimate prognosis (survival) and to monitor the result of treatment in patients with colorectal cancer. When the antigen appears in the adult circulation, it indicates (1) a response to healing and regeneration of cells of particular tissues or (2) malignancy. In healthy adults, the antigen is present in the serum only in minute amounts. In cancer patients, necrosis of the malignant tissue permits larger amounts of the antigen to escape through damaged cell membranes.

The test is not very specific because it demonstrates elevations for other malignancies, including gastric, pancreatic, and lung cancer (Lehmann, 1998). CEA is not very sensitive. This means that it does not always detect cases of early-stage cancer.

In recurrent colon cancer, however, the test is very helpful. With results greater than 5 ng/mL (SI >5 µg/L), 60% to 90% of the cases of recurrence are detected. At test values up to 15 ng/mL (SI up to 15 µg/L), 96% of the cases of advanced cancer are detected (Aziz, 1996). CEA is sensitive in detection of metastases to other organs, as well as extension or recurrence at the primary site. The elevations can occur as early as 36 months before clinical symptoms appear (Tietz, 1995).

Elevated CEA levels can occur in benign disease, but the test values are usually in a lower range (5 to 10 ng/mL; SI 5 to 10 µg/L). Smokers have elevated values without necessarily having a benign or malignant condition (Jacobs et al., 1996).

**Purpose of the Test**

Carcinoembryonic antigen is a tumor marker used to monitor for recurrence of colorectal cancer. It may also be used in the management of gastrointestinal, breast, lung, and pancreatic cancer (Fig. 18–1). The increase in the test value serves as an indicator for further diagnostic testing. Because of low specificity in distinguishing between benign and malignant conditions, the test is not used as a screening measure for the general population.

**Procedure**

A red-topped or lavender-topped tube is used to collect 5 to 10 mL of venous blood. The schedule for testing and monitoring the patient's condition is as

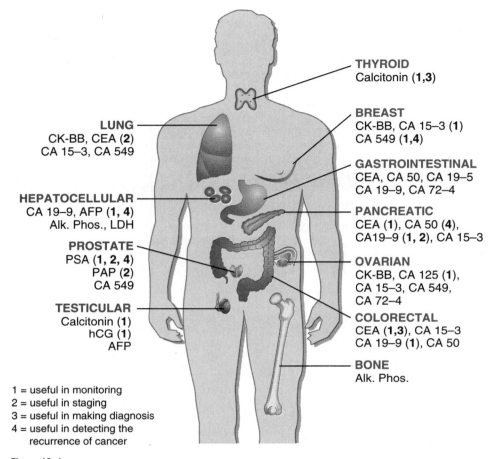

**THYROID**
Calcitonin (**1,3**)

**BREAST**
CK-BB, CA 15–3 (**1**)
CA 549 (**1,4**)

**GASTROINTESTINAL**
CEA, CA 50, CA 19–5
CA 19–9, CA 72–4

**PANCREATIC**
CEA (**1**), CA 50 (**4**),
CA19–9 (**1, 2**), CA 15–3

**OVARIAN**
CK-BB, CA 125 (**1**),
CA 15–3, CA 549,
CA 72–4

**COLORECTAL**
CEA (**1,3**), CA 15–3
CA 19–9 (**1**), CA 50

**BONE**
Alk. Phos.

**LUNG**
CK-BB, CEA (**2**)
CA 15–3, CA 549

**HEPATOCELLULAR**
CA 19–9, AFP (**1, 4**)
Alk. Phos., LDH

**PROSTATE**
PSA (**1, 2, 4**)
PAP (**2**)
CA 549

**TESTICULAR**
Calcitonin (**1**)
hCG (**1**)
AFP

1 = useful in monitoring
2 = useful in staging
3 = useful in making diagnosis
4 = useful in detecting the
      recurrence of cancer

**Figure 18–1**
Tumor markers. Various tumor markers are used in the diagnosis, monitoring, staging, and detection of recurrence of cancer. (Reproduced with permission from Lehmann, C. A. [1998]. *Saunders manual of clinical laboratory science.* Philadelphia: W. B. Saunders.)

follows: presurgery, 4 weeks postoperatively, monthly for 1 to 2 years, and at regular intervals thereafter for a total testing time of 5 years.

### Quality Control

Venipuncture technique must be smooth, with a blood flow that fills the vacuum tube readily. If the blood has excessive turbulence because of flawed venipuncture technique, the hemolysis of the erythrocytes will alter the test results.

The serum must be chilled immediately and radioimmunoassay analysis performed within 24 hours.

| **Findings** | **Elevated Values** | | |
| --- | --- | --- | --- |
| | MALIGNANT CONDITIONS | | |
| | Colorectal cancer | Lung cancer | Metastatic disease |
| | Stomach cancer | Thyroid medullary | (liver, bone, lung) |
| | Pancreatic cancer | cancer | |
| | Breast cancer | Ovarian cancer | |
| | BENIGN CONDITIONS | | |
| | Ulcerative colitis | Hepatitis | Pulmonary infection |
| | Crohn's disease | Cirrhosis | |

**Interfering Factors**

- Recent administration of radioisotopes
- Smoking
- Heparin
- Hemolysis

**Nursing Implementation**

Nursing actions are similar to those for other venipuncture procedures.

### Pretest

Schedule any radioisotope study for shortly after this test is performed.
If the patient is a smoker, indicate this information on the requisition slip.

### Posttest

The serum sample is packed in a container with ice and is sent directly to the laboratory.
Provide emotional support to the patient. Ongoing testing for cancer is upsetting because of the implications of a positive result.

## D-Xylose Absorption Test

**(Whole Blood, Urine)**     Synonyms: Xylose tolerance test, xylose absorption test

**Normal Values**

**Urine**
Child: 16%–33% of ingested dose/5 hr *or* SI 0.16–0.33 (fraction of ingested dose)
Adult (5-g dose): >1.2 g/5 hr *or* SI >8.00 mmol/L/5 hr
Adult (25-g dose): >4 g/5 hr *or* SI 126.64 mmol/L
Adult >65 years: 3.5 g/5 hr *or* SI >23.31 mmol/L
**Whole Blood**
Child (1 hour): >30 mg/dL *or* SI >2.0 mmol/L
Adult (2 hours, 5-g dose): >20 mg/dL *or* SI >1.33 mmol/L
Adult (2 hours, 25-g dose): >25 mg/dL *or* SI >1.67 mmol/L

## Background Information

Malabsorption and steatorrhea may originate from two different sources of pathophysiologic change. One is a luminal defect of the small bowel. This source of malabsorption may involve pancreatic disease, loss of bile salts, or Crohn's disease. The other source is a disorder caused by a defect in the epithelium or membrane of the small bowel. This source of malabsorption may involve gluten-sensitive enteropathy, celiac disease, or Whipple's disease. The D-xylose absorption test is used to investigate the cause of malabsorption and steatorrhea and helps to determine the origin of the problem.

D-Xylose is a carbohydrate (a pentose sugar) that does not require pancreatic enzymes for its absorption. In normal patients and in those with a lumen disorder such as pancreatic disease, a portion of ingested D-xylose is absorbed by the duodenum and jejunum and can be recovered later in the blood and urine.

When the amount of recovered D-xylose is less than normal, the most likely cause is malabsorp-tion caused by an epithelial or membrane disorder of the upper small bowel. Because more than one disease may cause this change, a follow-up endoscopic biopsy of small bowel tissue is needed to make the diagnosis.

**Physiologic Basis of the Test.**   Following a measured dose of D-xylose ingested orally, a portion should be absorbed by the duodenum and jejunum. The sugar reaches the bloodstream in 30 to 60 minutes, and the blood level is sustained for up to 2 hours. Thereafter, this sugar is filtered from the blood by the kidney. Within 5 hours, 16% to 23% of the initial dose should appear in the urine (Jacobs et al., 1996).

The D-xylose test is most accurate when both serum and urine specimens are analyzed at timed intervals. The accuracy of the test is dependent on the rate of absorption by the intestine and the rate of excretion by the kidneys. These and numerous other variables can interfere with the accuracy of the test results.

| Purpose of the Test | This test is used to investigate the cause of steatorrhea, to diagnose malabsorption syndrome, and to evaluate the functional ability of the duodenum and jejunum in the digestion of carbohydrates. |
|---|---|

| Procedure | To verify adequate renal function, blood specimens for blood urea nitrogen and creatinine determinations are drawn, and a urinalysis is obtained in the early morning before the D-xylose test begins. |
|---|---|

The recommended dose of D-xylose for adults and children older than 12 years is 25 g mixed in 250 mL of water. For children younger than 12 years, the recommended dose is 5 g or 0.5 g/kg of body weight.

A red-topped tube is used to collect 5 to 10 mL of venous blood for each specimen. In most institutions, a single blood sample is obtained 1 hour after the D-xylose is ingested. In some institutions, serial samples are obtained at 30, 60, and 120 minutes after the D-xylose is ingested.

For adults and children older than 12 years, all urine is collected for 5 hours.

For geriatric patients, those with some renal insufficiency, and infants or children younger than 12 years, the test may be limited to a single blood sample after 1 hour, with no urine collection.

■

*Critical Thinking 18–1*
The D-xylose test is under way. The 4-year-old patient had the morning blood tests, but she will not drink the D-xylose solution. How can you obtain the cooperation of the child?

### Quality Control

The full 25-g dose of D-xylose for adults is preferred because it will help detect less severe conditions. This dose, however, can cause diarrhea and vomiting. Hypermotility of the intestine interferes with absorption and results in lower-than-normal values.

**Findings**

**Decreased Values**

MALABSORPTION SYNDROMES

Tropical sprue
Lymphoma
Nontropical sprue
   (celiac disease,
   gluten-sensitive
   enteropathy)

Parasitic disease
   (hookworm,
   schistosomiasis,
   *Giardia lamblia*)
Whipple's disease
Gastroenteritis

Amyloidosis
Zollinger-Ellison
   syndrome
Scleroderma
Radiation enteritis
Small bowel ischemia

**Interfering Factors**

- Failure to maintain pretest dietary restrictions
- Physical activity during the test
- Poor renal function
- Ascites
- Vomiting or diarrhea
- Rapid or delayed gastric emptying
- Hypomotility or intestinal stasis
- Dehydration and hypovolemia

**Nursing Implementation**

**Pretest**

Instruct the patient on the following regarding preparation for the test:
The patient should discontinue all foods that contain pentose sugar (fruits, jellies, jams, fruit pastries) for 24 hours before the test.
The patient should discontinue all medications for 24 hours before the test (if possible).
Adults should refrain from ingestion of all food for 8 hours (children for 4 hours) before the test. Water intake is permitted and encouraged.
Ensure that early morning blood urea nitrogen, creatinine, and urinalysis results are posted in the patient's chart.

**During the Test**

At 8 AM, the patient drinks the prescribed dose of D-xylose mixed in 250 mL of water. This is followed by another 250 mL of water. At 9 AM, a third 250 mL of water is taken, with water intake as desired thereafter.
Instruct the patient to maintain bedrest in a supine position throughout the test period.
The patient voids at 8 AM, and this specimen is discarded. For the next 5 hours, all urine specimens are collected, using a brown or dark container. The urine is kept refrigerated.
After ingestion of the D-xylose, observe the patient for vomiting or diarrhea. Notify the physician and laboratory of the problem.

**Quality Control**

Hypermotility of the intestinal tract, physical activity, vomiting, and failure to collect all urine specimens can result in invalid test results.

### Posttest

All blood specimens are labeled, including the time and date of each sample. The refrigerated urine container is also labeled, including the time and date of the start and finish of the collection period.

The specimens are sent to the laboratory immediately. This prevents warming by the temperature of the room.

## Gastric Stimulation Test

**(Gastric Secretions)**      Synonyms: Tube gastric analysis, pentagastrin stimulation test, gastric acid stimulation test

| **Normal Values** | **Gastric pH:** 1.5–3.5 *or* SI 1.5–3.5 |
|---|---|
| | **Basal Acid Output (BAO)** |
| | Male: 0–10.5 mEq/hr *or* SI 0–10.5 mmol/hr |
| | Female: 0–5.6 mEq/hr *or* SI 0–5.6 mmol/hr |
| | **Peak Acid Output (PAO)** |
| | Male: 12–60 mEq/hr *or* SI 12–60 mmol/hr |
| | Female: 8–40 mEq/hr *or* SI 8–40 mmol/hr |
| | **BAO:MAO ratio:** <20% *or* SI <0.20 |

### Background Information

Gastric analysis is a laboratory measurement of the acid content of gastric secretions. The secretions are obtained by aspiration of the stomach contents via a nasogastric tube. The two phases of the test are basal acid output (BAO), which analyzes specimens obtained during a resting state, and maximal acid output (MAO), which analyzes specimens obtained after stimulation of the secretory flow of gastric secretions. The peak acid output (PAO) consists of the mathematical average of highest two values of poststimulation specimens. The BAO-to-MAO ratio is a numeric comparison of the results obtained at rest and after stimulation.

Because of different methods of collection and analysis, a rather wide range of normal values exists. Males, however, have higher acid values than do females, and aging results in lower acid values.

Patients who have marginal ulcers or duodenal ulcers tend to have higher-than-normal acid output. Patients who have gastric cancer or gastric ulcers tend to have lower-than-normal acid output. In Zollinger-Ellison syndrome (gastrinoma), massive acid hypersecretion exists, usually >60 mEq/L (SI >60 mmol/L). Additionally, in Zollinger-Ellison syndrome, the BAO-to-MAO ratio is elevated beyond 60% (0.6). The gastric stimulation test is used to support a diagnosis but cannot be used as the sole measure to confirm a diagnosis of Zollinger-Ellison syndrome.

The normal pH of gastric secretions ranges from 1.5 to 3.5 as the measure of acidity. When the pH value is greater than 6 after maximal stimulation, the condition is called *anacidity*. This finding supports the diagnosis of pernicious anemia.

The gastric stimulation test has problems associated with accuracy in the technique of specimen collection and the methods of analysis. Gastric biopsy specimens and serum gastrin radioimmunoassay techniques may be used with or in place of the gastric stimulation test.

### Purpose of the Test

Gastric analysis is used to evaluate the ability of the stomach to produce acid secretions in a resting state and after maximal stimulation.

## Procedure

■
*Critical Thinking 18–2*
The nasogastric tube is in place,
but before the procedure starts, no
gastric secretions are aspirated
by intermittent intestinal suction.
What can you do to investigate
and correct the problem?

The nasogastric tube is passed into the stomach until the tip of the tube rests in the distal portion of the stomach. Secretion removal is performed by manual aspiration with a Toomey syringe or machine aspiration with intermittent intestinal suction. The stomach is emptied of accumulated secretions before the timed collections begin.

**Basal Acid Output.**   Secretions are removed during four 15-minute consecutive intervals. The secretions from each collection interval are stored in separate containers and labeled correspondingly as "BAO 1," "BAO 2," and so on. On completion of the first hour of specimen collection, the MAO phase follows directly.

**Maximal Acid Output.**   The patient is given a subcutaneous injection of pentagastrin (Peptavlon), 6 mcg/kg of body weight. The medication stimulates gastric acid secretion. In the next hour, four more specimens are collected at 15-minute intervals. The containers are labeled correspondingly as "MAO 1," "MAO 2," and so forth.

### Quality Control

> The proper placement of the tip of the nasogastric tube in the distal portion of the stomach may be confirmed by fluoroscopy. This helps ensure complete collection of gastric acids and avoids inadvertent collection of bile from the duodenum.

## Findings

### Elevated Values

| | | |
|---|---|---|
| Zollinger-Ellison syndrome | Retained antrum syndrome | G cell hyperplasia |
| Vagal hyperfunction | Basophilic leukemia | Systemic mastocytosis |
| | | Duodenal ulcers |

### Decreased Values

| | | |
|---|---|---|
| Pernicious anemia | Chronic gastritis | Postsurgical antrectomy or vagotomy |
| Gastric ulcer | Myxedema | |
| Cancer of the stomach | | |

## Interfering Factors

- Failure to maintain a nothing-by-mouth status
- Failure to collect a complete sample of secretions
- Esophageal disease, aortic aneurysm
- Gastric hemorrhage

## Nursing Implementation

### Pretest

Explain the procedure to the patient so that fear and apprehension are minimized.

Obtain an informed consent from the patient or the person designated to make health care decisions for the patient.

For 24 hours before the test, alcohol, tobacco, and medications that affect gastric acid secretion are discontinued.

Food is discontinued for 12 hours and water for 8 hours before the test. Until the test is completed, the sight and smell of food is avoided.

### Quality Control

Psychological, physiologic, and environmental stimuli are reduced to avoid additional gastric acid secretion and to improve the reliability of the test results.

### During the Test

To collect the secretions with a Toomey syringe, aspirate gently every 5 minutes.

After administration of pentagastrin, assess for side effects of nausea, dizziness, headache, tachycardia, palpitations, and diaphoresis. If they occur, they should be mild and of short duration.

### Posttest

Remove the nasogastric tube, and allow the patient to resume eating.

Ensure that each specimen container has a lid and is labeled appropriately.

## Gastrin

**(Serum)**                          Synonyms: None

| **Normal Values** | Adult (16–60 years): 25–90 pg/mL *or* SI 25–90 ng/L |
|---|---|
| | Adult (>60 years): <100 pg/mL *or* SI <100 ng/L |
| | Child: <10–125 pg/mL *or* SI <10–125 ng/L |
| | Infant (0–4 days): 120–183 pg/mL *or* SI 120–183 ng/L |

### Background Information

The three forms of gastrin in the blood are G-34 (big gastrin), G-17 (little gastrin), and G-14 (mini gastrin). The gastrins are small but powerful peptides that stimulate gastric and pancreatic secretions.

The gastrins are produced primarily by the G cells in the antrum of the stomach. Once manufactured, the gastrins are first secreted into the bloodstream and then return to the body of the stomach, where they stimulate gastric acid production, antral motility, and the secretion of pepsin and intrinsic factor. The gastrins also stimulate pancreatic acinar and ductular cell secretions.

Gastrin secretion is increased by vagal stimulation and inhibited by the presence of hydrochloric acid. The normal gastrin levels fluctuate daily and in relationship to meals.

A gastrinoma, a pancreatic or duodenal endocrine tumor, produces and secretes large amounts of gastrin and serum; values are usually >500 pg/L (SI >500 ng/L). This can result in increased gastric acid secretion and formation of multiple peptic ulcers. The patient with this triad of findings is diagnosed with Zollinger-Ellison syndrome.

### Purpose of the Test

Serum gastrin is a helpful adjunctive test to diagnose Zollinger-Ellison syndrome and pernicious anemia.

| | |
|---|---|
| **Procedure** | A red-topped tube, without anticoagulant, is used to collect 10 mL of venous blood. |

**Findings**

**Elevated Values**

Zollinger-Ellison syndrome
Chronic atrophic gastritis
Pernicious anemia

Gastric ulcer
Antral G cell hyperplasia
Vagotomy without gastric resection

Pyloric obstruction
Chronic renal failure
Gastric cancer

**Decreased Values**

Antrectomy with vagotomy

Hypothyroidism

**Interfering Factors**

- Failure to maintain a nothing-by-mouth status
- Recent radioisotope administration
- Gastroscopy
- Heparin anticoagulant in the vacuum tube

**Nursing Implementation**

Nursing actions are similar to those for other venipuncture procedures. In addition, review the following:

**Pretest**

Schedule this test before gastroscopy and any radioisotope procedures.
Instruct the patient to discontinue all food intake for at least 12 hours before the test.

**Quality Control**

Recent ingestion of protein causes an elevation of the serum gastrin level.

**Posttest**

Ensure that the specimen is sent to the laboratory without delay.

**Quality Control**

Gastrin is unstable at room temperature, and delay will cause invalid results.

## *Helicobacter pylori* Tests

Synonyms: None

| Normal Values | **Serologic Test**<br>    IgG: Negative; <15 AU<br>**Urea breath test:** Negative<br>**Tissue Biopsy**<br>    Histology: Negative for *Helicobacter pylori*<br>    Rapid urease (CLO) test: Negative<br>    PCR: Negative<br>    Tissue culture: No *Helicobacter pylori* growth |
| --- | --- |

## Background Information

*Helicobacter pylori* is a gram-negative bacillus that infects the gastric epithelium or the gastric mucosal cells of the esophagus, duodenum, or rectum. The bacillus penetrates the mucosa and resides between the mucosal layer and the epithelial layer, where it causes inflammation (gastritis). It is the cause of most cases of peptic ulcers of the stomach and duodenum and is a definite human carcinogen. It plays a pivotal role in the growth of gastric carcinoma and primary B cell gastric lymphoma (Klein, Hoda, & Martin, 1996).

Six different tests confirm the diagnosis of *H. pylori* infection. The serologic test and the urea breath test are considered noninvasive because they do not require an endoscopy procedure. When tissue biopsy is required, it is done during an esophagogastroduodenoscopy (EGD) procedure. To identify *H. pylori* infection, four additional tests can be done on the tissue samples. All these tests are quite sensitive and specific, meaning that they are very accurate in the identification of the infection (Thijs et al., 1996).

**Serologic Test.** This test identifies the elevated level of the immunoglobulin G (IgG) antibody to *H. pylori* in the blood of the infected patient. The positive test result is considered a marker of active infection. The antibody remains elevated in the patient's blood for 6 to 12 months after treatment. For this reason, it cannot be used as a follow-up test to determine if the infection has been eliminated (Brooks, Maxson, & Rubin, 1996; Jacobs et al., 1996).

**Urea Breath Test.** $^{13}C$-labeled urea is administered to the patient orally. If *H. pylori* is present, the organism produces a unique enzyme called *urease*. The urease converts the radiolabeled urea to ammonia and radiolabeled carbon dioxide ($CO_2$).

The lungs clear the body of the radiolabeled $CO_2$ in exhaled air, and the $^{13}CO_2$ can be measured. The presence of $^{13}CO_2$ in the patient's breath is proof that *H. pylori* is present in the stomach (Fay & Jaffe, 1996). After treatment, this test can be used to confirm that the infection has been eradicated.

**Tissue Biopsy.** During an endoscopy procedure, the gastric and duodenal mucosa are examined, and suspicious lesions and areas of inflammation or ulceration are biopsied. Four different tests can be performed on the tissue samples. The endoscopy procedure is invasive and more involved than the noninvasive tests, but the extent of the gastritis, ulceration, or other gastric pathology can be determined at the same time as the tissue samples are obtained.

**Histology.** Biopsy tissue slides are prepared and stained for microscopic examination. When present, the characteristic *H. pylori* bacteria are visualized and identified.

**Rapid Urease Test.** The *H. pylori* bacillus produces a unique enzyme called urease. The urease can be detected by chemical analysis (such as the *Campylobacter*-like–organism [CLO] test) of the tissue sample. When urease is present, it is presumed that *H. pylori* is present.

**PCR.** From the tissue specimen, polymerase chain reaction (PCR) technique amplifies the DNA sequence of *H. pylori* bacillus. The microbe is identified by its genetic blueprint.

**Tissue Culture.** The tissue from several biopsy specimens is ground up and plated on culture medium. The plates are read at 1, 3, and 5 days to identify the presence of colonies of *H. pylori* (Onders, 1997). Although the positive results are very accurate, this procedure is not as effective as other test methodologies because of lower sensitivity. The *H. pylori* may not be in the exact location where the tissue samples were obtained. In addi-tion, if antimicrobial therapy is tried before the bi-opsy is done, it can cause a false-negative result.

**Procedure**

**Serologic Test.**  A red-topped tube is used to obtain 10 mL of venous blood. Some laboratories use a lavender-topped (EDTA) tube or a green-topped (heparin) tube.

**Urea Breath Test.**  The patient ingests a dose of $^{13}C$ urea in a pretest meal (e.g., pudding) or as a capsule. After 10 to 30 minutes, exhalation breath samples are collected in a special collection bag or in an aluminized balloon. The breath samples are sent or mailed to a laboratory that has mass spectrome-try. Analysis of the breath identifies the radiolabeled carbon dioxide content (Klein et al., 1996; Peura et al., 1996).

**Tissue Biopsy.**  During an esophagogastroduodenoscopy procedure, biopsy specimens are obtained.

**Findings**

**Abnormal Values**

| | |
|---|---|
| *H. pylori* infection | B cell gastric lym- |
| Gastric cancer | phoma |
| Gastritis | Peptic ulcer disease |

**Interfering Factors**

- Recent antimicrobial therapy

**Nursing Implementation**

**Pretest**

For the serology tests, nursing actions are similar to those for other venipunc-ture procedures.

For the breath tests, no special nursing measures are needed.

For tests that require gastric tissue biopsy, the reader is referred to the esopha-gogastroduodenoscopy procedure located in this chapter.

## 5-Hydroxyindoleacetic Acid, Quantitative

(Urine)    Synonym: 5-HIAA

**Normal Values**

Adult: 1–9 mg/24 hr *or* SI 5–48 µmol/24 hr

## Background Information

5-Hydroxyindoleacetic acid (5-HIAA) is a urinary metabolite of serotonin. The elevated value serves as a marker for malignancy. The parent hormone, sero-tonin, and this urinary metabolite are produced by most carcinoid tumors.

Carcinoid tumors are neuroendocrine tumors that arise from neural crest cells. During fetal devel-opment, these neural crest cells migrate to many organs throughout the body. If they become malig-nant in later life, they are classified as neuroendo-crine tumors because they secrete hormones. In addition to serotonin secretion, carcinoid tumors of the foregut may also secrete adrenocorticotropic hormone, insulin, growth hormone, calcitonin, and gastrin.

One method of classifying carcinoid tumors is by their anatomic location in the intestinal tract (Table 18–1). Some of these tumors remain small, and although they secrete serotonin and the 5-HIAA metabolite, they cause no problems. Others, how-ever, become aggressive. They increase in size, hor-mone output, and 5-HIAA output; they can metas-tasize to distant sites of the bone, brain, cervical nodes, and liver.

**Elevated Value.** A test result greater than 25 mg/24 hr (SI 131 μmol/24 hr) indicates a diagnosis of carcinoid tumor.

---

**Purpose of the Test**

The quantitative measure of 5-HIAA in the urine is used to diagnose carcinoid tumor and provide ongoing evaluation of the stability of the tumor mass.

---

**Procedure**

For a 24-hour period, all urine is collected in a large container.

**Quality Control**

The bottled specimen is cooled in the refrigerator during the collection period.

---

**Findings**

**Elevated Values**

| | | |
|---|---|---|
| Midgut carcinoid | Ovarian carcinoid | Chronic intestinal |
| Foregut carcinoid | Cystic fibrosis | obstruction |
| Oat cell carcinoma of | Tropical sprue | Celiac disease |
| the bronchus | Whipple's disease | |

**Decreased Values**

| | | |
|---|---|---|
| Mental depression | Mastocytosis | Hartnup disease |
| Small bowel resection | Phenylketonuria | |

---

**Interfering Factors**

- Numerous foods that contain serotonin
- Numerous medications that react with the laboratory reagent

---

**Nursing Implementation**

**Pretest**

Instruct the patient to avoid all foods that are high in serotonin for 48 hours before the test. These foods falsely elevate the test results and include avo-cados, tomatoes, bananas, plums, walnuts, pineapples, and eggplants.

**Table 18–1    Classification of Carcinoid Tumors**

| Intestinal Classification | Anatomic Location |
|---|---|
| Foregut carcinoid tumors | Bronchus, stomach, duodenum, pancreas |
| Midgut carcinoid tumors | Jejunum, ileum, ascending colon |
| Transverse carcinoid tumors | Transverse colon, descending colon, rectum |

For 48 hours before the test, discontinue all medications that interfere with the analysis procedure, because they falsely elevate the results.

### Quality Control

> The specific medication list depends on the method of laboratory analysis. To identify these medications, the nurse should call the laboratory beforehand.

### During the Test

For the 24-hour period of urine collection, the container is kept in the refrigerator.

### Posttest

Arrange for transport of the cooled specimen immediately.

## Lactose Tolerance Test

**(Blood, Urine)**                    Synonym: Oral lactose tolerance test

| Normal Values | |
|---|---|
| | **Adult** |
| | Blood glucose: >30 mg/dL *or* SI >1.7 mmol/L (increase over fasting value) |
| | Urine lactose (24-hour): 12–40 mg/dL *or* SI 0.7–2.2 mmol/L |
| | **Child** |
| | Urine lactose (24-hour): <1.5 mg/100 dL |

### Background Information

Lactose is a disaccharide that is present in milk and milk products. For absorption to occur, the lactose is hydrolyzed in the small intestine by the enzyme *lactase*. As a result, the lactose disaccharide is split into the monosaccharides *glucose* and *galactose*. These simple sugars are then absorbed through the microvilli and pass into the portal venous system by diffusion.

In the normal physiology of lactose metabolism, the absorption results in a slight rise in blood glucose, with small amounts of lactose present in the urine.

When lactase is deficient, the lactose disaccharide cannot be absorbed, and this sugar remains in the intestine. The sugar attracts water into the bowel lumen, causing osmotic diarrhea. Bacterial fermentation causes bloating, cramps, gas formation, and abdominal distention.

Lactose intolerance–lactase deficiency may be congenital and can affect the neonate as soon as the ingestion of milk begins. It also may be an acquired condition that develops in later life, or it can be caused by intestinal disease that damages the tissue integrity of the microvilli in the small bowel.

The basis of the lactose tolerance test is to provide an oral source of lactose to the fasting patient. In lactose intolerance–lactase deficiency, the serial blood samples will show a flat glucose curve rather than the mild elevation that is expected. A flat glucose curve is an increase of greater than 20 mg/dL (SI <1.1 mmol/L) above the patient's baseline value. Higher levels of lactose appear in the urine within 24 hours.

| | |
|---|---|
| **Purpose of the Test** | This test identifies lactose intolerance–lactase deficiency. It is used in the work-up for abdominal distention, chronic diarrhea, and abdominal cramps associated with the ingestion of milk. It is also used to investigate the cause of malabsorption syndrome. |
| **Procedure** | The fasting patient takes an oral dose of lactose with 200 to 300 mL of water. The usual dose is 50 g or 0.75 to 1.5 g/kg of body weight, but a smaller dose is used for children or for patients suspected of having severe disease. Diagnostic results are obtained from the analysis of serial blood samples or a 24-hour urine collection. In some cases, the blood test may be combined with the urine test. |

**Blood.**   Gray-topped (fluoride) tubes or capillary tubes are used to collect small venous samples that include the fasting, baseline specimen and additional specimens at timed intervals (30, 60, 120, 180, and 240 minutes).

**Urine.**   After ingestion of the lactose, all urine specimens are collected in a glass container for 24 hours.

**Findings**

**Positive Values**

| | | |
|---|---|---|
| Lactose intolerance–lactase deficiency | Small bowel resection | Whipple's disease |
| | Jejunitis | Cystic fibrosis |
| | Nontropical sprue | Viral or bacterial |
| Crohn's disease | Giardiasis | bowel infection |
| Ulcerative colitis | Tropical sprue | Abetalipoproteinemia |

**Interfering Factors**

- Failure to maintain dietary and exercise restrictions
- Delayed emptying of the stomach
- Vomiting
- Diabetes mellitus

**Nursing Implementation**

For glucose testing, nursing actions are similar to those for other venipuncture procedures. In addition, review the following.

**Pretest**

Instruct the patient regarding the following pretest restrictions:
No food intake for 8 hours before or during the test
No smoking or gum chewing before or during the test

**Quality Control**

Alterations in gastric motility and gastric emptying will affect the rate of absorption and alter test results.

**During the Test**

Assess for any signs of watery diarrhea, abdominal cramps, or nausea, because the lactose dosage can exacerbate symptoms.

Notify the physician of any vomiting, because this could affect the amount and
rate of lactose absorption.
Some laboratories require activity restriction during the test. This can be verified by the laboratory personnel.

## Posttest

After 4 hours, when the blood tests are completed, the patient can resume
normal activity and diet.
Remind the patient to continue with collection of the urine for 24 hours.

### Quality Control

All tubes and containers must be labeled and include the date and time of each specimen collection. This is because the blood glucose levels will vary during the test period. The laboratory
slip should indicate the time of lactose administration as well as the times of specimen collection.

## Occult Blood

**(Feces)**                    Synonyms: Fecal occult blood test, FOBT, FOB

**Normal Values**    Negative
Home testing: No color change in the test area of the pad

## Background Information

Occult blood refers to blood that is present in the
feces but is not visible. The feces are unchanged
in color and consistency despite the presence of
blood. In some cases, the blood is not seen because
the amount is too small. In other cases, the slow but
steady leakage of blood mixes with the feces. Fecal
occult blood can originate anywhere from the upper
to the lower gastrointestinal tract. Bleeding from the
rectal or anal area, however, produces bright red
blood that is visible on the surface of the fecal
matter.

A number of commercial tests are available to
detect fecal occult blood (Hemoccult II, Hemoccult
II Sensa, HemeSelect, Colo-Rect, Colo-Screen), but
problems of reliability exist because of false-positive
and false-negative results. Some of the tests are very
sensitive to minute amounts of blood and therefore
have a higher rate of false-positive results. Others
are more accurate in identifying an abnormal, larger
amount of blood. Because they are less sensitive,
however, they have a higher rate of false-negative
results. They do not detect the small abnormal

amount. Other factors that affect accuracy are
flawed technique of stool collection and the pretest
dietary regimen (Jacobs et al., 1996).

The test is used to screen for adenocarcinoma
and premalignant polyps in the colon. Less than
30% of adenocarcinomas and polyps in the colon
bleed enough to be detected (Jacobs et al., 1996).
This means that the pathology can be present, but
the fecal occult blood test alone does not identify
about 70% of cases. Despite these problems, annual
screening for fecal occult blood is strongly recommended, beginning at age 50 years. Successful detection and treatment of earlier-stage cancer result
in increased survival after treatment (Winawer,
Flehinger, Schottenfeld, & Miller, 1993).

Most of the tests of fecal occult blood are based
on chemical detection of the enzyme activity of
peroxidase or pseudoperioxidase present in erythrocytes, hemoglobin, and myoglobin. Dietary intake of meat will cause false-positive results because
meat contains both hemoglobin and protein. Ascorbic acid (vitamin C) depresses peroxidase activity;

dietary intake of this vitamin causes false-negative results. Some medications and alcohol irritate the intestinal mucosa and cause their own source of occult blood.

A positive fecal occult blood test is taken seriously. If any one of the three specimens contains occult blood, the test is considered positive. Because of the potential risk of cancer, particularly in the colon, physicians recommend that a positive test be followed up with a routine colonoscopy. As illustrated in Figure 18–2, benign polyps, arteriovenous malformations, and cancer are among the more common causes of occult blood in the lower gastrointestinal tract.

| **Purpose of the Test** | This test detects fecal occult blood from a gastrointestinal source and is used as a screening tool for an early diagnosis of bowel cancer. |
|---|---|

| **Procedure** | Three different stool specimens are collected in plastic containers. |
|---|---|

**Home Testing**

After fecal evacuation, wait 1 to 5 minutes without flushing the toilet. Drop the test paper into the water with the stool. After waiting 30 seconds to 2 minutes, observe the test area for a color change. Repeat the test on the next two bowel movements, for a total of three tests on three different specimens.

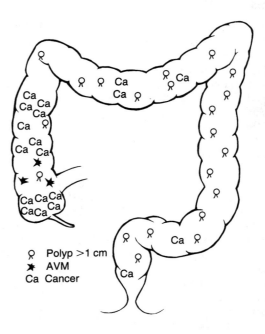

**Figure 18–2**
Sites of occult bleeding in the colon. Cancer, benign polyps, and arteriovenous malformations are three causes of occult bleeding. Their location and characteristic pathologic features are identified in follow-up colonoscopy. (Reproduced with permission from Church, J. M. [1992]. Colonoscopy for the diagnosis and treatment of colorectal bleeding. *Seminars in Colon and Rectal Surgery, 3,* 43.)

| **Findings** | **Positive Values** | | |
| --- | --- | --- | --- |
| | Esophageal varices | Peptic ulcer | Crohn's disease |
| | Dysentery | Arteriovenous | Hemorrhagic disease |
| | Mallory-Weiss tears | malformation of | Kaposi's sarcoma |
| | Parasitic disease | the colon | Intussusception |
| | Hiatal hernia | Adenocarcinoma of | |
| | Diverticular disease | the colon | |
| | Gastritis | | |
| | Benign polyps of the | | |
| | colon | | |

**Interfering Factors**

- Recent dietary intake of animal protein, vegetable peroxidase, or vitamin C
- Failure to refrigerate the specimens
- Presence of toilet bowl cleaner that contains chlorine

**Nursing Implementation**

### Pretest

Instruct the patient to avoid the foods presented in Table 18–2 for 3 days before the test. Red meat increases the amount of hemoglobin in the feces and causes a false-positive result.

Vitamin C supplement must be omitted for 5 days before the testing period. This vitamin suppresses peroxidase and results in false-negative findings. Fruits and vegetables that contain peroxidase cause a false-positive result.

Inform the patient to discontinue the medications listed in Table 18–2 for seven days before the test because they irritate the gastrointestinal mucosa and may be a source of occult blood.

Until the test is completed, alcohol should be avoided because it can be a gastrointestinal irritant.

Instruct the patient regarding correct fecal collection procedure (see also Chapter 2). Three consecutive stool specimens are placed in separate plastic containers with lids. The specimens are refrigerated and then taken promptly to the laboratory.

### During the Test

In performing the test, note that the directions vary somewhat according to the manufacturer. Basically, an applicator stick is used to place a thin smear of feces on the filter paper. Wait the prescribed time (3 to 5 minutes) to allow the specimen to penetrate the filter paper. Then, on the reverse side of the paper, place a few drops of reagent on the area with the specimen. Wait the designated time (30 seconds to 1 minute) and read the result. The appearance of color (usually blue) is considered a positive result (Dammel, 1997; Henry, 1996).

### Posttest

The nurse can educate and encourage healthy people older than 50 years to have an annual fecal occult blood test.

**Table 18–2 Food and Medication Restrictions for Fecal Occult Blood Tests**

| Foods | Medications |
|---|---|
| Horseradish | Aspirin |
| Turnips | Nonsteroidal anti-inflammatory drugs |
| Red meat | Iron replacement |
| Artichokes | Vitamin C |
| Broccoli | Steroids |
| Cauliflower | Reserpine |
| Grapes (black) | |
| Melon | |
| Bananas | |
| Plums | |
| Pears | |

To illustrate the need for education, one research study (Lipkus, Rimer, & Lyna, 1996) focused on low-income, older African Americans. The respondents had limited understanding of colorectal cancer, minimized the risk factors, and generally believed that "if they were in good health, they did not need a screening test." The population in general, and older African Americans in particular, need assistance to make better-informed decisions regarding health and use of early detection screening procedures such as fecal occult blood testing.

**Home Testing**

Teach the patient to follow the instructions exactly. The instructions can be complicated and detailed, making them hard to understand.

A positive result is the emergence of a blue (or blue-green) color or large blue plus sign in the test area of the paper.

If any of the three results is positive, the patient should see his or her physician.

Alert the patient that the presence of toilet bowl cleaner, disinfectant, or deodorizer will interfere with the results. Before testing, these products must be removed and the toilet flushed twice for a final cleansing. Some of the home tests will have a false-positive result because of a recent intake of red meat. Aspirin and anti-inflammatory drugs also can cause a false-positive result. Vitamin C, rectal ointments, and mineral oil can cause a false-negative result.

## Serotonin

**(Blood)** Synonym: 5-Hydroxytryptamine, blood

**Normal Values** 50–200 ng/mL *or* SI 0.28–1.14 µmol/L (Tietz, 1995)
Values vary among laboratories, depending on the method of analysis.

### Background Information

Serotonin is a hormone that is normally present in many tissues of the body. When it is present in the blood, the serotonin is concentrated in platelets and is released during coagulation processes.

Specific cells in the gastrointestinal mucosa provide one source of serotonin production.

**Elevated Values.** Carcinoid tumors are malignant growths that secrete excess serotonin. They 2cause carcinoid syndrome, with symptoms of flushing, diarrhea, cardiac valvular disease, bronchoconstriction, and hepatomegaly. Primary carcinoid tumors are usually located in the ileum or stomach, but they may also be located in the pancreas, duodenum, bronchus, and ovary. These malignancies may also grow aggressively and metastasize to the liver, brain, bone, and cervical glands.

## Purpose of the Test

The blood level of serotonin is used to diagnose carcinoid syndrome and to detect carcinoid tumor in patients who have normal or borderline 5-HIAA laboratory values.

## Procedure

A chilled vacuum tube that contains EDTA and sometimes ascorbic acid is used to collect 10 mL of venous blood. Laboratory policy will determine the specific tube and preservative, based on the method of analysis used.

## Findings

### Elevated Values

| | | |
|---|---|---|
| Carcinoid syndrome | Dumping syndrome | Acute myocardial |
| Abdominal carcinoid | Acute intestinal | infarction |
| tumor with | obstruction | Celiac disease |
| metastases | Cystic fibrosis | |

### Decreased Values

| | |
|---|---|
| Down syndrome | Parkinson's disease |
| Phenylketonuria | Severe mental |
| (untreated) | depression |

## Interfering Factors

- Monoamine oxidase inhibitors
- Radioisotopes
- Foods rich in serotonin

## Nursing Implementation

The nursing actions are similar to those for other venipunctures.

### Pretest

Schedule this test before any scans or other tests that use radioisotopes. The radioisotopes would interfere with the radioimmunoassay method of analysis.

Monoamine oxidase inhibitors should be discontinued for 1 week before the test because they elevate the serum level of serotonin.

Some laboratory methods require several days of avoidance of foods that are rich in serotonin (avocados, bananas, eggplants, tomatoes, pineapples, walnuts, and red plums).

### Posttest

Pack the blood sample in ice and arrange for immediate transport of the specimen to the laboratory.

### Quality Control

Because serotonin is unstable, the collection tube must contain the proper preservative and be chilled on ice before and after the test.

## Diagnostic Procedures

## Barium Enema

**(Radiology)**          Synonym: BE

| **Normal Values** | No lesions, deficits, or abnormalities of the colon are noted. |
|---|---|

### Background Information

Barium enema is a basic radiographic test that is performed when disease of the large bowel is suspected. It is used to investigate the cause of a change in elimination patterns, melena, obstruction of the colon, or the presence of an abdominal mass that has a suspected location in the colon.

Barium serves as an excellent contrast medium because it is radiopaque, has a different density than body tissue, and can be instilled into hollow organs such as the colon (Fig. 18–3). It coats the mucosa with a thin layer of contrast medium so that x-rays provide a clear view of the interior surfaces. In a barium enema, the entire colon and the distal portion of the ileum can be visualized.

When barium is the only contrast material used, the technique is called a single-contrast study. A double-contrast technique uses barium in conjunction with air or carbon dioxide as the contrast medium. After barium is instilled, the air or gas is introduced by insufflation. This dilates the lumen and provides a clearer view of the mucosal surface. During the barium enema procedure, fluoroscopy is used to monitor filling by the contrast medium and guide the selection of areas that require x-ray filming.

If colonic perforation or fistula is suspected, this test either is contraindicated or is performed cautiously using a water-soluble contrast medium. Ulcerative colitis, severe diverticulitis, acute bloody diarrhea, or pneumatosis cystoides intestinalis all have potential complications, such as perforation of the bowel. If barium enters the venous circulation via ulcerated mucosa, cardiac arrest will occur.

### Purpose of the Test

The barium enema is used to investigate and identify pathologic conditions that change the structure or function of the colon (Fig. 18–4).

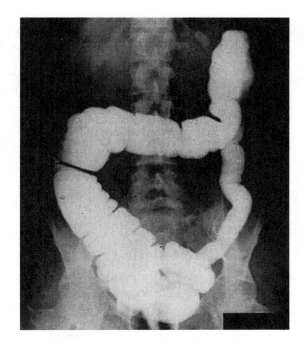

**Figure 18–3**
Barium enema. Radiopaque barium sulfate fills the colon in this lower gastrointestinal study. (Reproduced with permission from Adler, A. M., & Carlton, R. R. [1994]. *Introduction to radiography and patient care* [Vol. 1, Slide 200]. Philadelphia: W. B. Saunders.)

**Mural or mucosal lesions**

| AP | Lateral | AP | Lateral | AP | Lateral |

Polyp on stalk          Diverticulum          Apple core cancer
                        or ulcer

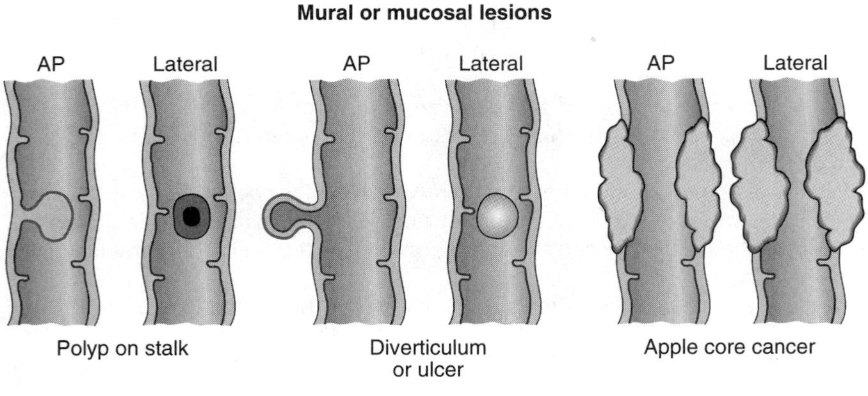

**Figure 18–4**
Schematic appearance of various gastrointestinal lesions on contrast examination. A polyp seen in profile will show a stalk. Seen end-on, it will be darkest in the center, with an ill-defined, fading edge. A diverticulum seen in tangent will project outside the lumen and, when seen end-on, will have very sharp edges. Cancer can be in one wall or, if circumferential, can leave contrast in the lumen that resembles an apple core. (Reproduced with permission from Mettler, F. A. [1996]. *Essentials of radiology* [p. 213]. Philadelphia: W. B. Saunders.)

**Procedure**

After the colon is completely emptied of feces, the contrast medium is instilled. The patient's positional changes (supine, prone, lateral) are used to enhance the gravity flow of the contrast material throughout the entire colon. Fluoroscopic and x-ray images are taken to identify the abnormalities. The procedure takes approximately 45 minutes to 1 hour to complete.

**Findings**

**Abnormal Values**

| | | |
|---|---|---|
| Adenocarcinoma | Polyps | Sigmoid torsion |
| Diverticulitis | Gastroenteritis | Crohn's disease |
| Sarcoma | Chronic amebic | Intussusception |
| Hirschsprung's | dysentery | |
| disease | Intestinal structural | |
| Carcinoma | change | |
| Idiopathic megacolon | Ulcerative colitis | |

**Interfering Factors**

- Upper gastrointestinal series within 3 days before the test
- Inability to retain barium
- Incomplete cleansing of the colon

**Nursing Implementation**

**Pretest**

Schedule the barium enema before any other barium studies.

Residual barium from the upper gastrointestinal tract will interfere with visualization of the colon.

Provide a complete explanation of the procedure for bowel cleansing. When the patient is very young or very old and the procedure is to be performed in an outpatient setting, the caregiver or a second person should be present and included in the teaching. Written instructions will help ensure thorough bowel preparation.

Posttest instructions should also be given in the pretest period. At this time, patients will be able to learn and to ask questions because they are mentally clear and rested.

Patients who report awakening frequently on the night before the test can experience greater energy expenditure during the test. Because they are tired or weak, the posttest period is not the best time to teach about follow-up care (Pieper, 1992).

Obtain a signed consent form from the patient or the person legally responsible for the patient's health care decisions.

For bowel preparation, the exact cleansing procedure is defined by the protocol of the radiologist. Because variations in procedure exist, the common methods of preparation are presented here.

A clear liquid diet begins 12 to 24 hours before the test to reduce the amount of fecal matter.

A cathartic such as castor oil, magnesium citrate, or senna extract (X-Prep) is taken on the afternoon before the test. Bisacodyl (Dulcolax) tablets are taken on the evening before the test, and a bisacodyl suppository is inserted on the morning of the test.

A warm tap water enema (1,500 mL for adults) is given on the night before the test or at 6 AM on the day of the test. When all fecal matter has been removed, the enema returns will be clear.

Extra oral fluids are taken in the pretest period to prevent dehydration or excess absorption from the barium solution in the colon. Some protocols require extra fluids in the afternoon and evening, but a nothing-by-mouth status is started by midnight before the test.

For children younger than 4 years, the bowel preparation is prescribed on an individualized basis.

### Quality Control

To obtain a clear and accurate visualization of the lumen, all fecal matter, residual gas, and mucus must be removed.

**■**

*Critical Thinking 18–3*
An elderly patient is scheduled for a barium enema to be done as an outpatient procedure. When you provide the pretest instruction, the patient tells you that she lives alone and that her severe arthritis prevents her from administering the cleansing enema. What alternatives can you suggest?

### Posttest

The patient is assisted to the toilet or in the use of a commode or bedpan to evacuate the contrast medium.

A laxative is prescribed to eliminate the residual barium and to prevent constipation caused by the barium. Residual barium changes the feces to a gray or whitish color for 24 to 72 hours after the test.

Encourage the patient to rest for the remainder of the day, because this test is tiring. Elderly patients are vulnerable to weakness and may experience a fall. They also may become mentally confused because of dehydration, so increased fluid intake is important.

## Barium Swallow

**(Radiology)**                    Synonym: Esophagography

### Normal Values

No structural or functional abnormalities are visualized.

### Background Information

The barium swallow procedure may be performed as a separate barium study or as a routine part of the upper gastrointestinal series. Dysphagia is the most common problem investigated by the barium swallow. The cause can be an obstruction in a part of the esophagus or a neuromuscular deficit that interferes with swallowing and slows the transit time for the passage of food to the stomach. The normal transit time from the oropharynx to the stomach is 6 to 15 seconds.

### Purpose of the Test

The barium swallow is used to identify abnormalities in the structure or function of the esophagus (Fig. 18–5).

### Procedure

The patient takes repeated swallows of barium liquid to provide views of the passage of contrast medium during swallowing and peristaltic movement of the

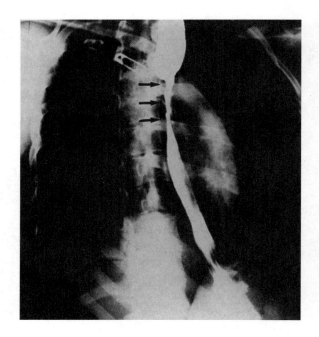

**Figure 18–5**
Benign esophageal stricture. This upper esophageal stricture
(*arrows*) was due to attempted suicide by lye ingestion.
(Reproduced with permission from Mettler, F. A. [1996].
*Essentials of radiology* [p. 185]. Philadelphia: W. B. Saunders.)

esophagus. Fluoroscopy and x-rays are used for visualization as the patient is
in vertical, semivertical, and horizontal positions on the tilting x-ray table.

| **Findings** | **Abnormal Values** | | |
| --- | --- | --- | --- |
| | Swallowed foreign body | Esophageal spasm | Plummer-Vinson syndrome |
| | Achalasia (neuromuscular incoordination) | Hiatal hernia | Varices |
| | | Pharyngeal neuromuscular weakness | Ulcers or peptic esophagitis |
| | Esophageal stricture | Polyps, tumors, carcinoma | |

**Interfering Factors**    • Failure to maintain a nothing-by-mouth status

**Nursing Implementation**    **Pretest**

Provide an explanation of the procedure and obtain written consent from the
patient or the person legally responsible for the patient's health care decisions.
Instruct the patient to fast from all food and liquids for 12 hours before the test.
At the radiology setting, have the patient remove all clothes, jewelry, and
metallic objects. A surgical gown is worn.

**Posttest**

A laxative is given to help eliminate the barium from the intestinal tract.

Inform the patient that the feces will appear gray or whitish for 24 to 72 hours until all barium is expelled.

## Colonoscopy
**(Endoscopy)**                    Synonym: Lower panendoscopy

| Normal Values | No abnormalities of structure or mucosal surface are observed in the colon or terminal ileum. |
|---|---|

## Background Information

Colonoscopy refers to the endoscopic visualization of the colon. With improvement in the equipment and newer technique, the endoscope also can explore the total colon and 20 to 30 cm of the ileum. When the ileum is included in the visualization, the procedure is called a *lower panendoscopy*.

The flexible endoscope is a long tube filled with thousands of ultrathin glass fibers. By reflection and refraction, these fibers transmit the light and visualized image from the distal lens to the viewer's eyepiece, even when the tube is curved. The flexibility of the tube enables it to be passed beyond each flexure of the colon (Fig. 18–6). The distal segment of the tube can be rotated through 360 degrees so that all aspects of the lumen are observed. Columns within the instrument allow for irrigation, suction, instrumentation, and instillation of air or gas.

**Psychological Issues.**    When the procedure is done as a routine measure to screen for colorectal cancer, the patient may experience some anxiety and feelings of embarrassment about the procedure. When symptoms exist that require investigation by colonoscopy, the denial, fear, or anxiety can be greatly increased. The average patient with colorectal symptoms delays for about 7 months before seeing the physician for an initial examination. Many factors contribute to the delay,

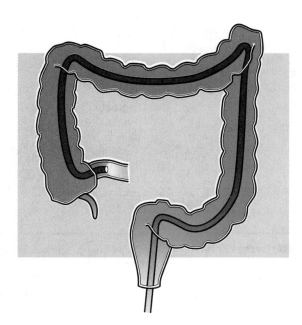

**Figure 18–6**
Lower panendoscopy. The endoscopic instrument is passed through the entire colon and into the distal segment of the ileum. The examination is used to identify sites of bleeding, inflammation, tissue irregularity, or abnormality, including polyps and tumor.

but once the decision is made to have a colonoscopy, denial is no longer operational and the patient may experience overt fear of cancer or death or may worry about disabling illness. It is important for the nurse and physician to support the patient emotionally before, during, and after the diagnostic tests. Maximizing hopefulness and maintaining an empathetic approach are ways to enhance the patient's ability to cope (Wagner, Kenrick, Rojas, & Woodward, 1995).

## Purpose of the Test

The purposes of colonoscopy are to perform a routine screening of the colon for detection of polyps or tumor and to investigate the cause of chronic diarrhea or other unexplained gastrointestinal complaints. The procedure may be done to further investigate an abnormal result of a barium enema, sigmoidoscopy, or fecal occult blood test. When suspicious lesions are found, biopsy is done (Robinson, 1995).

The purpose of lower panendoscopy is to examine the terminal ileum, particularly for sources of inflammation or bleeding, as well as to examine the colon for the purposes described above.

## Procedure

Virtually all patients have the procedure performed with conscious sedation (Phillips, 1995), although infants and small children may require general anesthesia. The tip of the endoscope is inserted into the rectum and passed through the sigmoid, descending, transverse, and ascending colon, including the cecum. When the ileum is included in the examination, the ileocecal valve is visualized and the tip of the instrument is passed through and advanced into the distal ileum. As the endoscope is withdrawn slowly, the tissue is examined and biopsy samples are taken as needed.

### Quality Control

The colonoscope and accessory parts must be mechanically cleansed and then disinfected after each procedure. The goal is to remove organic matter and infectious agents, thus minimizing the potential transmission of infection (Favero & Pugliese, 1996; Muscarella, 1996; Rutala, 1996).

## Findings

### Abnormal Values

| | | |
|---|---|---|
| Diverticulitis | Site of lower intestinal bleeding | Proctitis |
| Crohn's disease | | Pneumatosis cystoides intestinalis |
| Granulomatous disease | Colitis (radiation, ischemia, infection) | Gay bowel syndrome |
| Ulcerative colitis | | |
| Polyps | | |
| Carcinoma of the bowel | | |

## Interfering Factors

- Massive bleeding in the colon
- Toxic colitis
- Inflammatory bowel disease or stricture
- Peritonitis or bowel perforation

- Acute diverticulitis
- Recent myocardial infarction, pulmonary embolus, or acute cardiopulmonary disease
- Recent pelvic or colon surgery
- Large aortic or iliac aneurysm
- Pregnancy, second or third trimester
- Uncooperative patient behavior
- Poor bowel preparation
- Retained barium
- Failure to maintain pretest dietary restrictions

**Nursing Implementation**

### Pretest

Schedule this test before any barium studies.

Explain the procedure to the patient and obtain written consent from the patient or the person legally responsible for the patient's health care decisions.

Provide instructions about bowel cleansing. Because the protocol varies among institutions, follow the endoscopist's particular requirements. General guidelines are presented here. For bowel cleansing, the patient should follow a low-residue or clear liquid diet for 24 hours before the test, to reduce the amount of feces. The patient should drink the polyethylene glycol-electrolyte lavage solution (GoLYTELY or Colyte) starting at about 5 PM on the afternoon before the procedure. The volume is 2 to 4 L to be taken in 8 oz doses every 10 minutes until the patient has clear watery stool that is free of solid matter (Robinson, 1995). Clear liquids can be resumed until midnight, but no further liquids are permitted thereafter.

On the morning of the test, take the patient's baseline vital signs and record the results in the patient's chart.

### During the Test

Premedicate the patient with intravenous meperidine (Demerol), 25 to 50 mg, for analgesia and relaxation. This may be followed by intravenous diazepam (Valium), 1 to 3 mg, or intravenous midazolam (Versed), 1 mg for adults and 0.5 mg for elderly patients. To prevent apnea, respiratory depression, or cardiac arrest, these medications must be given slowly over a period of 5 minutes.

Naloxone (Narcan) is kept on hand to reverse the respiratory depressive effect of meperidine, but it is ineffective against diazepam.

Oxygen by nasal cannula increases the patient's oxygen reserves and helps prevent hypoxia. About 40% of the patients develop an oxygen saturation of <90% after intravenous sedation begins (Phillips, 1995).

Monitor the vital signs at frequent intervals throughout the procedure. In hospitals, automated blood pressure, pulse oximetry, and cardiac monitoring may be used for all endoscopy patients or for selected patients who are more vulnerable. This group includes elderly individuals and those with a history of cardiac disease.

Monitor for the vasovagal reflex that can occur during the procedure. Atropine sulfate is kept on hand to overcome the effects of sudden bradycardia.

Provide comfort and emotional support to help reduce anxiety and promote relaxation. Embarrassment, anxiety, stress, and fear are all common feelings for patients who undergo colonoscopy.

During insufflation and manipulation of the endoscope, the patient also can be restless or uncomfortable and may require additional medication.

Assist with the collection of tissue specimens, as described in the section on gastrointestinal cytologic studies in another part of this chapter.

### Posttest

Monitor vital signs every 15 minutes or continue automated monitoring until the results are stable.

Check the rectal area for signs of blood.

Send the properly identified tissue specimens to the laboratory without delay.

As soon as the patient is more responsive, the intake of food and liquids can resume.

On discharge from an ambulatory care setting, the patient must be accompanied by a responsible person who will provide transportation home.

Because of the effects of the intravenous medication, the patient cannot drive a car for 8 to 12 hours, until thinking is clear and memory is restored.

■
*Critical Thinking 18–4*
An elderly patient is scheduled for colonoscopy. In your care plan, what nursing measures will help ensure the safety of the patient before, during, and after the procedure?

### Complications

During the procedure, the patient can experience respiratory depression or respiratory arrest because of the sedative anesthetics or narcotic analgesics. Intravenous diazepam can cause thrombophlebitis in the small vein used for administration of medication.

The vasovagal reflex is thought to be caused by the stretching of the mesentery as the endoscope is advanced through the colon. Up to 16.5% of the patients will experience this problem during colonoscopy, but most of the reactions do not require treatment and have no long-lasting consequence (Robinson, 1995). Other patients will demonstrate electrocardiographic abnormality during colonoscopy, and serious arrhythmia or myocardial infarction can occur during or just after the procedure (Phillips, 1995; Robinson, 1995).

Hemorrhage and perforation are serious but infrequent complications. They are caused by manipulation of the endoscope and the use of force when advancing the endoscope. Patients with diverticular disease, adhesion, stricture, or severe inflammatory disease are most vulnerable. The nursing assessment of complications of colonoscopy is presented in Table 18–3.

## Computed Tomography of the Gastrointestinal Tract

**(Scan)**    Synonyms: CT scan, CAT, computerized axial tomography

The computed tomographic (CT) scan uses x-rays to provide multidimensional scanning of the body tissue. This procedure provides a view of the bowel wall, mesentery, peritoneum, and organs adjacent to the gastrointestinal tract. CT is used to detect intra-abdominal masses, including abscess, tumor, infarct, perforation, obstruction, inflammation, and diverticulitis. It is also useful in detection of metastases and in the staging of abdominal malignancy. Intravenous or oral contrast medium can be used to improve the visualization of the bowel loops and the blood supply of the bowel walls (Gore & Ghahremani, 1995). A complete discussion of computed tomography is presented in Chapter 12.

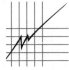

## Table 18–3   Complications of Colonoscopy

| Complication | Nursing Assessment |
| --- | --- |
| Respiratory depression, apnea | Infrequent, irregular, shallow breathing<br>Respiratory rate <12 breaths per minute<br>Hypotension<br>Bradycardia or tachycardia<br>Hypoxemia<br>Diaphoresis<br>Nausea, vomiting |
| Vasovagal reflex | Bradycardia (pulse <60 beats/min)<br>Hypotension<br>Cold, clammy skin |
| Cardiac arrhythmia | Premature atrial contractions<br>Premature ventricular contractions<br>Sinus tachycardia<br>ST-T depression<br>Chest pain<br>Hypotension<br>Atrial or ventricular fibrillation<br>Cardiac arrest |
| Hemorrhage, perforation | Rectal bleeding<br>Abdominal distention<br>Persistent abdominal pain<br>Abdominal tenderness on palpitation<br>Malaise<br>Decreased hematocrit<br>Hypotension<br>Tachycardia |

## Esophageal Function Tests

**(Manometry)**      Synonyms: Esophageal manometry, esophageal acidity test (Tuttle test), acid perfusion test (Bernstein test)

**Normal Values**

**Esophageal Manometry**
Lower esophageal sphincter (LES) pressure: Mean value 19.2 ±6.9 mm Hg
% LES relaxation (wet swallow): 96% ±10%
Primary peristalsis esophageal body (wet swallow): Mean amplitude 65–71 mm Hg; mean duration 3.3–6.2 sec
Primary peristalsis esophageal body (dry swallow): Mean amplitude 45 mm Hg; mean duration 4.7–4.8 sec
Esophageal body (tertiary contractions): Present (frequently to infrequently); mean amplitude 12 ±3 mm Hg; mean duration 2.9–3.1 ±0.4–0.5 sec
**Esophageal acidity test:** Alkaline (esophageal pH of 6 or higher)
**Acid perfusion test:** Negative

## Background Information

The esophagus is a muscular segment of the alimentary tract that propels food from the pharynx to the stomach by peristalsis. In peristaltic activity, smooth muscle contraction causes the intraluminal pressure to rise, and smooth muscle relaxation causes the intraluminal pressure to fall. The alternating waves of contraction and relaxation continuously move the bolus of food downward from high-pressure to low-pressure areas.

The final portion of the esophagus is called the lower esophageal segment (LES). Its functions are to accept the bolus of food, transport it to the stomach, and prevent regurgitation of gastric contents back into the esophagus. When at rest, the LES pressure is higher than that of the stomach. The combination of the pressure gradient and the LES sphincter or sphincterlike function prevents gastroesophageal reflux.

**Esophageal Manometry.**   The pressure within the body of the esophagus and at the lower esophageal segment can be measured at rest and during swallowing to provide information about peristalsis. The measures of the amplitude, frequency, and duration of the pressure define the effectiveness of esophageal motor function.

Patients who require this test have a history of unexplained dysphagia or chronic heartburn. The cause of the dysphagia may be progressive systemic sclerosis or esophageal motor dysfunction. The origin of the heartburn may be hiatal hernia. The manometry test helps rule out angina or other cardiac problems as the source of chest pain.

**Esophageal Acidity Test.**   During manometry testing, the esophageal acidity test is used to measure the pH within the esophagus. The normal esophageal pH is 6 or higher, an alkaline environment. The normal pH of the stomach is 1 to 3, an acidic reading. A lower-than-normal esophageal pH is caused by the regurgitation of gastric acids into the esophagus. The regurgitation is called gastroesophageal reflux and is caused by an incompetent LES.

**Acid Perfusion Test.**   During manometry testing, the acid perfusion test may be performed to identify the patient's subjective response to heartburn pain in the presence of dilute hydrochloric acid. In a positive result, the patient's esophagus is the source of the pain; it is sensitive to the presence of gastric acid.

## Purpose of the Test

Esophageal manometry is used to diagnose and evaluate esophageal motor disorders, including the evaluation of dysphagia. It is also used to evaluate pre- or postoperative esophageal surgery designed to improve esophageal motility and prevent esophageal reflux.

The esophageal acidity test is used to document gastroesophageal reflux or to evaluate the results of medical-surgical antireflux treatment. The acid perfusion test is used to determine that the heartburn is of esophageal rather than cardiac origin.

## Procedure

A triple-lumen catheter is passed into the esophagus via the nose or mouth. The procedure is performed while the patient is awake. A local anesthetic is used to numb the nose and throat so that the catheter-manometer can be passed without discomfort. The patient is then put into a supine position with a swallowing sensor attached to the neck.

In *esophageal manometry,* all channels of the catheter record pressures from the esophagus during a series of wet swallows (5 mL of water delivered by syringe) and dry swallows. The pressure readings give data about LES pressure, LES relaxation, peristalsis, and spontaneous contractions of the esophagus.

Provocative testing is performed to clarify the source of the dysphagia or chest pain, or both. A cholinergic drug, edrophonium hydrochloride (Tensilon), is given intravenously, and the pressure readings are repeated.

In the *esophageal acidity test*, the pH probe on the tip of the catheter records the pH values in the esophagus and stomach. Acidity readings from the esophagus are taken after swallowing, Valsalva maneuvers, straight leg-raising maneuvers, and abdominal compressions. If necessary, an infusion of 300 mL of 0.1 N hydrochloric acid is instilled into the stomach, and the preceding maneuvers are repeated.

In the *acid perfusion test,* a drip of 0.1 N hydrochloric acid is instilled through the esophageal manometry catheter or a nasogastric tube until the patient complains of heartburn or until 30 minutes have passed without symptoms. The solution is alternated with normal saline flow to confirm that the heartburn occurs in the presence of hydrochloric acid and disappears in the presence of normal saline.

### Quality Control

Before the start of the procedure, the entire system of components must be connected and checked for accurate function. This includes calibration of the recording system and confirmation of the accuracy of the pressure transducers, the pressure response rates, and the pH sensor and its equipment.

---

**Findings**

**Abnormal Values**

Achalasia
Esophageal spasm
Progressive systemic
  sclerosis (sclero-
  derma)

Gastroesophageal
  reflux
Hiatal hernia

---

**Interfering Factors**

- Unstable cardiac status
- Uncooperative patient

---

**Nursing Implementation**

### Pretest

Inform the patient about the procedure and obtain a written consent from the patient or the person legally responsible for the patient's health care decisions.

Instruct the patient to maintain a fasting state and to abstain from smoking for 8 hours before the start of the test. Medications that alter the acidity of the stomach are withheld for 24 hours. These include antacids, anticholinergics, cholinergics, steroids, cimetidine, and reserpine. If the physician wants them to be taken, the medications are noted on the requisition slip (Massoni, 1997a).

### During the Test

Monitor and record the vital signs at frequent intervals. Observe for signs of respiratory or cardiac change.

### Posttest

Once the gag and swallow reflexes return, the patient may resume the medication schedule and oral intake.

**Table 18–4    Complications of Esophageal Manometry Tests**

| Complication | Nursing Assessment |
| --- | --- |
| Vasovagal response | Bradycardia (pulse <60 beats/min)<br>Hypotension<br>Cold, clammy skin |
| Cholinergic reaction (side effects of edrophonium chloride) | Dizziness<br>Diaphoresis<br>Flushing<br>Nausea and vomiting<br>Muscle cramps<br>Urinary urgency<br>Bradycardia (pulse <60 beats/min) |

## Complications

Patients who have an unstable cardiac status, particularly with poor tolerance to vagal stimulation, should not undergo this test. A vasovagal reflex can occur, and atropine sulfate should always be on hand during the test.

When provocation testing is carried out with edrophonium chloride, side effects can occur. Atropine sulfate must be on hand for the reversal of the side effects and to counteract the cholinergic effect of the drug. The nursing assessment of complications of esophageal manometry is presented in Table 18–4.

# Esophagogastroduodenoscopy

**(Endoscopy)**    Synonyms: EGD, upper gastrointestinal endoscopy

## Normal Values

No abnormal structures or functions are observed in the esophagus, stomach, or duodenum.

## Background Information

In upper gastrointestinal endoscopy, the fiberoptic endoscope provides visualization of the lumen and mucosal lining of the esophagus, stomach, and upper duodenum.

The flexible fiberscope is a long tube filled with tens of thousands of thin glass fibers. By refraction and reflection, the fibers transmit light and the visualized image from the distal lens to the examiner's eyepiece, even when the tube is curved or flexed. Because of the ability to bend and rotate its distal segment, the fiberscope can be directed to view each segmented area until the entire lumen of each organ has been seen (Fig. 18–7). Within the instrument, columns exist to irrigate, suction, instill air or gas, and insert instruments.

In the diagnostic uses of esophagogastroduodenoscopy, tissue abnormalities are observed for their location, size, contour, shape, position, mobility, and surface appearance. Tissue or secretion samples are obtained by biopsy, scrapings, or aspiration and are sent for laboratory analysis.

## Purpose of the Test

The many purposes of upper gastrointestinal endoscopy include (1) identification and biopsy of tissue abnormality, (2) determination of the exact site and

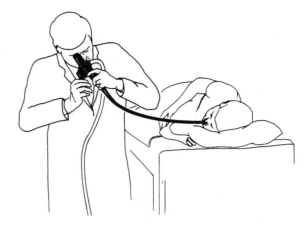

**Figure 18–7**

Esophagogastroduodenoscopy. Once the endoscope is inserted, the tube is moved around and rotated to obtain visualization of the lumen of the upper intestine. (Reproduced with permission from Sivak, M. V. [1987]. *Gastrologic endoscopy.* Philadelphia: W. B. Saunders.)

cause of upper gastrointestinal bleeding, (3) evaluation of the healing of gastric ulcers, (4) evaluation of the stomach and duodenum after gastric surgery, and (5) investigation for the cause of dysphagia, dyspepsia, gastric outlet obstruction, or epigastric pain.

**Procedure**

Virtually all patients have the procedure performed under conscious sedation and a local anesthetic spray to the throat. The goals of conscious sedation are to promote the patient's cooperation and tolerance of the procedure (Lugay, Otto, Kong, Mason, & Wilets, 1996). Infants and small children may require general anesthesia.

Once the patient is medicated, the endoscope is passed through the mouth and into the esophagus. As the tube is advanced distally and then withdrawn, the esophagus, stomach, pylorus, and upper duodenum are visualized. As the scope is moved around, and with 360-degree rotation and flexion of the tip, the surface of the entire lumen is visualized (Fig. 18–8). Tissue or cell samples are obtained for cytologic studies as indicated.

**Quality Control**

The endoscope and accessory parts must be mechanically cleansed and then disinfected after each procedure. The goals are to remove organic matter and infectious agents, thus minimizing the potential for transmission of infection (Favero & Pugliese, 1996; Muscarella, 1996; Rutala, 1996).

**Findings**

**Abnormal Values**

Ulcers, acute or chronic, gastric or duodenal
Tumors, benign or malignant
Diverticula
Stenosis, esophageal or pyloric

Hiatal hernia
Esophageal rings
Inflammation (esophagitis, gastritis, duodenitis)
Mallory-Weiss syndrome

Varices, esophageal or gastric

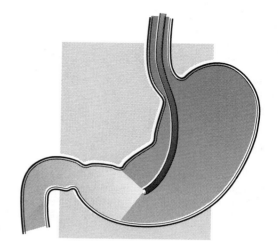

**Figure 18–8**
Endoscopic visualization of the upper gastrointestinal tract. The flexible tube, fiberoptic filaments, and a light are used to examine the mucosal surface of the esophagus, stomach, and duodenum for inflammation, erosion, ulceration, bleeding sites, stricture, and abnormal tissue.

**Interfering Factors**

- Failure to maintain a nothing-by-mouth status
- Unstable or life-threatening cardiac or pulmonary condition
- Known or suspected perforation of the stomach or intestine
- Shock
- Recent myocardial infarction

**Nursing Implementation**

**Pretest**

Schedule this test at least 2 days after an upper gastrointestinal series so that the barium will not interfere with visualization.

Inform the patient about the procedure and obtain written consent from the patient or the person legally designated to make health care decisions for the patient.

Provide written posttest instructions, because temporary memory loss will occur after sedative administration.

When the procedure is to be performed in an ambulatory setting, someone must accompany the patient and provide transportation after discharge.

Instruct the patient to take nothing by mouth for 6 to 8 hours before the procedure.

Obtain the pretest coagulation profile, which includes prothrombin time, partial thromboplastin time, bleeding time, and platelet count. Place the results in the patient's chart.

On the morning of the test, obtain and record the vital signs, including blood pressure, pulse, and respirations.

Assist the patient with the removal and storage of eyeglasses, dentures, jewelry, hairpins, and clothing. Provide a surgical gown for the patient to wear.

**During the Test**

Position the patient on the examination table in the left lateral recumbent position. An intravenous line is established, and the topical anesthetic is sprayed in the throat.

Intravenous medication is given for relaxation and analgesia. Meperidine (Demerol), 25 to 50 mg, is often followed by diazepam (Valium), 1 to 15 mg, or midazolam (Versed), 1 to 10 mg in adults. Smaller doses are often used for the elderly patient. To prevent apnea, respiratory depression, or cardiac arrest, these medications are given slowly over a period of 5 minutes (Norris, 1997). Naloxone (Narcan) is kept on hand to reverse any respiratory depressive effect of meperidine, but it is ineffective with diazepam.

Oxygen delivered by nasal cannula will increase the patient's oxygen reserves and help prevent hypoxia. Some protocols do not provide oxygen routinely but have it available for use as needed.

Monitor vital signs at 5-minute intervals throughout the procedure and observe the patient for signs of hypoxia or loss of consciousness. In most hospitals and outpatient settings, automated blood pressure, pulse oximetry, and cardiac monitoring are used for all endoscopy patients or for selected patients who are more vulnerable. These are elderly patients and those with a history of cardiac disease (Norris, 1997).

Assist with the collection of specimens obtained by biopsy, brush technique, or washing technique (see also Gastrointestinal Cytologic Studies). Tissue samples are placed in a jar with preservative and labeled appropriately. The requisition slip includes the source of the tissue, the procedure, and the date.

### Posttest

Continue to assess the vital signs and level of consciousness until the patient is stable for at least 30 minutes.

Once the patient is coherent and the vital signs are stable, permit the patient to ambulate. Minimal dizziness may occur, but there should be no postural hypotension or fainting (Marley & Moline, 1996).

Oral fluids can be started as soon as the swallow and gag reflexes have returned. Fluids should not be forced, however, because of possible nausea and the potential for vomiting.

Review the posttest instructions with the patient, as follows: Use of throat lozenges or saline gargle to relieve the discomfort in the throat, no driving for 12 hours, and full resumption of fluids and food, as desired.

---

**Complications**

The incidence of overall complications in esophagogastroduodenoscopy is quite low, and the procedure is considered reasonably simple (Norris, 1997). Complications can occur, however, and require ongoing assessment during and after the procedure.

Aspiration pneumonia associated with oversedation and transient bacteremia are the most likely sources of infection. Bacteremia may result from a variety of microorganisms from the patient's intestine or from contaminated instruments; the bacteria are introduced into the bloodstream during the procedure.

Mild hypoxemia and hypoventilation occur fairly often during the EGD procedures. The respiratory insufficiency is attributed to a combination of premedication with sedative-narcotics, the presence of the endoscope in the hypopharynx, and aspiration of fluids into the trachea. Elderly patients and those with chronic obstructive pulmonary disease are most vulnerable (Lugay et al., 1996).

Serious cardiac complications are rare, but arrhythmias are common

### Table 18–5 Complications of Esophagogastroduodenoscopy

| Complication | Nursing Assessment |
| --- | --- |
| Infection | Fever |
| | Malaise |
| | Shaking chills |
| | Elevated white blood cell count |
| | Cough |
| | Dyspnea |
| Respiratory depression | Bradypnea <12 breaths/min |
| | Shallow breathing |
| | Pallor, cyanosis |
| | Tachycardia |
| Cardiac arrhythmia | Irregular pulse |
| | Premature ventricular contractions |
| | Premature atrial beats |
| | Atrial fibrillation |
| Perforation, bleeding | Hematemesis |
| | Melena |
| | Persistent pain in the esophagus, mediastinum, or epigastric area |
| | Persistent dysphagia |
| | Fever |

during the procedure. The triggering factors are not fully understood, but hypoxia and anxiety are contributing factors. Elderly patients and those with a history of cardiac or chronic lung disease are most vulnerable.

Perforation of the pharynx, esophagus, or stomach can occur with uncooperative patient behavior or because of anatomic abnormality. Bleeding may be the result of perforation, a dislodged clot, or a coagulation disorder. The nursing assessments for complications of esophagogastroduodenoscopy are presented in Table 18–5.

## Gallium Scan

**(Radionuclide Scan)**  Synonyms: Gallium 67 imaging, total body scan

### Normal Values

No anatomic or functional abnormalities are visualized.

### Background Information

When the radiopharmaceutical gallium 67 is injected into the bloodstream, it will bind to transferrin and other plasma proteins. As the gallium 67 is transported through the bloodstream, it will concentrate in neoplastic tumors and sites of inflammation or infection. The uptake mechanism is not fully understood but may be related to transferrin receptor sites in malignant tissue and an attraction to neutrophils, bacteria, and purulent matter contained in inflamed or infected tissue.

Gallium 67 is a radioactive isotope that emits gamma rays. As the radiopharmaceutical circulates throughout the plasma and then concentrates in areas of abnormality, it is detected by the scintillation scanner. The nuclear scan may be performed as a total body scan or may concentrate on spot imaging of a particular body region, or it may be used in both ways.

The gallium 67 radioisotope has a half-life of 78 hours. It is partially excreted from the body by the kidneys and colon over a period of 3 days.

## Purpose of the Test

The gallium scan is used to locate malignancy, metastases, and sites of inflammation, infection, and abscess (Fig. 18–9).

## Procedure

The radionuclide is injected intravenously. Four to six hours later, images are taken to identify infectious or inflammatory disease; 24 hours later, images are taken to identify tumors. Additional images may be taken at 24-hour intervals for up to 72 hours for the imaging of infection. A single body region requires 45 minutes, and a total body scan takes 90 minutes for completion.

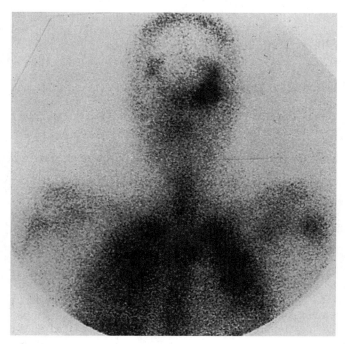

**Figure 18–9**

Gallium scan. An anterior image obtained 48 hours after injection of a dose of gallium 67 citrate. Intense uptake of radiotracer occurs in the left maxillary sinus. Also, diffuse, bilateral, moderately intense pulmonary uptake occurs in an HIV-positive patient with *Pneumocystis carinii* pneumonia and clinically unsuspected left maxillary sinusitis. (Reproduced with permission from Wagner, H. N., Szabo, Z., & Buchanan, J. W. [1995]. *Principles of nuclear medicine* [2nd ed., Figure 36–1, p. 733]. Philadelphia: W. B. Saunders.)

Because gallium 67 will accumulate in the colon, the presence of feces can interfere with the visualization of the abdominal region. On the day before the test, bowel preparation usually is required to remove fecal matter (Winchester, Dhekne, Moore, & Murphy, 1994). The nurse should consult with the nuclear medicine department for specific instructions.

| Findings | Abnormal Values | | |
|---|---|---|---|
| | Peritonitis | Abdominal abscess | *Pneumocystis carinii* |
| | Malignancy of the head, neck, bronchus, thorax, liver, genitourinary tract, and lymphatic system | Metastatic disease | Sarcoidosis |
| | | Osteomyelitis | |
| | | Amebiasis | |
| | | Granulomatous disease | |
| | | Pneumonia | |

**Interfering Factors**

- Barium in the intestinal tract
- Recent lymphangiography
- Pregnancy

**Nursing Implementation**

**Pretest**

Schedule this test before any barium studies or lymphangiography. The gamma rays of the gallium 67 scan cannot penetrate the retained barium. Recent lymphangiography will increase the gallium uptake in the lungs, giving a false-positive reading.

Explain the procedure to the patient and obtain an informed consent form from the patient or the person legally responsible for the patient's health care decisions.

Instruct the patient regarding the specific bowel preparation required.

The patient may experience fear and anxiety about the undiagnosed illness. While waiting for the procedure to begin, the nurse can provide empathy and reassurance in verbal and nonverbal ways. A pat on the shoulder and a supportive smile are ways to express caring. Asking the patient, "How are you feeling?" is one way to assess the patient's emotional status. If the patient is concerned about the procedure or the radiation exposure, the nurse can respond with information and explanations (Davidhizar & Dowd, 1996).

**Posttest**

Use gloves to dispose of fecal matter and wash hands immediately after removing gloves.

Teach the patient to flush the toilet promptly after evacuation and to wash the hands promptly. The radioactive dosage is small, and the exposure is minimal for 72 hours. Because the fecal matter contains the excreted radioisotope, handwashing and hygiene measures prevent additional radiation contact with the skin.

## Gastric Emptying Scan

**(Radionuclide Scan)**          Synonyms: None

| Normal Values | No delay in gastric emptying<br>Half-time emptying of liquid phase: 40 minutes (range: 12–65 min)<br>Half-time emptying of solid phase: 90 minutes (range: 45–110 min) |
| --- | --- |

## Background Information

In normal physiology of gastric emptying, solid foods first undergo churning and grinding activity until the solids consist of small particles. Peristalsis causes the emptying of the solid matter through the pylorus into the duodenum. Liquids are emptied from the stomach by gravity, with some assistance from peristalsis.

The rate of gastric emptying depends partially on the quality of muscle tone and the opening of the pylorus. The emptying rate is also influenced by the foods that have been ingested. Large meals and fatty or high-calorie foods also slow the emptying rate.

**Abnormal Results.**   In this test, when the patient has a rapid gastric emptying rate, the time for half the test meal to exit the stomach is only a few minutes, below the acceptable range of normal values. When the patient has gastric stasis and a slow emptying rate, the time for half the meal to exit the stomach is prolonged beyond the upper range of normal values.

The stomach empties at a faster rate when peristalsis increases. Inflammation, malabsorption, and gastric surgical procedures such as a subtotal gastrectomy or vagotomy are common causes of rapid gastric emptying.

*Gastroparesis* is the term for a delay in gastric emptying from a nonobstructive cause. The gastric stasis is caused by reduced muscle contractility, often due to diabetes mellitus, other metabolic or electrolyte disturbances, or gastric ulcer disease (Wagner, Szabo, & Buchanan, 1995).

## Purpose of the Test

Because the gastric emptying scan can measure the precise rate of emptying of the stomach, the test is used to investigate the cause of a rapid or slow rate of gastric emptying. It is also used to evaluate the effect of treatment of conditions of abnormal gastric motility.

## Procedure

The test meal consists of a radionuclide, such as technetium 99 sulfur colloid, mixed with a liquid and a food. These are given to the patient for oral intake. With the patient in a sitting position, the scintillation scanner takes images of the stomach and duodenum at 10- to 15-minute intervals for about 3 hours. The images and the measurements of the radionuclide that empty from the stomach are calculated with computer assistance. The computer images demonstrate the gastric-emptying function over time (Fig. 18–10).

## Findings

### Elevated Values

Delayed gastric emptying is caused by the following:

| | | |
| --- | --- | --- |
| Diabetes mellitus (diabetic gastroparesis) | Gastric ulcer | Anorexia nervosa |
| | Post gastric surgery | Gastric outlet obstruction |
| | Gastritis | |
| Hypokalemia, hypomagnesemia | Postoperative ileus | Scleroderma |
| | Gastroesophageal reflux | Amyloidosis |
| Gastroenteritis | | |

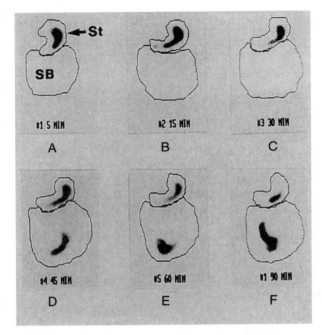

**Figure 18–10**
Gastric emptying scan. Regions of interest are drawn about the stomach (St) and small bowel (SB). By 45 minutes, the stomach is beginning to empty, and by 90 minutes, more than half the activity is in the small bowel. (Reproduced with permission from Mettler, F. A. [1996]. *Essentials of radiology* [p. 194]. Philadelphia: W. B. Saunders.)

**Decreased Values**

Rapid gastric emptying is caused by the following:

| | |
|---|---|
| Duodenal ulcer | Malabsorption |
| Zollinger-Ellison | syndromes |
|  syndrome | Dumping syndrome |

---

**Interfering Factors**

- Failure to maintain a nothing-by-mouth status
- Pregnancy or lactation

---

**Nursing Implementation**

**Pretest**

Teach the patient about the procedure and obtain an informed consent form from the patient or the person legally designated to make health care decisions for the patient.

Reassure the patient that the test is painless and easily tolerated. No special radiation precautions are needed, because the dose of the radioisotope is small and the half-life is short.

Advise the patient to fast from food and liquids for 8 hours before the start of the test.

### Posttest

No specific patient instruction or intervention is needed.

## Gastroesophageal Reflux Scan

(Radionuclide Scan)                    Synonym: GE reflux scan

| Normal Values | The gastroesophageal reflux is 3% or less. |
| --- | --- |

### Background Information

Gastroesophageal reflux is the passive backflow of gastric juices into the esophagus. When the gastric acids are in contact with the esophageal mucosa of adults, they cause reflux esophagitis with ulcers, stricture, or shortening of the esophagus. The patient experiences the symptom of heartburn. In infants and children, the consequences are much more significant. The reflux can rise up the esophagus and enter the trachea. The child can develop failure to thrive, apnea, aspiration pneumonia, esophageal stricture, or esophagitis (O'Hara, 1996).

Normally, the pressure gradient, sphincter activity, and anatomic angle at which the esophagus connects with the stomach all act to prevent the regurgitation of acid into the esophagus. The abnormal reflux of gastric acids occurs when (1) the pressure of the LES is lower than that of the stomach, (2) the sphincter activity is impaired, or (3) the esophagogastric angle is wider or more open. Under these conditions, gastroesophageal reflux occurs when the body is in a supine position or when increased intra-abdominal pressure exists. A gastroesophageal reflux result that is 4% or higher is considered abnormal.

This nuclear scan is more precise than esophageal barium studies in the diagnosis of gastroesophageal reflux. Unlike esophageal manometry tests, it does not require intubation.

### Purpose of the Test

This scan uses a radionuclide and computer-assisted scintigraphy to identify and measure gastroesophageal reflux. It can also be used to measure the response to treatment, including the surgical repair of a hiatal hernia.

### Procedure

An abdominal binder with an inflatable cuff is applied to the patient's abdomen. The adult patient drinks the radiopharmaceutical technetium 99m sulfur colloid mixed in a solution of orange juice and dilute hydrochloric acid. For the infant, the radiopharmaceutical is mixed in formula and given by bottle or nasogastric tube. An additional ounce of water is then given to clear the esophagus of any residual radiopharmaceutical.

The gamma camera takes pictures while the patient is in a supine position and as the binder is gradually tightened by the inflatable cuff. Body position, abdominal pressure, and the presence of acid are used to aggravate the reflux. Images of the reflux of the radiopharmaceutical are taken, and the computer linkage provides graphic data to measure the degree of gastroesophageal reflux (Fig. 18–11). Each spike on the graph indicates an episode of reflux. The height of the spike indicates the amount of reflux, and the width of

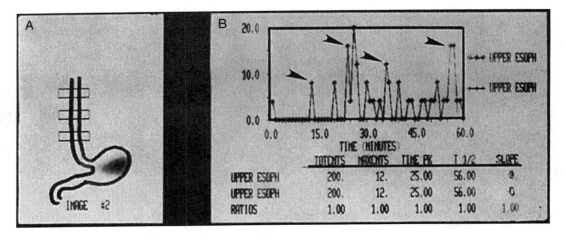

**Figure 18–11**

Gastroesophageal reflux scan. *A,* Anterior view of the chest and upper abdomen shows activity within the stomach and three computer regions of interest. *B,* Computer-generated graph of activity over the upper esophagus shows multiple spikes indicating significant reflux. (Reproduced with permission from Mettler, F. A., & Guiberteau, M. J. [1991]. *Essentials of nuclear medicine imaging* [3rd ed., p. 205]. Philadelphia: W. B. Saunders.)

the spike indicates the duration of the reflux (O'Hara, 1996). The procedure requires 2 hours of imaging time.

| **Findings** | **Elevated Values** |
|---|---|

Gastroesophageal reflux is caused by the following:

| | |
|---|---|
| Hiatal insufficiency | Achalasia |
| Hiatal hernia | Failed antireflux |
| Systemic progressive | surgery |
| sclerosis (sclero- | Esophageal spasm |
| derma) | |

**Interfering Factors**

- Failure to maintain a nothing-by-mouth status

**Nursing Implementation**

**Pretest**

Inform the patient about the procedure and obtain written consent from the patient or the person legally designated to make health care decisions for the patient.

Instruct the patient to discontinue all foods and fluids for 8 hours before the test. An alternative protocol is to fast from food for 8 hours and from fluids for 2 hours before the test (Mettler & Guiberteau, 1991).

**Posttest**

No special patient instruction or intervention is needed.

## Gastrointestinal Bleeding Scan

(Radionuclide Scan)          Synonyms: Gastrointestinal scan to investigate blood loss, GI scintigraphy

| Normal Values | No evidence of a focal area of bleeding |
|---|---|

### Background Information

The source of gastrointestinal (GI) bleeding (melena) is sometimes difficult to locate, particularly in the small bowel or colon. Endoscopic examination is often used but is not always successful. Heavy bleeding obscures the viewing tip of the endoscope, intermittent bleeding may not be active at the time, and the small bowel is too narrow and long for endoscopic visualization.

The GI bleeding scan uses nuclear imaging to identify the location of the bleeding. The intravenous radionuclide circulates through the vasculature until it reaches the site of the bleeding. There, it leaks through the break in the vascular wall and intestinal mucosa and accumulates in the intestinal lumen. The pooled blood and radionuclide is called a *focal area of increased activity*. The nuclear imaging process records the image of the pooled blood and the start of its peristaltic flow in the intestinal tract. This test is sensitive to small amounts of bleeding; it can detect a bleeding rate of 0.2 mL/min. The usual time required for this procedure is 30 to 45 minutes.

### Purpose of the Test

Technetium 99m sulfur colloid or technetium 99m–labeled red blood cells are administered to the patient intravenously. When tagged red blood cells are used, the source is the patient's own blood.

Using a scintillation camera, images of the abdomen and pelvis are taken at 5-minute intervals for 45 minutes and at 15- to 60-minute intervals thereafter as needed. With technetium 99m–labeled red blood cells, reimaging can be performed for up to 24 hours. The prolonged study time is used when early results are negative and bleeding is intermittent.

### Findings

**Abnormal Values**

| | | |
|---|---|---|
| Diverticula | Inflammatory bowel | Polyps |
| Ulcers | disease | Meckel's diverticulum |
| Angiodysplasia | Neoplasm | Intussusception |

### Interfering Factors

- Recent upper GI series or barium enema
- Pregnancy
- Hemodynamic instability due to blood loss

### Nursing Implementation

**Pretest**

Schedule this test before any barium studies are performed. Explain the procedure to the patient. Except for the venipuncture, the procedure is painless.

Obtain a written consent from the patient or the person legally designated to make health care decisions for the patient.

Take the vital signs and record the data in the patient's chart.

### Posttest

On return to the unit, take the patient's vital signs and assess for shock. Potential exists for acute bleeding while the patient is in the nuclear medicine unit or during transport back to the nursing unit.

## Gastrointestinal Cytologic Studies

**(Cytology)** Synonyms: None

| **Normal Values** | Within normal limits; no evidence of abnormal cells or infectious organisms |
|---|---|

### Background Information

Cytologic examination of tissue from the GI tract is dependent on the ability to collect cells from a specific lesion or precise area. Once the cells are collected, cytologic study and microscopic analysis provide information about cellular changes.

Specimens of the GI tract for cytologic study are usually obtained during an endoscopic procedure, including esophagogastroduodenoscopy, endoscopic retrograde cholangiopancreatography, and colonoscopy.

### Purpose of the Test

Cytologic study identifies benign or malignant growth that is evident in the biopsy specimen. It helps identify particular infections that cause characteristic cell changes. In some cases, the results are nonspecific. These results describe new epithelial tissue, also called *epithelial repair*. The presence of healing or repair implies that the new cellular activity is in response to an injury to the tissue.

### Procedure

During the endoscopic examination, specimens of tissue can be obtained by biopsy, brush technique, or washing technique. The specific methods of handling the biopsy tissue, the cytologic specimen, and the type of fixative can vary from one hospital to another. Generally, the endoscopy personnel coordinate the activity and procedure with the laboratory so that the tissue is not damaged or destroyed.

**Quality Control**

To avoid confusion from mislabeling, the laboratory requisition slip, the slides, and the specimen containers must include the patient's name and the source of the tissue.

**Biopsy Technique.** This is performed by passing a forceps through the endoscope and obtaining several small samples of suspicious tissue. The tissue samples are placed on a filter paper, and the paper is placed into a specimen jar with fixative solution.

**Brush Technique.** This involves the use of a disposable brush that is sent through the endoscope and passed over a suspicious area of tissue to obtain a sample of cells. The brush, with its cells and exudate, is placed in a jar of fixative solution. An alternative method is to pass the brush over a slide that is moistened with normal saline. The slide is then placed in preservative in a container, or it is sprayed with fixative.

**Washing Technique.**   This involves the use of the endoscope to inject 25 mL of normal saline onto the lesion, with subsequent aspiration of the fluid, cells, and exudate into a specimen cup.

### Quality Control

The specimen collected by washing technique must be placed in ice and sent to the laboratory immediately. Because no fixative is used, heat or time delay would result in lysis of the cells.

---

**Findings**

**Abnormal Values**

ESOPHAGUS

| | | |
|---|---|---|
| Herpes simplex virus | Epithelial repair | Large cell malignant |
| *Candida albicans* | Squamous cell | lymphoma |
| Cytomegalovirus | carcinoma | |
| Barrett's metaplasia | Adenocarcinoma | |

STOMACH

| | |
|---|---|
| *Candida albicans* | Large cell malignant |
| Intestinal metaplasia | lymphoma |
| Epithelial cell repair | |

COLON

| | |
|---|---|
| Cytomegalovirus | Squamous cell |
| Herpes simplex virus | dysplasia |
| Adenocarcinoma | Infectious colitis |

---

**Interfering Factors**

- Barium study within 2 to 3 days before endoscopy
- Failure to properly label or transport the specimen
- Food or particulate matter near the lesion

---

**Nursing Implementation**

Nursing measures are the same as those for the particular endoscopic procedure used in the collection of the tissue specimen.

---

## Paracentesis and Peritoneal Fluid Analysis

**(Peritoneal Fluid)**      Synonyms: Abdominal paracentesis, abdominal tap

---

**Normal Values**

**Peritoneal Fluid Analysis**
Appearance: Clear, odorless, pale yellow, scanty
Ammonia: <50 µg/dL
Amylase: 138–404 amylase units/L

*Continued on following page*

*Continued*

Bacteria and fungi: None present
Cells: No malignant cells present
Glucose: 70–90 mg/dL *or* SI 3.89–4.99 mmol/L
Protein: 0.3–4.1 g/dL *or* SI 3–41 g/L
Red blood cells: None
White blood cells: <300 cells per µL

## Background Information

Normal patients have less than 50 mL of peritoneal fluid and no distention of the abdominal cavity. Peritoneal fluid is an ultrafiltrate of plasma; the small amount is constant because the fluid formation and resorption are in homeostatic balance.

The accumulation of serous fluid in the peritoneal cavity is called *ascites*. This may occur because of increased hydrostatic or oncotic pressure in capillaries, altered permeability of the capillaries, or failure of the lymphatic system to reabsorb the fluid in sufficient amounts.

The peritoneal fluid is aspirated by paracentesis. The laboratory analysis of the fluid includes cytologic study, chemistry analysis, and microbiologic examination as requested.

In visual assessment of an abnormal specimen,

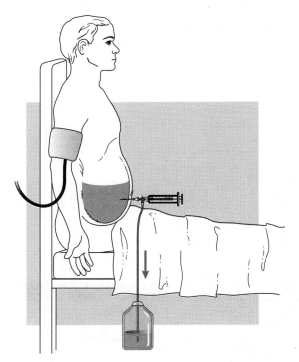

**Figure 18–12**
Paracentesis. The three-way stopcock controls the direction of the peritoneal fluid into the syringe or the drainage tubing and collection container.

the fluid can appear bright red and bloody, indicating rupture of an organ from blunt trauma. Cloudy fluid is often due to infection, strangulated bowel, or organ rupture. Greenish fluid can result from perforation of the duodenum or gallbladder, causing bile peritonitis. Milky fluid may be the result of blockage of the thoracic duct from causes such as malignancy, hepatic cirrhosis, adhesions, and infection from tuberculosis or parasites. When the ascites is advanced, the fluid volume can increase to 750 to 1,500 mL or more.

## Purpose of the Test

Abdominal paracentesis is used to obtain peritoneal fluid as part of the investigation of ascites, the effect of blunt abdominal trauma, or the cause of an acute abdomen when perforation is suspected.

## Procedure

**Paracentesis.** Under local anesthesia, a long, thin needle or trochar and stylet is inserted through the skin and into the peritoneal cavity. The insertion site is midline, about 2 inches below the umbilicus (Colodny, 1995). Either a syringe or a three-way stopcock with polyethylene tubing is used to draw off the fluid (Fig. 18–12). The procedure takes about 30 to 45 minutes to complete.

**Peritoneal Fluid.** For cell counts, a lavender-topped tube is used to collect 5 mL of fluid. For culture specimens, blood culture bottles are used. For cytology studies, at least 100 mL of fluid is collected in a sterile jar or collection bag (Henry, 1996).

## Findings

**Abnormal Values**

| | | |
|---|---|---|
| Peritonitis, bacterial | Chyle from a blocked | Tumor (benign, |
| Duodenal ulcer, | thoracic duct | malignant) |
| perforated | Pancreatitis | Infectious peritonitis |
| Traumatic rupture of | Hepatic cirrhosis | (tuberculous, |
| the bowel, gall- | Strangulated, infarcted | fungal, parasitic) |
| bladder, spleen, | bowel | Congestive heart |
| liver, or bladder | Hypoproteinemia | failure |
| Perforated intestine | Appendicitis | |

## Interfering Factors

- Contamination of the fluid by urine, feces, blood, or bile
- Pregnancy
- Coagulation disorder
- Intestinal obstruction
- Abdominal wall infection
- Uncooperative behavior
- History of multiple abdominal surgical procedures
- Portal hypertension

## Nursing Implementation

**Pretest**

Because of the risk of bleeding in the posttest period, obtain the hematocrit, prothrombin time, partial thromboplastin time, and platelet values within 48 hours of the test.

Explain the procedure to the patient and obtain written consent from the patient or the person legally responsible for making health care decisions for the patient.

Record baseline vital signs, temperature, weight, and measure of the abdominal girth.

When removal of a large volume of fluid is anticipated, the installation of a central venous pressure (CVP) line may be indicated. Record baseline CVP readings.

Just before the procedure, have the patient void to completely empty the bladder. This helps prevent an inadvertent puncture of the organ during the procedure.

Position the patient in a full Fowler's position. Some modification of position may be necessary according to the physician's preference.

### During the Test

Reassure the patient to alleviate fear. Some pain or a jolting sensation is felt when the needle or trochar penetrates the peritoneum. Encourage the patient to remain immobile during the procedure.

Assist with the collection of the fluid specimens.

Monitor vital signs every 15 minutes. Observe for pallor, dizziness, diaphoresis, or other signs of impending shock.

On removal of the needle, an adhesive bandage is applied to the puncture site. On removal of the trochar, a suture or two are used to close the abdomen, and a small dressing is applied to the incision.

### Posttest

Vital signs, a CVP reading, and an abdominal girth measurement are recorded. Thereafter, the vital signs and the CVP readings are taken every hour for 6 hours or until the patient is stable. When large amounts of fluid and albumin are removed from the peritoneal cavity, a rapid shift of fluid, potassium, and albumin from the circulation into the peritoneal cavity may occur. This can result in hypovolemia, hypokalemia, and hypotension or shock.

The dressing is checked frequently for excessive drainage or blood.

The nurse's note about the procedure describes the patient's tolerance of the test, the amount of fluid removed, and the color, odor, and characteristics of the fluid. The amount of peritoneal fluid is entered as output on the input-output record.

All specimens are appropriately labeled, including identification of the specimen as peritoneal fluid. The requisition slip states the specific laboratory analyses to be performed. The specimen bottles and collection tubes are all sent to the laboratory without delay.

---

**Complications**

The two complications of diagnostic paracentesis are hemorrhage and perforation of the bowel. Additionally, patients who have severe liver disease are at risk for the development of hepatic coma. A summary of the complications of paracentesis and the associated nursing assessments are found in Table 18–6.

## Percutaneous Peritoneal Biopsy

**(Cytology)**                    Synonyms: None

## Table 18–6   Complications of Abdominal Paracentesis

| Complication | Nursing Assessment |
|---|---|
| Hemorrhage | Hypotension<br>Tachycardia<br>Dyspnea<br>Diaphoresis and pallor<br>Acute abdomen or abdominal distress<br>Ecchymosis<br>Decreased hematocrit<br>Decreased CVP |
| Perforation of the bowel | Acute abdominal pain<br>Abdominal distention<br>Boardlike abdomen<br>Shock (hypotension, tachycardia)<br>Sepsis (fever) |
| Hepatic coma | Mental confusion<br>Lethargy<br>Drowsiness, stupor<br>Elevated serum ammonia |

## Background Information

The peritoneal biopsy is used to help evaluate un-explained ascites. It provides a tissue sample of the peritoneum and helps rule out tuberculosis, fungal infection, and metastatic carcinoma. The procedure used to obtain the sample is essentially the same as that for paracentesis. The specimen is obtained using a trochar, biopsy shaft, and snare. Once the biopsy shaft is in the peritoneal cavity, the snare is introduced down the shaft and is then drawn back until it touches the inner lining of the peritoneum. With rotation of the shaft, the snare removes a small scraping of tissue. This is repeated in several directions to obtain three to four tissue samples.

After withdrawal of the trochar, the tissue samples are placed in a jar with formalin preservative. The jar is labeled appropriately, including the tissue source and procedure used. The specimen is sent to the laboratory without delay (see also Gastrointestinal Cytologic Studies).

Following the test, the patient remains on bedrest for 6 hours. The vital signs are taken every hour for the 6 hours or until the signs are stable. The abdomen and dressing are assessed for swelling, ecchymosis, or leakage of peritoneal fluid.

## Roentgenography of the Abdomen

(Radiology)              Synonyms: Abdominal flat plate, flat plate of the abdomen

## Background Information

Plain radiographs of the abdomen provide information about gas patterns, air fluid levels in the GI tract, possible free air in the peritoneal cavity or retroperitoneal space, and areas of calcification.

Tumors, swelling of the mucosa, abscess formation, and fluid in the intestinal lumen can be identified by gas patterns. Air fluid levels can indicate intestinal obstruction. Calcifications inside or outside the intestinal tract are usually due to parasites or infections such as *Echinococcus, Cysticercus,* tuberculosis, and *Brucella.* Some tumors are calcified, such as Wilms' tumor, mucinous carcinoma of the stomach, and colloid carcinoma of the colon.

Other calcifications can be visualized in the kidneys, bladder, genital tract, and abdominal wall. Calcium salt deposits are visible in chronic inflammation of the gallbladder, pancreatitis, and myoma of the uterus. Additional discussion of plain roentgenography is presented in Chapter 9.

## Sigmoidoscopy and Anoscopy

**(Endoscopy)**          Synonyms: None

| Normal Values | No tissue abnormalities are seen in the sigmoid colon, rectum, or anus. |
|---|---|

### Background Information

*Sigmoidoscopy* uses a flexible, fiberoptic endoscope (sigmoidoscope) to examine the sigmoid colon and rectum. *Anoscopy* uses a short, blunt anoscope to examine the anus and rectum. Anoscopy is usually performed in conjunction with sigmoidoscopy or colonoscopy.

### Purpose of the Test

Sigmoidoscopy is used to screen for cancer of the colon in individuals age 50 years and older. It is also used to investigate the source of unexplained rectal bleeding, to evaluate the postoperative anastomosis of the colon, and to diagnose or monitor inflammatory bowel disease. Anoscopy is used to investigate anal symptoms such as bleeding, pain, discomfort, or prolapse.

### Procedure

The patient is placed in a lateral or knee-chest (jackknife) position (Fig. 18–13). No sedative or analgesic is needed, because the mucosa of the colon is relatively insensitive to pain. The well-lubricated instrument is inserted into the anus and advanced to the desired depth. A tissue biopsy or culture specimen may be obtained during the procedure. The time needed for the examination is 5 to 10 minutes.

**Quality Control**

The endoscope and accessory parts must be mechanically cleansed and then disinfected after each procedure. The goal is to remove organic matter and infectious agents, thus minimizing the potential for transmission of infection (Favero & Pugliese, 1996; Muscarella, 1996; Rutala, 1996).

### Findings

**Abnormal Values**

SIGMOIDOSCOPY

| | | |
|---|---|---|
| Colitis | Irritable bowel | Intestinal ischemia |
| Polyps | syndrome | Parasitic disease |
| Colorectal cancer | Sigmoid volvulus | |
| Gay bowel syndrome | Crohn's disease | |

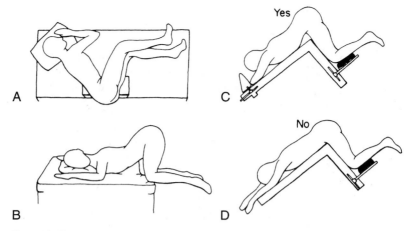

**Figure 18–13**

Three major positions for anoscopy and sigmoidoscopy. *A,* Left lateral (Sims') position. *B,* Knee-chest position. *C,* Prone, inverted jackknife position. *D,* An improper jackknife position is shown; the knee rest is too low, and no elbow rest is provided. (Reproduced with permission from Drossman, D. A. [1987]. *Manual of gastrointestinal procedures* [2nd ed., p. 128]. New York: Raven Press.)

ANOSCOPY

| | | |
|---|---|---|
| Hemorrhoids | Abscess formation | Perianal hematoma |
| Fissure | Adenomatous polyps | Prolapsed rectum |
| Fistula in ano | Anal herpes | |
| Crohn's disease | Squamous cell | |
| Pilonidal sinus with | carcinoma | |
| abscess | Anal condylomas | |

**Interfering Factors**

- Uncooperative patient behavior
- Severe bleeding
- Suspected bowel perforation
- Peritonitis
- Toxic megacolon
- Acute diverticulitis
- Paralytic ileus

**Nursing Implementation**    **Pretest**

Explain the procedure to the patient and obtain written consent from the patient or the person legally responsible for making the patient's health care decisions.

Because the protocol for bowel preparation varies, the examining physician should be consulted for specific instructions. The preparation usually consists of administering a combination of laxative and one or two Fleet enemas. The goal is to empty the lower colon of fecal matter.

### During the Test

Position and drape the patient.

Provide reassurance and promote relaxation during the procedure. A few deep breaths help to relax sphincter muscles. The patient may also feel cramping pain as air is instilled during the passage of the instrument.

Assist with the collection of tissue or other specimens.

### Posttest

Label any specimen containers, including the name of the procedure and the tissue source. Send specimens to the laboratory without delay.

Inform the patient that flatulence and mild gas pain may be experienced from the air that was put into the colon during the examination. When a biopsy is performed, it is normal to see a small amount of blood in the stool. Both these aftereffects are temporary. Advise the patient to contact the physician for problems of severe pain, nausea, vomiting, or heavy bleeding (Harper & Pope, 1997).

## Upper Gastrointestinal Series and Small Bowel Series

**(Radiology)**    Synonyms: Upper GI series, small bowel follow-through

| Normal Values | No structural or functional abnormalities are found. |
|---|---|

### Background Information

The upper GI series involves a radiologic examination from the oral part of the pharynx to the duodenojejunal junction. When the small bowel requires examination, the small bowel series often follows the upper GI series directly, but it can be performed as a single procedure.

The barium liquid is a chalky contrast medium that is taken orally. Because it is radiopaque, it outlines the size, shape, and contour of the intestinal lumen. Air may be instilled to provide double contrast and better visualization of the lumen of the esophagus, stomach, and duodenum (Levine, 1995). Fluoroscopy and x-ray films are used at intermittent intervals to obtain the gastrointestinal images.

The common sources of abnormality in the upper GI tract are stricture, inflammation, swelling, ulcers, tumors, motility disorders, or structural changes in the wall of the intestine.

### Purpose of the Test

The upper GI series detects disorders of structure or function of the esophagus, stomach, and duodenum. One week postoperatively, it is used to evaluate the results of gastric surgery, particularly when an anastomotic leak is suspected. As an extension of the upper GI series, the small bowel series detects disorders of the jejunum and ileum.

### Procedure

The patient drinks a barium solution to provide contrast views during swallowing and peristaltic action in the esophagus. As the barium coats the mucosal lining of the stomach, additional films are taken to outline the shape and contour of the organ (Fig. 18–14). The patient's positional changes (vertical, supine, prone, and lateral) help coat the mucosa throughout the organ.

When a small bowel series is included in this radiologic study, the transit time of the barium can be from 30 minutes to 6 hours before it reaches the colon. At the start of the small bowel series, additional barium is taken orally. The transit time can be shortened by having the patient drink 200 mL of iced water or eat a light meal after all the additional barium has left the stomach. Fluoroscopic views are taken three times in the first hour and every 30 minutes thereafter. Radiographic films are taken of any abnormality.

When the small bowel series is performed separately, enteroclysis may be used to instill the barium. A radiopaque catheter is passed through the nose or mouth and advanced past the pylorus and into the duodenum. Barium, followed by methylcellulose solution, is instilled by the catheter route directly into the small bowel. Views of the total small bowel can be completed in 20 to 30 minutes.

In a small bowel series, the barium may also be administered as an enema. As the barium moves in a retrograde direction through the ileocecal valve, the distal ileum can be better visualized. Alternatively, if the patient has

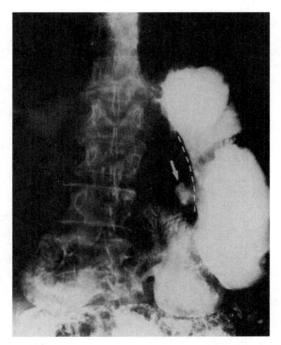

**Figure 18–14**
Upper gastrointestinal series view of a benign gastric ulcer. A large ulcer (*arrow*) is seen along the lesser curvature of the stomach. Notice that the ulcer projects out beyond the normal expected lesser curvature (*dotted line*). (Reproduced with permssion from Mettler, F. A. [1996]. *Essentials of radiology* [p. 191]. Philadelphia: W. B. Saunders.)

a mature ileostomy, the barium and air contrast can be instilled via a tube inserted into the ileostomy, for visualization of the distal bowel. In both these techniques, an intravenous injection of 1 mg of glucagon hydrochloride must be administered before instilling the barium (Herlinger, 1995). The action of the glucagon is to relax the smooth muscle of the bowel.

---

**Findings**

**Abnormal Values**

ESOPHAGUS

| | |
|---|---|
| Reflux esophagitis | Barrett's esophagus |
| Esophageal scarring or stricture | Infectious esophagitis |

STOMACH–DUODENUM

| | | |
|---|---|---|
| Peptic ulcer (gastric, duodenal) | Pyloric obstruction | Perforation |
| | Benign tumor | Diverticula |
| Cancer (stomach, duodenum) | Gastric inflammatory disease | |

SMALL BOWEL

| | | |
|---|---|---|
| Malabsorption | Lymphosarcoma | Disaccharidase deficiency |
| Crohn's disease | Diffuse sclerosis | |
| Chronic appendicitis | Surgical resection | Intussusception |
| Stricture | Congenital abnormality | Perforation |
| Hodgkin's disease | | |

---

**Interfering Factors**

- Failure to maintain nothing-by-mouth status
- Excess air in the small bowel

---

**Nursing Implementation**

**Pretest**

Explain the procedure to the patient and obtain written consent form the patient or the person legally responsible for making health care decisions for the patient.

Instruct the patient to fast from all food for 8 hours and all liquids for 4 hours before the test. Most oral medications are withheld in the 8 hours before the test. Narcotics and anticholinergics are withheld for 24 hours before the test because they slow the motility of the intestinal tract.

**During the Test**

The hospitalized patient may return to the nursing unit for an interval before the small bowel filming begins. Obtain instructions from the radiology department about the nothing-by-mouth status or about a prescribed meal.

**Posttest**

A laxative is given to help evacuate the barium promptly. Retained barium can cause constipation, obstruction, or fecal impaction.

Inform the patient that the feces will be gray or whitish for 24 to 72 hours until all barium has been evacuated.

The patient should plan to rest for the remainder of the day because the test is tiring.

## References

Allison, J. E., Tekawa, I. S., Ransom, L. J., & Adrain, A. L. (1996). A comparison of fecal occult-blood tests for colorectal cancer screening. *New England Journal of Medicine, 334*(3), 155–159.

Auringer, S. T., Sharling, E. S., & Summer, T. E. (1996). CT of the pediatric gastrointestinal tract. *Radiologic Clinics of North America, 34*(4), 701–715.

Aziz, D. C. (1996). Clinical use of tumor markers based on outcome analysis. *Laboratory Medicine, 27*(12), 817–821.

Breuninger, K. (1996). The utility of flexible sigmoidoscopy as a screening tool for colon cancer. *Journal of the American Academy of Nurse Practitioners, 8*(9), 431–432.

Brooks, M. J., Maxson, C. J., & Rubin, W. (1996). The infectious etiology of peptic ulcer disease. Diagnosis and implications for therapy. *Primary Care, 23*(3), 443–455.

Burt, R. W. (1997). Screening of patients with a positive family history of colorectal cancer. *Gastrointestinal Endoscopy Clinics of North America, 7*(1), 65–79.

Burtis C. A., & Ashwood, E. R. (1999). *Tietz textbook of clinical chemistry* (3rd ed.). Philadelphia: W. B. Saunders.

Church, J. M. (1992). Colonoscopy for the diagnosis and treatment of colorectal bleeding. *Seminars in Colon and Rectal Surgery, 3*, 42–46.

Cohen, L. B. (1996). Colorectal cancer: A primary care approach to screening. *Geriatrics, 51*(12), 45–50.

Cohen, S. M., Wexner, S. D., Binderow, S. R., Nogueras, J. J., Daniel, N., Ehrenpreis, E. D., Jensen, J., Bonner, G. F., & Ruderman, W. B. (1994). Prospective randomized endoscopic-blinded trial comparing precolonoscopy bowel cleansing methods. *Diseases of the Colon and Rectum, 37*(7), 689–696.

Collins, P. A., & Wright, M. S. (1997). Emerging intestinal protozoa: A diagnostic dilemma. *Clinical Laboratory Science, 10*(5), 273–278.

Colodny, C. S. (1995). Paracentesis and peritoneal lavage. *Patient Care, 29*(13), 137–138, 140, 145.

Corley, J., Yoder, J., Raibon, S., & Burke, G. (1995). Nuclear medicine's new role in peptic ulcer disease management. *Journal of Nuclear Medicine Technology, 23*(4), 299–300.

Dammel, T. (1997). Fecal occult-blood testing: Looking for hidden danger. *Nursing, 27*(7), 44–55.

Davidhizar, R., & Dowd, S. B. (1996). Fear in the patient with undiagnosed symptoms. *Journal of Nuclear Medicine Technology, 24*(4), 325–328.

DiMarino, A. J. (1996). Special report. Reprocessing of flexible endoscopes—an American society for gastrointestinal endoscopy white paper. *Gastroenterology Nursing, 19*(3), 109–112.

Eisenberg, P., & Muhs, S. M. J. (1996). QI study in the ICU: Bedside testing of gastric contents. *Nursing Management, 27*(3), 48J, 48L–48M.

Favero, M. S., & Pugliese, G. (1996). Infectious transmitted by endoscopy: An international problem. *American Journal of Infection Control, 24*(5), 343–345.

Fay, M., & Jaffe, P. E. (1996). Diagnostic and treatment guidelines for *Helicobacter pylori. Nurse Practitioner: American Journal of Primary Care, 21*(7), 28, 30, 33–34.

Fuchs, P. C. (1993). Infant stool specimens. *Medical Laboratory Observer, 25*(2), 11.

Garrett, C. T., Liscia, D. S., Nasim, S., & Ferreira-Gonzalez, A. (1995). Genetics of colorectal and breast cancer. *Clinics in Laboratory Medicine, 15*(4), 957–971.

Gore, R. M., & Ghahremani, G. G. (1995). Radiologic investigation of acute inflammatory and infectious bowel disease. *Gastroenterology Clinics of North America, 24*(2), 353–384.

Graham, D. Y., Evans, D. J., Peacock, J., Baker, J. T., & Schrier, W. H. (1996). Comparison of rapid serological tests (Flexsure HP and Quick Vue) with conventional ELISA for detection of *Helicobacter pylori* infection. *American Journal of Gastroenterology, 91*(5), 942–948.

Hageman, M., & Goei, R. (1993). Cleansing enema prior to double-contrast barium enema examination: Is it necessary? *Radiology, 187*(1), 109–112.

Harper, M. B., & Pope, J. B. (1997). Flexible sigmoidoscopy. *Primary Care, 24*(2), 341–357.

Hartwig, P. A. (1993). Patient education for endoscopy. *Seminars in Perioperative Nursing, 2*(3), 187–192.

*Helicobacter pylori.* (1997). *Laboratory Medicine, 28*(6), 405.

Henry, J. B. (1996). *Clinical diagnosis and management by laboratory methods* (19th ed.). Philadelphia: W. B. Saunders.

Herlinger, H. (1995). Guide to imaging of the small bowel. *Gastroenterology Clinics of North America, 24*(2), 309–329.

Jacobs, D. S., Dermott, W. R., Grady, H. J., Horvat, R. T., Huestis, D. W., & Kasten, B. L. (Eds.). (1996). *Laboratory test handbook* (4th ed.). Baltimore: Williams & Wilkins.

Klein, P. D., Hoda, M. M., & Martin, R. F. (1996). Non invasive detection of *Helicobacter pylori* infection in clinical practice: The $^{13}$C urea breath test. *American Journal of Gastroenterology, 91*(4), 690–695.

Lefton, H. B., Pilchman, J., & Harmatz, A. (1996). Colon cancer screening and the evaluation and follow-up of colonic polyps. *Primary Care, 23*(3), 515–524.

Lehmann, C. A. (1998). *Saunders manual of clinical laboratory science.* Philadelphia: W. B. Saunders.

Levine, M. S. (1994). The upper GI series: A call to arms. *Applied Radiology, 23*(4), 8.

Levine, M. S. (1995). Role of the double-contrast upper gastrointestinal series in the 1990's. *Gastroenterology Clinics of North America, 24*(2), 289–308.

Lipkus, I. M., Rimer, B. K., & Lyna, A. (1996). Colorectal screening patterns and perceptions of risk among African American users of a community health center. *Journal of Community Health, 21*(6), 409–427.

Lugay, M., Otto, G., Kong, M., Mason, D. J., & Wilets, I. (1996). Recovery time and safe discharge of endoscopy patients after conscious sedation. *Gastroenterology Nursing, 19*(6), 194–200.

Marley, R. A., & Moline, B. M. (1996). Patient discharge from the ambulatory setting. *Journal of Post Anesthesia Nursing, 11*(1), 39–49.

Massoni, M. (1997a). Gastrointestinal care. In: *Illustrated handbook of nursing care.* Springhouse, PA: Springhouse Corporation.

Massoni, M. (1997b). Gastrointestinal disorders. In *Diseases* (2nd ed.). Springhouse, PA: Springhouse Corporation.

Mettler, F. A. (1996). *Essentials of radiology.* Philadelphia: W. B. Saunders.

Mettler, F. A., & Guiberteau, M. J. (1991). *Essentials of nuclear medicine imaging* (3rd ed.). Philadelphia: W. B. Saunders.

Muscarella, L. F. (1996). High-level disinfection or "sterilization" of endoscopes? *Infection Control and Hospital Epidemiology, 17*(3), 183–187.

Noerr, B. (1995). Pointers in practical pharmacology. Midazolam (Versed). *Neonatal Network: Journal of Neonatal Nursing, 14*(1), 65–67.

Norris, T. E. (1997). Esophagogastroduodenoscopy. *Primary Care, 24*(2), 327–340.

O'Hara, S. M. (1996). Pediatric gastrointestinal nuclear imaging. *Radiologic Clinics of North America, 34*(4), 845–862.

Onders, P. P. (1997). Detection methods of *Helicobacter pylori:* Accuracy and costs. *American Surgeon, 63*(8), 665–668.

Pepe, J. L. (1993). Diagnostic techniques in blunt and penetrating trauma. *Topics in Emergency Medicine, 15*(1), 8–21.

Peterson, W. L., Barnett, C. C., Evans, D. J., Feldman, M., Carmody, T., Richardson, C., Walsh, J., & Graham, D. Y. (1993). Acid secretion and serum gastrin in normal subjects and patients with duodenal ulcer: The role of *Helicobacter pylori. American Journal of Gastroenterology, 88,* 2038–2043.

Peura, D. A., Pambianco, D. J., Dye, K. R., Lind, C., Frierson, H. F., Hoffman, S. R., Combs, M. J., Guilfoyle, E., & Marshall, B. J. (1996). Microdose 14C-urea breath test offers diagnosis of *Helicobacter pylori* in 10 minutes. *American Journal of Gastroenterology, 91*(2), 233–238.

Phillips, M. S. (1995). Drugs and sedation for colonoscopy. *Primary Care, 22*(3), 433–443.

Pieper, B. (1992). A study of persons undergoing outpatient gastrointestinal radiography. *Journal of ET Nursing, 19*(2), 54–58.

Podolski, J. L. (1996). Recent advances in peptic ulcer disease: *Helicobacter pylori* infection and its treatment. *Gastroenterology Nursing, 19*(4), 128–136.

Redei, I., & Rubin, R. N. (1995). Techniques for evaluating the cause of bleeding in the ICU. *Journal of Critical Illness, 10*(2), 133–137.

Robinson, R. (1995). Colonoscopy. *Primary Care, 22*(3), 399–409.

Rothstein, R. I., & Littenberg, B. (1995). Disposable, sheathed, flexible sigmoidoscopy: A prospective, randomized trial. *Gastrointestinal Endoscopy, 41*(6), 566–572.

Rutala, W. A. (1996). APIC guidelines for infection control practices. *American Journal of Infection Control, 24*(Suppl. 4), 313–342.

Saunderlin, G. (1995) Mechanical bowel preparation in review. *MEDSURG Nursing, 4*(4), 267–278, 304.

Seifert, B. (1997). *Helicobacter pylori. AORN Journal, 65*(3), 614–616, 619–620.

Selby, J. V. (1993). Disease prevention. Screening sigmoidoscopy for colorectal cancer. *Lancet, 341,* 728–729.

Spiegal, T. (1995). Flexible sigmoidoscopy training for nurses. *Gastroenterology Nursing, 18*(6), 206–209.

Sumner, T. E., & Auringer, S. T. (1996). Pediatric gastrointestinal radiology. *Radiologic Clinics of North America, 34*(4), 701–717.

Thijs, J. C., van Zwet, A. A., Thijs, W. S., Oey, H. B., Karrenbeld, A., Stellaard, F., Luijt, D. S., Meyer, B. C., & Kleibeuker, J. H. (1996). Diagnostic tests for *Helicobacter pylori.* A prospective evaluation of their accuracy, without selecting a single test as the gold standard. *American Journal of Gastroenterology, 91*(10), 2125–2129.

Tietz, N. W. (Ed.) (1995). *Clinical guide to laboratory tests* (3rd ed.). Philadelphia: W. B. Saunders.

Wagner, H. N., Szabo, Z., & Buchanan, J. W. (1995). *Principles of nuclear medicine* (2nd ed.). Philadelphia: W. B. Saunders.

Wagner, P. J., Kenrick, J. B., Rojas, T., & Woodward, L. D. (1995). Psychological considerations in colonoscopy. *Primary Care, 22*(3), 479–489.

Waltz, G. M., Ellett, M., Winchester, M., Horn, D., & Fitzgerald, J. (1996). A quality assurance monitor on preparation for outpatient lower endoscopic procedures. *Gastroenterology Nursing, 19*(5), 162–166.

Which test for occult fecal blood in children? (1994). *Emergency Medicine, 26*(7), 125–126.

Winawer, S. J. (1993). Colorectal cancer screening comes of age. *New England Journal of Medicine, 328*(19), 416–417.

Winawer, S. J., Flehinger, B. J., Schottenfeld, D., & Miller, D. G. (1993). Screening for colorectal cancer with fecal occult blood testing and sigmoidoscopy. *Journal of the National Cancer Institute, 85*(16), 1311–1318.

Winchester, C. B., Dhekne, R. D., Moore, W. H., & Murphy, P. H. (1994). Clinical applications of nuclear medicine in gastroenterology. *Gastroenterology Nursing, 17*(1), 1994.

# CHAPTER 19

# Hepatic, Biliary, Pancreatic, and Splenic Function

This chapter discusses the laboratory tests and diagnostic procedures used to identify dysfunction or abnormality in the liver, gallbladder, and pancreas (Table 19–1). These organs are in close proximity in the upper abdomen and share the biliary tree for drainage of bile. Because of the common location and shared structure, abnormalities can start in one organ and directly extend to the others. Usually, several laboratory tests and diagnostic procedures are needed to identify the specific source of the problem and to detect any extension of disease into the other organs.

The laboratory tests generally measure the metabolic functions of the liver, the exocrine functions of the pancreas, the effects of cholestasis in the liver or biliary system, and the presence of cellular damage or necrosis. No one laboratory test gives a specific diagnosis of, for example, cirrhosis of the liver; however, a combination of tests and a pattern of abnormal results provide strong indicators of organ damage and its cause.

The diagnostic procedures provide visualization of the structure and function of the liver, biliary system, and pancreas. With the use of radiography, radionuclide scanning, computed tomography scanning, endoscopy, and ultrasound, the size, shape, and contour of the organs and their ducts are revealed. From a biopsy specimen, microscopic analysis of tissue samples also provides data about the quality of the cells, their ability to function, and the cause of abnormality.

## Laboratory Tests

**Table 19–1 Laboratory Tests According to Organ Involvement**

| Organ | Test |
|---|---|
| Liver | Alanine aminotransferase |
| | Albumin, serum |
| | Albumin-globulin ratio |
| | Alkaline phosphatase |
| | Alkaline phosphatase isoenzymes |
| | Alpha$_1$-fetoprotein |
| | Ammonia |
| | Aspartate aminotransferase |
| | Bilirubin, total, serum |
| | Bilirubin, direct |
| | Bilirubin, indirect |
| | Carbohydrate antigen 19–9 |
| | Fat, fecal |
| | Gamma-glutamyltransferase |
| | Globulin, serum |
| | Hepatitis virus tests |
| | Lactate dehydrogenase |
| | Leucine aminopeptidase |
| | 5′-Nucleotidase |
| | Protein electrophoresis, serum |
| | Protein, total, serum |
| | Prothrombin time |
| | Urobilinogen, fecal |
| | Urobilinogen, urine |
| Gallbladder | Alkaline phosphatase |
| Biliary ducts | Alkaline phosphatase isoenzymes |
| | Alpha$_1$-fetoprotein |
| | Bilirubin, total, serum |
| | Bilirubin, direct |
| | Fat, fecal |
| | Gamma-glutamyltransferase |
| | Leucine aminopeptidase |
| | Lipase |
| | 5′-Nucleotidase |
| | Urobilinogen, fecal |
| | Urobilinogen, urine |
| Pancreas | Amylase, serum |
| | Amylase, urine |
| | Carbohydrate antigen 19–9 |
| | Gamma-glutamyltransferase |
| | Leucine aminopeptidase |
| | Lipase |
| | Trypsinogen, immunoreactive assay |
| | Sweat test |

## Alanine Aminotransferase

**(Serum)**    Synonyms: ALT, glutamic-pyruvic transaminase, SGPT, GPT, transaminase

**Normal Values**

Average adult range: 10–35 IU/L at 37°C
Male >60 years: 13–40 IU/L at 37°C
Female >60 years: 10–28 IU/L at 37°C
Male infant–adult <60 years: 15–35 IU/L at 37°C
Female infant–adult <60 years: 15–35 IU/L at 37°C
Male newborn–1 year: 13–45 IU/L at 37°C
Female newborn–1 year: 15–45 IU/L at 37°C

### Background Information

Alanine aminotransferase (ALT) is a transaminase enzyme that is found predominantly in the liver and to a lesser extent in the kidneys, heart, skeletal muscle, and pancreas. Some ALT is always present in the blood. Within the liver cells, the ALT is located in the cytoplasm of each hepatocyte.

When injury or necrosis of the liver cells occurs, the ALT enzyme leaves the cytoplasm, passes through the damaged cell membrane, and enters the serum. When acute hepatitis occurs, the serum level can rise to 20 times the normal value or more. In cases of obstructive jaundice, cirrhosis, and liver tumor, the ALT values will be mildly to moderately elevated, or two to four times the normal value.

The ALT enzyme value also rises slightly as a result of myocardial infarction, congestive heart failure, and shock. It is believed that in these conditions, an impaired blood supply and lack of adequate oxygenation to the liver exist, causing some liver damage and a rise in the hepatic source of the transaminase enzyme.

### Purpose of the Test

The ALT test is used to detect hepatocellular injury. It is the most specific of the transaminase enzyme tests in the detection of acute hepatitis from viral, toxic, or drug-induced causes. ALT values are usually compared to aspartate aminotransferase (AST) values (*ALT-to-AST ratio*) to help differentiate among the different forms of liver disease.

### Procedure

A red-topped, sterile tube is used to collect 10 mL of venous blood.

**Quality Control**

Venipuncture technique must be smooth, with a blood flow that fills the vacuum tube readily. If the blood has excessive turbulence because of flawed venipuncture technique, the hemolysis of the erythrocytes will alter the test results.

### Findings

**Elevated Values**

| | | |
|---|---|---|
| Acute or chronic hepatitis | Shock | Infectious mononucleosis |
| Myocardial infarction | Acute pancreatitis | Obstructive jaundice |
| Liver cell necrosis | Dermatomyositis | Muscular dystrophy |
| | Cirrhosis | |

| | | |
|---|---|---|
| Biliary obstruction | Fatty liver | Hemolytic anemia |
| Muscle trauma | Pregnancy-induced | Chronic alcohol |
| Liver tumor | hypertension | abuse |
| Recent surgery | Reye's syndrome | |

## Interfering Factors

- Hemolysis

## Nursing Implementation

Nursing actions are the same as for other venipuncture procedures.

### Pretest

Many medications cause an elevated test result. If they cannot be discontinued for 12 hours, list the medications on the requisition slip.

## Alkaline Phosphatase

(Serum)  Synonyms: ALP, total alkaline phosphatase, T-ALP

## Normal Values

Adult: 4.5–13 King-Armstrong units/dL *or* SI 32–92 U/L; 1.4–4.4 Bodansky units
Child: 15–30 King-Armstrong units/dL *or* SI 107–213 U/L; 5–14 Bodansky units
Infant: 10–30 King-Armstrong units/dL *or* SI 71–213 U/L

## Background Information

Serum alkaline phosphatase (ALP) is an enzyme that is located in the osteoblast cells of bone, in liver cells, and also in the intestines, kidney, and placenta. This enzyme is excreted via the biliary tract.

The function of any enzyme is to activate particular chemical reactions of cells in the region in which the enzyme is located. A high level of any enzyme usually means that a specific organ or tissue has increased synthesis or manufacture of the enzyme. Thus, the ALP enzyme will rise with increased osteoblast activity in bones during the healing of a fracture. The normally high level in children and adolescents is related to vigorous bone growth.

In the presence of a lesion or disease in tissue that contains the ALP enzyme, the level will also rise. Thus, the serum value of ALP will rise with biliary tract obstruction or hepatic malignancy as the affected tissue manufactures additional ALP enzymes.

## Purpose of the Test

Serum ALP testing provides a nonspecific indicator of liver disease, bone disease, or hyperparathyroidism. It is part of a battery of tests that evaluate liver function. It also serves as a nonspecific tumor marker, indicating rapid cell growth or accelerated function due to malignancy of the liver or bone.

## Procedure

A red-topped sterile tube is used to collect 10 mL of venous blood.

**Quality Control**

The serum must be kept refrigerated until analyzed, because heat or warmth will falsely elevate the results. The specimen should be analyzed within 4 hours, because the value will rise during the storage period.

**Findings**

**Elevated Values**

Cancer of the liver
Paget's disease
Biliary obstruction
  (gallstones or
  pancreatic cancer)
Osteogenic sarcoma
Bone metastases
Cholestasis
Osteomalacia

Sclerosing cholangitis
Rickets
Cirrhosis
Healing bone fracture
Acute fatty liver
Leukemia
Infectious mononu-
  cleosis
Myelofibrosis

Infiltrating liver
  disease (abscess,
  sarcoid, tubercu-
  losis, amyloidosis)
Acromegaly
Hyperthyroidism
Hyperparathyroidism
Tumors (such as
  hypernephroma)

**Decreased Values**

Malnutrition (protein
  deficiency, magne-
  sium deficiency, or
  both)

Hypophosphatemia
Hypothyroidism

**Interfering Factors**

- Pregnancy
- Healing bone fracture
- Fatty food intake 2 to 4 hours before the test

**Nursing Implementation**

Nursing actions are the same as for other venipuncture procedures.

**Pretest**

Instruct the patient to discontinue food intake for 12 hours before the test as indicated by laboratory policy. Foods in general, and fatty foods in particular, can elevate the test results in some individuals (Jacobs et al., 1996).

## Alkaline Phosphatase Isoenzymes

**(Serum)**          Synonym: I-ALP

**Normal Values**

Percent Inactivation after 16 Minutes at 55°C
  Liver isoenzymes: 50%–70%
  Bone isoenzymes: 90%–100%
  Intestine isoenzymes: 50%–60%
  Placental isoenzymes: 0%
  Regan isoenzymes: 0%

*Continued on following page*

*Continued*

> Fractional Inactivation after 16 Minutes at 55°C
> Liver isoenzymes: 0.5–0.7
> Bone isoenzymes: 0.9–1.0
> Intestine isoenzymes: 0.5–0.6
> Placental isoenzymes: 0
> Regan isoenzymes: 0

## Background Information

The isoenzymes of ALP are measurements of the components of the liver, bone, intestinal, placental, and Regan isoenzymes to the total ALP. The tests are not fully developed for clinical use, because interpretation is difficult and better methodology is still under development (Tietz, 1995).

The value of each isoenzyme is expressed as the percentage of isoenzyme that is inactivated after 16 minutes of exposure to heat at 55°C. Thus, the remainder of the total ALP is attributed to one of the other isoenzymes. This heat method is combined with serum electrophoresis to attain more specific results without overlap of values. In the older adult, the total ALP is composed of 40% bone isoenzymes and 60% liver isoenzymes.

## Purpose of the Test

When the total ALP level is elevated, the alkaline phosphatase isoenzymes help identify the source of the pathologic change in enzyme activity. Generally, the goal is to distinguish between liver and bone pathology.

## Procedure

A red-topped sterile tube is used to collect 10 mL of venous blood. It is not necessary for the patient to fast before the test.

### Quality Control

> The specimen is to be kept refrigerated until the analysis is performed.

## Findings

### Elevated Values

Bone isoenzyme: Increased osteoblastic activity
Liver I isoenzyme: Hepatic congestion, pregnancy
Liver II isoenzyme: Parenchymal cell damage

Biliary ALP: Cholestasis
Intestine ALP: Intestinal disease, patients with type O or type B blood
Placental ALP: Third trimester of pregnancy

Unidentified isoenzymes (Regan, Nagao): Neoplasm

## Interfering Factors

• Exposure of serum sample to heat

| Nursing Implementation | **Pretest** |
|---|---|
| | Nursing actions are the same as for other venipunctures. No additional preparation or intervention is needed. |

## Alpha₁-Fetoprotein

(Serum)    Synonyms: AFP, α₁-fetoprotein

| **Normal Values** | Adult: <10 ng/mL *or* SI <10 µg/L <br> Normal pregnancy: 5–50 ng/mL *or* SI 5–50 µg/L (Result rises to this maximum value in third trimester of pregnancy.) |
|---|---|

### Background Information

Alpha₁-fetoprotein (AFP) is synthesized by the fetal yolk sac and fetal liver. During pregnancy, it is found in fetal plasma, amniotic fluid, and maternal circulation. The normal value rises as the pregnancy progresses to term.

In normal, nonpregnant adults, AFP exists at low levels. The value will rise in liver disorders because of hepatocyte regeneration. Thus, some elevations are a result of healing activity after trauma to the liver, exposure to hepatotoxins, or exposure to the hepatitis virus.

### Purpose of the Test

In nonpregnant adults, this test serves as a tumor marker. AFP provides a strong indication of the diagnosis of primary hepatocellular carcinoma (hepatoma). In this condition, the value will rise to greater than 1,000 ng/mL (SI 1,000 µg/L) or even dramatically higher. Additionally, the test is diagnostic for testicular germinal carcinoma, including endodermal sinus tumor (yolk sac tumor), embryonal carcinoma, teratocarcinoma, and choriocarcinoma. These tumors can exist in nongonadal sites, as in the retroperitoneum and mediastinum. Additional procedures, such as scanning or biopsy, will be needed to confirm the diagnosis.

In patients who are being treated for hepatoma or germinal tumor, AFP values will be used to monitor the response to antineoplastic medications. A rising AFP level indicates increased tumor growth, and a falling value indicates a favorable response to the medications.

In the pregnant female, AFP is used for intrauterine screening, optimally in the 16th to 18th weeks of pregnancy. Abnormally elevated values are often present in cases of open neural tube deficits, which include spina bifida, myelomeningocele, and anencephaly. Other congenital defects may also cause an elevation of AFP.

Because this test can have false-positive results in pregnancy, the abnormal elevation is considered to be only suggestive of abnormality in the fetus. Other tests, such as ultrasound of the fetal spine and analysis of the amniotic fluid, are needed to provide additional data.

**Procedure**

A red-topped, sterile tube is used to collect 10 mL of venous blood. The patient does not need to fast for this test.

**Quality Control**

The specimen is kept refrigerated until the analysis is performed.

**Findings**

**Elevated Values**

NONPREGNANT STATE

| | | |
|---|---|---|
| Liver cancer | Cancer of the stomach | Necrosis of the liver |
| Gonadal germinal tumor | Cancer of the gallbladder | Hepatitis |
| Cancer of the pancreas | Cancer of the bile ducts | Cirrhosis |
| | | Liver trauma |

PREGNANT STATE

| | | |
|---|---|---|
| Spina bifida | Oligohydramnios | Pregnancy-induced hypertension |
| Myelomeningocele | Esophageal atresia | Abruptio placentae |
| Fetal death | Congenital nephrosis | |
| Anencephaly | Multiple pregnancy | |

**Interfering Factors**

• Recent radioisotope scan

**Nursing Implementation**

**Pretest**

Nursing actions are the same as for other venipuncture procedures. In addition, include the following data on the requisition slip: gestational age, maternal weight, race, and diabetic status. These are variables that affect the interpretation of the results.

## Ammonia

(Serum)    Synonym: $NH_3$

**Normal Values**

Adult: 15–45 µg/dL *or* SI 11–32 µmol/L
Child: 29–70 µg/dL *or* SI 21–50 µmol/L
Neonate: 90–150 µg/dL *or* SI 64–107 µmol/L

## Background Information

Ammonia, a byproduct of protein catabolism, is manufactured during the process of deamination of amino acids. It is made by the metabolizing tissues of the body and by bacterial activity that acts on protein in the intestine. As ammonia enters and circulates in the bloodstream, the liver pulls it out of the portal vein circulation. In hepatic metabolic function, the ammonia is used in the urea synthesis cycle and is converted to urea. The kidneys remove the urea from the circulation and excrete it in the urine. The two most common causes of an elevated ammonia level are the failure of hepatic cells to function in the conversion of ammonia to urea and the impairment of the portal vein circulation, which prevents ammonia from reaching the liver tissue (Fig. 19–1).

## Purpose of the Test

The ammonia level test is used to evaluate or monitor severe liver failure, hepatoencephalopathy, and the effects of impaired portal vein circulation. It is used in the preliminary identification of rare types of inborn errors of metabolism that affect the urea synthesis cycle of the neonate (aminoaciduria). It is also used to help diagnose Reye's syndrome, a childhood disorder that results in an acute fatty liver and encephalopathy.

## Procedure

A gray-, lavender-, or green-topped sterile tube is used to collect 7 to 10 mL of venous blood.

### Quality Control

The vacuum tube must be completely filled and then kept sealed to prevent a false-positive result. Once the blood is drawn, the vial must be placed on ice and rotated immediately to chill the specimen.

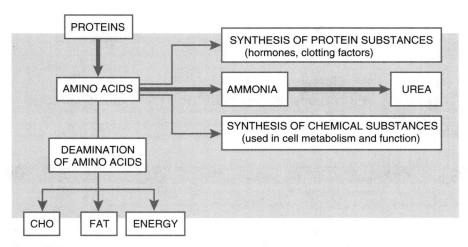

**Figure 19–1**
The synthesis of proteins by the liver. Ammonia is a toxic chemical byproduct created by the utilization of amino acids. Ammonia should be converted to urea by the liver and the urea excreted in urine. When ammonia is retained, the level rises in the blood. After it crosses the blood-brain barrier, the elevated ammonia level affects cerebral function and results in hepatic encephalopathy. CHO = carbohydrate.

| **Findings** | **Elevated Values** | |
| --- | --- | --- |
| | Liver failure (hepatic necrosis, terminal cirrhosis) | Inborn errors of metabolism that affect the urea synthesis cycle (some aminoacid-uria) |
| | Hepatoencepha-lopathy | |
| | Portal hypertension | Reye's syndrome |
| | Portacaval shunting of the blood | |

**Interfering Factors**

- Tobacco smoke
- High protein intake
- Gastrointestinal hemorrhage
- Hyperalimentation (total parenteral nutrition)
- Ureterosigmoidostomy

**Nursing Implementation**

Nursing actions are the same as for other venipuncture. In addition, review the following specific measures.

**Pretest**

Instruct the patient to fast from food for 8 hours before the test, because protein intake raises the ammonia level. Water intake is permitted.
Instruct the patient not to smoke before the test, because the smoke itself will alter the results.

**Posttest**

Ensure that the vial of blood is kept on ice and is sent to the laboratory immediately.

**Quality Control**

> The blood must be delivered to the laboratory in its ice container to avoid false-positive results.

## Amylase, Serum

**(Serum)**                                           Synonyms: None

**Normal Values**

> Adults: 27–131 U/L *or* SI 0.46–2.23 µkatal (µkat)/L
> Children >2 years: Same as adult values
> Neonates: 5–65 U/L *or* SI 0.09–1.11 µkat/L
> The normal values depend on the method of analysis. Use the reference values provided by the laboratory that performs the test (Jacobs et al., 1996).

## Background Information

Amylase is a group of enzymes manufactured in the exocrine pancreas and parotid glands. The digestive function is to hydrolyze starch and convert it to maltose. The alpha-amylase present in saliva converts some of the starch, but the vast majority of the activity results from pancreatic amylase. The lack of pancreatic amylase results in poor digestion of dietary starch.

When the acinar cells of the pancreas produce the amylase, the enzymes normally flow out through the pancreatic ducts, common bile duct, and ampulla of Vater to empty into the duodenum.

**Elevated Values.**   Inflammation or obstruction in any part of the pancreatic ducts or the common bile duct causes regurgitation of the amylase back into pancreatic tissue. The amylase is then absorbed into the bloodstream via the pancreatic venules and the lymphatics. In acute pancreatitis, the serum amylase value starts to rise in 2 to 12 hours, peaks in 12 to 72 hours, and returns to normal in 3 to 4 days (Lehmann, 1998). The elevated level in the blood is called *hyperamylasemia.*

Intestinal diseases such as perforated peptic ulcer, intestinal obstruction, mesenteric infarct, and other serious intestinal disorders can cause pancreatic inflammation or obstruction of the common duct and result in an elevated serum amylase value. Serum absorption of salivary amylase can occur with acute inflammation of the parotid glands, as in parotitis (mumps).

**Decreased Values.**   Mucoviscidosis is a congenital pancreatic disease that causes dysfunction of mucus-secreting glands. Thick, viscid mucus obstructs the pancreatic ductal system, causing acinar cell atrophy and cystic fibrosis of the pancreas. In children or adults who have advanced cystic fibrosis, the serum amylase levels are decreased.

## Purpose of the Test

The serum amylase test is used to investigate the cause of abdominal pain or epigastric pain, with the goal of differentiating between acute pancreatitis and a surgical emergency such as perforation of the stomach or infarct of the bowel. It helps in the diagnosis of acute pancreatitis, traumatic injury to the pancreas, or a surgical complication that affects the pancreas.

## Procedure

A red-topped, sterile tube is used to collect 10 mL of venous blood.

### Quality Control

Personnel should not talk, sneeze, or cough near an open collection tube. Their saliva will add to the amylase content of the specimen.

## Findings

### Elevated Values

| | | |
|---|---|---|
| Acute pancreatitis | Obstruction of the common bile duct | Pancreatic pseudocyst |
| Trauma to the pancreas | Intestinal obstruction | Aortic aneurysm |
| Obstruction of the ampulla of Vater | Pancreatic cancer | Pancreatic ascites |
| Parotitis (mumps) | Perforated peptic ulcer | Traumatic shock |
| | | Pancreatic abscess |

### Decreased Values

| | | |
|---|---|---|
| Chronic pancreatitis | Cirrhosis | Hepatitis |
| Pancreatic cancer | Toxemia of pregnancy | Cystic fibrosis |

| | |
|---|---|
| **Interfering Factors** | • Ingestion of alcohol before the test<br>• Recent use of morphine, which closes Oddi's sphincter |

| | |
|---|---|
| **Nursing Implementation** | Nursing actions are the same as for other venipuncture procedures. In addition, include the following information in the nursing plan. |

### Pretest

Instruct the patient not to ingest alcohol for 24 hours before the test. Alcohol stimulates the secretion of salivary amylase. No other fasting measures are required.

Before the test, morphine, codeine, meperidine (Demerol), and other drugs that affect amylase levels may be omitted.

| | |
|---|---|
| **Critical Value** | **An increase of greater than three times the upper limit of the normal value**<br><br>Severe increases are significant, and the physician must be notified. The sudden rise in the serum amylase value is usually a result of acute pancreatitis or of an acute surgical condition of the abdomen. Assess the patient for signs of acute abdominal pain. Describe the pain, including any increase in severity. Assess the vital signs, looking for indications of shock. |

## Amylase, Urine

**(Urine)**                Synonyms: None

| | |
|---|---|
| **Normal Values** | Adults<br>    2–19 U/hr (1-hr test)<br>    4–37 U/2 hr (2-hr test)<br>    170–2,000 U/24 hr (24-hr test) *or* SI 2.89–34.0 μkat/L |

### Background Information

Amylase is excreted or cleared from the body in the urine. When the serum amylase level is elevated, the glomerular filtration rate increases, and a greater amount of amylase clearance occurs. The amount of amylase clearance is measured in units per volume in a specified period.

| | |
|---|---|
| **Purpose of the Test** | Urine amylase testing can help diagnose acute pancreatitis when the serum levels are borderline or normal. The urinary amylase levels remain elevated for up to 2 weeks after the onset of acute pancreatitis, as compared with the serum level that declines after 3 to 4 days. |

| | |
|---|---|
| **Procedure** | Urine is collected in a clean container for a specific period. The most common time span is 1 or 2 hours, but 6-, 8-, or 24-hour collection periods are sometimes used. |

**Findings**

**Elevated Values**

Acute pancreatitis
Cancer of the head of
   the pancreas
Pancreatic pseudocyst
Gallbladder disease

Obstruction (pancre-
   atic ducts,
   intestine, salivary
   glands)
Parotitis (mumps)

**Decreased Values**

Alcoholism
Hepatitis

Hepatic abscess
Chronic pancreatitis

Cirrhosis
Cancer of the liver

**Interfering Factors**

- Heavy menstrual flow
- Bacterial contamination of the urine
- Salivary amylase contamination of the specimen
- Omission of any voided specimen
- Failure to cool the specimen

**Nursing Implementation**

**Pretest**

Instruct the patient not to ingest alcohol for 24 hours before the test. Alcohol stimulates the secretion of salivary amylase.

Just before the start of the test, instruct the patient to void and discard the specimen. This urine has been in the bladder for an unknown period of time.

All subsequent specimens are collected and added to the clean urine container, including the final voided urine of the period.

During the test, refrigerate the container of urine or place the container in a basin of ice. Amylase is unstable in acidic urine.

On the specimen label and the requisition slip, write the date and time for the start and finish of the test.

## Aspartate Aminotransferase

**(Serum)**    Synonyms: AST; glutamate oxaloacetate transaminase, serum; SGOT; GOT; transaminase

**Normal Values**

Average adult range: 8–20 U/L
Male adult >60 years: 11–26 U/L
Female adult >60 years: 10–20 U/L
Child <5 years: 19–28 U/L
Infant: 16–72 U/L
Newborn: 16–72 U/L

## Background Information

Aspartate aminotransferase (AST) is a transaminase enzyme found predominantly in the heart, but it is also highly concentrated in the liver. It is present to a lesser extent in skeletal muscle, kidney, brain, pancreas, spleen, and lungs. Some concentration of AST is always found in the blood. Most of the AST within the liver cells is located in the mitochondria of hepatocytes. The discussion of the AST test as a laboratory test in heart disease is presented in Chapter 15.

When mild injury, inflammation, or necrosis of liver cells occurs, the AST is released through damaged cell membranes and results in rising levels within the serum. With severe damage, the mitochondria of the hepatocytes are destroyed, and greater amounts of AST are released. In severe or fulminant viral hepatitis, the AST value can rise to 20 to 100 times the normal value.

Because AST is also present in skeletal muscle tissue and other organs, the serum AST value will rise because of inflammation, injury, or necrosis of those tissues. Generally, these elevations are slight to moderate, although shock, acute pancreatitis, and infectious mononucleosis occasionally cause a severe elevation of the serum value.

**AST-to-ALT Ratio.**   Comparisons of AST to ALT are sometimes used to differentiate among the causes of hepatocellular damage. The results are expressed as a ratio of AST to ALT. Because the amounts of each enzyme are about equal, the ratio is expressed as AST = ALT, or the normal value of AST:ALT = 1.

In alcoholic hepatitis, the AST value is greater than the ALT value (AST >ALT), or the ratio is expressed numerically. For example, AST:ALT = 3:1 means that the AST value is three times greater than the ALT value. It is proposed that alcohol is toxic to the mitochondria of the hepatocytes and that therefore the AST level rises to more than the ALT level. Conversely, the ALT value can rise to greater than the AST value (ALT >AST). This is often true in viral hepatitis.

---

### Purpose of the Test

AST is an indicator of inflammation, injury, or necrosis of the tissues that contain the enzyme. It shows moderate elevation for a timed interval after myocardial infarction. In liver disease, it is an indicator of hepatocellular damage from any cause.

The AST test is also used to monitor liver function in patients who receive medication that is potentially hepatotoxic.

---

### Procedure

A red-topped sterile tube is used to collect 10 mL of venous blood.

**Quality Control**

Venipuncture technique must be smooth, with blood flow that fills the tube readily. If the blood has excessive turbulence because of flawed venipuncture technique, the hemolysis of erythrocytes will alter the results.

---

### Findings

**Elevated Values**

| | | |
|---|---|---|
| Myocardial infarction | Cardiac arrhythmias | Heart failure |
| Renal infarction | Legionnaires' disease | Cerebral necrosis |
| Pericarditis | Post–cardiac surgery, | (trauma, cerebro- |
| Pulmonary infarction | catheterization | vascular accident, |
| | Acute pancreatitis | craniotomy) |

Dermatomyositis
Polymyositis
Muscular dystrophy
Hepatitis (viral,
   toxic)
Hemochromatosis
Cirrhosis

Trichinosis
Cancer of the liver
Delirium tremens
Obstructive jaundice
Gangrene
Infectious mononu-
   cleosis

Severe injury to
   skeletal muscle
   tissue
Shock

**Decreased Values**

Pregnancy

---

**Interfering Factors**

- Hemolysis
- Failure to maintain a nothing-by-mouth status
- Intense exercise before the test

---

**Nursing Implementation**

Nursing actions are the same as for other venipunctures. In addition, review the following.

**Pretest**

Instruct the patient to fast for 12 hours before the test.
Advise the ambulatory patient to avoid strenuous exercise before the test.

---

**Critical Value**

**An AST value greater than three times the upper limit of normal or an AST-to-ALT ratio greater than 1**

Notify the physician of this very elevated result. Many commonly prescribed medications have a potential for hepatotoxicity. The rise above the critical value is usually an indicator to discontinue the medication. Patients who are alcoholic and take only moderate doses of acetaminophen are vulnerable to severe hepatotoxicity, demonstrated by dramatic elevations of the AST value (Jacobs et al., 1996).

---

## Bilirubin

**(Serum)**

Synonyms: Total bilirubin: Blood bilirubin, serum bilirubin, plasma bilirubin
Direct bilirubin: Conjugated bilirubin
Indirect bilirubin: Unconjugated bilirubin, free bilirubin
Neonatal bilirubin: Total bilirubin, neonatal; baby bilirubin; microbilirubin

---

**Normal Values**

**Total Bilirubin**
Child–adult: 0.3–1.2 mg/dL *or* SI 5–21 µmol/L
Full-term neonate (by 24 hours after birth): 1.4–8.7 mg/dL *or* SI 24–149 µmol/L

*Continued on following page*

*Continued*

**Direct Bilirubin**
  Adult: 0–0.2 mg/dL *or* SI <3.4 µmol/L
**Indirect Bilirubin**
  Adult: <1.1 mg/dL *or* SI <19 µmol/L

---

## Background Information

**Production.**  Bilirubin is produced in the reticuloendothelial cells, primarily Kupffer's cells of the liver. It is also produced in the reticuloendothelial cells of the spleen, bone marrow, and lymph nodes. Most bilirubin is formed from the hemoglobin as the reticuloendothelial cells break down senescent erythrocytes that have reached the end of their 120-day life span. The remainder of bilirubin formation is from the enzymes that contain heme and from the destruction of damaged, abnormal erythrocytes that have a short life span.

**Transport.**  Once bilirubin is produced, it is transported in plasma to the liver. In this transport process, bilirubin is bound to molecules of albumin and is called *indirect* or *unconjugated* bilirubin. A small amount of the unconjugated bilirubin remains in the plasma circulation, but the rest of it is acted on by the liver to convert it to direct, conjugated bilirubin.

**Conjugation.**  Within the liver cells, indirect bilirubin is first separated from the albumin. It is then acted on by the enzyme glucuronyl transferase, is conjugated with glucuronic acid, and is transformed into direct, conjugated bilirubin. The conjugated bilirubin is a water-soluble, yellow-green pigment that can now cross the cell membrane and enter bile canaliculi. As it mixes with fluid, the conjugated bilirubin becomes a component of bile.

**Excretion.**  The excreted bile flows from canaliculi and hepatic ducts within the liver to the biliary ductal system. Bile and its conjugated bilirubin component are concentrated and then stored in the gallbladder. The bile exits to the duodenum via the cystic and common ducts for ultimate elimination in feces. The physiologic basis for the bilirubin diagnostic tests is presented in Table 19–2.

**Jaundice.**  This is a clinical term that describes the yellow discoloration of the skin and sclera caused by excess bilirubin in the blood and body tissues. The jaundice becomes visible when the total serum bilirubin level rises to greater than 2 mg/dL. The elevated serum bilirubin level is called *hyperbilirubinemia.*

One method of classification of jaundice is based on the predominant type of elevation of bilirubin in the blood. A rise in the unconjugated bilirubin is usually a result of excessive hemolysis of red blood cells and is sometimes called *hemolytic jaundice.* A rise in the conjugated bilirubin is usually a result of obstruction in the flow of bile and is sometimes referred to as *cholestasis.* The obstruction can occur at any level, from bile canaliculi to the ampulla of Vater or from intrahepatic to extrahepatic sites.

A second method of classification is based on three possible locations of the problem. They are the *prehepatic, hepatic,* and *posthepatic* categories of jaundice.

**Prehepatic Jaundice.**  This means that the problem occurs before the bilirubin reaches the liver. The causes are all hemolytic, and more erythrocytes are hemolyzed than can be transported or conjugated. Thus, the elevation of bilirubin is a result of the rise in the indirect or unconjugated component.

**Hepatic Jaundice.**  This means that the origin of the problem is within the liver. Some of the abnormalities are due to an inability to transport or conjugate bilirubin within hepatocytes, resulting in an elevation of indirect, unconjugated bilirubin. Other abnormalities are a result of blockage in the excretion of the bile within the liver, and the problem is referred to as *intrahepatic cholestasis.* The blockage can occur at the cell level when injured or diseased hepatocytes cannot permit conjugated bilirubin to cross the cell membranes or exit from the bile canaliculi and hepatic ducts. When conjugated bilirubin cannot be excreted, a resultant rise in the serum values occurs.

**Posthepatic Jaundice.**  This means that the origin of the problem is outside or beyond the liver;

### Table 19–2    Physiologic Basis for Bilirubin Diagnostic Tests

| Anatomic Sites | Physiology of Bilirubin: Formation, Transport, and Excretion | Diagnostic Tests |
|---|---|---|
| Reticuloendothelial system | Hemolysis of senescent and abnormal erythrocytes | |
| Circulation | Transport of unconjugated bilirubin to the liver | Indirect serum bilirubin |
| Liver | Conversion of unconjugated to conjugated bilirubin Excretion of bilirubin in bile salts and bile | Total serum bilirubin and direct serum bilirubin |
| Biliary ductal system | Concentration, transport, storage, and excretion of bile | |
| Intestine | Conversion of direct bilirubin to urobilinogen Excretion of urobilinogen | Fecal urobilinogen |
| Kidney | Filtration and excretion of urobilinogen and bilirubin | Urine urobilinogen Urine bilirubin |

■

*Critical Thinking 19–1*
A 2-day-old infant is to be discharged from the newborn nursery. The value of the neonate's total bilirubin has risen to 10 mg/dL (SI 171 μmol/L). What are important parts of a discharge plan for this baby and her parents?

it is sometimes called *extrahepatic cholestasis.* The bile flow is obstructed somewhere in the biliary ductal system, including at the head of the pancreas, within the ampulla of Vater, and in the common bile duct. In these cases, a rise in the direct, conjugated bilirubin value also occurs. A summary of the classifications of jaundice is presented in Table 19–3.

**Neonatal Jaundice.**   Newborn infants experience varying levels of elevated bilirubin in the first few days of life. The condition is called *physiologic jaundice.* It is not clear why this condition occurs, but it is temporary. The condition may be a result of excess hemolysis of red blood cells, a transient defect in glucuronyl transferase enzyme activity, or a reabsorption of unconjugated bilirubin from the intestine.

Other causes of neonatal jaundice are considered abnormal or pathologic, including ABO or Rh incompatibility that causes a great increase in unconjugated bilirubin. If the bilirubin level is greater than 20 mg/dL, potential exists for bilirubin encephalopathy or kernicterus. In kernicterus, bilirubin is deposited in the brain, and permanent damage can occur. The possible causes include hemolysis of erythrocytes, impaired ability of the liver to conjugate bilirubin, impaired ability of the unconjugated bilirubin to bind to albumin for transport, and impairment in the conjugation of bilirubin.

If the infant is born with biliary atresia, the extrahepatic biliary ducts are blocked. A rapid, severe rise in conjugated bilirubin will occur.

---

**Purpose of the Test**

Total serum bilirubin is the sum total of indirect unconjugated bilirubin and direct conjugated bilirubin in the blood. The purpose of the total bilirubin test is to evaluate liver function, diagnose jaundice, monitor the progression of jaundice, and determine whether an infant needs treatment to prevent kernicterus.

The purpose of the indirect and direct bilirubin tests is to help identify the underlying cause of hyperbilirubinemia.

**Table 19–3    Classification of Jaundice**

| Category of Jaundice | Origin of the Problem | Type of Bilirubin Elevation |
|---|---|---|
| Prehepatic | Excessive hemolysis of erythrocytes<br>Hemolytic jaundice | Indirect (unconjugated) |
| Hepatic | Defect in transport or conjugation in hepatocytes<br>Physiologic jaundice | Indirect (unconjugated) |
| | Injury to or disease of hepatocytes<br>Blockage of intrahepatic bile ducts<br>Intrahepatic cholestasis | Direct (conjugated) |
| Posthepatic | Blockage in the biliary ductal system<br>Extrahepatic cholestasis | Direct (conjugated) |

**Procedure**

**Adult.**   A red-topped, sterile tube is used to collect 10 mL of venous blood.
**Infant.**   A blue capillary tube is used to draw drops of blood from the heel, which has been pricked by a sterile lancet.

**Quality Control**

Venipuncture technique must be smooth, with a blood flow that fills the vacuum tube readily. If the blood flow has excessive turbulence because of flawed venipuncture technique, hemolysis of the erythrocytes will alter the test results.

**Findings**

**Elevated Values**

TOTAL SERUM BILIRUBIN

Hepatocellular damage (toxic or neoplastic)
Biliary tree obstruction (intra- or extrahepatic)

Neonatal (physiologic jaundice)
Hemolytic diseases
Gilbert's disease (familial hyperbilirubinemia)

Dubin-Johnson syndrome

DIRECT BILIRUBIN

Hepatotoxins causing necrosis
Cirrhosis
Cancer of the liver, gallbladder, ampulla of Vater, or pancreas

Dubin-Johnson syndrome
Pregnancy
Medications
Sclerosing cholangitis
Lymphoma
Primary biliary cirrhosis

Parasites
Biliary atresia
Acute pancreatitis
Biliary stones
Infection of liver

INDIRECT BILIRUBIN

Familial defects of
   erythrocytes
   (spherocytosis,
   sickle cell disease)
Hodgkin's disease
Malaria
Medications
Traumatic tissue
   injury with
   hemorrhage or
   hematoma

Familial enzyme
   disorders (glucuro-
   nyl transferase
   deficiency, Gilbert's
   disease)
Neonatal jaundice
Rh or ABO incom-
   patibility
Blood transfusion
   reaction due to
   incompatibility

## Interfering Factors

- Sunlight
- Hemolysis
- Failure to maintain a nothing-by-mouth status (adults only)

## Nursing Implementation

Nursing care for capillary puncture and venipuncture is presented in Chapter 2.

### Pretest

Instruct the patient to fast from food for 8 to 12 hours (overnight), because serum lipids will alter results.

### Posttest

Ensure that the vial of blood or microcapillary tube is covered and sent to the laboratory without delay.

### Quality Control

Because bilirubin is photosensitive, the blood sample must be protected from exposure to light or prolonged time in a lighted environment.

## Critical Value

**Neonatal Bilirubin**
   **Term infants: >15 mg/dL *or* SI >257 μmol/L**
   **Premature infants: >10–15 mg/dL *or* SI 171–257 μmol/L**

Notify the physician of this very elevated result. The elevation is considered pathologic, rather than physiologic, jaundice. The baby must be reevaluated medically to determine the cause of the hyperbilirubinemia. Phototherapy will be considered at this blood level. If the level goes higher, phototherapy will be initiated, and exchange blood transfusion may also become necessary (Berrios & Jain, 1996).

# Carbohydrate Antigen 19–9

**(Serum)**                           Synonym: CA 19–9

| **Normal Values** | Adult: <37 U/mL *or* SI <37 kU/L |
| --- | --- |

## Background Information

Carbohydrate antigen 19–9 (CA 19–9), an oncofetal antigen, is a tumor marker found in the blood. This antigen appears in the serum of adults when (1) the cells of particular organs undergo healing and regeneration and (2) malignant cells that are known to produce the antigen proliferate in tumors.

As a tumor marker, CA 19–9 is most accurate for pancreatic cancer, with a positive result in 72% to 100% of cases (Aziz, 1996). It is also highly accurate in many cases of cancer of the liver, some cases of colorectal cancer, and some cancers in other locations. In pancreatic cancer, the test does not identify an early onset of the disease. The accuracy rate is highest in a late stage of tumor growth and in recurrence (Jacobs et al., 1996).

Malignancy causes this result to rise dramatically. Large tumors of the pancreas can cause the result to rise to >1,000 U/mL. To stage the cancer (i.e., to determine whether surgical removal of the tumor is an option), a CA 19–9 test result greater than 300 U/mL is an indicator that the pancreatic tumor may not be resectable. In the patient with colorectal cancer, elevation of CA 19–9 is an ominous finding (Aziz, 1996).

After surgical removal of a malignancy, the CA 19–9 may be used to monitor or predict recurrence, particularly for pancreatic, liver, gastrointestinal, head and neck, gallbladder, biliary duct, and gynecologic cancer (Jacobs et al., 1996). After treatment, a recurrent rise in CA 19–9 is an indicator that a relapse has occurred. The test result rises before clinical symptoms exist.

Benign conditions, such as hepatic cirrhosis, or conditions that cause pancreatitis or jaundice can cause a false-positive elevation of the CA 19–9. Benign disease tends to produce a lower elevation than does cancer, with a test value greater than 70 U/mL (Lehmann, 1998).

## Purpose of the Test

CA 19–9 is a tumor marker that is used in preoperative staging of cancer of the pancreas. It is also used to monitor the course of the disease and the success of therapy and to predict the recurrence of cancer. Because of problems with sensitivity and specificity, CA 19–9 is not used as a screening tool for asymptomatic patients.

## Procedure

A red-topped tube with a serum separator is used to obtain 5 to 10 mL of venous blood.

## Findings

**Elevated Values**

MALIGNANCY

| | |
| --- | --- |
| Cancer of the pancreas | Hepatobiliary cancer |
| Cancer of the stomach | Cancer of the lung |
| | Cancer of the head and neck |
| Cancer of the colon | Gynecologic cancer |

BENIGN CONDITIONS

| | |
| --- | --- |
| Hepatobiliary disease | Acute pancreatitis |

| **Interfering Factors** | • None |

| **Nursing Implementation** | **Pretest** |

Nursing care for venipuncture is presented in Chapter 2.
Provide emotional support for the patient. Ongoing testing for cancer and
tumor markers is upsetting because of the implications of a positive result.

## Ceruloplasmin
**(Serum)**                              Synonyms: None

| **Normal Values** | Adult: 18–45 mg/dL *or* SI 180–450 mg/L<br>Neonate–3 months: 5–18 mg/dL *or* 50–180 mg/L |

### Background Information

Ceruloplasmin, an alpha$_2$ globulin, is a copper-binding protein that is synthesized by the liver. Its exact function is unknown, but the serum ceruloplasmin contains most of the total plasma copper. As an enzyme, it may be important in the release of iron from ferritin so that the iron can bind to transferrin.

**Elevated Values.**   Ceruloplasmin is one of a group of serum proteins that are part of the body's response designed to handle extensive insult or injury. The serum ceruloplasmin level rises in condi-tions of inflammation, infection, surgery, trauma, and malignancy.

**Decreased Values.**   A low level of ceruloplasmin is associated with malabsorption, protein loss, and advanced liver disease that results in inadequate manufacture of all serum proteins. A low ceruloplasmin level is specifically associated with Wilson's disease, an autosomal recessive disease that results in the deposit of copper in all body tissues, including the brain and liver.

| **Purpose of the Test** | Ceruloplasmin testing is used to evaluate chronic active hepatitis, cirrhosis, and other liver diseases. Because low levels can indicate Wilson's disease, the test is also used to help diagnose unexplained central nervous system disorders that affect coordination. |

| **Procedure** | A red-topped, *chilled,* sterile tube is used to collect 10 mL of venous blood. |

**Quality Control**

Venipuncture technique must be smooth, with a blood flow that fills the vacuum tube readily. If the blood has excessive turbulence because of flawed venipuncture technique, the hemolysis of the erythrocytes will alter the results.

**Findings**

### Elevated Values

| | | |
|---|---|---|
| Inflammation | Trauma | Systemic lupus |
| Leukemia | Malignancy |   erythematosus |
| Tissue necrosis | Primary biliary | Rheumatoid arthritis |
| Hodgkin's disease |   cirrhosis | |

### Decreased Values

| | | |
|---|---|---|
| Wilson's disease | Malabsorption | Hepatocellular |
| Menkes' disease |   syndrome |   disease |
| Nephrotic syndrome | | |

**Interfering Factors**

- Pregnancy
- Hemolysis
- Failure to maintain a nothing-by-mouth status

**Nursing Implementation**

Nursing actions are similar to those used in other venipuncture procedures. In addition, review the following information.

### Pretest

Instruct the patient to fast from food and fluids for 12 hours before the test. High levels of serum lipids will affect the results.

Inform the laboratory when the patient is pregnant or taking oral contraceptives. High levels of estrogen will cause high levels of ceruloplasmin.

### Posttest

Ensure that the vial of blood is placed on ice and sent to the laboratory immediately.

### Quality Control

| |
|---|
| Prolonged exposure to room temperature will result in a falsely depressed value. |

## Fecal Fat

**(Feces)**

Synonyms: Fecal lipids; fat, quantitative; 72-hour stool collection; stool fat, quantitative

**Normal Values**

Adult: <7 g/24 hr
Adult (fat-free diet): <4 g/24 hr
Child (newborn–6 years): <2 g/24 hr
Infant (breast-fed): <1 g/24 hr

## Background Information

In normal digestive processes, dietary fats undergo digestion and absorption in the small intestine. The first stage is emulsification of the neutral fats or triglycerides by bile acids and bile salts. In this emulsification process, the bile acts as a detergent and breaks the globules of fat into tiny droplets. This provides a large surface for lipolytic activity by the pancreatic enzyme lipase.

In the second stage, the pancreatic lipase splits the fat molecule into free fatty acids, glycerol, and glyceride (monoglycerides and diglycerides), the end products of fat digestion. Bile salts then surround some of these end products and carry them to the mucosal cell membranes for absorption by the small intestine. The free fatty acids and mono-glycerides are soluble and are absorbed directly into the small intestine without the assistance of the carrier mechanism.

In normal digestion, virtually all fatty acids, monoglycerides, and triglycerides are absorbed. The normal adult excretes only a small portion of fat in the feces. When malabsorption of fat occurs, a high level of fat appears in the feces and is called steatorrhea. The possible causes are (1) a lack of bile flow into the intestine, (2) pancreatic insufficiency, and (3) damage to the mucosal cells of the small intestine.

| | |
|---|---|
| **Purpose of the Test** | The fecal fat test is the definitive test to identify steatorrhea. It does not define the cause of the problem but rather evaluates the ability to digest fat from dietary intake. Abnormal results support evidence of hepatobiliary, pancreatic, or small intestinal disease. |
| **Procedure** | For 3 days preceding the test and during the 3 days of specimen collection, the patient eats a standard, high-fat diet (100 g of fat per day). The 72-hour collection of feces is performed on days 4, 5, and 6 of the diet. All fecal matter in the 72-hour period is collected in a clean, heavy plastic, screw-capped container. The specimen is refrigerated during the collection period. |

## Findings

**Elevated Values**

| | | |
|---|---|---|
| Pancreatic insufficiency | Cystic fibrosis | Intestinal tuberculosis |
| Regional enteritis | Gastroduodenal fistula | Impaired hepatic function |
| Pancreatic obstruction | Chronic pancreatitis | Dumping syndrome |
| Celiac disease | Extensive small bowel resection | Thyrotoxicosis |
| Pancreatic resection | Biliary tract obstruction | Psoriasis |
| Tropical sprue | Scleroderma | Addison's disease |
| Whipple's disease | Liver cirrhosis | Lymphomas |
| Radiation enteritis | | |

| | |
|---|---|
| **Interfering Factors** | • Use of improper collection container<br>• Contamination of the sample<br>• Failure to follow the dietary prescription<br>• Incomplete collection—omission of any specimen |

- Alcohol ingestion before or during the test
- Ingestion of mineral oil before or during the test

---

**Nursing Implementation**

### Pretest

Instruct the patient to follow the prescribed diet for 3 days before and 3 days during the test. Ingestion of alcohol is omitted for 24 hours before collection and during the 3 days of collection.

Instruct the patient about proper collection procedure, including the correct type of container (see Chapter 2).

### Quality Control

Improper containers include coffee cans, paper cartons, waxed containers, or plastic bags. The specimen must be free of urine, toilet paper, tongue depressors, and plastic spoons.

### During the Test

Ensure that the specimen is refrigerated for the entire collection period and until it is transported to the laboratory.

■
*Critical Thinking 19–2*
When the patient is told to keep the specimen in the refrigerator, she refuses. How can you resolve this problem?

### Posttest

Write the time and date for the start and finish of the collection period on the container label and on the requisition slip.

---

## Gamma-Glutamyltransferase

**(Serum)** Synonyms: γ-Glutamyltransferase, γ-glutamyl transpeptidase, GGT, GGTP, GTP, GT

---

**Normal Values**

Male adult: 22.1 ±11.7 U/L *or* SI 0.38 ±0.020 µkat/L
Female adult: 15.4 ±6.58 U/L *or* SI 0.26 ±0.11 µkat/L
Male child >6 months: 2–30 U/L *or* SI 0.03–0.51 µkat/L
Female child >6 months: 1–24 U/L *or* SI 0.02–0.41 µkat/L

---

### Background Information

Gamma-glutamyltransferase is a biliary enzyme that is present in cell membranes and microsomes of cells. It is most predominant in the kidneys, but it is also amply present in the liver and pancreas. The enzyme's probable functions are to assist in the transport of amino acids across cell membranes and in glutathione metabolism.

The serum level of gamma-glutamyltransferase rises when intrahepatic or posthepatic biliary obstruction exists. This laboratory value will rise early and remain elevated as long as the dysfunction persists.

---

### Purpose of the Test

The gamma-glutamyltransferase test is used to detect hepatobiliary disease. The gamma-glutamyltransferase values will rise parallel with the values of ALP, leucine aminopeptidase, and 5′-nucleotidase in conditions of posthepatic jaundice and in diseases of the liver and pancreas.

In the presence of elevated ALP, the gamma-glutamyltransferase level is used to differentiate between hepatobiliary and bone sources of abnormality.

The gamma-glutamyltransferase test is also used to diagnose and evaluate chronic alcoholic liver disease. It can detect the resumption of drinking in the alcoholic patient.

| | |
|---|---|
| **Procedure** | A red-topped sterile tube is used to collect 10 mL of venous blood. |

**Findings**

**Elevated Values**

Obstructive biliary disease

Infectious mononucleosis

Obstructive liver disease

Hyperthyroidism

Acute liver disease

Systemic lupus erythematosus

Acute pancreatitis

Myocardial disease

Hepatoma

Following renal transplantation

Cancer of the pancreas

**Decreased Values**

Hypothyroidism

**Interfering Factors**

- Intake of alcohol within 60 hours before the test
- Use of medications such as barbiturates, phenytoin, and oral contraceptives

**Nursing Implementation**

Nursing actions are similar to those used in other venipuncture procedures. In addition, review the following information.

**Pretest**

Instruct the patient to abstain from alcohol for 72 hours before the test. Inform the patient to fast from food and fluids for 12 hours before the test. Inform the physician or laboratory staff of the use of medications that interfere with the results. Patients who must continue to take these medications should not suspend the dosage schedule. An alternative test such as leucine aminopeptidase or 5′-nucleotidase may be preferable.

## Hepatitis Virus Tests

In acute and chronic hepatitis, at least six distinct viruses can cause the infection, inflammation, and cell necrosis in the liver. The viruses are identified as hepatitis viruses A (HAV), B (HBV), C (HCV), D (HDV), E (HEV), and G (HGV). Hepatitis G virus, recently discovered, is transmitted parenterally, particularly by blood transfusion. Its role in posttransplant hepatitis is not yet understood (Belli, Ideo, & Silini, 1997; Bryan, 1995; Lehmann, 1998; Rodriguez Inigo et al., 1997).

To confirm the exact cause of the infection, many of the laboratory tests detect the presence of the specific viral antigen or antibody in the patient's blood. These tests are commercially available for all the hepatitis viruses except the hepatitis G virus. The tests for detection of the hepatitis B virus are confusing, because antigen and antibody tests are available for the core, the surface, and the degradation products of this virus. The patterns of emergence and disappearance of these antigens and antibodies are used to identify the virus and the stage of the illness.

Molecular analysis is the most recent technologic development and is used to identify and measure the amount of the hepatitis B and C viruses. In molecular analysis, polymerase chain reaction (PCR) technique amplifies or multiplies the DNA sequence of the hepatitis B virus, and a specific nucleic acid probe identifies the virus by matching the genetic sequence (Jacobs et al., 1996). In similar methodology, the reverse transcriptase-polymerase chain reaction (RT-PCR) technology is used to identify the RNA in the genetic material of the hepatitis C and E viruses. The technique of molecular assay is still at a research stage for hepatitis E and G viruses, and the tests are not commercially available (Lehmann, 1998; Rodriguez Inigo, 1997).

The diagnosis of hepatitis is usually based on the clinical manifestations and on liver function test results. These hepatitis virus tests are used to determine which of the viruses has caused the infection. Once the specific virus is identified, the patient's treatment and epidemiologic interventions are more accurate.

## Hepatitis A Antibody

**(Serum)**                     Synonyms: HAV, Ab; HAVAb; anti-HAV

| **Normal Values** | Hepatitis A antibody: Negative<br>IgM type: Negative<br>IgG type: Negative |
| --- | --- |

### Background Information

The hepatitis A virus is transmitted by the fecal-oral route, primarily after ingestion of virus-contaminated water, food, milk, or shellfish. Although the antigen has been found in fecal matter, the serologic diagnosis is based on the presence of hepatitis A antibodies in the blood.

Two types of hepatitis A antibodies exist: the immunoglobulin M (IgM) type and the immuno-globulin G (IgG) type. The IgM type, also called anti-HAV IgM, appears early. It is present in the blood within 1 week after symptoms begin. It peaks within 3 months and subsides in 4 to 6 months during convalescence. The IgG type, also called anti-HAV total or hepatitis A antibody IgG, begins to rise after 4 weeks of infection and persists for life (Fig. 19–2).

### Purpose of the Test

The hepatitis A virus antibodies identify the hepatitis A virus as the cause of infection. The specific antibody type distinguishes between current and past infections.

### Procedure

A red-topped, sterile tube is used to collect 10 mL of venous blood.

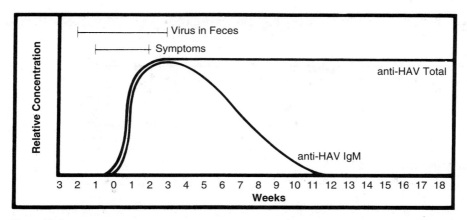

**Figure 19–2**
Hepatitis A diagnostic profile. (Reproduced with permission from Abbott Laboratories. [1992].
*Principles in practice: Testing for viral hepatitis.* North Chicago, IL: Author.)

**Quality Control**

Venipuncture is always performed with gloves, and needles should be used and disposed of carefully. When hepatitis is suspected, extra attention to technique should help prevent needlestick injury or contact with blood from splashes.

---

**Findings**

**Elevated Values**

Hepatitis A virus antibody: Hepatitis A infection
IgM: Current hepatitis A infection, acute or convalescent stage

IgG: Old hepatitis A infection with permanent immunity to reinfection by the hepatitis A virus

---

**Interfering Factors**

• Recent administration of radioisotopes

---

**Nursing Implementation**

Nursing actions are similar to those used in other venipuncture procedures, with the following additional measures.

**Pretest**

To alert the laboratory personnel, write on the requisition slip that hepatitis is suspected.
Until the specific virus type is identified, apply standard precautions. This infection is contagious before symptoms of the illness exist.

## Hepatitis B Core Antibody

**(Serum)**    Synonyms: Anti-HBc, AHBC, antibody to hepatitis B core antigen, core antibody HBcAb

---

**Normal Values**    Hepatitis B core antibody: Negative
Type IgM: Negative
Type IgG: Negative

---

### Background Information

The hepatitis B core antibody is a marker of hepatitis B infection in the acute or chronic phase of illness or is a marker of past illness. This hepatitis B core antibody appears after 1 to 2 weeks of infection, before symptoms appear. It rises during the acute stage, with a peak and plateau during convalescence several months later. It remains elevated for months to years and is considered a lifetime marker of past infection (Fig. 19–3). When the subtypes are tested, a positive IgM result indicates an acute infection, and a positive IgG result indicates a chronic infection or carrier state.

---

**Purpose of the Test**    The hepatitis B core antibody test is used to assess the stage of hepatitis B infection.

---

**Procedure**    A red-topped, sterile tube is used to collect 10 mL of venous blood.

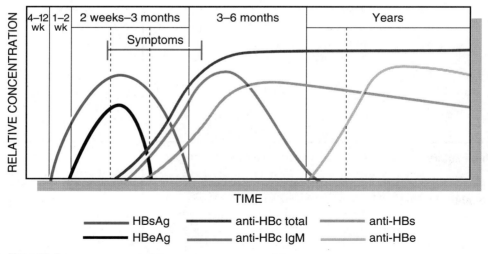

**Figure 19–3**
Viral markers in hepatitis B infection. The various antigen and antibody responses are present at specific times in the course of the infection. (Reproduced with permission from Lehmann, C. A. [1998]. *Saunders manual of clinical laboratory science.* Philadelphia: W. B. Saunders.)

**Quality Control**

> Venipuncture is always performed with gloves, and needles should be used and disposed of carefully. When hepatitis is suspected, extra attention to technique helps prevent needlestick injury or contact with splashing blood.

| **Findings** | **Elevated Values** | | |
|---|---|---|---|
| | Hepatitis B core antibody: Hepatitis B infection | IgM: Acute or convalescent stage | IgG: Chronic stage or past infection |

**Interfering Factors**

- Recent administration of radioisotopes

**Nursing Implementation**

Nursing actions are similar to those used in other venipuncture procedures, with the following additional measures.

**Pretest**

To alert the laboratory personnel, write on the requisition slip that hepatitis is suspected.
Until the specific virus type is identified, institute standard precautions.

## Hepatitis B e Antibody

**(Serum)**    Synonyms: Anti-HBe, HBeAb

**Normal Values**    Anti-HBe: Negative

## Background Information

In hepatitis B infection, the hepatitis B e antibody indicates reduced infectivity with lower potential for the transmission of infection to others. The antibody usually appears after the hepatitis B e antigen disappears, or about 3 months after the onset of infection (see Fig. 19–3). This antibody to the hepatitis B e antigen can persist for years but by itself is not considered a marker for hepatitis B infection.

**Purpose of the Test**

The hepatitis B e antibody test helps stage the course of the illness and is a prognostic indicator.

**Procedure**

A red-topped, sterile tube is used to collect 10 mL of venous blood.

**Quality Control**

Venipuncture is always performed with gloves, and needles should be used and disposed of carefully. When hepatitis is suspected, extra attention to technique should help prevent needlestick injury or contact with the blood from splashing.

| **Findings** | **Elevated Values** | | |
|---|---|---|---|
| | Reduced infectivity in convalescence | Reduced infectivity in a carrier state | Reduced infectivity in chronic infection |

**Interfering Factors**

• Radioactive scan in the preceding week

**Nursing Implementation**

Nursing actions are similar to those used in other venipuncture procedures, with the following additional measures.

**Pretest**

To alert the laboratory personnel, write on the requisition slip that hepatitis is suspected.
Until the specific virus is identified, institute standard precautions.

## Hepatitis B e Antigen

**(Serum)** Synonym: HBeAg

**Normal Values**

Hepatitis B e antigen: Negative

### Background Information

The hepatitis B e antigen is found in patients infected with the hepatitis B surface antigen. The hepatitis B e antigen appears in the serum about 1 week after the hepatitis B surface antigen appears, persists for 3 to 6 weeks, and disappears about 1 week before the hepatitis B surface antigen disappears (see Fig. 19–3).

In the acute stage of hepatitis B infection, the hepatitis B e antigen indicates the period of greatest infectivity and ability to transmit the infection to others. The presence of the hepatitis B e antigen beyond 12 weeks is an indication of a chronic carrier state with potential for chronic liver disease.

**Purpose of the Test**

The hepatitis B e antigen determination is used in the diagnosis and prognosis of hepatitis B infection.

**Procedure**

A red-topped sterile tube is used to collect 10 mL of venous blood.

**Quality Control**

Venipuncture is always performed with gloves, and needles should be used and disposed of carefully. When hepatitis is suspected, extra attention should be paid to technique so that needlestick injury or contact with blood from splashes is avoided.

| Findings | **Elevated Values** | | |
|---|---|---|---|
| | Increased infectivity in acute stage | Increased infectivity and chronic carrier of hepatitis B | Chronic liver disease |

**Interfering Factors**

- Radioactive scan in the preceding week

**Nursing Implementation**

Nursing actions are similar to those used in other venipuncture procedures, with the following additional measures.

**Pretest**

To alert the laboratory personnel, write on the requisition slip that hepatitis is suspected.
Until the specific virus is identified, institute standard precautions.

## Hepatitis B Surface Antibody

**(Serum)**    Synonyms: HBsAb, anti-HBs, antibody to hepatitis B surface antigen, HBsAgAb, hepatitis B s antibody

**Normal Values**    Hepatitis B surface antibody: Negative

### Background Information

The hepatitis B surface antibody appears several weeks to several months after the hepatitis B surface antigen has disappeared. It remains during convalescence and may or may not disappear after recovery (see Fig. 19–3). The presence of this antibody usually, but not always, indicates that recovery is complete and that immunity now exists to any recurrent hepatitis B infection. If this antibody and the hepatitis B core antibody are present simultaneously, immunity to recurrent hepatitis B infection is definite.

**Purpose of the Test**

The hepatitis B surface antibody test is used to evaluate possible immunity or the need for vaccination in individuals at high risk for the development of hepatitis B infection. It is also used to evaluate the need for hepatitis B immune globulin after a needlestick incident.

**Procedure**

A red-topped, sterile tube is used to collect 10 mL of venous blood.

**Quality Control**

Venipuncture is always performed with gloves, and needles should be used and disposed of carefully. When hepatitis is suspected, extra attention to technique should help prevent needlestick injury or contact with splashing blood.

---

**Findings**

**Elevated Values**

Convalescent stage of hepatitis B infection

Clinical recovery from hepatitis B infection

---

**Interfering Factors**

• Recent administration of radioisotopes

---

**Nursing Implementation**

Nursing actions are similar to those used in other venipuncture procedures, with the following additional measures.

**Pretest**

To alert the laboratory personnel, write on the requisition slip that hepatitis is suspected.

Until the specific virus is identified and stage of infectivity is known, institute standard precautions.

---

## Hepatitis B Surface Antigen

**(Serum)**                    Synonyms: HBsAg, HAA, hepatitis-associated antigen

---

**Normal Values**

Hepatitis B surface antigen: Negative

---

### Background Information

The hepatitis B virus is transmitted by a parenteral route, for example, exposure to infected blood or blood products, sexual transmission, and perinatal exposure. The best markers indicating the presence of hepatitis B infection are the hepatitis B surface antigen and the hepatitis B e antigen.

The hepatitis B surface antigen is present 2 to 4 weeks before liver enzyme levels become elevated and up to 5 weeks before the patient demonstrates clinical symptoms. During the course of the illness, the values of the hepatitis B surface antigen rise, peak, and then decline steadily over a 12-week period as the infection resolves (see Fig. 19–3). In a different pattern, if the hepatitis B surface antigen rises to a plateau and remains elevated for 4 to 6 months or more, the patient is probably a carrier of hepatitis B virus or has a chronic hepatitis B infection.

---

### Purpose of the Test

The hepatitis B surface antigen test is used to identify the specific type of hepatitis and to diagnose the infection in its acute or chronic stage. It is used to screen the blood of potential donors, with rejection of those with positive results. It is also used to evaluate risk in needlestick incidents involving health care personnel.

| | |
|---|---|
| **Procedure** | A red-topped tube is used to obtain 10 mL of venous blood. |

**Quality Control**

Venipuncture is always performed with gloves, and needles should be used and disposed of carefully. When hepatitis is suspected, extra attention to technique helps prevent contact with the blood from a needlestick injury or splashing.

| | |
|---|---|
| **Findings** | **Elevated Values** |

| | | |
|---|---|---|
| Active acute hepatitis B infection | Active chronic hepatitis B infection | Chronic carrier of hepatitis B surface antigen |

| | |
|---|---|
| **Interfering Factors** | • Recent administration of radioisotopes |

| | |
|---|---|
| **Nursing Implementation** | Nursing actions are similar to those used in other venipuncture procedures, with the following additional measures. |

**Pretest**

To alert the laboratory personnel, write on the requisition slip that hepatitis is suspected.
Until the specific virus is identified, institute standard precautions.

## Hepatitis B Viral DNA Assay

**(Serum, Liver Tissue)** Synonym: HBV DNA probe test

| | |
|---|---|
| **Normal Values** | Negative; no hepatitis B virus DNA detected |

## Background Information

The DNA of the hepatitis B virus can be detected by molecular analysis of the nuclear material. Polymerase chain reaction (PCR) technique is used to amplify or multiply the genetic material of the virus. A specific target probe is used to identify the DNA sequence of the hepatitis B virus.

This test is used when the antigen and antibody results are negative in a patient suspected of having hepatitis B infection. The amount of virus (viral load) also can be quantified by this test (Jacobs et al., 1996).

| | |
|---|---|
| **Purpose of the Test** | This test helps diagnose the chronic carrier state of hepatitis B infection and helps establish the stage of the disease. |

**Procedure**

**Serum.** A lavender- or red-topped tube is used to obtain 7 or 10 mL of venous blood.

**Tissue.** A sample of liver biopsy tissue is placed in a sterile container. The container is sealed in a plastic bag.

**Quality Control**

Venipuncture and liver biopsy are always performed with gloves, and needles should be used and disposed of carefully. When hepatitis is suspected, extra attention to technique helps prevent contact with the blood from a needlestick injury or splashing.

**Findings**

**Elevated Values**

Hepatitis B infection

**Interfering Factors**

• Recent radioactive isotope scan

**Nursing Implementation**

Nursing actions are similar to those used in other venipuncture procedures, with the following additional measures.

**Pretest**

To alert the laboratory personnel, write on the requisition slip that hepatitis is suspected.

Until the specific virus is identified, institute standard precautions.

## Hepatitis C Antibody

**(Serum)**  Synonym: Anti-HCV

**Normal Values**

Hepatitis C antibody: Negative

**Background Information**

The hepatitis C virus is responsible for most cases of posttransfusion hepatitis. The virus is spread via a blood transfusion from an infected donor; parenterally through the use of contaminated needles, as in intravenous drug use; and by exposure to the blood and body fluids of an infected person.

The hepatitis C antibody appears in the blood some time after the patient is infected. The antibody appears from 3 to 9 weeks after infection and disappears with full recovery. If the infection is chronic, the antibody will persist at an elevated level.

**Purpose of the Test**

The hepatitis C antibody determination is used to diagnose hepatitis and the specific virus involved. The test is also used to screen the blood of potential donors, with rejection of those with positive results.

| **Procedure** | A red-topped, sterile tube is used to collect 10 mL of venous blood. |
|---|---|

### Quality Control

Venipuncture is always performed with gloves, and care is taken in the use and disposal of contaminated needles. When hepatitis is suspected, one should be especially careful to prevent needlestick injury or contact with splashing blood.

| **Findings** | **Elevated Values** |
|---|---|

Hepatitis C infection,
   acute or chronic

| **Interfering Factors** | • Recent administration of radioisotopes |
|---|---|

| **Nursing Implementation** | Nursing actions are similar to those used in other venipuncture procedures, with the following additional measures. |
|---|---|

### Pretest

To alert the laboratory personnel, write on the requisition slip that hepatitis is
   suspected.
Until the specific virus is identified, institute standard precautions.

## Hepatitis C-RNA Assay

**(Serum, Liver Tissue)**    Synonyms: None

| **Normal Values** | Negative; no hepatitis C viral RNA is detected. |
|---|---|

## Background Information

Hepatitis C is responsible for most cases of post-transfusion hepatitis. It may be the causative agent in hepatitis associated with hemodialysis and often causes infection in the intravenous drug user. Until recently, the hepatitis C antibody test was the only test available, but it did not show a positive result for 3 to 9 months after infection (Lehmann, 1998). The molecular analysis method of identifying the hepatitis C-RNA shows a positive result when only a small amount of virus is present. It also detects the virus within 1 to 2 weeks of exposure (Neiblum & Boynton, 1996).

In this test, the RNA is extracted from viral nuclei in the serum or liver biopsy tissue of the infected individual. The viral RNA is changed to DNA by reverse transcriptase (RT). Then, polymerase chain reaction (PCR) technique is used to amplify or make copies of the DNA material. A special nucleic acid probe identifies the DNA of the hepatitis C virus and can quantify the amount of the virus (viral load) that is present (Kuhns, 1995).

| **Purpose of the Test** | This test is used to diagnose hepatitis C virus and monitor the response to treatment. |
|---|---|

**Procedure**

**Serum.**   A red-topped tube is used to obtain 10 mL of venous blood.

**Tissue.**   A sample of liver biopsy tissue is placed in a sterile container. The container is sealed in a plastic bag.

**Quality Control**

Venipuncture and liver biopsy are always performed with gloves, and needles should be used and disposed of carefully. When hepatitis is suspected, extra attention to technique helps prevent contact with the blood from a needlestick injury or splashing.

**Findings**

**Elevated Values**

Hepatitis C infection, acute, convalescent, or chronic

**Interfering Factors**

- Recent radioactive isotope scan
- Delay in separating the serum from the blood sample
- Warming of the tissue specimen

**Nursing Implementation**

Nursing actions are similar to those used in other venipuncture procedures, with the following additional measures.

**Pretest**

To alert the laboratory personnel, write on the requisition slip that hepatitis is suspected.

Until the specific virus is identified, institute standard precautions.

**Posttest**

Send the blood or tissue sample to the laboratory promptly.

**Quality Control**

The serum must be separated from the blood cells within 2 hours, because HCV-RNA degrades quickly. A delay results in a false-negative test result. If the specimen is stored at room temperature, the RNA signal is reduced, and this can lead to a false-negative test result. If the tissue specimen is shipped to a different laboratory, the specimen must be frozen and the cold temperature maintained throughout the transit time (London & Evans, 1996).

## Hepatitis D Antibody

**(Serum)**                    Synonym: Anti-delta, anti-HD

**Normal Values**

Anti-HD: Negative
Type IgM: Negative
Type IgG: Negative

## Background Information

The hepatitis D (delta) virus is an incomplete RNA virus that cannot survive alone. This virus is transmitted primarily by the parenteral route and coinfects or superinfects a liver that is already infected with the hepatitis B virus. The hepatitis D virus depends on the synthesis of the hepatitis B surface antigen surface coat to infect and multiply within the individual. When the hepatitis D virus coinfects with the hepatitis B virus, the infection is more severe or relapsing. Superinfection occurs in the chronic carrier stage of hepatitis B. This results in chronic hepatitis D infection, with severe acute illness.

A positive reaction occurs to the hepatitis D antibody and its subtypes, which appear 5 to 7 weeks after the onset of infection. A positive IgM result indicates acute illness by the hepatitis D virus. A positive IgG result indicates the chronic carrier stage of hepatitis D.

| Purpose | The purpose of the test is to diagnose hepatitis D and identify the stage of infection. |
|---|---|

**Procedure**

A red-topped, sterile tube is used to collect 10 mL of venous blood.

**Quality Control**

Venipuncture is always performed with gloves, and needles should be used and disposed of carefully. When hepatitis is suspected, extra attention should be paid to technique, avoiding needlestick injury or splashing blood.

**Findings**

**Elevated Values**

Hepatitis D infection
Type IgM: Acute
  hepatitis D

Type IgG: Chronic
  carrier, hepatitis D

**Interfering Factors**

• Recent administration of radioisotopes

**Nursing Implementation**

Nursing actions are similar to those used in other venipuncture procedures, with the following additional measures.

**Pretest**

To alert the laboratory personnel, write on the requisition slip that hepatitis is suspected.
Until the specific virus is identified, institute standard precautions.

## Hepatitis E Antibody

(Serum)

Synonym: Anti-HEV

| Normal Values | Hepatitis E antibody: Negative<br>IgM type: Negative<br>IgA type: Negative<br>IgG type: Negative |
|---|---|

## Background Information

The hepatitis E virus (HEV) is transmitted via the fecal-oral route. Although hepatitis E infection is not widely prevalent in the United States, travelers to endemic areas, including Mexico, Asia, and Africa, may acquire the infection (Lehmann, 1998).

The HEV can be indentified in the feces, liver tissue, or bile sample, but the usual method of indentification of the virus is to test the blood sample for the presence of HEV antibodies.

## Purpose of the Test

The presence of HEV antibodies identifies the HEV as the source of the infection. The specific antibody type distinguishes between acute or recent infection and past infection.

## Procedure

A red-topped, sterile tube is used to collect 10 mL of venous blood.

### Quality Control

Venipuncture is always performed with gloves, and needles should be used and disposed of carefully. When hepatitis is suspected, extra attention should be paid to technique, avoiding needle-stick injury or splashing blood.

## Findings

### Elevated Values

Hepatitis E infection
Types IgM and IgA:
    Acute or recent
    HEV infection

Types IgG: Past HEV
    infection

## Interfering Factors

- Recent administration of radioisotopes

## Nursing Implementation

Nursing actions are similar to those used in other venipuncture procedures, with the following additional measures.

### Pretest

To alert the laboratory personnel, write on the requisition slip that hepatitis is suspected.
Until the specific virus infection is identified, institute standard precautions.

## Lactate Dehydrogenase

(Serum)          Synonym: LDH

Total lactate dehydrogenase and its isoenzyme LDH5 will be mildly elevated in the presence of primary hepatic disease. The most common causes are hepatitis, cirrhosis, congestion of the liver, and hepatic anoxia. These tests are costly to perform and are not part of a liver function screen. A complete discussion of lactate dehydrogenase and its isoenzymes is presented in Chapter 15.

## Leucine Aminopeptidase

(Serum)          Synonym: LAP

| Normal Values | 55.2 ±10.6 U/L *or* SI 0.94 ±0.18 µkat/L |
|---|---|

### Background Information

Leucine aminopeptidase is a proteolytic enzyme that is produced for further breakdown of peptides and amino acids. The enzyme is produced in the cells of virtually all human tissue, but a larger concentration exists in the biliary epithelium of the liver, biliary tract, pancreas, and mucosa of the intestine. The source of the serum level of leucine aminopeptidase is probably liver tissue.

During pregnancy, the serum value rises progressively, peaks at the end of the third trimester, and subsides in the postpartum period. In this instance, the origin of the leucine aminopeptidase enzyme appears to be the placenta.

The leucine aminopeptidase test is not widely used, but it is part of the group of tests that evaluate hepatobiliary disease. In purpose, it is similar to ALP, GGP, and 5'-nucleotidase, but it is more specific than ALP because it does not become elevated in bone disorders.

| Purpose of the Test | The leucine aminopeptidase test is used to detect hepatobiliary disease and biliary obstruction. It also helps differentiate hepatobiliary disorders from bone disease. |
|---|---|

| Procedure | A red-topped, sterile tube is used to collect 10 mL of venous blood. |
|---|---|

**Findings**

**Elevated Values**

Obstructive hepato-
    biliary disease
Metastatic cancer of
    the liver and
    pancreas

Pregnancy-induced
    hypertension
Acute intoxication
Hepatitis

Chronic alcohol
    abuse
Cirrhosis
Biliary atresia

**Interfering Factors**

- Pregnancy

| | |
|---|---|
| **Nursing Implementation** | Nursing actions are similar to those used in other venipuncture procedures, with the following additional measure. |

### Pretest

When fasting is required by an individual laboratory, instruct the patient to discontinue all food and fluids for 12 hours before the test.

## Lipase

| | |
|---|---|
| (Serum) | Synonyms: None |

| | |
|---|---|
| **Normal Values** | Adult: <200 U/L *or* SI <3.4 µkat/L<br>The normal value varies with the method of analysis. |

### Background Information

Lipase is an enzyme manufactured primarily by the pancreas. The function of this digestive enzyme is to hydrolyze fatty acids. Lipolysis by lipase increases in the presence of bile salts because the bile emulsifies the fat and creates a greater surface area for the lipase activity. If bile is not present, the lipase is ineffective.

In pancreatic disorders, the serum value of lipase is usually parallel and complementary to amylase, but clinically lipase is considered more sensitive and specific in the diagnosis of acute pancreatitis.

| | |
|---|---|
| **Purpose of the Test** | The serum lipase test is used to diagnose pancreatitis and pancreatic disease. |

| | |
|---|---|
| **Procedure** | A red-topped, sterile tube is used to collect 10 mL of venous blood. |

### Quality Control

Venipuncture must be smooth, with a blood flow that fills the vacuum tube readily. If the blood has excessive turbulence because of flawed venipuncture technique, the hemolysis of the erythrocytes will alter the test results.

| | |
|---|---|
| **Findings** | **Elevated Values** |

| | | |
|---|---|---|
| Acute pancreatitis | Primary biliary | Strangulated or |
| Colic from gallstone | cirrhosis | perforated bowel |
| Pancreatic cyst or | Pancreatic ductal | Peritonitis |
| pseudocyst | obstruction | |

| | |
|---|---|
| **Interfering Factors** | • Heparin<br>• Narcotics |

- Hemolysis
- Failure to maintain a nothing-by-mouth status

**Nursing Implementation**

Nursing actions are similar to those used in other venipuncture procedures, with the following additional measures.

### Pretest

For dialysis patients, ensure that the lipase blood sample is obtained before a dialysis treatment. The heparin used during dialysis would cause a false rise in the lipase value.

Instruct the patient to discontinue all food and fluid for 12 hours before the test.

## 5'-Nucleotidase

**(Serum)**          Synonyms: 5'-N, 5'-NT

**Normal Values**

Adults: 2–17 IU/L *or* SI 0.03–0.29 µkat/L

### Background Information

5'-Nucleotidase is an enzyme found in the plasma membranes of all cells; its function is to assist in the catabolism of nucleic acids. The enzyme is active in the liver because of the multiple metabolic functions of that organ. 5'-Nucleotidase is mostly inactive in bone tissue, because bone cells are relatively stable and undergo few metabolic changes.

**Purpose of the Test**

5'-Nucleotidase demonstrates a dramatic rise in the presence of extrahepatic or intrahepatic biliary obstruction and cancer of the liver. It parallels the values of gamma-glutamyltransferase, leucine aminopeptidase, and ALP in the presence of hepatobiliary disease. Unlike ALP, it remains at normal levels in the presence of bone disease.

**Procedure**

A red-topped, sterile tube is used to collect 10 mL of venous blood.

### Quality Control

Venipuncture technique must be smooth, with a blood flow that fills the vacuum tube readily. If the blood has excessive turbulence because of flawed venipuncture technique, the hemolysis of the erythrocytes will elevate the test results.

| Findings | Elevated Values | | |
|---|---|---|---|
| | Common bile duct obstruction | Hepatitis (viral, toxic) | Metastatic cancer of the liver |
| | Lymphoma of the liver | Biliary cirrhosis | |
| | Hepatic cirrhosis | Pregnancy (third trimester) | |

| Interfering Factors | • Failure to maintain a nothing-by-mouth status<br>• Hemolysis |
|---|---|

| Nursing Implementation | Nursing actions are similar to those used in other venipuncture procedures, with the following additional measure. |
|---|---|

**Pretest**

Because lipemia will elevate the serum value, instruct the patient to fast from food and fluids for 12 hours before the test.

## Protein Electrophoresis

(Serum)                          Synonym: Serum protein electrophoresis

| Normal Values | **Adults**<br>Albumin: 3.5–5 g/dL *or* SI 35–50 g/L<br>Alpha$_1$-globulin: 0.1–0.3 g/dL *or* SI 1–3 g/L<br>Alpha$_2$-globulin: 0.6–1 g/dL *or* SI 6–10 g/L<br>Beta-globulin: 0.7–1.1 g/dL *or* SI 7–11 g/L<br>Gamma-globulin: 0.8–1.6 g/dL *or* SI 8–16 g/L<br>**Children**<br>Albumin: 3.6–5.2 g/dL *or* SI 36–52 g/L<br>Alpha$_1$-globulin: 0.1–0.4 g/dL *or* SI 1–4 g/L<br>Alpha$_2$-globulin: 0.5–1.2 g/dL *or* SI 5–12 g/L<br>Beta-globulin: 0.5–1.1 g/dL *or* SI 5–11 g/L<br>Gamma-globulin: 0.5–1.7 g/dL *or* SI 5–17 g/L |
|---|---|

## Background Information

Total serum consists of albumin and globulins. The process of electrophoresis uses an electric field to separate out the fractional protein components in greater detail and to measure the quantity of each component. It is possible to quantify more than 100 plasma proteins by electrophoresis.

**Albumin.** This is the largest component and constitutes up to two thirds of the total plasma proteins. The functions of albumin are to (1) maintain oncotic pressure (the pressure that holds water within vascular walls), (2) sustain a reserve nitrogen pool for tissue growth and repair, and (3) serve as a transport or carrier protein for numerous substances such as medications, lipids, bilirubin, hormones, minerals, and fat-soluble vitamins.

**Globulins.** Three main subgroups of globulins exist: alpha-, beta-, and gamma-globulins. In each of these subgroups, numerous component fractions have distinct functions. The main fractions are presented here, but numerous additional fractions are present in the blood.

The largest of the *alpha₁*-globulins is alpha₁-antitrypsin, a protease inhibitor that inactivates trypsin in the blood.

*Alpha₂*-globulins consist of two important plasma proteins: haptoglobin and alpha₂-macroglobulin. Haptoglobin binds the hemoglobin that has been released from the lysis of erythrocytes. This hemoglobin-binding capacity preserves iron and additional protein. Alpha₂-macroglobulin is a protease inhibitor. Because of its large size relative to other globulins, it cannot pass into glomerular filtrate. In nephrotic syndrome, when other smaller globulins are lost via the glomerular filtrate, the concentration of alpha₂-macroglobulin increases dramatically and allows the serum globulins to rise to a level that equals or exceeds the albumin level. Alpha₂-globulin can also sustain the oncotic pressure within the vascular system.

**Beta₁-Globulins.** These globulins consist mainly of transferrin, the iron-transporting protein. It carries ferric ions from intracellular storage to the bone marrow.

**Beta₂-Globulins.** These globulins consist primarily of the low-density lipoprotein that transports cholesterol to the cells. Other beta-globulins are fibrinogen and complement factors.

**Gamma Globulins.** These globulins consist of the immunoglobulins G, A, D, E, and M. They are usually identified as IgG, IgA, IgD, IgE, and IgM. Each of these plasma proteins is designed to carry out antibody activity by binding with and neutralizing specific antigens (Fig. 19–4).

## Purpose of the Test

Serum protein electrophoresis is used in the detection of hepatobiliary disease, in the evaluation of nutritional status, and to detect monoclonal gammopathy. The latter refers to the presence of a pattern of spikes of the M protein in monoclonal gammopathies.

## Procedure

A red-topped, sterile tube is used to collect 10 mL of venous blood.

### Quality Control

Once the blood has been centrifuged in the laboratory, the serum is kept refrigerated until the analysis is performed.

## Findings

### Elevated Values

ALBUMIN

Dehydration

ALPHA₁-GLOBULINS

Inflammatory disease
Neoplastic disease

ALPHA₂-GLOBULINS

Nephrotic syndrome     Rheumatic fever
Neoplasm               Acute infection

BETA-GLOBULINS

Hyperlipoproteinemia
Monoclonal gam-
    mopathies

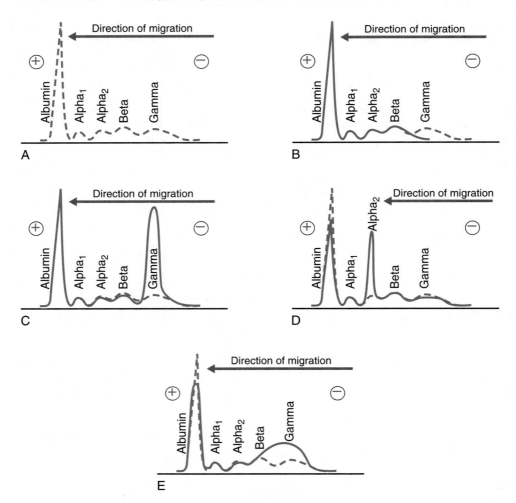

**Figure 19–4**

Serum protein electrophoresis: Normal versus abnormal patterns. *A*, Normal pattern. *B*, Hypogammaglobulinemia indicated by an almost absent gamma region. *C*, Monoclonal gammopathy, marked by a single spike in the gamma region. *D*, Nephrotic syndrome, indicated by a loss of most serum proteins and a rise in alpha₂-macroglobulin. *E*, Active hepatocellular damage (cirrhosis) marked by fusion of the beta and gamma regions and an increase in immunoglobulin A in that region. (Adapted with permission from Lehmann, C. A. [1998]. *Saunders manual of clinical laboratory science*. Philadelphia: W. B. Saunders.)

GAMMA-GLOBULINS

| | | |
|---|---|---|
| *Polyclonal Gammopathies* | Collagen diseases (systemic lupus erythematosus, rheumatoid arthritis) | Infection |
| Chronic liver diseases (hepatitis, cirrhosis) | | Inflammation (sarcoidosis) |
| | | Neoplasm |

| *Monoclonal Gam-* *mopathies* | Waldenström's macroglobulinemia | Malignant lymphoma |
| Multiple myeloma | Primary amyloidosis | |

**Decreased Values**

ALBUMIN

See section on serum protein.

ALPHA₁-GLOBULINS

Hereditary alpha₁-antitrypsin deficiency

ALPHA₂-GLOBULINS

Hemolysis
Hepatocellular damage

BETA-GLOBULINS

Hypobetalipoproteinemia

GAMMA-GLOBULINS

| Response to cytoxic or immunosuppressive medication | Lymphocytic leukemia | Immunodeficiency syndrome |
| | Lymphosarcoma | |
| | Multiple myeloma | |

---

**Interfering Factors**

• None

---

**Nursing Implementation**

Nursing actions are similar to those used in other venipuncture procedures. No other specific preparation is necessary.

---

## Serum Proteins

**(Serum)**

Synonyms: Total protein: TP, serum total protein; albumin: Alb; globulin: globulins, calculated; albumin-to-globulin ratio: A:G ratio

---

**Normal Values**

Total Protein
    Adult, ambulatory: 6.4–8.3 g/dL *or* SI 64–83 g/L
    Adult, recumbent: 6–7.8 g/dL *or* SI 60–78 g/L
    Child >3 years: 6–8 g/dL *or* SI 60–80 g/L
    Newborn: 4–7 g/dL *or* SI 40–70 g/L

*Continued on following page*

*Continued*

> Albumin
>     Adult >60 years: 3.4–4.8 g/dL *or* SI 34–48 g/L
>     Adult 18–60 years: 3.5–5 g/dL *or* SI 35–50 g/L
>     Child: 3.2–5.4 g/dL *or* SI 32–54 g/L
>     Newborn: 2.8–4.4 g/dL *or* SI 28–44 g/L
> Globulin: 2.8–4.4 g/dL *or* SI 28–44 g/L
> Albumin-to-globulin ratio: >1

## Background Information

The parenchymal cells of the liver are responsible for the manufacture of the serum proteins albumin and fibrinogen, other coagulation factors, and most of the alpha- and beta-globulins. The only exceptions are the gamma-globulins that are manufactured by the reticuloendothelial system.

Plasma proteins are amino acids that function to (1) maintain oncotic pressure within the walls of blood vessels; (2) provide a reserve source of protein for tissue growth and repair; (3) provide transport for lipids, lipid-soluble substances, iron, copper, magnesium, and calcium; (4) act as immunologic agents; (5) provide factors for coagulation; and (6) provide numerous enzymes for a variety of activities.

**Total Serum Protein.** Total serum protein provides a broad indicator of the quantity and concentration of all plasma proteins except fibrinogen. The total serum protein value measures the amount of albumin and globulins combined. The test value is nonspecific in that it does not provide details about the individual globulin components or the cause of the abnormal value. A low total serum protein of less than 4.0 g/dL (SI 40 g/L) together with a low serum albumin level causes edema to occur (Jacobs et al., 1996).

**Albumin.** This is the largest component of the plasma proteins and is responsible for about 80% of the colloidal osmotic pressure within the blood (Gosling, 1995). Albumin also serves as a reserve nitrogen source for tissue growth and healing, and it is a transport vehicle for many substances.

A high albumin level results from a loss of vascular fluid. Because of a reduced volume of fluids, the albumin shows a relative rise from more concentrated blood.

A low albumin level can occur for a variety of reasons. Decreased synthesis of serum protein may exist because of liver disease or malnutrition. Losses of serum albumin may occur in renal disease, ascites, or inflammatory intestinal disease or through the skin as in advanced dermatitis or thermal injury. Lastly, the albumin level may be decreased because of a hypermetabolic disorder that consumes the protein at a very fast rate.

A low serum albumin level causes a low osmotic pressure of the blood. Normally, a low osmotic pressure stimulates the liver to synthesize sufficient albumin to restore fluid and pressure in the vasculature. If the liver is unable to respond adequately or the albumin loss is severe or rapid, fluid will leak out of the vasculature and the blood pressure will fall because of hypovolemia. Edema will result from a serum albumin level of 2.0 to 2.5 g/dL (SI 20 to 25 g/L) or less (Jacobs et al., 1996). A decrease in serum albumin also causes decreased serum concentrations of calcium and magnesium. These ions must be bound to albumin for transport in the blood (Henry, 1996).

**Globulin.** This measurement refers to the total of all the globulin proteins: alpha-, beta-, and gamma-globulins. Each component globulin has a specific function, but generally the globulins are either enzymes or immunologic agents.

**Albumin-to-Globulin Ratio.** This is a calculation obtained by dividing the value of albumin by the value of the globulins. Normally, an equal or greater amount of albumin than globulins is in the blood, with a ratio result equal to or greater than 1. If a severe loss of albumin or a greater amount of globulin synthesis occurs, the ratio drops to less than 1.

**Purpose of the Tests**

Total serum protein testing provides general information about the patient's nutritional status and the severity of diseases of the liver, bone marrow, and kidneys. The test is also used to investigate the cause of edema.

The serum albumin test is used to evaluate the nutritional status, the oncotic pressure of the blood, and the losses of protein associated with some severe renal, hepatic, skin, or intestinal diseases.

The globulin value identifies the need for additional testing to determine which globulins are elevated or decreased.

The albumin-to-globulin ratio identifies the proportionate amounts of these two proteins in the blood.

**Procedure**

A red-topped, sterile tube is used to collect 10 mL of venous blood. A capillary tube is used for newborns.

**Quality Control**

Venipuncture technique must be performed skillfully, because prolonged application of a tourniquet and hemolysis will give a false elevation of the total protein value. If intravenous fluids are being administered, the blood sample is drawn from the opposite arm. This avoids local hemodilution and a false decrease in all serum protein values.

**Findings**

**Elevated Values**

TOTAL PROTEIN

Dehydration
Hyperimmunoglobu-
    linemia

Polyclonal or mono-
    clonal
    gammopathies

ALBUMIN

Dehydration

GLOBULIN

Inflammatory
    conditions
Waldenström's
    macroglobulinemia

Multiple myeloma
Collagen diseases
Sarcoidosis
Cirrhosis

Chronic active
    hepatitis

**Decreased Values**

TOTAL PROTEIN

Protein-losing
    gastroenteropathies
    (Crohn's disease,
    ulcerative colitis,
    intestinal fistula)
Acute burns (thermal
    injury)

Nephrotic syndrome
Severe protein
    deficiency
Chronic liver disease
Malabsorption
    syndrome
Agammaglobulinemia

Pregnancy (third
    trimester)

ALBUMIN

| | | |
|---|---|---|
| Rapid hydration or overhydration with intravenous fluids | Nephrotic syndrome Malignancy Protein-losing enteropathies (Crohn's disease, ulcerative colitis, draining fistula) | Burns (thermal injury) Severe skin disease Thyroid disease Heart disease Peptic ulcer |
| Infection and fever Malnutrition Cirrhosis Chronic alcoholism | | |

GLOBULIN

| | |
|---|---|
| Agammaglobulinemia Hypogammaglobulin- emia | Protein-losing enteropathies Multiple myeloma |

ALBUMIN-TO-GLOBULIN RATIO

| | | |
|---|---|---|
| Cirrhosis and other liver diseases Chronic glomerulo- nephritis Nephrotic syndromes Waldenström's macroglobulinemia | Sarcoidosis Collagen diseases Severe infections Severe or chronic inflammatory diseases Ulcerative colitis | Cachexia Multiple myeloma Burns |

---

**Interfering Factors**
■

*Critical Thinking 19–3*
The patient with liver damage has decreased serum values for total protein and albumin. What types of problems can occur, and how does the nurse assess for them?

- Hemolysis
- Prolonged bedrest
- Massive intravenous infusion
- Venous stasis
- Peripheral vascular collapse
- Hyperlipidemia
- Hyperbilirubinemia

---

**Nursing Implementation**    **Pretest**

Nursing actions are similar to those used in other venipuncture procedures. No other specific preparation is necessary.

---

**Critical Value**

**Albumin <1.5 g/dL (SI <15 g/L)**

At this severely low level, the patient is so depleted of albumin that oncotic pressure cannot be maintained.
  Hypovolemia and hypotension occur when the fluid shifts out of the blood vessels. Notify the physician of the test result and the measurements of the vital signs that were just taken. Generally, a decline in the albumin value tends to be gradual over time, but at this critical level the patient is likely to be in hypovolemic shock and could develop a vascular collapse, leading to death.

## Prothrombin Time

**(Serum)**                     Synonyms: None

The prothrombin time test is a measure of clotting ability. Severe liver disease results in depressed values of plasma prothrombin and factors II, VII, IX, and X. The injured hepatocytes are unable to use fat-soluble vitamin K to manufacture the clotting factors. When these clotting factors are inadequate or depressed, the serum prothrombin time is prolonged, and it takes longer for a clot to form. Liver diseases that can cause a prolonged or elevated prothrombin time include advanced cirrhosis, infectious hepatitis, liver failure, Wilson's disease, hemochromatosis, and hepatoma.

Conditions that impair the absorption of fat-soluble vitamin K from the intestine also cause a prolonged prothrombin time. The reason is that a deficiency exists in the supply of vitamin K for the liver to use in the manufacture of clotting factors. Conditions that inhibit the absorption of vitamin K include obstructive jaundice, biliary cirrhosis, and cancer of the head of the pancreas. A full discussion of this test is presented in Chapter 6.

## Sweat Test

**(Sweat)**                     Synonyms: Chloride, sweat; cystic fibrosis sweat test; iontophoresis sweat test

**Normal Values**          Adults and children: 5–40 mEq/L *or* SI 5–40 mmol/L

### Background Information

Cystic fibrosis (mucoviscidosis) of the pancreas is an autosomal recessive disease that is characterized by abnormal secretion of pancreatic exocrine glands and the other distinct exocrine glands of the body. In cystic fibrosis, increased sodium and chloride content exists in the sweat gland secretions.

In children up to the age of 20 years, a sweat chloride concentration greater than 60 mEq/L (SI >60 mmol/L) is considered abnormal, and a value of 40 to 60 mEq/L (SI 40 to 60 mmol/L) is considered a borderline result. In adults, values up to 70 mEq/L (SI 70 mmol/L) may be normal (Henry, 1996).

This test can produce false results because of poor technique, but it remains the definitive diagnostic test for cystic fibrosis. The diagnosis is based on at least two positive sweat test results and the presence of clinical manifestations of the disease. Genetic testing is useful in identifying the presence of cystic fibrosis mutations (Constantinescu & Hilman, 1996).

### Purpose of the Test

The chloride sweat test is used to diagnose cystic fibrosis in children.

### Procedure

Sweat is obtained by stimulating skin sweat production with pilocarpine and low-voltage electric current in a process called *iontophoresis*. The pads of pilocarpine and sodium chloride are placed on cleansed skin of the volar aspect of the right arm, and the electrodes are strapped on over the pads. For infants, the skin of the back may be used. For 5 minutes, the low-voltage electric current introduces small amounts of pilocarpine into the skin. Pilocarpine is a cholinergic drug that evokes a sweat response. On removal of the electrodes, the sweat is collected on sterile gauze pads or filter paper, weighed, and then analyzed for chloride content.

| **Findings** | **Elevated Values** |
|---|---|

Cystic fibrosis            Fucosidosis                      Mucopolysacchari-
Hypothyroidism             Renal insufficiency              dosis
Adrenal insufficiency      Glucose-6-phosphate
Malnutrition                  deficiency
Ectodermal dysplasia       Diabetes insipidus

**Decreased Values**

Edema
Hypoproteinemia

**Interfering Factors**

- Dermatitis or skin lesion
- Improper placement of electrodes
- Inadequate sweat collection
- Salt depletion in the body
- Excessive sweating with fever or exercise just before the test

**Nursing Implementation**

**Pretest**

Explain the procedure to the parents and the child.

Reassure them that the electrodes produce a mild tingling sensation but do not cause shock or pain.

Encourage the parents to accompany the child during the test and to bring a book or favorite toy for the child. These distractions will help pass the time and minimize the child's apprehension.

Before placement of the electrodes, the skin area must be cleansed with soap and water and dried thoroughly.

This test must not be performed on the child who is receiving oxygen or who is in a mist tent. Danger of explosion exists as well as probability of false test results.

**Quality Control**

Earlier deposits of salt and perspiration must be removed to ensure that results are valid. The palm of the hand is never used as a site for electrode placement. The electrodes must be placed correctly to avoid burning the skin.

**During the Test**

At the start of the test, ask the child if he or she feels any burning sensation. If this occurs, the test is stopped and the electrodes are checked and repositioned.

### Posttest

The skin may appear reddened at the site of the electrodes.
Reassure the patient and the parents that the redness will disappear in a few
hours.

## Trypsinogen, Immunoreactive Assay

**(Serum)**                    Synonyms: IRT, immunoreactive trypsin assay

| **Normal Values** | CIS method: <80 µg/L<br>ELISA Method<br>    Neonate 1–4 days: 55–109 µg/L<br>    Infant 4–6 weeks: 70–104 µg/L |
| --- | --- |

## Background Information

Trypsinogen, an inactive digestive proenzyme, is
manufactured in the pancreas. When it is secreted
into the duodenum, it converts to the active
enzyme, trypsin. In normal infants, a small amount
of trypsinogen is secreted into the blood, but this
decreases over time. In infants with cystic fibrosis,
the serum level of trypsinogen is higher. To screen
for cystic fibrosis, this test should be performed in
the first month of life.

This test is used to identify cystic fibrosis at a
very early age, before any symptoms of illness
appear. Several states in the United States, as well
as Australia and New Zealand, have made this
test mandatory to screen all newborn children for
cystic fibrosis (Baroni, Anderson, & Mischler,
1997).

Controversies exist related to the test and the
mandatory aspect of testing. One problem is that
the test has a false-positive rate of 86% to 90%
(Baroni et al., 1997; Gregg et al., 1993). This is to
say that most of the infants who test positive do not
have cystic fibrosis and are not genetic carriers of
the disease. The goal of mandatory testing is to
make an early diagnosis and provide prompt and

accurate treatment before or as soon as the infant
becomes ill. The problem is that early treatment
may improve the initial health of the child but not
necessarily change the long-term outcome of the
disease.

**Elevated Values.**   In an older protocol, the
neonate with a CIS assay test result that is 140 µg/L
or higher is retested at 2 to 8 weeks. If that test
result is 80 µg/L or higher, a sweat test is ordered to
provide a definitive diagnosis. To reduce the false-
positive rate, the newer screening protocol recommends that the initial positive immunoreactive trypsinogen assay be followed by DNA analysis of the
initial dried blood sample. If this test is positive, the
infant either is a carrier of cystic fibrosis or has the
disease. The parents are then notified, and the child
has a sweat test to make a definitive diagnosis (Balnaves, Bonaquisto, & Francis, 1995; Tietz, 1995).
The DNA test for cystic fibrosis is presented in
Chapter 13.

**Procedure.**   The heelstick method is used to
obtain sufficient drops of blood to fill a circle wider
than 4 mm on filter paper. This technique is explained in Chapter 2.

## Findings

**Elevated Values**

Possible cystic
   fibrosis
   disease

Possible cystic
   fibrosis carrier
   status

| | |
|---|---|
| **Interfering Factors** | • None |

**Nursing Implementation**

**Pretest**

The test is done by heelstick capillary puncture at the same time that the neonate (1 to 4 days old) has a mandatory test for phenylketonuria (PKU) and hypothyroidism. The procedure and nursing care for the heelstick method are presented in Chapter 2.

**Posttest**

When the parents learn that the trypsinogen test result is positive, it is necessary to provide additional information about the need for follow-up testing with a repeat trypsinogen test or a DNA analysis. The nurse provides emotional support because parents often feel anxiety until they know the ultimate outcome (Balnaves et al., 1995; Williams, 1995). If the test result was a false-positive one, the parents sometimes react with anger or irritation (Gregg et al., 1993).

When the ultimate outcome is of carrier status or cystic fibrosis disease for the neonate, the nurse in the genetic counseling center may participate with other professionals in providing additional testing and accurate information to the family members (Williams, 1995).

## Urobilinogen, Fecal

**(Fecal)**    Synonym: Fecal urobilinogen

**Normal Values**    Adult: 40–280 mg/day *or* SI 0.068–0.470 nmol/day; 80–280 Ehrlich units/day
Random stool: Positive

### Background Information

Conjugated bilirubin becomes a component of bile and enters the duodenum via biliary tract drainage. In the intestine, the bilirubin is converted to urobilinogen by the action of bacterial flora. Most of the urobilinogen is excreted from the body in the fecal matter.

Excess urobilinogen in the feces usually is caused by excess production of bilirubin and bile pigment. The excess production occurs because of a rapid, abnormal rate of erythrocyte hemolysis. Laboratory analysis may demonstrate a dramatic excess of more than 400 mg/day.

Diminished urobilinogen in the feces is usually a result of severe biliary tract obstruction or hepatocellular damage. Laboratory analysis may demonstrate a marked decrease to less than 5 mg/day.

**Purpose of the Test**    Fecal urobilinogen is used to help detect disorders of erythrocytes and to help confirm the diagnosis of liver disease or biliary tract obstruction.

**Procedure**    The procedure may be based on a single stool specimen, several consecutive daily stool specimens, or a pooled 4-day specimen. Because the amount of urobilinogen in feces is not always consistent from one day to the next, multiple specimens are often required (see also Chapter 2).

| Findings | | | |
|---|---|---|---|

**Elevated Values**

| | | |
|---|---|---|
| Hemolytic anemia | Thalassemia | Hemorrhage into |
| Sickle cell anemia | Pernicious anemia | body tissues |

**Decreased Values**

| | | |
|---|---|---|
| Cirrhosis with hepatocellular jaundice | Depressed erythro-poiesis, as in aplastic anemia | Tumors (head of the pancreas, ampulla of Vater, bile duct) |
| Hepatitis | Choledocholithiasis | |

**Interfering Factors**

- Exposure of specimen to sunlight or warmth
- Antibiotic reduction of intestinal flora
- Contamination of the specimen

**Nursing Implementation**

**Pretest**

Instruct the patient to place all the stool in one or more special darkened containers, as required by the particular method of collection. The stool specimen must not be contaminated with toilet paper or urine.

**Quality Control**

When it is exposed to sunlight or the warmth of room temperature, urobilinogen will convert to urobilin. Therefore, all specimens are kept refrigerated in dark containers until they are transported to the laboratory.

**Posttest**

The requisition slip and container or containers for pooled or multiple specimens are labeled with the dates of specimen collection.

The single, fresh specimen is sent to the laboratory immediately. Refrigeration is required when a delay in transport of 30 minutes or more occurs.

## Urobilinogen, Urine

(Urine)                     Synonyms: Urinary urobilinogen, 2-hour urine urobilinogen

**Normal Values**

Male: 0.3–2.1 mg/2 hr *or* SI 0.5–3.6 μmol/2 hr
Female: 0.1–1.1 mg/2 hr *or* SI 0.2–1.9 μmol/2 hr

## Background Information

Conjugated bilirubin exits from the liver as a component of bile. It passes through the biliary ductal system and enters the intestinal tract at the duodenum. In the intestine, bilirubin is converted to urobilinogen by the action of bacterial flora.

Most of the urobilinogen is excreted from the body in the fecal matter. The small remainder is absorbed by the portal vein system. From this circulatory portion, most will return to the liver via the enterohepatic circulation and will be recycled

in bile. The remainder of the circulatory portion is filtered out of the blood by the kidney and is excreted in the urine (Fig. 19–5).

Urinary urobilinogen increases when the following exist: (1) excessive bilirubin formation as in excessive hemolysis of erythrocytes, (2) constipation that increases the time that urobilinogen is in contact with bacterial flora, (3) bacterial intestinal infection, and (4) liver disease that interferes with the enterohepatic circulation.

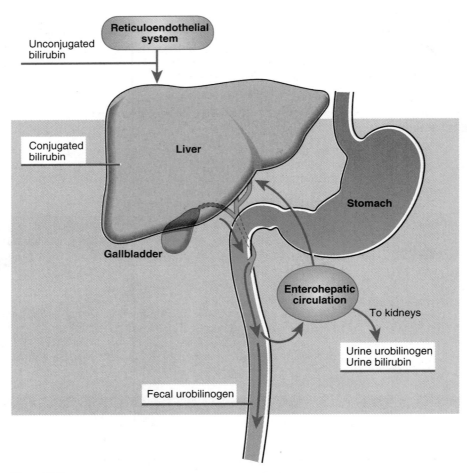

**Figure 19–5**

Pathways for bilirubin metabolism. Several organs and organ systems make different forms and amounts of bilirubin and urobilinogen.

Urobilinogen decreases when the following exist: (1) obstruction or impairment of the flow of bile into the intestine, (2) reduction in the intestinal flora, (3) rapid intestinal transit time, and (4) renal insufficiency.

---

**Purpose of the Test**

The test is used to screen for evidence of hemolytic anemia or as an early indicator of moderate damage to the parenchymal cells of the liver.

---

**Procedure**

The 2-hour urine collection is scheduled for the afternoon, between 2 PM and 4 PM, because of the diurnal pattern of excretion of urine urobilinogen.

---

**Findings**

**Elevated Values**

| | | |
|---|---|---|
| Moderate hepatocellular damage (hepatitis, hepatotoxicity from drugs or toxins, hepatic hypoxia) | Hemolytic anemia<br>Hemorrhage into tissues<br>Intravascular hemolysis<br>Portal vein cirrhosis | Congestive heart failure<br>Pernicious anemia<br>Constipation<br>Hemolysis of erythrocytes |

**Decreased Values**

| | | |
|---|---|---|
| Biliary tract obstruction | Massive hepatocellular damage | Renal insufficiency |

---

**Interfering Factors**

- Failure to collect all specimens in the time allotted
- Exposure of the specimen to light or warmth
- Recent or current use of antibiotics

---

**Nursing Implementation**

**Pretest**

Explain the procedure to the patient to maximize cooperation and accuracy in the collection of the specimen.

Schedule the test from 2 to 4 PM. The patient voids just before 2 PM, and this specimen is discarded because the urine has been in the bladder for an unknown period.

Give the patient 500 mL of water to drink all at once. From 2 to 4 PM, place all voided urine in a dark-colored, sterile urine container. As an alternative, a clear container can be covered with aluminum foil to protect the urine from light.

Keep the urine in the refrigerator during the test period.

**Quality Control**

The urine specimen must not be exposed to sunlight or remain at room temperature. Urobilinogen is unstable and will convert to urobilin in the presence of sunlight, fluorescent light, or warmth.

### Posttest

On completion of the test, send the urine container to the laboratory immediately. The analysis will be performed within 30 minutes, or the specimen will be frozen for longer storage.

## Diagnostic Procedures

## Cholangiography, Percutaneous Transhepatic

**(Radiography)**   Synonyms: Transhepatic cholangiography, PTC, PTHC

**Normal Values**   The biliary ducts are patent and demonstrate normal anatomic structure. No evidence of tumor, stone, or stricture is found.

### Background Information

When obstructive jaundice is present and the ultrasound test reveals dilated biliary ducts, the site of the obstruction may be intrahepatic or extrahepatic. The usual causes of the obstruction are gallstone, parasites, or tumor. If endoscopic cholangiopancreatoscopy is incomplete, or if the endoscopic examination cannot be performed, a percutaneous approach may be used to visualize the biliary tract and the location of the obstruction. Percutaneous transhepatic cholangiography allows contrast medium to be instilled into the biliary tree via percutaneous needle insertion into the hepatic ducts of the liver. Fluoroscopy and x-ray films are used to assist the physician in the placement of the needle and in obtaining multiple views of obstruction in the biliary ductal system.

**Purpose of the Test**   Percutaneous transhepatic cholangiography is used to diagnose the cause of obstructive jaundice, visualize the anatomic structure of intrahepatic and extrahepatic ducts, and evaluate changes in the biliary tree.

**Procedure**   Percutaneous transhepatic cholangiography is performed in a fluoroscopy room. The patient is sedated with intravenous diazepam and placed in a supine position on the fluoroscopy table.

The skin is prepared, draped, and anesthetized locally. The site of the needle insertion is in the lower right lateral surface or angled toward the dorsal surface at the level of the eighth or ninth intercostal space. The patient is instructed to inhale deeply, exhale fully, and hold his or her breath on expiration. At that point, the needle is inserted into the liver near the hepatic ducts. As the patient resumes shallow breathing, the needle is repositioned until its tip is well into one of the hepatic ducts (Fig. 19–6). The placement of the needle is guided by visualization with fluoroscopy, but many passes may be needed until the position is correct.

Contrast medium is injected slowly into the duct until the entire biliary tree is filled with contrast material. If excess bile is present in dilated ducts, the bile is aspirated slowly and is gradually replaced with an equal amount of contrast medium. A specimen of bile is sent to the laboratory for culture and cytologic analysis.

A tilt table is used to take multiple x-ray films of the patient in various positions until the total biliary tree is visualized. At the end of the procedure, the biliary ducts are aspirated of contrast medium, and the dilated ducts are decompressed. The entire procedure takes 45 minutes to 1 hour.

| Findings | **Abnormal Values** | |
| --- | --- | --- |
| | Gallstones | Nonobstructive |
| | Biliary tract obstruc- | jaundice |
| | tion | Hepatitis |
| | Cancer of the pan- | Cirrhosis |
| | creas | |

**Interfering Factors**

- Obesity
- Ascites
- Gas in the intestinal tract
- Failure to maintain a nothing-by-mouth status
- Bleeding abnormalities
- Sepsis, peritonitis
- Allergy to iodine-based contrast medium

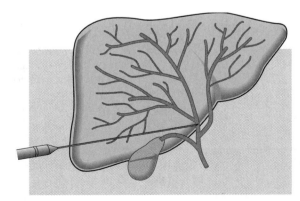

**Figure 19–6**
Percutaneous transhepatic cholangiography. The aspirating needle is passed through the patient's skin and liver tissue until the tip penetrates one of the hepatic ducts. Radiopaque medium is then instilled into the biliary tree to enhance radiographic visualization.

**Nursing Implementation**

### Pretest

Schedule this test before any barium studies are performed.

Question the patient about any history of allergy to iodine or seafood or a previous allergic reaction to iodine-based contrast medium.

An informed consent form must be signed by the patient or the person legally responsible for the patient's health care decisions.

To prevent sepsis, antibiotics may be prescribed in the pretest period and continued into the posttest period.

Instruct the patient to take the prescribed laxative on the night before the test and a cleansing enema on the morning of the test.

Tell the patient to discontinue all food and fluids for 12 hours before the test.

Additional pretest instructions include information about the procedure. The patient is informed that pain control is provided by intravenous medication and a local anesthetic to numb the skin. The breathing instructions of deep inspiration, expiration, and holding the breath should be practiced.

The nurse assesses and records baseline vital signs, including blood pressure, pulse, respiratory rate, and temperature. Any elevation of the temperature is reported to the physician and radiologist, because sepsis and peritonitis are absolute contraindications to performing the test.

Ensure that the recent prothrombin time and complete blood count reports are in the patient's chart. Poor clotting ability is an absolute contraindication.

Moderate to severe anemia may be a contraindication to performance of this test. Alert the radiologist of abnormal test results.

### Quality Control

> The prothrombin time should be no more than 3 seconds greater than the control time. The platelet count should be greater than 100,000 cells/mm³.

### Posttest

Take vital signs regularly and frequently because of the risk of hemorrhage or hypotension. Generally, the pattern is every 15 minutes for 1 hour, every hour for 4 hours, and every 4 hours thereafter, until the patient is stable. The temperature is taken initially and every 4 hours thereafter because of the risk of sepsis and cholangitis.

Place the patient on his or her right side, with a pillow or sandbag pressed against the lower ribs and abdomen. The gentle pressure and immobility help promote clotting. Bedrest is maintained for 6 hours after the test.

Since hemorrhage or biliary leakage could require surgery, nothing-by-mouth status is maintained until the patient is stable.

Observe the lower right area of the rib cage for signs of bleeding, hematoma formation, ecchymosis, or leakage of bile. Some small leakage of blood is expected.

**Complications**

Complications from percutaneous transhepatic cholangiography occur more from dilation of the biliary ducts than from the number of passes with the needle. Sometimes, bleeding complications begin during the test, and emer-

**Table 19–4    Complications of Percutaneous Transhepatic Cholangiography**

| Complication | Nursing Assessment |
| --- | --- |
| Cholangitis (bacterial infection of the biliary tree) | Leukocytosis<br>Moderate abdominal pain<br>Abnormal test results of liver function<br>Fever and chills<br>Jaundice |
| Peritonitis | Acute abdominal pain<br>Abdominal distention<br>Boardlike abdomen<br>Hypotension, shock<br>Fever |
| Bleeding | Hypotension, shock<br>Tachycardia<br>Dyspnea<br>Diaphoresis and pallor<br>Acute abdomen<br>Localized ecchymosis in the lower right lateral area of the ribs or side of the abdomen just below the ribs |

gency surgery will be required to control or correct it. Other complications tend to appear within hours after the test is completed. Cholangitis and sepsis often occur when the underlying problem is gallstones, cancer of the bile duct, or cancer of the pancreas. A summary of the complications and appropriate nursing assessments is presented in Table 19–4.

## Cholangiography, T-Tube and Intravenous

**(Radiography)**          Synonyms: T-tube cholangiography, postoperative cholangiography, intravenous cholangiography, IVC

**Normal Values**          The bile ducts are patent, with no evidence of retained gallstones, obstruction, or other abnormality.

### Background Information

Using radiopaque dye and x-rays to provide visualization of the biliary ductal system, four possible ways exist to perform cholangiography. The T-tube route and the intravenous route are presented in this section. Percutaneous transhepatic cholangiography and endoscopic retrograde cholangiopancreatography are discussed as separate procedures in this chapter.

**T-Tube Cholangiography.**    When stones are in the gallbladder, it is also possible to have one or more small calculi in the biliary tract. Every effort is made to remove any biliary stones in the ducts during surgical removal of the gallbladder, but sometimes the stone is tiny and is discovered postoperatively. If the early postoperative patient develops jaundice or a fistula, a T-tube cholangiogram is performed.

**Intravenous Cholangiography.**   This test may be used for the patient who has a cholecystectomy and at a later date has a possible stone in the cystic or common duct. It may be used for patients who cannot undergo an oral cholecystogram.

---

**Purpose of the Test**

The cholangiogram is used to visualize the biliary ductal system in an effort to identify calculi and other causes of obstruction of bile.

---

**Procedure**

**T-Tube Cholangiogram.**   Radiopaque contrast medium is instilled slowly into the T-tube. X-rays are taken to visualize the lumen of the cystic and common bile ducts.

**Intravenous Cholangiogram.**   In the radiology department, an intravenous dose of radiopaque iodine-based dye is administered to the patient. Starting about 20 minutes later, x-rays films are taken at intervals until the visualization of the ducts is completed in 1 to 2 hours.

For visualization of the gallbladder of the nonsurgical patient, a fatty meal is given to stimulate contraction of the gallbladder. An additional series of x-ray films is then taken. The total time for the intravenous cholangiography is 1 to 8 hours, depending on the extent of the study and the filming that is desired.

---

**Findings**

**Abnormal Values**

T-TUBE CHOLANGIOGRAM

| | | |
|---|---|---|
| Biliary duct stone | Neoplasm | Fistula |

INTRAVENOUS CHOLANGIOGRAM

| | |
|---|---|
| Stone in the cystic or common duct | Nonfunctional gallbladder |
| Gallbladder stones | Polyps or benign |
| Inflammatory disease of the gallbladder | tumors of the biliary ducts |

---

**Interfering Factors**

- Obesity
- Pregnancy (first trimester)
- Failure to maintain nothing-by-mouth status
- Retained barium or gas in the intestine

---

**Nursing Implementation**

**Pretest**

**T-Tube and Intravenous Methods**

Question the patient about any history of allergy to iodine or seafood or previous allergic reaction to iodine-based contrast medium.

An informed consent form must be signed by the patient or the person legally responsible for the patient's health care decisions.

Instruct the patient to discontinue all oral fluids and food for 12 hours before the test.

### Intravenous Method

To clear the bowel of fecal matter and gas, the patient takes 2 bisacodyl (Dulco-lax) tablets on the morning of the day before the test and has nothing by mouth after midnight on the night before the test. On the morning of the test, a saline enema may be given.

Advise the patient that sensations of heat and flushing of the skin may be felt at the time of the injection. Reassure the patient that this is common and will last for only a short while.

### Posttest

#### T-Tube Cholangiogram

Reapply a sterile dressing on the wound area of the T-tube. Reconnect the T-tube to its drainage collection system.

#### T-Tube and Intravenous Cholangiogram

Take vital signs and examine the skin for signs of flushing or urticaria. Record the results. A reaction to the contrast material can occur after the test is completed.

| | |
|---|---|
| **Complications** | Occasionally, a reaction can occur because of allergy to the iodinated contrast medium. The severity of the reaction can range from mild itching and swelling to anaphylaxis, respiratory arrest, and death. Depending on the patient's sensitivity to iodine, the reaction can be mild and delayed in onset or sudden, intense, and potentially catastrophic within minutes after the contrast medium is injected. The medical and nursing personnel of the radiology department observe for any signs of allergic response so that immediate intervention can be initiated. A summary of the complications and the appropriate nursing assessments is provided in Table 19–5. |

## Cholecystography, Oral

(Radiography)     Synonyms: Gallbladder series, GB series, oral cholecystogram

| | |
|---|---|
| **Normal Values** | The gallbladder and biliary ductal system are able to fill, concentrate, contract, and empty, with no evidence of stone, obstruction, or other abnormality. |

### Background Information

Bile is manufactured in the liver and excreted via the intrahepatic ducts, the hepatic ducts, and the cystic duct. It is then stored and concentrated in the gallbladder. As ingested fat reaches the duodenum, the gallbladder is stimulated to contract and expel the bile. The bile flows out through the cystic and common ducts into the duodenum, where it will emulsify fats in digestive processes.

Stones can form in the gallbladder and also lodge in the cystic or common duct (Fig. 19–7). Most stones are made of bile pigment and cholesterol, and some are made of calcium carbonate. Stones in the gallbladder cause acute pain as the gallbladder contracts and squeezes down on them. Stones in the ducts will obstruct the flow of bile and cause posthepatic jaundice.

**Table 19–5   Complications of Cholecystography and Cholangiography**

| Complication | Nursing Assessment |
|---|---|
| Moderate allergic reaction | Urticaria (hives)<br>Angioedema (diffuse swelling of the skin)<br>Edema of the larynx and oropharynx<br>Wheezing and coughing<br>Apprehension<br>Nausea and vomiting |
| Severe allergic reaction (anaphylaxis) | Urticaria<br>Angioedema<br>Pallor or cyanosis<br>Bronchospasm<br>Respiratory failure<br>Tachycardia<br>Hypotension<br>Shock<br>Seizures<br>Coma<br>Death |

The oral cholecystogram is not always precise because of a number of problems that can occur. Visualization of the gallbladder is dependent on an adequate amount of contrast medium reaching these areas. The patient may not ingest the complete amount of the contrast material. Additionally, vomiting, diarrhea, or malabsorption will interfere with the intestinal absorption of the contrast medium. Severe liver disease or biliary obstruction will impair the uptake and excretion of the contrast me-dium, and an inflamed gallbladder cannot concentrate the contrast medium sufficiently to provide for radiographic visualization. When nonvisualization occurs, the test must be repeated with a double dose of contrast medium.

This test is used less widely today because of the better diagnostic alternatives available. CT and ultrasound are more sensitive and consistent in the detection of gallstones.

**Purpose of the Test**     The oral cholecystogram is used to visualize the gallbladder and biliary ductal system in an effort to identify stones and other causes of obstruction. It also is used to evaluate the gallbladder's ability to function in the storage and excretion of bile.

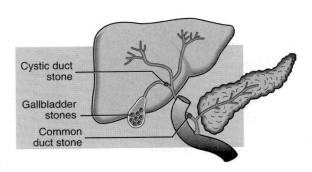

**Figure 19–7**
Common anatomic locations of gallstones.

## Procedure

The patient eats a fat-free meal on the evening before the test and thereafter ingests nothing by mouth (no food or fluids except water). Two or 3 hours after eating, the patient takes the prescribed number of tablets of iopanoic acid (Telepaque) or other prescribed iodinated contrast medium. In some radiology settings, a saline enema may be required in the early morning of the test to remove any gas or feces that can obscure the view.

*Critical Thinking 19–4*
The Hispanic patient speaks little English. His oral cholecystogram could not be completed because the undissolved iopanoic acid (Telepaque) tablets were wrapped in their foil papers in his stomach. How can pretest instruction be improved?

During the test, the patient will undergo a series of initial x-ray studies over a period of 45 to 60 minutes. These films will identify the gallbladder filled with contrast material and any stones that are present. The patient is then given a fatty meal or a synthetic fat substance (Bilevac) that causes the gallbladder to contract within 10 to 30 minutes. A second series of x-ray films demonstrates the contrast material in the cystic and common ducts and its entry into the duodenum. This second phase of the test takes an additional 1 to 2 hours to complete.

## Findings

**Abnormal Values**

Gallstones
Nonfunctioning
  gallbladder

Polyp or benign
  tumor of biliary
  duct

Cholecystitis

## Interfering Factors

- Failure to maintain a fat-free diet followed by nothing-by-mouth status before the test
- Failure to take all the contrast tablets
- Intestinal loss of the contrast material
- Pregnancy (first trimester)
- Retained barium in the intestine
- Impaired hepatic function
- Biliary obstruction and jaundice

## Nursing Implementation

**Pretest**

Schedule this test before any required barium tests, because retained barium in the intestinal tract would obscure the view of the gallbladder and biliary tree.

Question the patient about any history of allergy to iodine or seafood or a previous allergic reaction during a diagnostic test that used an iodine-based dye.

Obtain an informed consent form signed by the patient or the person legally responsible for the patient's health care decisions.

Instruct the patient regarding pretest procedure. The patient must eat a fat-free meal the night before the test, with no further intake of food or beverages, except water. Two or 3 hours after dinner, the patient begins to take the six tablets of iopanoic acid with 8 oz of water. One tablet is taken every 5 minutes until all six tablets have been ingested. The patient may continue to drink water as desired until midnight and follows a completely nothing-by-mouth protocol thereafter. A saline enema in the morning may be required.

After the ingestion of the contrast medium, any vomiting or diarrhea must be reported to the radiologist.

**Quality Control**

> The patient must understand the pretest instructions and be willing to comply. Failure to take the iopanoic acid as prescribed results in inadequate visualization of the gallbladder and ducts.

**Posttest**

If a repeat test must be performed the next day, instruct the patient to maintain a low-fat diet until the pretest procedure begins again.

**Complications**

Occasionally, a reaction can occur because of allergy to the iodinated contrast medium. The severity of the reaction can range from mild and delayed in onset to sudden, intense, and potentially catastrophic. The medical and nursing personnel observe for any sign of allergic response so that immediate intervention can be initiated. (See Table 19–5 for a summary of the complications and the appropriate nursing assessments.)

## Computed Tomography of the Liver, Biliary Tract, Pancreas, and Spleen

**(Tomography)**

Synonym: CT scan

Images of the liver, gallbladder, pancreas, and spleen are clearly demonstrated by computed tomographic (CT) scan. In liver disease, the CT scan is used to detect abnormal size or shape and the presence of tumor, abscess, cyst, or bleeding in the liver. It also can help identify the source of jaundice due to liver disease or obstruction of the biliary ducts. In pancreatic disease, the CT scan identifies tumors, cysts, and pseudocysts. An enlarged, edematous pancreas is an indication of acute pancreatitis. Intravenous contrast medium is used to evaluate the liver and pancreas (Seeram, 1994).

A CT scan of the spleen can reveal a cyst, abscess, hematoma, bleeding, infarct, or malignancy. The CT scan is the procedure of choice in the evaluation of abdominal trauma because it has an accuracy rate of 91% (Chintapalli & Schnitker, 1994).

**Helical (Spiral) Computed Tomography.**   This technology has become the best CT method to image the liver. Because multiple images can be obtained rapidly as the patient holds his or her breath, no movement in the abdomen occurs during the moments of imaging. Because of the speed of the imaging, the iodinated contrast medium can be delivered in short bursts and the images of the liver can be obtained shortly thereafter while the contrast material is very concentrated in the liver tissue. The images are of high quality and clarity, so that it is possible to visualize small tumors, sites of early infection or abscess, fibrosis, and fatty deposits. Vascular imaging with contrast medium is also possible. Examination for obstruction of the hepatic artery and portal veins is also done (Bluemke, Soyer, & Fishman, 1995).

The advantages of helical CT in liver imaging are also true for imaging of the pancreas and biliary system. Helical CT provides greater detail and accuracy in the imaging of small tumors or stones in these organs. The vascular structures may be reproduced in three-dimensional images, particularly as part of presurgical assessment (Zeman et al., 1995).

A complete discussion of CT scanning is presented in Chapter 12.

## Endoscopic Retrograde Cholangiopancreatography and Pancreatic Cytology

**(Endoscopy)**                    Synonym: ERCP

**Normal Values**

> **ERCP:** The anatomy of the ductal systems of the gallbladder, liver, and pancreas are patent, with no evidence of obstruction from stone, stricture, or tumor.
> **Pancreatic cytology:** No malignant cells are present.

### Background Information

When obstruction occurs in any part of the biliary system or at the head of the pancreas, bile flow is impeded and obstructive jaundice develops. If obstruction of the pancreatic ductal system exists, pancreatitis occurs. Pancreatic obstruction that extends into the ampulla, the common duct, or both also causes jaundice. Because of the close proximity of the organs and the common bile duct that drains both bile and pancreatic secretions, it is difficult to determine the precise problem and location. ERCP provides direct visualization and radiographic views of the biliary and pancreatic ducts.

### Purpose of the Test

ERCP is used to investigate the cause of obstructive jaundice, persistent abdominal pain, or both associated with a biliary or pancreatic disorder. The most common findings are a retained stone in the common bile duct, chronic pancreatitis, and cancer.

### Procedure

A side-viewing duodenoscope or other type of fiberoptic endoscope is passed through the mouth, esophagus, and stomach and into the duodenum. At the ampulla of Vater, a small cannula is inserted into the ampulla and then, in turn, into the common duct and pancreatic duct (Fig. 19–8). An intrave-

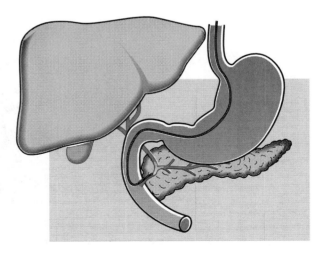

**Figure 19–8**
Endoscopic retrograde cholangiopancreatography. At the level of the duodenum, the papilla is located and the cannula is inserted through it. The cannula is passed first into the common bile duct (endoscopic retrograde cholangiography) and then into the pancreatic duct (endoscopic retrograde pancreatography).

nous bolus of glucagon may be given for its antispasmodic effect on the intestine and Oddi's sphincter. Fluoroscopic views are used to guide the placement of the instrument. Once the cannula is in the common duct, radiopaque contrast is instilled and multiple x-ray films are taken (Fig. 19–9). To enhance the gravity flow of the contrast medium, the patient is assisted in changing positions, and the table is tilted so that all branches of the biliary tree are filled and visible. Once the biliary duct examination is completed, the

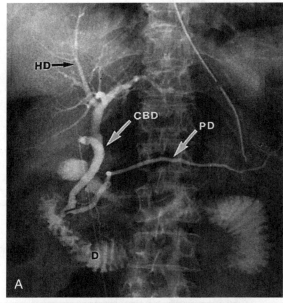

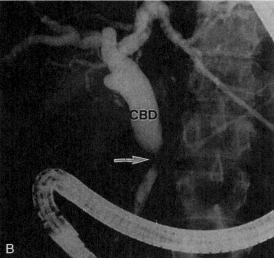

**Figure 19–9**

Normal versus abnormal radiologic findings during endoscopic retrograde cholangiopancreatography (ERCP). *A*, ERCP radiographic view of the normal common bile duct (CBD), pancreatic duct (PD), and hepatic ducts (HD). *B*, ERCP radiographic view of stricture and proximal dilation of the common bile duct. (Reproduced with permission from Mettler, F. A. [1996]. *Essentials of radiology*. Philadelphia: W. B. Saunders.)

cannula is relocated to the pancreatic duct, and the radiographic procedure with contrast medium is repeated.

**Pancreatic Cytology.** When cytologic examination of the pancreatic secretions is indicated, it is performed during the endoscopic retrograde pancreatography phase of the procedure. The patient is given an intravenous bolus of secretin to stimulate the flow of pancreatic secretions. A sample of the secretion is aspirated from the duct and is sent to the laboratory for cytologic analysis.

### Quality Control

The endoscope and its accessories must be cleaned, disinfected, and dried meticulously to reduce the number of microorganisms (Favero & Pugliese, 1996). ERCP is a deeply invasive endoscopic procedure that can easily result in sepsis.

---

**Findings**

**Abnormal Values**

BILIARY

| | | |
|---|---|---|
| Biliary stone | Cholangiocarcinoma | Primary biliary |
| Papillary stenosis | Caroli's disease | cirrhosis |
| Fibrosis or stricture | (cystic dilation of | Lymphoma |
| Sclerosing cholangitis | the ducts) | Liver metastases |

PANCREATIC

| | | |
|---|---|---|
| Acute, recurring | Cancer, adenocarci- | Fistula |
| pancreatitis | noma | Abscess |
| Chronic pancreatitis | Pseudocyst | |

---

**Interfering Factors**

- Uncooperative patient behavior
- Severe, acute pancreatitis
- Acute biliary obstruction
- Septic cholangitis (unless biliary drainage is performed)
- Acute myocardial infarction
- Pancreatic pseudocyst
- Esophageal or gastric outlet obstruction
- Hepatitis B infection

---

**Nursing Implementation**

**Pretest**

Provide preprocedure teaching so that the patient can relax during the 1-hour examination. Because ERCP is uncomfortable, intravenous medication will promote relaxation and analgesia. The patient will be aware enough to assist in changing from a lateral to a prone position and to remain immobile during the viewing process.

An informed consent form must be signed by the patient or the person legally responsible for the patient's health care decisions.

Take vital signs and record these baseline values. Question the patient regarding any history of allergy to iodine, seafood, or iodine-based dye used during a previous diagnostic study. Inform the physician of a positive history.

Instruct the patient to discontinue all foods and fluids for 12 hours before the test.

Before the examination starts, the endoscopy nurse tests all equipment for correct mechanical function and proper illumination.

One hour before the start of the procedure, an intravenous infusion is started in the patient's arm or hand. When cholangitis or infection is suspected, systemic antibiotics are started and continued into the postprocedure period.

Intravenous diazepam (Valium), meperidine, and atropine are given to the patient to provide relaxation, analgesia, and reduced motility of the intestinal tract.

Alternatively, a bolus dose of midazolam (Versed) exerts a powerful, rapid enhancement of the narcotic. It also provides sedation and amnesia. The side effects of diazepam and midazolam are central nervous system and respiratory depression (Noerr, 1995).

Once the administration of medication begins, the nurse monitors the vital signs and respiratory status frequently. In many endoscopy units, automated blood pressure, pulse oximetry, and cardiac monitoring are used. Because a risk of apnea exists, resuscitation equipment must be readily available.

Before insertion of the endoscope, the patient's mouth and throat are anesthetized with a topical spray. After that, the tongue feels thick, and swallowing is difficult. An oral brace is inserted into the mouth to keep it open; a suction catheter is inserted to remove saliva.

The patient wears a lead shield over the thyroid gland. Personnel in the room must wear a lead body shield and a thyroid shield because of repeated exposure to radiation during the procedure.

### During the Test

Continue to assess the patient's cardiovascular and respiratory status frequently. Oxygen administered by nasal cannula helps prevent hypoxemia. Sudden bradycardia from a vasovagal reflex can occur as the endoscope is manipulated.

### Quality Control

> To prevent respiratory depression or cardiac arrest, intravenous analgesics are given slowly over a 1- to 2-minute period. Naloxone (Narcan) is kept on hand to reverse the respiratory depressive effect of meperidine, but it is ineffective against diazepam. Atropine sulfate is kept on hand to overcome the effects of bradycardia.

Assist the patient with positioning and relaxation.

Two vials of pancreatic secretions are collected for cytologic examination. The first is discarded because the initial flow of secretions also contains the contrast medium. The second specimen is identified, labeled, packed in ice, and sent to the laboratory quickly. The cooling process minimizes the deterioration of any cells within the fluid.

### Posttest

The nurse monitors the cardiovascular and respiratory status at 15-minute intervals until the patient is stable.

The patient ingests nothing by mouth until the gag reflex and swallowing ability return, at which point clear fluids are started; a light meal can follow shortly thereafter. In the first hour or so, colicky abdominal pain can occur because of the air that was inserted during the test. It will disappear as food intake resumes.

The nurse instructs the patient to use throat lozenges or warm saline gargles to relieve soreness in the throat.

Discharge teaching includes informing the patient to notify the physician of any severe or prolonged symptoms of abdominal pain, fever, nausea, or vomiting.

| | |
|---|---|
| **Complications** | Because of tissue manipulation during the procedure and the already compromised state of the patient's health, complications can occur. Sepsis is the most significant problem, affecting either the biliary tract or the pancreas. Pancreatitis is the problem that occurs most frequently. Sometimes the complication begins within hours, and other times it takes a day or two to develop. Table 19–6 provides a summary of the complications and the appropriate nursing assessments. |

## Laparoscopy, Abdominal

**(Endoscopy, Tissue Biopsy)**      Synonym: Diagnostic laparoscopy

| | |
|---|---|
| **Normal Values** | The size, shape, and structure of the abdominal organs are normal. No bleeding or ascitic fluid loss occurs, and the tissue biopsy is normal. |

## Background Information

Diagnostic laparoscopy provides direct visualization of the organs in the abdominal cavity, the diaphragm, the abdominal wall, and the peritoneum. Once placed in the abdominal cavity, the laparoscope illuminates and magnifies the image so that the various tissues can be assessed visually. The instrument also is used to biopsy specific tissue sites. A video camera is attached to the instrument to document the findings.

**Laparoscopic Liver Biopsy.**   When biopsy of a specific site in the liver is needed, the laparoscopic approach has a very high rate of accuracy in diagnosis. The first part of the procedure is to visualize the surface of the liver, assessing for possible abnormality. Once a specific area of tumor, fibrosis, or infection is located, the biopsy specimen is taken.

**Staging for Cancer.**   Preoperative staging of cancer can be done for hepatobiliary, pancreatic, and ovarian malignancy. Using the laparoscope, the staging process determines the extent of the primary cancer site and identifies any metastasis in the organ and surrounding tissues of the abdominal cavity.

Biopsy specimens are obtained when indicated by the findings.

**Laparoscopic Ultrasound.**   During the laparoscopic staging of the malignancy, the laparoscopic ultrasound (LUS) instrument is inserted through a separate small incision. It uses sound waves to locate areas of different tissue density, or tumors, within the organ. The purpose is to assist with the accuracy of the biopsy and to identify small sites of malignancy that may be hidden beneath the tissue surface, in lymph nodes, or within vascular walls. Laparoscopic ultrasound detects tumors that are smaller than 1 cm in size. Often, these tumors are too small to be detected by CT, magnetic resonance imaging (MRI), or ultrasound (Callery, Strasberg, Doherty, Soper & Norton, 1997).

**Abdominal Trauma.**   In cases of penetrating trauma to the abdomen, as from a stab wound, diagnostic laparoscopy can determine whether or not the peritoneum was penetrated. In blunt abdominal trauma, the laparoscopy is used to investigate suspected intra-abdominal bleeding

**Table 19–6   Complications of Endoscopic Retrograde Cholangiopancreatography**

| Complication | Nursing Assessment |
|---|---|
| Pancreatitis | Acute epigastric pain<br>Abdominal distention<br>Ecchymosis of the skin in the left flank or periumbilical area<br>Boardlike abdomen<br>Nausea and vomiting |
| Cholangitis (bacterial infection of the biliary tree) | Moderate abdominal pain<br>Leukocytosis and abnormal liver function test results<br>Fever and chills<br>Jaundice |
| Cardiovascular change | Hypotension<br>Tachycardia<br>Shock<br>Angina<br>Arrhythmia<br>Tachypnea or dyspnea<br>Diaphoresis |
| Perforation | Acute epigastric pain<br>Abdominal distention<br>Boardlike abdomen<br>Shock<br>Sepsis |
| Bleeding | Hypotension<br>Tachycardia<br>Dyspnea<br>Diaphoresis and pallor<br>Acute abdomen or abdominal distention<br>Ecchymosis<br>Melena |

and injury to the internal organs. This procedure is helpful, particularly with injury to the liver or spleen, because initial clinical symptoms do not always reveal the extent of the damage. Diagnostic laparoscopy is helpful in cases when a nonsurgical treatment approach may be possible. It is not used when an obvious and urgent need to repair the damage surgically exists (Pepe, 1993).

**Purpose of the Test**   Laparoscopy provides direct visualization and the means to biopsy organs of the abdominal cavity when hepatobiliary, pancreatic, ovarian, or splenic disease is suspected. In cancer, the procedure can be used to help stage the disease and determine the feasibility of surgical removal of the tumor.

In cases of blunt or penetrating trauma to the abdomen, laparoscopy is done to assess for intraperitoneal bleeding and to define the location and the extent of the damage (Collin & Bianchi, 1997; Pepe, 1993).

| | |
|---|---|
| **Procedure** | While the patient is under local anesthesia and intravenous sedation, the peritoneal cavity is filled with gas (nitrous oxide or carbon dioxide) to provide space for the instruments and viewing of the organs. The laparoscope and the laparoscopic ultrasound instrument are inserted through small incisions in the abdomen. Ultrasound recordings and biopsy of affected tissue may be done in addition to the direct visualization. |

**Findings**

### Abnormal Values

| | | |
|---|---|---|
| Primary or metastatic cancer | Cirrhosis of the liver | Tuberculosis |
| Trauma to the spleen, liver, or colon | Hodgkin's disease | |
| | Penetration of the peritoneum | |

**Interfering Factors**

- Severe, symptomatic cardiac or respiratory disease
- Uncooperative patient behavior

**Nursing Implementation**

### Pretest

Obtain a signed consent form from the patient or the person legally responsible for the patient's health care decisions.

Instruct the patient to discontinue all food and fluids for 8 hours before the test.

Check that the results of a recent prothrombin time test, partial thromboplastin time test, complete blood count, platelet count, and possible electrocardiogram are posted in the patient's chart. The physician is notified of abnormal values.

### Quality Control

Patients with liver disorders may also have poor clotting ability. The prothrombin time should not be more than 3 seconds longer than the control time, and the platelet count should be greater than 100,000 cells/mm³. This procedure is contraindicated for patients with an acute cardiac or respiratory condition.

Take baseline vital signs and record them in the patient's chart.

Administer the prescribed pretest medication about 1 hour before the test. Meperidine (Demerol) and midazolam (Versed) are often used for analgesia and relaxation.

Establish the intravenous line for fluid replacement and as the route for intravenous sedation.

To monitor for adequate oxygenation, place the pulse oximeter on the patient's finger and connect the equipment for monitoring of vital signs.

Set up the laparoscopic instrument system, ensuring that it is sterile and functional.

Prepare the abdomen with povidone-iodine, and drape the area with sterile cloth.

### During the Test

Stand near the patient to provide reassurance and to give instructions. Despite the use of local anesthesia, sedation, and narcotics, the patient feels some pain in the abdomen and the top of the shoulder as gas is instilled in the abdominal cavity and as the instruments are manipulated.

Monitor the vital signs and the oxygen saturation regularly. The oxygen saturation should remain in the normal range of greater than 95% (>0.95). The oxygen level can drop by as much as 10% (to the mid-80 range) because of the sedation and narcotics. In addition, the pneumoperitoneum and Trendelenburg's position put pressure on the diaphragm and lungs, making it harder to breathe (Slowey, Slowey, & Cato, 1996). To prevent hypoxemia during the procedure, supplement the breathing with oxygen administration by nasal cannula (Haydon, Dillon, Simpson, Thomas, & Hayes, 1996).

Observe for a vasovagal response, as indicated by a sudden drop in the pulse. This can occur as the abdominal contents are manipulated.

Place the biopsy tissue into the specimen container with formalin, and label it with the source of the tissue and the patient's name (Jacobs et al., 1996).

Once the procedure is completed, cover the incisions with sterile dressings and take vital signs.

### Quality Control

> The endoscope and accessory parts must be mechanically cleansed and disinfected after each procedure. The goal is to remove organic matter and infectious agents, thus minimizing the potential for transmission of infection (Rutala, 1996).

### Posttest

Take vital signs frequently and regularly.

Observe the dressings and the surrounding tissue for ascites fluid, bleeding, or hematoma formation. Some blood is expected on the dressing, but it should be minimal.

Administer the prescribed pain medication for incisional pain.

Maintain the intravenous fluid replacement until the patient begins to drink clear fluids, usually in 2 to 4 hours. A light diet is usually started in 6 hours.

If the patient is to be discharged after 6 hours, provide instructions to remain in the regional area for 24 hours in case of problems. The patient should call the physician regarding problems of bleeding, intense abdominal pain, fever, leakage of fluid, malaise, or respiratory difficulty (Coles & Caldwell, 1995; Jacobs et al., 1996). (Table 19–7 provides a summary of the complications of liver biopsy and the corresponding nursing assessments.)

## Liver-Biliary Scan

**(Radionuclide Imaging)**   Synonyms: Biliary tree scan, hepatobiliary imaging, hepatobiliary scintigraphy, DISDA scan, HIDA scan

**Normal Values**   Homogeneous uptake of the radionuclide throughout the liver occurs, with excretion into the biliary tree and gallbladder and emptying into the duodenum. The liver and biliary tract are normal in structure and function.

## Background Information

Technetium 99m sulfur colloid is bonded with imi-nodiacetic acid (IDA) agent for the radionuclide imaging of the liver and biliary tract. After the intravenous injection of the radionuclide imaging agent, the hepatocytes clear the agent from the blood and concentrate it within the liver. Shortly thereafter, clearance of the radionuclide agent from the liver occurs. It will enter hepatic ducts, biliary ducts, and the gallbladder and finally exit via the duodenum.

When the gallbladder is inflamed, the radiopharmaceutical cannot enter. With obstruction in the biliary tract, good visualization of the liver and part of the biliary tree is possible, but no radiopharmaceutical enters beyond the point of obstruction. The patient who is scheduled for this test is usually jaundiced and has an elevated serum bilirubin level.

## Purpose of the Test

The liver-biliary scan is used for visualization of the biliary ductal system for the purpose of diagnosis of an acute or chronic biliary tract disorder.

## Procedure

After the intravenous dose of the radiopharmaceutical is administered, a gamma camera takes serial images of the abdomen at 5- to 10-minute intervals. In a normal hepatobiliary system, the gallbladder and biliary tree are visible within 30 minutes (Fig. 19–10). If the common bile duct and the duodenum are not visualized within 1 hour, delay images are taken every hour for 4 hours.

The uptake and excretion of the isotope are recorded on x-ray film, video screen, or photographic film. The procedure takes 1 to 4 hours.

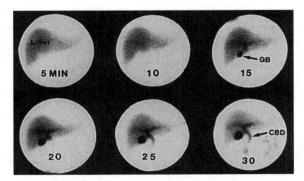

**Figure 19–10**
Normal hepatobiliary scan. With normal function of the liver and biliary system, the radionuclide provides visualization of the liver and gallbladder (GB) within 15 minutes and visualization of the common bile duct (CBD) within 30 minutes. (Reproduced with permission from Mettler, F. A. [1996]. *Essentials of radiology*. Philadelphia: W. B. Saunders.)

| **Findings** | **Abnormal Values** | |
|---|---|---|
| | Cholecystitis, acute or chronic | Biliary atresia |
| | | Stenosis of the |
| | Obstruction of the biliary tract | ampulla of Vater |

**Interfering Factors**

- Failure to maintain a nothing-by-mouth status
- Prolonged fasting or hyperalimentation
- Pregnancy
- Hepatocellular disease

**Nursing Implementation**    **Pretest**

Obtain informed consent from the patient or the person legally responsible for the patient's health care decisions.

For an elective procedure, instruct the patient to discontinue all food and fluids for 8 hours before the test. When this test is performed on an urgent basis, a minimum of a 2-hour fast is desirable.

**Quality Control**

The patient must fast before the test to prevent food stimulation of the gallbladder. When food is in the stomach, the gallbladder contracts intermittently and will not fill with the radiopharmaceutical. This causes a false-positive result. Paradoxically, prolonged fasting can also cause a false-positive result, so the maximum time for the patient to fast is 8 hours.

## Liver Biopsy, Percutaneous

**(Tissue Biopsy)**      Synonym: Percutaneous liver biopsy

**Normal Values**

The liver cells are normal, with no evidence of inflammation, scarring, degeneration, tumor, or other pathologic condition.

### Background Information

The liver biopsy is performed by percutaneous needle aspiration or needle excision of a small sample of liver tissue. Microscopic examination of the stained tissue provides specific and detailed information about the tissue cells, structure, and any pathologic change that is identified.

Some diagnostic data have already been obtained, and the abnormal results are indicators that a liver biopsy is needed to identify the cause. The abnormal findings often include an unexplained enlargement of the liver, persistent elevation of liver function test results, jaundice, or a history of infiltrating disease that commonly affects the liver.

### Purpose of the Test

The biopsy is used to diagnose pathologic changes in the liver and to help evaluate the extent of the disease process.

**Procedure**

Liver biopsy is performed by using needle aspiration to obtain a small sample of liver tissue for microscopic examination. After administration of local anesthesia, the aspirating needle is placed between the anterior and midaxillary lines, usually in the sixth or seventh intercostal space (Fig. 19–11). While the patient holds his or her breath on expiration, the needle is inserted quickly and a 10-mL syringe is used to aspirate a small sample of liver tissue. Once the needle is removed, the patient resumes breathing.

When the aspiration is completed, the tissue is placed in a specimen container filled with formalin or saline. The specimen is labeled and sent to the pathology laboratory for microscopic examination.

**Quality Control**

The aspiration must be coordinated with breathing because during expiration, the liver and diaphragm are at their highest position. When the patient holds his or her breath, the liver tissue is immobile. Both these factors help prevent laceration of the liver and diaphragm.

**Findings**

**Abnormal Values**

| | | |
|---|---|---|
| Cirrhosis | Sarcoidosis | Wilson's disease |
| Hemochromatosis | Chronic hepatitis B | Metastatic cancer |
| Alcoholic liver disease | Amyloidosis | Miliary tuberculosis |
| | Hepatoma | Cyst of the liver |

**Interfering Factors**

- Obesity
- Infection in right pleural cavity or right upper quadrant of the abdomen
- Uncooperative patient behavior
- Abnormal clotting ability

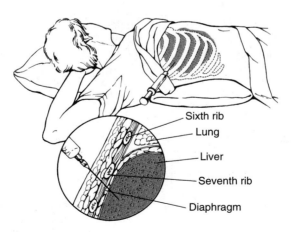

Sixth rib
Lung
Liver
Seventh rib
Diaphragm

**Figure 19–11**
Liver biopsy. The patient is positioned for liver biopsy in a supine or left lateral position with the right arm abducted. (Reproduced with permission from Burden, N. [1993]. *Ambulatory surgical nursing* [p. 576]. Philadelphia: W. B. Saunders.)

**Nursing Implementation**

### Pretest

Obtain a signed consent form from the patient or the person legally responsible for the patient's health care decisions.

Provide pretest teaching about the procedure, positioning, breathing instructions, and posttest instructions. Because patients tend to experience anxiety about this test, provide reassurance and support as needed.

Instruct the patient to discontinue all food and fluids for 8 hours before the test.

Check that a recent prothrombin time test, partial thromboplastin time test, hematocrit, and platelet count have been obtained and that the results are within safety guidelines for this procedure. The laboratory reports are placed in the chart, and the physician is notified of abnormal values.

### Quality Control

Patients with liver disorders may also have poor clotting ability. The prothrombin time should not be more than 3 seconds longer than the control time, and the platelet count should be greater than 100,000 cells/mm³.

Take baseline vital signs and record them in the patient's chart.

Administer any prescribed pretest medication about 1 hour before the test. Meperidine, 50 mg, or diazepam, 10 mg, is commonly used for analgesia and relaxation.

Position the patient on the left side or in the supine position with the arm under the head. The skin is cleansed with antiseptic and draped with a sterile cloth.

### During the Test

Stand beside the patient to provide reassurance and help in remaining immobile. Despite the use of local anesthesia, the patient feels some pain in the side and the top of the shoulder as the needle passes through phrenic nerves and into the liver.

Assist with the placement of the tissue in the specimen container and label it appropriately.

Cover the aspiration site with a sterile dressing, take vital signs, and position the patient on the right side.

Record assessment data and make a note about the procedure in the patient's chart.

### Posttest

For 1 to 2 hours, the patient remains positioned on the right side with a pillow pressing on the waist area. This helps the liver remain somewhat compressed against the rib cage and will help promote clotting.

Vital signs are monitored frequently until they are stable. It is customary to take them every 15 minutes for 1 hour, every hour for 4 hours, and every 4 hours thereafter.

The nurse observes for signs of bleeding on a frequent or regular basis. The dressing is not removed, however. If bleeding occurs, it is likely to appear as leakage at the needle puncture site, to flow into the peritoneal cavity, or to appear as ecchymosis in a nearby area.

The patient can resume food and fluid intake as soon as desired. Bedrest is maintained for 12 to 24 hours. If the patient is to be discharged to the home, he or she remains on bedrest in the recovery area for 6 hours before discharge (Neidzwick & Stringer, 1994).

For discharge to the home, instruct the patient to notify the physician of any malaise, fever, pain, or shortness of breath. For 2 weeks, the patient must avoid aspirin and medicines that contain aspirin. He or she must also avoid heavy lifting until healing is complete. Removal of the bandage is done, and bathing may be resumed in 24 hours (Neidzwick & Stringer, 1994).

**Complications**

Usually, complications do not occur, but potential exists for bleeding, pneumothorax, and peritonitis. If a small blood vessel is punctured inadvertently during the procedure, blood loss will be greater than normal. Because coagulation ability may be limited, the blood loss can be considerable to severe. If a bile duct is punctured inadvertently, bile will leak into the peritoneal cavity and cause severe peritonitis. If the needle was angled too high, the diaphragm or lung can be punctured or lacerated, resulting in pneumothorax. A summary of the complications and the appropriate nursing assessments is presented in Table 19–7.

**Table 19–7     Complications of Liver Biopsy**

| Complication | Nursing Assessment |
| --- | --- |
| Bleeding | Tachycardia |
| | Hypotension, shock |
| | Pallor and diaphoresis |
| | Dyspnea |
| | Distended abdomen |
| | Boardlike abdomen |
| | Ecchymosis |
| | Decreased hematocrit |
| | Abdominal pain |
| Peritonitis | Persistent, severe pain in the abdomen or shoulder |
| | Boardlike abdomen |
| | Fever |
| | Tachycardia |
| | Hypotension, shock |
| Pneumothorax | Dyspnea |
| | Cyanosis |
| | Hypotension |
| | Restlessness, apprehension |

## Liver-Spleen Scan

(Radionuclide Imaging)   Synonym: Liver scan

**Normal Values**   Homogeneous uptake of the radionuclide throughout the liver and spleen occurs. The organs are normal in their structure and function.

### Background Information

Technetium 99m sulfur colloid is a radioactive nuclide used to scan the liver and spleen. Each of these organs contains reticuloendothelial cells. Because of their phagocytosis capability, the reticuloendothelial cells accumulate the isotope and allow simultaneous imaging of both organs.

Space-occupying lesions such as tumor, abscess, hematoma, or scarring do not fill with radioisotope. The image created by the radioisotope reveals the deficit and demonstrates the decreased activity in a particular area. The abnormal finding is called a filling defect or "cold" spot. Additional information about nuclear scanning is found in Chapter 10.

The liver and spleen are evaluated for size, shape, position, function, and the presence of defects in the uptake of the radionuclide (Mettler, 1996).

**Purpose**   The liver-spleen scan is used to confirm and evaluate suspected hepatocellular disease and enlargement of the liver or spleen and to detect space-occupying lesions in either organ.

**Procedure**   After the technetium 99m sulfur colloid is injected intravenously, it is cleared from the blood by the liver within minutes. The liver will absorb 80% to 90% of the radionuclide, and the spleen will absorb most of the remainder. Once the radionuclide is concentrated in the organ, it emits impulses that are converted into images. Within 15 to 30 minutes after injection, a rotating gamma camera or scintillation scanner is used to obtain anterior, posterior, and lateral views of the liver and spleen. The images are recorded on x-ray film, video screen, or photographic film. The procedure takes 1 to 2 hours to complete.

**Findings**   **Elevated Values**

| | | |
|---|---|---|
| Hepatomegaly, splenomegaly | Cirrhosis | Cyst formation |
| Abscesses | Hematoma of liver or spleen | |
| Hepatitis | Metastatic liver cancer | |
| Tumor of liver or spleen | Hemangioma | |

**Interfering Factors**   • Pregnancy
• Breastfeeding

| | |
|---|---|
| **Nursing Implementation** | **Pretest** |

Obtain an informed consent form from the patient or the person legally responsible for the patient's health care decisions.

Ask the female patient if she is pregnant or breast-feeding. The radiation from the radionuclide would enter the infant via the breast milk, and radiation can harm the fetus.

**Posttest**

The radionuclide is eliminated from the body in the urine within 24 hours. Instruct the patient to flush the toilet and wash the hands immediately after voiding to minimize exposure to the small amount of radiation present in the urine.

## Ultrasound of the Liver, Gallbladder, Biliary Tract, Spleen, and Pancreas

**(Ultrasonography)**      Synonyms: None

Ultrasound uses high-frequency sound waves to visualize the size and structure of internal organs. When the sound waves pass through skin and muscle and then reach an organ or tissue surface of a different texture, the sound waves are reflected back. The echoes are changed, amplified, and demonstrated on a cathode ray tube (CRT).

Ultrasound is a major diagnostic tool for the examination of the liver, hepatobiliary tract, spleen, and pancreas. In the liver, it can detect a cyst, abscess, hematoma, primary neoplasm, and metastatic tumor. It is the best diagnostic tool to detect gallstone. It detects 95% of the stones in the gallbladder, but only 50% of those located in the common bile duct (Nahrwold, 1993). It also may show thickening of the gallbladder walls associated with acute cholecystitis or dilation of the biliary tract associated with obstruction. An enlarged or edematous pancreas is measurable by ultrasound. Pancreatic abscess, pseudocyst, and pancreatic tumor are readily identified. Ultrasound identifies a congenital absence of the spleen or the existence of multiple spleens. It can also identify the presence and size of space-occupying lesions such as cysts or tumors and is accurate in the measurement of the size of the spleen. A complete discussion of ultrasound is presented in Chapter 8.

## References

Abbott Laboratories. (1992). *Principles in practice: Testing for viral hepatitis.* North Chicago, IL: Author.

Abnormal cholangiograms don't mean exploration is necessary. (1996). *Laparoscopic Surgery Update, 4*(8), 91–93.

Aziz, D. C. (1996). Clinical use of tumor markers based on outcome analysis. *Laboratory Medicine, 27*(12), 817–821.

Baer, D. (1995). Assays on bile specimens. *Medical Laboratory Observer, 27*(10), 17–18.

Baer, D. (1995). Fecal fat. *Medical Laboratory Observer, 27*(11), 18, 20.

Baer, D. M. (1995). Elevated lipase. *Medical Laboratory Observer, 27*(9), 12.

Balnaves, M. E., Bonaquisto, L., & Francis, I. (1995). The impact of newborn screening on cystic fibrosis testing in Victoria, Australia. *Journal of Medical Genetics, 32*(7), 537–542.

Baroni, M. A., Anderson, Y. E., & Mischler, E. (1997). Cystic fibrosis newborn screening: Impact of early screening results on parenting stress. *Pediatric Nursing, 23*(2), 143–151.

Belli, L. S., Ideo, G., & Silini, E. (1997). Hepatitis G and post transplantation hepatitis. *New England Journal of Medicine, 335*(18), 1394–1395.

Berrios, F., & Jain, L. (1996). Current concepts in neonatal hyperbilirubinemia. *Neonatal Intensive Care, 9*(3), 48–52.

Blackburn, S. (1995). Hyperbilirubinemia and neonatal jaundice. *Neonatal Network: Journal of Neonatal Nursing, 14*(7), 15–25.

Bluemke, D. A., Soyer, P., & Fishman, E. K. (1995). Helical (spiral) CT of the liver. *Radiologic Clinics of North America, 33*(5), 863–886.

Bryan, J. P. (1995). Viral hepatitis: Update on hepatitis D and E. *Consultant, 35*(12), 1846–1850.

Burtis, C. A., & Ashwood, E. R. (1999). *Tietz textbook of clinical chemistry* (3rd ed.). Philadelphia: W. B. Saunders.

Callery, M. P., Strasberg, S. M., Doherty, G. M., Soper, N. J., Norton, J. A. (1997). Staging laparoscopy with laparoscopic ultrasonography: Optimizing resectability in hepatobiliary and pancreatic malignancy. *American College of Surgeons, 185,* 33–39.

Chintapalli, K. N., & Schnitker, J. B. (1994). Spleen imaging. *Applied Radiology, 23*(12), 29–37.

Coles, M., & Caldwell, S. H. (1995). Diagnostic laparoscopy of the liver and peritoneum, using conscious sedation. *Gastroenterology Nursing, 18*(2), 62–66.

Collin, G. R., & Bianchi, J. D. (1997). Laparoscopic examination of the traumatized spleen with blood salvage for autotransfusion. *American Surgeon, 63*(6), 478–480.

Colodny, C. S. (1995). Paracentesis and peritoneal lavage. *Patient Care, 29*(13), 137–138, 140, 145.

Constantinescu, M., & Hilman, B. C. (1996). The sweat test for quantitation of electrolytes: A challenge in precision. *Laboratory Medicine, 27*(7), 472–477.

Covington, C., Gieleghem, P., Board, F., Madison, K., Nedd, D., & Miller, L. (1996). Family care related to alpha fetoprotein screening. *Journal of Obstetric, Gynecologic and Neonatal Nursing, 25*(2), 125–130.

Favero, M. S., & Pugliese, G. (1996). Infections transmitted by endoscopy: An international problem. *American Journal of Infection Control, 24*(5), 343–345.

Favorov, M. O. (1992). Serological diagnosis of hepatitis E infection. *Journal of Medical Virology, 36,* 246–250.

Ginsberg, A. L. (1996). Liver enzymes: How to interpret the diagnostic implications. *Consultant, 36*(3), 575–578.

Gosling, P. (1995). Albumin in the critically ill. *Care of the Critically Ill, 11*(2), 57–61.

Gregg, R., Wilford, B., Farrell, P., Laxova, A., Hassemer, D., & Mischler, E. H. (1993). Application of DNA analysis in a population-screening program for neonatal diagnosis of cystic fibrosis (CF): Comparison of screening protocols. *Journal of Human Genetics, 52,* 616–626.

Gretch, D. R. (1997). Diagnostic tests for hepatitis C. *Hepatology, 26*(9), 48S–56S.

Harisinghani, M. G., Saini, S., & Schima, W. (1996). Computed tomography and magnetic resonance imaging of focal hepatic masses. *Applied Radiology, 25*(11), 15–16, 19–20, 25–26.

Haydon, G. H., Dillon, J., Simpson, K. J., Thomas, H., & Hayes, P. C. (1996). Hypoxemia during diagnostic laparoscopy: A prospective study. *Gastrointestinal Endoscopy, 44*(2), 124–128.

Henry, J. B. (1996). *Clinical diagnosis and management by laboratory methods* (19th ed.). Philadelphia: W. B. Saunders.

Hepatitis G discovery raises new worries. (1996). *Hospital Infection Control, 23*(5), 62–63.

Herlong, H. F. (1994). Approach to the patient with abnormal liver enzymes. *Hospital Practice, 29*(11), 32–38.

Hu, K. Q., & Vierling, J. M. (1994). Molecular diagnostic techniques for viral hepatitis. *Gastroenterology Clinics of North America, 23*(3), 479–498.

Jackson, M., & Rymer, T. E. (1994). Commentary on viral hepatitis: Anatomy of a diagnosis. *American Journal of Nursing, 94*(1), 43–48.

Jacobs, D. S., DeMott, W. R., Grady, H. J., Horvat, R. T., Huestis, D. W., & Kasten, B. L. (Eds.). (1996). *Laboratory test handbook* (4th ed.). Baltimore: Williams & Wilkins.

Kant, J. A., Mifflin, T. E., McGlennen, R., Rice, E., Naylor, E., & Cooper, D. L. (1995). Molecular diagnosis of cystic fibrosis. *Clinics in Laboratory Medicine, 15*(4), 877–898.

Kuhns, M. C. (1995). Viral hepatitis. Part I: The discovery, diagnostic tests and new viruses. *Laboratory Medicine, 26*(10), 650–659.

Lehmann, C. A. (1998). *Saunders manual of clinical laboratory science.* Philadelphia: W. B. Saunders.

London, W. T., & Evans, A. A. (1996). The epidemiology of viruses B, C, and D. *Clinics in Laboratory Medicine, 16*(2), 251–271.

Lum, G. (1995). Low activities of aspartate and alanine aminotransferase: Their significance in alcoholic liver disease. *Laboratory Medicine, 26*(4), 273–276.

Mettler, F. A. (1996). *Essentials of radiology.* Philadelphia: W. B. Saunders.

Nahrwold, D. L. (1993). Gallstone disease update: Diagnostic dilemmas, therapeutic options. *Consultant, 33*(8), 27–29, 31, 35.

Neiblum, D. R., & Boynton, R. F. (1996). Evaluation and treatment of hepatitis C infection. *Primary Care, 23*(3), 535–549.

Neidzwick, L., & Stringer, C. (1994). Liver biopsy and nursing intervention. *Gastroenterology Nursing, 17*(1), 17–19.

Noerr, B. (1995). Pointers in practical pharmacology: Midazolam (Versed). *Neonatal Network: Journal of Neonatal Nursing, 14*(1), 65–67.

Norris, M. K. G. (1993). Measuring serum amylase levels. *Nursing, 23*(11), 28.

One quick test for acute pancreatitis. (1994). *Emergency Medicine, 26*(7), 119.

Pepe, J. (1993). Diagnostic techniques in blunt and penetrating abdominal trauma. *Topics in Emergency Medicine, 15*(1), 8–21.

Rodriguez Inigo, E., Thomas, J. F., de Soria, V. G. G., Bartolomé, J., Pinilla, I., Amaro, M. J., Carreño, V., Fernández-Rañada, J. M. (1997). Hepatitis C and G virus infection and liver dysfunction after allogeneic bone marrow transplantation: Results from a prospective study. *Blood, 90*(3), 1326–1331.

Rutala, W. A. (1996). APIC guidelines for infection control practices. *American Journal of Infection Control, 24*(Suppl. 4), 313–342.

Saxena, S., Korula, J., Fong, T., & Schulman, I. A. (1995). Are gender-specific ALT cutoff values necessary? *Laboratory Medicine, 26*(10), 682–686.

Scheig, R. (1996). Evaluation of tests to screen patients with liver disorders. *Primary Care, 23*(3), 551–561.

Schwartz, J. G. (1997). A lesson in the ABCs of hepatitis. *Medical Laboratory Observer, 29*(1), 30–32, 36–38, 40–41.

Schwoebel, A., & Sakraida, S. (1997). Hyperbilirubinemia: New approaches to an old problem. *Journal of Perinatal and Neonatal Nursing, 11*(3), 78–97.

Seeram, E. (1994). *Computed tomography. Physical principles, clinical applications & quality control.* Philadelphia: W. B. Saunders.

Siconolfi, L. A. (1995). Clarifying the complexity of liver function tests. *Nursing, 25*(5), 39–44, L2.

Sjogren, M. H. (1994). Serologic diagnosis of viral hepatitis. *Gastroenterology Clinics of North America, 23*(3), 457–478.

Slowey, K. B., Slowey, M. J., & Cato, J. (1996). Cardiac complications of laparoscopy: Anesthetic implications. *CRNA: The Clinical Forum for Nurse Anesthetists, 7*(1), 9–13.

Statland, B. E. (1995). ALT and blood donors. *Medical Laboratory Observer, 28*(8), 86.

Statland, B. E. (1995). High alkaline phosphatase. *Medical Laboratory Observer, 27*(10), 17.

Statland, B. E. (1995). Increased GGT. *Medical Laboratory Observer, 27*(7), 12.

Stepp, C. A., & Woods, M. A. (1998). *Laboratory procedures for medical office personnel.* Philadelphia: W. B. Saunders.

Tietz, N. W. (Ed.). (1995). *Clinical guide to laboratory tests* (3rd ed.). Philadelphia: W. B. Saunders.

When to order serum amylase in children. (1995). *Emergency Medicine, 27*(2), 59.

Williams, J. K. (1995). Genetics and cystic fibrosis: A focus on carrier testing. *Pediatric Nursing, 21*(5), 444–448.

Zeman, R. K., Silverman, P. M., Ascher, S. M., Patt, R. H., Cooper, C., & al-Kawas, F. (1995). Helical (spiral) CT of the pancreas and biliary tract. *Radiologic Clinics of North America, 33*(5), 887–902.

# CHAPTER 20

# Endocrine Function

Because the endocrine system influences all body systems, one of the most difficult diagnostic problems is recognizing clinical manifestations as possible endocrine dysfunction. Once symptoms are recognized as a potential endocrine disorder, the clinician must select from a wide variety of specific and nonspecific tests. Some of the tests are invasive, whereas others present no potential danger to the client. Other tests may have potential side effects that would be harmful to the patient unless they are assessed by the nurse, with appropriate action taken.

The endocrine system is confusing, because hormones often have more than one name and therefore more than one abbreviation. Also, with the scientific and medical technology available, something new is learned every day about human hormones. The way hormones interact does not make clinical differentiation or learning easy.

Radioimmunoassay (RIA) techniques have revolutionized the diagnostic evaluation of patients with endocrine problems. These techniques have replaced older tests, which lacked specificity and reliability. Computed tomography (CT) and magnetic resonance imaging (MRI) have permitted more confidence in the diagnostic evaluation of many patients with endocrine system dysfunction. However, most tests confirm rather than make a diagnosis. Many test results will support a diagnosis but not rule out other diagnoses.

Myriad tests are available to assess endocrine function. This chapter focuses on common tests used clinically. Some classic tests are no longer performed and are not included in this chapter. Although some tests are no longer performed in research institutions, they are performed in community hospitals and are included in this chapter.

Table 20–1 provides an easy reference for the varied laboratory tests, based on the endocrine gland involved.

## Laboratory Tests

## Table 20–1   Laboratory Tests According to Organ Involvement

| Endocrine Organ | Endocrine Test |
|---|---|
| Adrenal gland | ACTH, plasma<br>ACTH stimulation test<br>Aldosterone, serum<br>Aldosterone, urinary<br>Catecholamines, plasma<br>Catecholamines, urinary<br>Cortisol, plasma<br>Dexamethasone suppression test<br>Free cortisol<br>Metyrapone<br>17-Hydroxycorticosteroids<br>17-Ketogenic steroids<br>17-Ketosteroids, urinary |
| Kidney | Osmolality, plasma<br>Osmolality, urine<br>Renin, plasma |
| Pancreas | Fasting blood glucose<br>Glucagon<br>Glucose, capillary<br>Glucose, urinary<br>Glycosylated hemoglobin assay<br>2-hr postprandial glucose<br>Insulin, blood<br>Insulin tolerance test<br>Ketones, serum<br>Ketones, urinary<br>Oral glucose tolerance test<br>Tolbutamide stimulation test |
| Parathyroid gland | Calcium, ionized<br>Parathyroid hormone<br>Vitamin D, activated |
| Pituitary gland | Growth hormone<br>Growth hormone stimulation test<br>Growth hormone suppression test<br>Osmolality, serum<br>Osmolality, urinary<br>Vasopressin, plasma<br>Water deprivation test<br>Water-loading test |
| Thyroid gland | Calcitonin<br>Free thyroxine<br>Free triiodothyronine<br>Long-acting thyroid stimulation<br>Resin triiodothyronine<br>Thyroglobulin autoantibodies<br>Thyroid microsomal autoantibodies<br>Thyrotropin<br>Thyrotropin-releasing hormone<br>Thyroxine, serum<br>Thyroxine-binding globulin<br>Triiodothyronine |

ACTH = adrenocorticotropic hormone.

## Adrenocorticotropic Hormone, Plasma

**(Plasma)**                    Synonyms: ACTH, corticotropin

| **Normal Values** | **Adult** |
|---|---|
| | In morning: 25–100 pg/mL *or* SI 25–100 ng/L |
| | In evening: 0–50 pg/mL *or* SI 0–50 ng/L |

### Background Information

Adrenocorticotropic hormone (ACTH) is produced and secreted by the anterior pituitary gland. Its secretion is under the control of the hypothalamus and the central nervous system by neurotransmitters and corticotropin-releasing hormone (CRH). ACTH, in turn, regulates the secretion of the glucocorticoids and androgens from the adrenal cortex.

The mechanisms of regulation of CRH, ACTH, and the adrenal hormones are multiple, and patterns of secretion of these hormones vary within the individual and among individuals. CRH and ACTH are excreted episodically and by circadian rhythm. Increases in ACTH levels cause increased levels of glucocorticoids and androgens in the blood within minutes. Generally, CRH, ACTH, and cortisol (the major glucocorticoid) levels are low in the evening and continue to decline for the first few hours of sleep. After 3 to 5 hours of sleep, the levels of the hormones increase and then peak after 6 to 8 hours of sleep. On waking, the hormone levels begin to decline. Superimposed on this circadian rhythm are episodic secretions. The hormone levels increase with exercise, eating, and stress.

Multiple factors may interfere with the circadian rhythm of CRH, ACTH, and cortisol, including changes in one's sleep pattern, meal times, and emotional or physical stress as well as central nervous system disorders, hepatic disorders, and renal failure.

Stress will cause an increase in CRH levels and thus an increase in ACTH, which will stimulate an increase in plasma cortisol levels. The stress may be physical, such as serious illness, hypoglycemia, or surgery, or psychological, such as severe anxiety. The episodic secretion of the hormones may abolish their circadian rhythm if the stress response is chronic. When high-dose exogenous glucocorticoid therapy is administered, the hormonal stress response of CRH and ACTH is suppressed.

A feedback mechanism also regulates the hypothalamic-pituitary-adrenal hormonal responses. As the cortisol level increases in the plasma, it inhibits both ACTH secretion by the pituitary gland and CRH secretion by the hypothalamus (Fig. 20–1). It is this feedback inhibition of CRH and ACTH, which occurs with prolonged exogenous administration of glucocorticoids, that can cause atrophy of the adrenal glands.

An increase or decrease in the production of ACTH will cause an increase or decrease in the glucocorticoid levels. A deficiency of ACTH will cause secondary adrenal insufficiency. An increase in ACTH will cause Cushing's disease (Cushing's syndrome is a primary adrenal disorder).

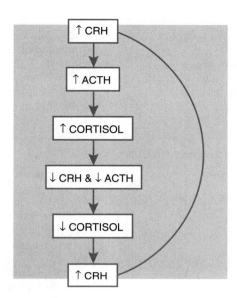

**Figure 20–1**

Hypothalamic-pituitary-adrenal axis. Hypothalamic control of adrenal hormone secretion occurs through release of corticotropin-releasing hormone (CRH), which stimulates the secretion of adrenocorticotropic hormone (ACTH) by the pituitary gland. ACTH stimulates the adrenals to increase their secretion of cortisol. By a negative feedback mechanism, the increase in serum cortisol level suppresses the release of CRH and ACTH.

---

**Purpose of the Test**

A plasma ACTH determination is obtained to diagnose Cushing's disease and differentiate primary and secondary adrenal insufficiency.

---

**Procedure**

Venipuncture is required to obtain 7 mL of venous blood in a heparinized green-topped tube. The plasma ACTH is measured by RIA.

---

**Findings**

**Elevated Values**

Primary adrenal insufficiency

Cushing's disease

Congenital adrenal hyperplasia

Ectopic ACTH syndrome

**Decreased Values**

Primary adrenal hypersecretion

Cushing's syndrome

Tumors of the adrenal gland may suppress the ACTH level if they produce glucocorticoids; however, not all adrenal tumors do.

## Interfering Factors

■

*Critical Thinking 20–1*
How will the ingestion of exogenous glucocorticoids affect
the results of an ACTH level test?

- Noncompliance with medication, diet, or activity restrictions
- Administration of radioactive scans within 7 days
- Pregnancy
- Traumatic venipuncture
- Ingestion of alcohol, amphetamines, calcium gluconate, corticosteroids, es-
  trogen, lithium, or spironolactone

## Nursing Implementation

### Pretest

Explain to the patient the need to obtain two specimens of blood, one in the
early morning (6 to 8 AM) and one in the evening (6 to 11 PM). The early
morning specimen reflects the peak secretion time and the evening specimen
the low secretion time for ACTH.

Instruct the patient to ingest nothing by mouth for 12 hours before the test.
Some physicians recommend a low-carbohydrate diet for 2 days before
the test.

Obtain a medication history and ask the prescriber if any interfering drugs
should be withheld.

Inquire and note on requisition slip if the patient is pregnant, because this may
affect test results.

### During the Test

Have a glass, heparinized syringe and ice available.

After blood is obtained by venipuncture, place the specimen on ice and immediately send it to the laboratory.

Notify laboratory personnel that the specimen is being transported, because it
should be frozen until an RIA can be performed.

### Posttest

The patient resumes a normal diet, activity, and medication regimen.

## Adrenocorticotropic Hormone Stimulation Test

**(Plasma, Serum)**  Synonyms: ACTH stimulation test, rapid ACTH testing, cosyntropin test, Cortrosyn stimulating test

## Normal Values

Within 30–60 minutes, plasma cortisol increases to ≥20 µg/dL *or* SI ≥276 nmol/L.

## Background Information

ACTH is secreted by the pituitary gland. Its target
organ is the adrenal cortex, where it stimulates
the secretion of the glucocorticoids, aldosterone,
and androgens. Synthetic ACTH, known as cosyntropin (Cortrosyn), normally has the same effect—
an increase in adrenal cortex hormones. A normal
response excludes the diagnosis of primary adrenocorticoid insufficiency, because the gland was able
to respond. A normal response will also rule out
complete ACTH deficiency (secondary adrenocorticoid failure), because complete lack of ACTH
causes adrenal atrophy, and the gland is unable to
respond.

In an abnormal response, primary or secondary

adrenal insufficiency may be present. To distinguish between the two forms, aldosterone levels levels may be measured (see pp. 555–559). If no change occurs in the aldosterone levels after cosyn-

tropin is given, primary adrenal insufficiency is present. With secondary adrenal insufficiency, aldosterone levels will increase by more than 4 µg/dL.

| **Purpose of the Test** | The ACTH stimulation test is performed to diagnose primary and secondary adrenal insufficiency. |
|---|---|

| **Procedure** | After baseline plasma cortisol levels are obtained, cosyntropin is given intravenously. Cosyntropin may be given intramuscularly if the patient is not hypotensive. After 30 to 60 minutes, another plasma cortisol level is obtained. Instead of cosyntropin, insulin may be used. |
|---|---|

**Findings**

**Elevated Values**

Normal response

**Unchanged Values**

| Addison's disease | Adrenal atrophy | Hypopituitarism |
|---|---|---|

**Interfering Factors**

- See section on plasma cortisol (pp. 564–566).

**Nursing Implementation**

See section on plasma cortisol (pp. 564–566).

■

*Critical Thinking 20–2*
The patient has been ill for many weeks, during which multiple intravenous injections and lines have been necessary. When it is time for the second blood collection for the ACTH stimulation test, the patient refuses. How can the nurse help?

**Pretest**

Explain to the patient the need for more than one venipuncture procedure. If insulin is being used as the stimulant, instruct the patient to fast overnight.

**During the Test**

If insulin is used as the stimulant, observe the patient for clinical manifestations of hypoglycemia.

**Posttest**

Ensure, especially if insulin was used as the stimulant, that the patient eats.

## Aldosterone, Serum

**(Serum)**  Synonyms: None

**Normal Values**

**Adult (Average Sodium Diet)**
Peripheral blood, supine position: 3–10 ng/dL *or* SI 0.08–0.27 nmol/L
Peripheral blood, upright position: 5–30 ng/dL *or* SI 0.14–0.83 nmol/L
After fludrocortisone acetate (Florinef) suppression or intravenous saline infusion:
    <4 ng/dL *or* SI <0.11 nmol/L
Adrenal vein: 200–800 ng/dL *or* SI 5.54–22.16 nmol/L

*Continued on following page*

*Continued*

**Child**
11–15 years: <5–50 ng/dL *or* SI <0.14–1.39 nmol/L
3–11 years: <5–80 ng/dL *or* SI <0.14–2.22 nmol/L
1–3 years: 5–60 ng/dL *or* SI 0.14–1.7 nmol/L
1 week–1 year: 1–160 ng/dL *or* SI 0.03–4.43 nmol/L

## Background Information

Aldosterone is a mineralocorticoid produced by the adrenal cortex and controlled primarily by the renin-angiotensin system (Fig. 20–2). Renin secreted by the kidneys acts on angiotensinogen to convert it to angiotensin I. Later, angiotensin I is converted to angiotensin II. Angiotensin II stimulates the adrenal cortex to produce and secrete aldosterone. The aldosterone acts on the renal tubules to (1) increase sodium retention and thus increase fluid retention, which increases plasma fluid volume and blood pressure, and (2) increase potassium excretion in the urine.

Another stimulant for aldosterone secretion is the serum potassium level. When serum potassium levels are elevated, increased secretion of aldosterone occurs, promoting greater urinary excretion of potassium.

The presence of high levels of aldosterone is called *aldosteronism*. Primary aldosteronism often is caused by adrenal adenoma (Conn's syndrome). This condition is characterized by hypertension with hypokalemia and urinary potassium loss. Secondary aldosteronism is caused by nonadrenal disease that stimulates the adrenal cortex to produce and secrete excessive aldosterone.

In testing for serum aldosterone levels, a number of variables must be controlled to provide accurate results. A low-salt diet, an upright position, and stress all produce increased levels of aldosterone. A high-salt diet and a supine position decrease the serum levels. With the administration of fludrocortisone acetate (Florinef) or intravenous saline, the secretion of aldosterone is suppressed in normal patients and in patients with secondary aldosteronism, but serum levels rise in patients with primary aldosteronism.

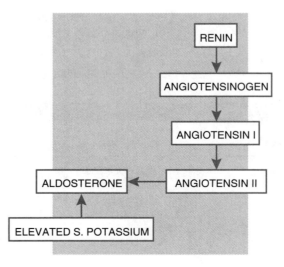

**Figure 20–2**
Primary regulation of aldosterone secretion.

**Purpose of the Test**    The aldosterone level is used in the work-up for hypertension and in the diagnosis of aldosteronism.

**Procedure**    A red-topped or green-topped heparinized tube is used to collect 7 to 10 mL of venous blood. The vascular site may be any peripheral vein. The patient may be in a supine or an upright position. A blood sample from the adrenal vein may be needed to confirm the diagnosis of adrenal adenoma.

Other diagnostic methods include administering 2 L of normal saline over 4 hours before the blood test or drawing the blood on the third day after the administration of fludrocortisone acetate, a synthetic mineralocorticoid.

**Findings**    **Elevated Values**

PRIMARY ALDOSTERONISM

Adrenal adenoma    Adrenal hyperplasia
  (Conn's syndrome)

SECONDARY ALDOSTERONISM

Laxative abuse    Renal juxtaglomerular    Bartter's syndrome
Excessive diuretic      hyperplasia    Toxemia of pregnancy
  therapy    Renin-producing
Nephrotic syndrome      renal tumor

**Decreased Values**

Addison's disease    Diabetes mellitus
Turner's syndrome    Renin deficiency
Aldosterone defi-    Acute alcoholic
  ciency      intoxication

**Interfering Factors**
- Licorice intake
- Uncontrolled sodium intake
- Postural changes
- Warming of the specimen
- Recent radioisotope administration
- Loop diuretics

**Nursing Implementation**    **Pretest**

Instruct the patient to follow a normal sodium intake (3 g/day) for 2 to 4 weeks, if not contraindicated by clinical status.
Instruct the patient to discontinue all diuretics, antihypertensives, cyclic progesterone, estrogens, and licorice for 2 to 4 weeks as ordered.
Administer potassium replacement, as needed.
Schedule any radioactive scans for after the aldosterone level is obtained.

■

*Critical Thinking 20–3*
As the night nurse, you note an empty pepperoni pizza box at the bedside of a patient scheduled for a serum aldosterone level test in the morning. What should you do?

## During the Test

### Supine Position

On the morning of the test, instruct the patient to remain flat in bed until the specimen is drawn.

### Upright Position

On the morning of the test, instruct the patient to remain seated in a chair for 2 hours until the blood is drawn.

### Posttest

Ensure that the requisition slip contains the following information: the time and date of the test, the venous source of the blood, the patient's position, the pretest diet, and the time and date of administration of fludrocortisone acetate or intravenous saline infusion.

Place the blood specimen on ice and arrange for its immediate transport to the laboratory.

## Aldosterone, Urinary

**(Urine)** Synonyms: None

**Normal Values**

2–26 µg/24 hr *or* SI 6–72 nmol/24 hr

## Background Information

Aldosterone is a mineralocorticoid produced by the adrenal cortex. Its synthesis and release are controlled primarily by the renin-angiotensin system. Aldosterone acts on the renal tubules to resorb greater quantities of sodium, and therefore water, and increases the excretion of potassium into the urine. Elevated levels of urinary aldosterone may be caused by excess secretion of aldosterone by the adrenal glands, excessive secretion of renin, or conditions that result in decreased kidney perfusion.

The normal value for this test varies among laboratories.

**Purpose of the Test**

The main use of the urine aldosterone test is to help identify primary hyperaldosteronism caused by adrenal adenoma.

**Procedure**

A 24-hour urine specimen is collected in a clean plastic container. Some laboratories add a measured quantity of preservative (boric, acetic, or hydrochloric acid) to the container before the start of the collection period.

**Findings**

### Elevated Values

| | | |
|---|---|---|
| Aldosterone-producing adrenal adenoma (Conn's syndrome) | Nephrotic syndrome | Renal hypertension |
| | Renin-producing renal hyperplasia or tumor | Bartter's syndrome |
| Adrenal hyperplasia | | Preeclampsia |

**Decreased Values**

| | | |
|---|---|---|
| Addison's disease | Renin deficiency | Acute alcoholic |
| Aldosterone defi- | Diabetes mellitus | intoxication |
| ciency | | |

---

**Interfering Factors**

- Excess salt intake
- Recent administration of radioisotopes
- Licorice intake
- Failure to collect all urine
- Warming of the specimen
- Diuretics (loop or thiazides)
- Lithium
- Oral contraceptives

---

**Nursing Implementation**

**Pretest**

Instruct the patient to follow a normal (3 g/day) sodium diet for 2 to 4 weeks. Excessive sodium intake suppresses sodium secretion and causes a false decrease in the aldosterone value.

Administer prescribed potassium to correct any deficiencies that may be present.

Instruct the patient to discontinue all diuretics, antihypertensives, and oral contraceptives for 2 weeks as ordered. These medications interfere with the test results.

Schedule any radioisotope scan for after the urine test is completed.

**During the Test**

At the start of the test, instruct the patient to void at 8 AM and discard this urine. The collection period starts at this time, and the patient collects all the urine for 24 hours, including the 8 AM specimen of the following morning.

On the requisition slip and specimen label, write the patient's name and the time and date of the start and finish of the test period.

Keep the urine refrigerated or on ice throughout the collection period.

**Posttest**

On the requisition slip, write the pretest sodium diet.

Arrange for prompt transport of the cooled specimen to the laboratory.

---

## Calcitonin

**(Serum, Plasma)**      Synonyms: CT, thyrocalcitonin

---

**Normal Values**

**Serum**
Adult: <150 pg/mL *or* SI <150 ng/L
Infant (cord blood): 25–150 pg/mL *or* SI 30–240 ng/L
Infant (7 days old): 77–293 pg/mL *or* SI 77–293 ng/L

*Continued on following page*

*Continued*

> **Plasma**
> Male: ≤19 pg/mL *or* SI ≤19 ng/L
> Female: ≤14 pg/mL *or* SI ≤14 ng/L

## Background Information

Calcitonin is a hormone produced and secreted by the parafollicular cells (C cells) of the thyroid gland. It may also be produced and secreted by ectopic sites such as the lungs, intestines, pituitary gland, and bladder. The action of calcitonin is to inhibit bone reabsorption, inhibit calcium absorption in the gastrointestinal tract, and increase calcium and phosphate excretion from the kidneys. It is believed that calcitonin is not secreted until plasma calcium levels reach 9.3 ng/dL.

## Purpose of the Test

A calcitonin determination is usually performed to diagnose medullary carcinoma of the thyroid gland.

## Procedure

Venipuncture is performed to obtain 7 mL of venous blood in a heparinized green-topped tube. Calcitonin is measured using RIA. To assess familial medullary cancer in relatives of patients with the cancer, a provocation test may be performed. Calcium chloride is given intravenously over 10 minutes, or pentagastrin is given intravenously over 5 to 10 minutes. Patients with medullary cancer will respond to these stimulants with excessive secretion of calcitonin. The normal values for a *calcitonin stimulation test* are ≤190 pg/mL or SI ≤190 ng/L in males and ≤130 pg/mL or SI ≤130 ng/L in females.

## Findings

### Elevated Values

| | |
|---|---|
| Cancer of the thyroid | Pernicious anemia |
| Chronic renal failure | Subacute Hashi- |
| Ectopic secretion by | moto's thyroiditis |
| malignant tumors | Parathyroid adenoma |
| Endocrine tumors of | or hyperplasia |
| the pancreas | Pregnancy |

## Interfering Factors

• Noncompliance with fasting requirement

## Nursing Implementation

Nursing actions are similar to those in other venipuncture procedures.

### Pretest

Instruct the patient not to eat or drink anything but sips of water for 8 hours before the blood is drawn.

### Posttest

Inform the laboratory personnel that a calcitonin level is being obtained, because the blood sample must be separated immediately.

The blood sample must be sent to the laboratory immediately after it is drawn. The patient may resume a normal diet.

## Catecholamines, Plasma

(Plasma)

Synonyms: Catecholamine fractionalization, plasma

**Normal Values**

**Catecholamine**

Epinephrine (supine): <50 pg/mL *or* SI <273 pmol/L
Epinephrine (standing): <900 pg/mL *or* SI <4,914 pmol/L
Norepinephrine (supine): 110–410 pg/mL *or* SI 650–2,423 pmol/L
Norepinephrine (standing): 125–700 pg/mL *or* SI 739–4,137 pmol/L
Dopamine (supine): <87 pg/mL *or* SI <475 pmol/L
Dopamine (standing): <87 pg/mL *or* SI <475 pmol/L

### Background Information

The catecholamines are three hormones produced and secreted by the adrenal medulla. This structure is the inner core of the adrenal glands, which lie at the superior pole of each kidney. The catecholamines are epinephrine, norepinephrine, and dopamine (a precursor of norepinephrine). The adrenal medulla secretes the catecholamines when stimulated by preganglionic neurons. The result mimics the effect of a mass discharge of the sympathetic nervous system. Their secretion is part of the "fight or flight" response. The catecholamines help maintain serum glucose levels by promoting liver glycogenolysis, by stimulating the secretion of insulin and glucagon, and by lipolysis. The catecholamines stimulate the reticular activating system, making the person more alert.

### Purpose of the Test

Plasma catecholamines are usually assessed to diagnose pheochromocytoma or to identify extra-adrenal tumors after abdominal surgery. Pheochromocytomas are tumors developing in the sympathetic nervous system. These tumors usually secrete epinephrine, norepinephrine, or both, and sometimes dopamine.

### Procedure

Plasma catecholamines are measured using radioenzymatic technique. A venous sampling of 10 mL of blood is drawn into a green-topped tube with ethylenediaminetetraacetic acid (EDTA), once while the patient is lying down and then once with the patient standing. The normal values vary among laboratories. Results may not reveal a tumor that secretes intermittently, so the test may be ordered for when the patient is symptomatic. To localize small tumors, percutaneous venous catheterization may be needed.

A *clonidine suppression test* may be performed to differentiate between pheochromocytoma and essential hypertension. With this test, clonidine is given 2 to 3 hours before a venous blood sample is taken. Clonidine suppresses neurogenic catecholamine release. If suppression occurs, the test result is consistent with the diagnosis of essential hypertension. If the catecholamines remain elevated, the diagnosis of pheochromocytoma is supported.

| Findings | Elevated Values | | |
|---|---|---|---|
| | Pheochromocytoma | Ganglioneuroma | Neuroblastoma |

| Interfering Factors | <ul><li>Noncompliance with diet and relaxation requirements</li><li>Amine-rich foods and drinks</li><li>Anger</li><li>Cold environment</li><li>Medications such as amphetamines, barbiturates, decongestants, epinephrine, levodopa, phenothiazines, reserpine, sympathomimetics, and tricyclic antidepressants</li><li>Severe anxiety</li></ul> |
|---|---|

| **Nursing Implementation** | **Pretest** |
|---|---|

■

*Critical Thinking 20–4*
The patient with newly diagnosed hypertension appears agitated as a heparin lock is about to be inserted for catecholamine levels. When questioned, the patient says that the test is unnecessary and implies distrust of his physician. How should the nurse respond?

**Pretest**

Instruct the patient to avoid amine-rich foods and drinks (e.g., avocados, bananas, beer, cheese, chianti wine, cocoa, coffee, tea) for 48 hours before the test.

Instruct the patient not to smoke for 4 hours before the test.

Explain to the patient that a venous catheter (heparin lock) is inserted 24 hours before the blood sample is drawn, because venipuncture may increase catecholamine levels.

Instruct the patient to lie down and relax for an hour before the blood is drawn.

**During the Test**

The nurse carries out duties similar to those of other venipuncture procedures, except that blood is drawn through the heparin lock. If the heparin lock has been flushed with heparin, withdraw 3 mL of blood and discard it before drawing the sample.

After the first sample is drawn, the patient stands for 10 minutes, and a second sample is drawn.

Include on the requisition slip the position of the patient when the blood was drawn.

Flush the heparin lock according to hospital protocol.

**Posttest**

The patient may resume pretest diet and activity. Notify the laboratory that the specimen is coming, because it must be frozen immediately.

## Catecholamines, Urinary

**(Urine)**                                  Synonyms: None

| Normal Values | Norepinephrine: 15–56 µg/24 hr *or* SI 88.6–331 nmol/24 hr<br>Epinephrine: <20 pg/mL *or* SI <109 nmol/24 hr<br>Dopamine: 100–400 pg/mL *or* SI 625–2,750 nmol/24 hr |
|---|---|

Vanillylmandelic acid: 2–7 mg/24 hr *or* SI 10–35 µmol/24 hr
Metanephrine: 24–96 µg/24 hr
Normetanephrine: 75–375 µg/24 hr
Homovanillic acid: 2–12 mg/24 hr *or* SI 10.98–65.88 µmol/24 hr

## Background Information

Catecholamines are excreted in the urine in conjugated and unconjugated (free) forms. Together these forms make up the total urinary catecholamines. As serum catecholamines are metabolized, several end product metabolites are created, which are excreted in the urine (Fig. 20–3). The primary metabolite is *vanillylmandelic acid* (VMA). Other major metabolites of epinephrine and norepinephrine are metanephrine and normetanephrine. Dopamine's metabolites are 3-methoxy-4-hydroxyphenylacetic acid (*homovanillic acid*, or HVA) and 3,4-dehydroxyphenylacetic acid (DOPA$_c$).

## Purpose of the Test

Urinary catecholamine determinations are usually obtained as a part of the work-up to identify the cause of hypertension and to diagnose pheochromocytoma.

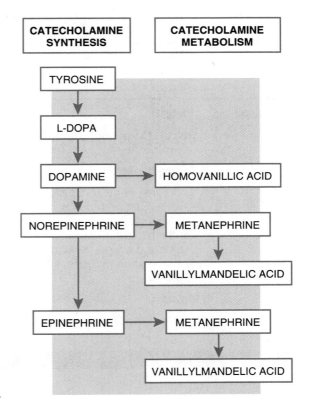

**Figure 20–3**
Catecholamine synthesis and metabolism.

| | |
|---|---|
| **Procedure** | A 24-hour urine specimen is collected, with a boric acid or potassium bisulfate preservative added to the container. |

**Findings**

**Elevated Values**

CATECHOLAMINES AND VANILLYLMANDELIC ACID

| | | |
|---|---|---|
| Pheochromocytoma | Neuroblastoma | Ganglioneuroma |

HOMOVANILLIC ACID

| | |
|---|---|
| Pheochromocytoma ruled out | Ganglioblastoma |
| Tumors of the autonomic nervous system | |

**Interfering Factors**

Factors vary with the specific laboratory technique used. Catecholamine-metabolite interfering factors include the following.

- Epinephrine: Stress
- Norepinephrine: Exercise
- Dopamine: Foods and drugs containing catecholamines, high-fluorescent compounds (e.g., tetracycline, quinidine), levodopa, or methyldopa
- Metanephrine: Catecholamines and monoamine oxidase (MAO) inhibitors
- Normetanephrine: Severe stress
- Vanillylmandelic acid: Catecholamines, foods with vanilla, levodopa, and MAO inhibitors

**Nursing Implementation**

**Pretest**

Instruct the patient to avoid chocolate, coffee, bananas, foods with vanilla, and citrus fruits.

**During the Test**

At the start of the test, instruct the patient to void at 8 AM and discard this urine. The collection period begins at this time, and all urine is collected for 24 hours, including the 8 AM specimen of the following morning.

On the requisition slip and specimen label, write the patient's name and the time and date of the start and finish of the test period.

Keep the urine specimen refrigerated or on ice throughout the collection period.

**Posttest**

Arrange for prompt transport of the cooled specimen to the laboratory.

## Cortisol, Total

**(Plasma, Serum)**

Synonyms: None

| **Normal Values** | **Adult** |
| --- | --- |
| | 8–10 AM: 5–23 µg/dL *or* SI 138–635 nmol/L |
| | 4–6 PM: 3–16 µg/dL *or* SI 83–441 nmol/L |

## Background Information

The adrenal cortex produces a group of hormones called *glucocorticoids*. The primary glucocorticoid is cortisol. Secretion of cortisol is regulated by ACTH, which is secreted by the anterior pituitary gland. When secreted, most of the cortisol in the plasma binds with corticosteroid-binding globulin (CBG). The free cortisol is the biologically active form, whereas the bound hormone acts as a storehouse to replace the free cortisol.

The actions of cortisol and the other glucocorticoids are multiple and relate to their plasma concentrations. At normal plasma levels, glucocorticoids, as the name implies, maintain glucose levels by promoting hepatic gluconeogenesis and glycogenolysis, prevent fatigue by making tissues more responsive to glucagon and catecholamines, reduce the secretion of antidiuretic hormone (ADH), increase glomerular filtration rates, and make the distal tubules of the kidneys more permeable to water reabsorption.

At elevated levels, for example, in times of stress or in pharmacologic doses, the glucocorticoids have an immunosuppressive and an anti-inflammatory effect.

Cushing's syndrome includes excessive secretion of the adrenal cortex hormones resulting from a primary adrenal dysfunction. When a pituitary or hypothalamic disorder causes an increase in the production of glucocorticoids, including cortisol, it is called Cushing's disease. The high cortisol levels may be dangerous for the individual, because the inflammatory response is suppressed. The inflammatory response is necessary to destroy invading microorganisms, to wall off infected areas, and to initiate normal wound healing.

Chang, Anderson, and Wood (1995) recommend testing saliva for newborns, instead of performing a heelstick or venipuncture when doing cortisol levels. If saliva is used to test for cortisol, no milk should be present in the infant's mouth.

| **Purpose of the Test** | Plasma cortisol levels are used to diagnose Cushing's syndrome, Cushing's disease, and primary and secondary adrenal insufficiency. Primary adrenal insufficiency is called Addison's disease. |
| --- | --- |

| **Procedure** | Venipuncture is performed to obtain 5 mL of blood in a green-topped tube. If a serum level is desired instead of a plasma level, 5 mL of blood is collected in a red-topped tube. Varied methods are used to measure cortisol, including RIA, competitive protein-binding assay, fluorimetric assay, and high-performance liquid chromatography. |
| --- | --- |

## Findings

**Elevated Values**

| | | |
| --- | --- | --- |
| Stress | Exogenous estrogen | Chronic renal failure |
| Acute illness | Anxiety | Adrenal hyperfunction |
| Surgery | Starvation | Excessive ACTH |
| Trauma | Anorexia nervosa | |
| Pituitary destruction | Alcoholism | |

### Decreased Values

| | |
|---|---|
| Addison's disease | Pregnancy |
| Hypophysectomy | Hepatitis |
| Postpartum pituitary necrosis | Cirrhosis of the liver |

---

### Interfering Factors
■

*Critical Thinking 20–5*
A patient with Cushing's syndrome awaits cortisol level test results. What medical diagnoses in potential roommates would make them inappropriate as roommates?

- Noncompliance with dietary or activity restrictions
- With RIA: Androgens, estrogens, phenytoin, hepatic dysfunction, and renal failure
- With competitive protein-binding assay: Prednisolone and 6-alpha-methylprednisolone
- With fluorimetric assays: Jaundice, renal failure, and medications (niacin, quinacrine, quinidine, spironolactone)
- With high-performance liquid chromatography: Prednisone, prednisolone

---

### Nursing Implementation

The nurse performs actions similar to those performed in plasma ACTH determinations (see pp. 552–554).

#### Pretest

Instruct the patient to limit physical activity for 12 hours before the test and to lie down for 30 minutes before the blood is drawn.

---

## Dexamethasone Suppression Test

**(Serum, Urine)**         Synonyms: None

---

### Normal Values

> Serum cortisol: <5 µg/dL *or* SI <138 nmol/L
> Urine 17-hydroxycorticosteroid (17-OHCS): <4 ng/24 hr
> Urine for free cortisol: <25 µg/24 hr

---

### Background Information

Dexamethasone (Decadron) is a potent glucocorticoid. It will normally suppress ACTH secretion by the pituitary gland via the normal hormonal feedback mechanism. With the suppression of ACTH, the stimulation for cortisol secretion is suppressed in the adrenal cortex, resulting in a decrease in plasma cortisol and urinary corticosteroid levels.

High-dose dexamethasone testing can be helpful in distinguishing Cushing's disease (pituitary hypersecretion of ACTH) from adrenal tumors or ectopic secretion of ACTH. With high-dose dexamethasone, pituitary secretion of ACTH can be suppressed, with a resulting decrease in plasma cortisol levels. No change will occur with adrenal tumors or ectopic ACTH production.

---

### Purpose of the Test

The dexamethasone suppression test assesses the hypothalamic-pituitary-adrenal axis. It is usually performed to identify Cushing's syndrome. With the dexamethasone test, Cushing's disease and ectopic production of ACTH and adrenal tumors can be differentiated.

| | |
|---|---|
| **Procedure** | A variety of dexamethasone procedures are possible. Low-dose dexamethasone testing may be carried out overnight or over 2 days. Overnight testing requires the oral administration of 1 mg of dexamethasone at night (10 to 11 PM). The next morning, a plasma cortisol level is determined. With the 2-day method, 0.5 mg of dexamethasone is given orally every 6 hours for 2 days. A 24-hour urine specimen is obtained before and after administration (see discussion of 17-OHCS on pp. 600–601), and a plasma cortisol test is performed 6 hours after the last dose of dexamethasone.

High-dose dexamethasone testing begins with a baseline plasma cortisol level being obtained and then 8 mg of dexamethasone being given orally at night, and the next morning another plasma cortisol level being obtained. Another technique requires 2 mg of dexamethasone being given orally every 6 hours for 2 days and a 24-hour urine specimen for 17-OHCS being collected on the second day of administration. A plasma cortisol or free cortisol level is also obtained. |

| | |
|---|---|
| **Findings** | **Unchanged Values**

Cushing's syndrome

**Decreased Values**

Cushing's disease |

| | |
|---|---|
| **Interfering Factors** | • Review discussion of 17-OHCS (pp. 600–601), free cortisol (pp. 570–571), and plasma cortisol (pp. 564–566). |

| | |
|---|---|
| **Nursing Implementation** | Review discussion of 17-OHCS (pp. 600–601), free cortisol (pp. 570–571), and plasma cortisol (pp. 564–566). |

## Fasting Blood Glucose

**(Blood, Serum, Plasma)**     Synonyms: Fasting blood sugar, FBS

| | |
|---|---|
| **Normal Values** | **Children 2 Years to Adult**<br>Whole blood: 60–110 mg/dL *or* SI 3.3–6.1 mmol/L<br>Plasma or serum: 70–120 mg/dL *or* SI 3.9–6.7 mmol/L<br>**Elderly individuals:** 80–150 mg/dL *or* SI 4.4–8.3 mmol/L<br>**Children <2 years:** 60–100 mg/dL *or* SI 3.3–5.6 mmol/L<br>**Infant:** 40–90 mg/dL *or* SI 2.2–5.0 mmol/L<br>**Neonate:** 30–60 mg/dL *or* SI 1.7–3.3 mmol/L |

## Background Information

To meet cellular needs, the body has developed complex mechanisms to take in, use, and store nutrients. A serum glucose level determination reflects the ability of the body to perform its metabolic tasks. Glucose levels are not static; they vary after eating, so a fasting blood glucose (FBS) level determination is desirable. Many factors influence blood glucose, but testing is most frequently used to diagnose and manage diabetes mellitus.

With age, the norms for blood and plasma glucose levels are adjusted by 1 mg/dL per year of life after age 60 years.

One elevated fasting blood glucose level is not considered diagnostic, but the test should be repeated. If the second fasting blood glucose level test result is elevated (>126 mg/dL or SI 6.99 mmol/L), it supports the diagnosis of diabetes mellitus. Previously, to be diagnosed with diabetes, a level of >140 mg/dL was needed. The newest guidelines by the American Diabetes Association have lowered the cutoff.

| | |
|---|---|
| **Purpose of the Test** | Fasting blood glucose is evaluated to diagnose and manage patients with diabetes mellitus. The fasting blood glucose level is also obtained as supportive data in many diagnoses, because metabolic factors will influence glucose use and storage. Certain therapies may be evaluated by checking the fasting blood glucose level, for example, hyperalimentation and exogenous glucocorticoid therapy. |
| **Procedure** | After a 12-hour fast, venipuncture is performed to obtain 5 mL of blood in a red-topped tube for a plasma or serum sample or in a green-topped tube for a whole blood sample. Usually serum or plasma sampling is performed, because these tests reflect glucose levels in interstitial tissue and are not affected by the hematocrit. |

**Findings**

**Elevated Values**

Acromegaly              Diabetes mellitus          Pheochromocytoma
Chronic pancreatitis    Hyperthyroidism            Stress
Cushing's syndrome      Hyperosmolar coma

**Decreased Values**

Addison's disease       Excessive exogenous
Advanced liver            insulin
  disease               Islet cell adenoma
Alcohol intake when     Leucine sensitivity
  fasting               Malnutrition

**Interfering Factors**

- Noncompliance with fasting
- Vigorous exercise
- Stress
- Medications such as acetaminophen, arginine, benzodiazepines, beta blockers, epinephrine, ethacrynic acid, furosemide, glucocorticoids, glucose, hypoglycemic agents, insulin, lithium, MAO inhibitors, oral contraceptives, phenothiazines, phenytoin, and thiazide diuretics

**Nursing Implementation**

The nurse's actions are similar to those in other venipuncture procedures.

**Pretest**

Instruct the patient to fast for 12 hours before the blood is drawn.
Instruct the patient who is taking insulin or hypoglycemic agents to withhold the medication until after the blood is drawn.
Observe the patient for clinical manifestations of hypoglycemia.

**Posttest**

Ensure that the patient receives food and medications that were withheld.
Send blood to the laboratory, because it needs to be centrifuged within 30 minutes for serum and plasma levels.

---

**Critical Values**

■

*Critical Thinking 20–6*
The patient's FBS is higher in the morning than was the late afternoon glucose level, which is not a fasting glucose level. How can this occur, even though insulin was given?

**<60 mg/dL *or* >400 mg/dL or, in neonates, <30 mg *or* >300 mg/dL**

Low FBS indicates hypoglycemia. Notify the physician. If the patient is alert and not in danger of aspiration, give glucose by mouth. If the patient is unconscious, or if aspiration is likely, prepare to give 50% glucose as ordered.

High FBS indicates hyperglycemia, usually related to diabetes ketoacidosis or hyperosmolar coma. Notify the physician. Change any glucose-containing infusion the patient is receiving to a nonglucose solution. Prepare to give short-acting insulin as ordered. Assess ketone levels.

---

**Complications**

Because a fasting blood glucose determination requires that the patient maintain a nothing-by-mouth status, hypoglycemia may occur (Table 20–2).

**Table 20–2    Complications of a Fasting Blood Sugar Test**

| Complication | Nursing Assessment |
|---|---|
| Hypoglycemia | Pallor |
| | Diaphoresis |
| | Tachycardia |
| | Palpitations |
| | Hunger |
| | Paresthesia |
| | Vagueness |
| | Confusion |
| | Slurred speech |
| | Somnolence |
| | Convulsions |
| | Coma |

## Free Cortisol

(Urine)                    Synonyms: None

**Normal Values**    20–90 µg/24 hr *or* SI 55–248 nmol/24 hr

### Background Information

When secreted by the adrenal cortex, cortisol binds with corticosteroid-binding globulin (CBG) and, to a much lesser degree, albumin. Only a small amount of cortisol circulates unbound or in the free state, which is the biologically active form. Free cortisol is normally excreted in the urine in small amounts.

If excessive secretion of cortisol occurs, the CBG binding sites are filled, causing an increase in free cortisol; therefore, the urinary excretion increases. Because of this, an increased secretion of urinary free cortisol is helpful in diagnosing Cushing's syndrome. It is not helpful in diagnosing adrenal insufficiency, because it is not sensitive at low levels, and low levels are relatively common in healthy individuals.

CBG is produced by the liver. Liver failure will affect CBG and, therefore, free cortisol levels. CBG is influenced by other factors. CBG levels increase in hyperthyroidism, diabetes, and high-estrogen states such as pregnancy. Genetic disorders may cause an increase or decrease in CBG. Hypothyroidism, protein deficiency, and renal failure may cause a decrease in CBG and influence free cortisol levels.

### Procedure

A 24-hour urine specimen is collected and assessed by RIA or by competitive protein-binding assay.

### Findings

**Elevated Values**

Cushing's syndrome          Ectopic ACTH
Adrenal or pituitary            production
   tumor

### Interfering Factors

- Stress
- Physical activity
- Failure to collect all the urine during the 24-hour period
- Failure to store urine on ice or in a refrigerator
- Medications such as amphetamines, morphine sulfate, phenothiazines, reserpine, and steroids

### Nursing Implementation

**Pretest**

Instruct the patient to avoid strenuous physical activity.

**During the Test**

At the start of the test, instruct the patient to void at 8 AM and discard this urine. The collection period starts at this time, and all urine is collected for 24 hours, including the 8 AM specimen of the following morning.

On the requisition slip and specimen label, write the patient's name and the time and date of the start and finish of the test period.

Keep the urine refrigerated or on ice throughout the collection period.

### Posttest

Arrange for prompt transport of the cooled specimen to the laboratory.

## Free Thyroxine

(Serum)                                    Synonym: FT$_4$

| Normal Values | 0.9–1.7 mg/dL *or* SI 11.5–21.8 nmol/L |
|---|---|

### Background Information

The majority of thyroxine (see section on thyroxine, pp. 607–609) is carried by thyroid-binding globulin, albumin, and prealbumin. It is free thyroxine (FT$_4$), which is not bound, that is biologically active and converts to triiodothyronine (T$_3$) in the peripheral circulation. The ability to measure free thyroxine has replaced a classic test called *protein-bound iodine*.

Frequently, because of the expense of an FT$_4$ test, free thyroxine may be evaluated by the *free thyroxine index* (FT$_4$I), which is an estimated value. The FT$_4$I is calculated by multiplying the total T$_4$ by the thyroid hormone-binding ratio (THBR). The normal value for an adult is 4.2 to 13.0 (no units of value).

### Purpose of the Test

Free thyroxine is used to diagnose hyper- and hypothyroidism. It is especially helpful when abnormal thyroxine-binding globulin levels exist.

### Procedure

Venipuncture is performed to collect 5 mL of blood in a red-topped tube. Laboratory procedures vary in assessing free thyroxine. If RIA is performed, albumin levels and a radionuclide scan within 7 days will affect the results.

### Findings

**Elevated Values**

Acute psychiatric           Hyperthyroidism
  disorders

**Decreased Values**

Anorexia nervosa            Hypothyroidism

### Interfering Factors

- Medications such as carbamazepine, exogenous thyroid therapy, heparin, phenytoin, salicylates, and radioisotopes

### Nursing Implementation

The nurse takes actions similar to those taken in other venipuncture procedures.

## Free Triiodothyronine

**(Serum)**   Synonym: FT$_3$

| **Normal Values** | 260–480 pg/dL *or* SI 4.0–7.4 pmol/L |
| --- | --- |

### Background Information

Triiodothyronine is a hormone secreted by the thyroid gland. Most of the hormone is bound to thyroid-binding globulin. Some triiodothyronine is in the free state, that is, unbound. The unbound or free triiodothyronine is the biologically active form of the hormone.

### Purpose of the Test

Free triiodothyronine is used to diagnose hyper- and hypothyroidism.

### Procedure

Venipuncture is performed to collect a specimen in a red-topped tube. Laboratory methods to assess free triiodothyronine vary. If RIA is used, albumin levels and a radionuclide scan within 7 days will affect results.

### Findings

**Elevated Values**

Hyperthyroidism

**Decreased Values**

Hypothyroidism

### Interfering Factors

- Exogenous thyroid therapy
- Radioisotopes

### Nursing Implementation

Nursing actions resemble those of other venipuncture procedures.

## Glucagon, Blood

**(Plasma)**   Synonyms: None

| **Normal Values** | Adult: 20–100 pg/mL *or* SI 20–100 ng/L<br>Child: 0–148 pg/mL *or* SI 0–148 ng/L<br>Infant: 0–1,750 pg/mL *or* SI 0–1,750 ng/L |
| --- | --- |

## Background Information

Glucagon is produced and secreted by the alpha cells of the islets of Langerhans of the pancreas. Glucagon stimulates the breakdown of stored glycogen and maintains gluconeogenesis. Glucagon is secreted in response to hypoglycemia, helping to meet glucose needs of tissues between intakes of food.

## Purpose of the Test

Glucagon levels are assessed in suspected pancreatic tumors, chronic pancreatitis, and familial hyperglucagonemia.

## Procedure

Venipuncture is performed to obtain 7 mL of blood in a lavender-topped tube with EDTA. The specimen is placed on ice and sent to the laboratory immediately to be centrifuged.

## Findings

### Elevated Values

| | | |
|---|---|---|
| Acute pancreatitis | Hypoglycemia | Renal failure, chronic |
| Cirrhosis | Parasympathetic | Stress, high levels |
| Diabetic ketoacidosis | stimulation | Sympathetic stimu- |
| Glucagonoma | Pheochromocytoma | lation |

### Decreased Values

| | | |
|---|---|---|
| Chronic pancreatitis | Hyperglycemia | Pancreatic tumors |
| High fatty acid levels | Insulinoma | |

## Interfering Factors

- Stress
- Prolonged fasting
- Radioactive scan within 2 days
- Medications such as catecholamines, insulin, and glucocorticoids

## Nursing Implementation

The nurse takes actions similar to those used in other venipuncture procedures.

### Pretest

Instruct the patient to fast for 10 to 12 hours before the blood is drawn.
Explain to the patient the need to rest for 30 minutes before the test.
Take a medication history and determine if any interfering drugs should be withheld until after the blood is drawn.
Schedule any radioactive scans for after the glucagon determination is obtained.
Place the specimen on ice and send it to the laboratory immediately. (Not all laboratories require the specimen to be placed on ice.)

### Posttest

The patient can resume a normal diet and medication regimen.

## Glucose, Capillary

**(Whole Blood)**   Synonyms: Self-blood glucose monitoring (SBGM), capillary bedside glucose monitoring (CBGM), capillary sugar monitoring

| Normal Values | 60–110 mg/dL *or* SI 3.3–6.1 mmol/L |
| --- | --- |

### Background Information

Capillary glucose monitoring has revolutionized the management of patients with insulin-dependent diabetes mellitus (IDDM). Capillary glucose monitoring determines the glucose level of whole blood (which is lower than serum or plasma levels). It evaluates current status, permitting more accurate management and therapy. It has replaced urine glucose testing as the preferred technique to determine insulin replacement requirements in hospitals and in the home.

To perform capillary glucose monitoring, a drop of capillary blood is dropped onto a reagent strip, and the glucose level is determined by the color changes on the strip. The color change can be compared to a color chart or assessed by a glucose meter. Because the visual method is subjective and some diabetics have visual impairment, glucose meters are frequently used. Newer meters are relatively affordable (less than $50). For the diabetic who is blind, "talking" meters are available, but they are more expensive.

Non–insulin-dependent diabetics may find the use of capillary glucose monitoring helpful in managing their diabetes. These patients can check their glucose level 2 hours after they eat to see how specific foods affect it and modify their intake by an objective measurement.

For insulin-dependent and non–insulin-dependent diabetics, regular capillary glucose testing will produce greater control, with more effective long-term treatment. Capillary glucose testing can help the diabetic maintain control during periods of stress, for example, illness, pregnancy, and surgery. Usually, the patient with IDDM will monitor the capillary glucose level before each meal and at bedtime. The patient with non–insulin-dependent diabetes (NIDDM) usually monitors the capillary glucose twice a day—before breakfast and 2 hours after dinner.

Nurses need to teach their patients how to monitor capillary glucose, including how to use and care for the glucose meter and reagent strips and how to check the reliability of the meter. This information needs to be reinforced periodically.

### Purpose of the Test

Capillary glucose monitoring is carried out to assess and manage patients with diabetes mellitus. It may be used in hospitals to monitor other hyperglycemic patients, such as those on hyperalimentation or high-dose glucocorticoid therapy. Capillary glucose evaluation is *not* used to diagnose diabetes mellitus, but it may indicate a need to perform a glucose tolerance test. It is usually used as part of aggressive treatment for diabetes, which requires the glucose to be checked at least four times per day. Controlling the blood glucose level in diabetes very strictly has been shown to lower the complications of the disease.

### Procedure

With a lancet, a fingerstick is performed, and a drop of blood is placed on a reagent strip. The intensity of the color change is proportional to the amount of glucose in the blood. The darker the color, the higher the glucose concentration. The color change is assessed visually by comparing it to a color chart or is assessed by the blood glucose meter. The meter may read the strip by the process of refractance photometry or by electrochemical technology. Either method will provide a digital readout of the glucose level.

## Nursing Implementation

Many different glucose meters are on the market. It is *essential* to follow the manufacturers' guidelines for their use. In addition, a number of lancing devices are available.

### Pretest

#### Quality Control

> Glucose meters should be checked daily in hospitals and once a week or when opening a new vial of strips at home, using quality control solution containing a known amount of dissolved glucose in water. The meter should also be tested if the meter is dropped or if the meter reading does not correlate with clinical assessments.

#### Quality Control

> When a fasting blood glucose determination is obtained, a capillary glucose level can also be obtained and the two measures compared. A variance of less than 15% is acceptable.

■

*Critical Thinking 20–7*
As part of the diabetic teaching plan, you instruct the patient on capillary glucose testing. What adaptations to the plan will be necessary if the patient has significant loss of vision?

If the battery in the meter has worn out, recalibrate the meter with the plastic calibration strip provided in the reagent vial according to the manufacturer's guidelines.

Check the code numbers on the glucose meter and on the reagent strip to ensure that they are the same. Check the expiration date on the reagent strip container and discard outdated strips.

Wear gloves for this procedure, because blood contact is possible.

## During the Test

■

*Critical Thinking 20–8*
On readmission of a diabetic patient, the patient demonstrates her technique for at-home capillary glucose testing. The patient makes two errors in technique. How do you correct these mistakes while maintaining the patient's self-esteem and confidence?

Instruct the patient to wash his or her hands in warm water and soap. The warm water will help dilate the vessels.

Hospital protocol may require the patient's finger to be wiped with an alcohol swab (this is usually not done in the home). If alcohol is used, it must be allowed to dry out or it will affect the results and increase the painfulness of the procedure.

Have the reagent strip on hand, and puncture the skin. The puncture site should be on the side of the fingertip. The middle of the fingertip is more sensitive to pain, and the side has more capillaries. Instruct the patient to rotate sites.

Milk the fingertip toward the puncture site until a large drop of blood forms.

Let the drop of blood fall on the reagent strip so that the entire pad at the tip is covered with blood. Do not smear the blood or try to add another drop.

Time the wiping of the strip, if required, and the insertion of the strip into the meter according to the manufacturer's guidelines. Timing is essential for accurate measurement. Some manufacturers require that a cotton ball be used to wipe the reagent strip.

Insert the strip into the meter (Fig. 20–4). Read and document the results.
Instruct the patient on how to dispose of the lancet in a heavy plastic container, for example, an empty detergent bottle.

### Posttest

Administer insulin as ordered.
Instruct the patient to keep an accurate record of the glucose level and insulin replacement. This record should be brought to the physician, diabetic nurse specialist, or clinic on the next visit.

### Home Testing

The procedure for home capillary glucose testing is the same as that for capillary bedside monitoring. The above nursing implementation integrates the teaching required. Emphasis must be placed on the patient's having an opportunity to practice self-blood glucose monitoring.

Inform the patient to follow the manufacturer's instructions exactly. Unfortunately, the hospital glucometer may not be the same as the one the patient will use at home. The community health nurse needs to assess the patient's ability to apply hospital learning to the home environment. Reinforce learning. Periodically, the community health nurse needs to observe the patient's technique to ensure accurate test results. If the patient is using a color chart to determine glucose levels, periodic visual evaluation is appropriate. Instruct the patient to document test results and any insulin administered based on the results and bring the record to the physician, nurse practitioner, or diabetic clinic on each visit.

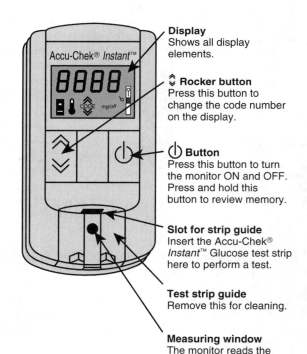

**Display**
Shows all display elements.

**Rocker button**
Press this button to change the code number on the display.

**Button**
Press this button to turn the monitor ON and OFF. Press and hold this button to review memory.

**Slot for strip guide**
Insert the Accu-Chek® Instant™ Glucose test strip here to perform a test.

**Test strip guide**
Remove this for cleaning.

**Measuring window**
The monitor reads the test strip through this window.

**Figure 20–4**
Glucometer. (Reproduced with permission from Stepp, C. A., & Woods, M. A. [1998]. *Laboratory procedures for medical office personnel* [p. 217]. Philadelphia: W. B. Saunders.)

# Glucose, Urinary

(Urine)

Synonyms: Self-monitoring of urine glucose, SMUG, urinary sugar

| Normal Values | Negative |
|---|---|

## Background Information

As serum glucose levels rise, the renal threshold for glucose will be reached and glucose will "spill out" into the urine. The presence of glycosuria (glucose in the urine) once played a major role in regulating the diet and insulin therapy of patients with diabetes mellitus. The urine was checked four times a day—before each meal and at bedtime—and insulin coverage given depending on how much glucose was spilled.

Today, patients with insulin-dependent diabetes mellitus (IDDM) and many patients with non–insulin-dependent diabetes mellitus (NIDDM) are regulated by self-capillary blood glucose monitoring. Capillary glucose monitoring is superior to urinary glucose testing because it reflects the patient's current glucose status, whereas urine reflects the blood glucose level at the time the urine was formed. Even when the patient performs a double void, complete emptying of the bladder is questionable, and old and fresh urine will mix. The *double-void* method of obtaining a urine sample requires the patient to void, attempting to empty the bladder. After 30 minutes, the patient voids again and uses this urine to check for glucose.

If the patient is planning to use self-monitoring of urinary glucose (SMUG) to manage his or her diabetes, the renal glucose threshold must be determined; otherwise, the patient may be overtreated or undertreated.

## Purpose of the Test

When capillary glucose monitoring is not possible, urinary glucose is measured to determine insulin and dietary requirements of patients with diabetes mellitus.

## Procedure

Two methods are commonly used to check for urinary glucose: Copper reduction tests (using Clinitest tablets) or the reagent strip method. The latter is more frequently used at home.

## Findings

Glucosuria may be a result of the following:

| | | |
|---|---|---|
| Diabetes mellitus | Thyroid disorders | Pregnancy |
| Chronic renal failure | Fanconi's syndrome | |
| Cushing's syndrome | Hyperalimentation | |

## Interfering Factors

- Failure to use fresh urine
- Urine heavily contaminated with bacteria
- Clinitest tablet or dipstick exposed to air, light, heat, or moisture
- Medications such as acetylsalicylic acid, chloral hydrate, glucocorticoids, isoniazid, levodopa, lithium, methyldopa, penicillin G, probenecid, salicylates, streptomycin, tetramycin, and thiazide diuretics

**Nursing Implementation**

Because this test is used for self-monitoring, patient education is an essential part of the nursing role.

### Pretest

Instruct the patient on the double-void technique.
Explain to the patient the need to collect the specimen in a clean container.
With the Clinitest tablets, heat is created by the chemical action. Warn the patient not to hold the test tube in the hand after dropping the tablet into it.

### During the Test

#### Clinitest Tablet

Add 5 drops of urine and 10 drops of water to a clean, dry test tube and then drop a Clinitest tablet into the test tube.
Compare the color change of the urine with the color chart that comes with the tablets.
Record results.

#### Dipstick Method (Clinistix, Diastix, Tes-Tape)

The dipstick is dipped in urine. The waiting time is indicated by the manufacturer.
Compare the color change with the chart provided.
Record results.

### Posttest

Clean the equipment with soap and water and rinse thoroughly.
Store the tablets and dipstick in a dry, cool place in their original containers.
Document the results on a flow sheet.
Adjust insulin dosage as ordered based on the results.

### Home Testing

Determine with the physician and the patient the method of SMUG that will be used at home. Instruct the patient on the double-void technique. Most patients choose to collect their urine in a disposable paper cup. Instruct the patient according to the chosen method (see Nursing Implementation). Provide the patient with the opportunity to practice SMUG.

The community health nurse needs to assess the patient's ability to apply hospital learning to the home. Reinforce learning. Periodically, the community health nurse needs to observe the patient's technique to ensure that test results are accurate. Periodic evaluation of the patient's visual acuity is necessary, because the patient must use a color chart to determine glucose level. Instruct the patient to document results and any insulin taken based on the results and bring the record to the physician, nurse practitioner, or diabetes clinic at each visit.

## Glycosylated Hemoglobin Assay

**(Blood)**                    Synonyms: Glycohemoglobin, GHB, hemoglobin A₁

**Normal Values**

**Glycosylated Hemoglobin Assay**
Normal, healthy person: 5.5%–8.8% of total hemoglobin *or* SI 0.05–0.08 (fraction of total hemoglobin)

> Diabetic under control: 7.5%–11.4% of total hemoglobin
> **Hemoglobin $A_{1a}$:** 1.8% of total hemoglobin
> **Hemoglobin $A_{1b}$:** 0.8% of total hemoglobin
> **Hemoglobin $A_{1c}$:** 3.56% of total hemoglobin

## Background Information

*Glycosylated hemoglobin* refers to hemoglobin that has hooked up with glucose. The major glycosylated hemoglobin is hemoglobin $A_{1c}$, which is approximately 4% to 6% of the total hemoglobin. The other glycosylated hemoglobins are phosphoxylated glucose ($A_{1a}$) and phosphoxylated fructose ($A_{1b}$). Usually, a laboratory will report the total glycosylated hemoglobin level (hemoglobin $A_1$).

The reaction between glucose and hemoglobin is based on the blood glucose concentration. The higher the glucose concentration, the higher the percentage of glycosylated hemoglobin. Because the reaction is not reversible, once the glucose adheres to the hemoglobin it remains glycosylated. Since the life span of a red blood cell is normally 120 days, measuring the glycosylated hemoglobin can assist in diabetic control assessment. It is not affected by recent changes in diet or medication, as fasting blood glucose levels are, so the physician can determine diabetic control over a period of weeks or months. Patients whose diabetes is poorly controlled will have a glycosylated hemoglobin value that is more than 12% of the total hemoglobin value.

The reliability of the test is based on normal hemoglobin levels. If a person has an abnormal hemoglobin value, the accuracy of the $HbA_{1c}$ is suspect. An example of this is the sickle cell trait. Also, any condition that shortens or lengthens the life of the red blood cells will make the results questionable.

| | |
|---|---|
| **Purpose of the Test** | A glycosylated hemoglobin determination is performed to measure a patient's diabetic control over a period of weeks or months. The maximum period for evaluation of control is the life span of the red blood cells (120 days). |
| **Procedure** | Venipuncture is performed to obtain 5 mL of blood in a test tube containing an anticoagulant (a lavender-topped tube with EDTA or a green-topped tube with heparin). |
| **Findings** | **Elevated Values**<br><br>Poorly controlled<br>   diabetes mellitus<br>Hyperglycemia |
| **Interfering Factors** | • Acetylsalicytic acid<br>• Anemia<br>• Chronic renal failure<br>• Clotting of specimen<br>• Fetal-maternal transfusion<br>• Hemodialysis<br>• Hemorrhage |

- Hemolytic disease
- Phlebotomies
- Thalassemias

**Nursing Implementation**   The actions of the nurse resemble those used in other venipuncture procedures.

■

*Critical Thinking 20–9*
The hemoglobin A$_1$ results indicate that the patient's glucose is poorly controlled. When informed, the patient angrily states that he never cheated on his diet and always took his insulin. How should you respond?

## Growth Hormone

**(Serum)**   Synonyms: Somatotropin, GH, STH

**Normal Values**

> Adult male: Undetectable–5 ng/mL *or* SI 0–5 µg/L
> Adult female: Undetectable–10 ng/mL *or* SI 0–10 µg/L
> Child: Undetectable–16 ng/mL *or* SI 0–16 µg/L

### Background Information

Growth hormone is synthesized and secreted by the anterior pituitary gland under the direction of the hypothalamus. The hypothalamus controls growth hormone secretion via somatostatin (growth hormone release-inhibiting hormone) and growth hormone releasing hormone. The primary function of growth hormone is the promotion of linear growth, which it does by stimulating the production of somatomedin, which is produced by a variety of organs. It is believed that growth hormone also has a direct effect on tissues.

During linear growth and afterward, growth hormone influences protein, carbohydrate, and fat metabolism. It increases protein synthesis, decreases protein catabolism, and activates lipolysis. Excessive growth hormone will decrease carbohydrate use and glucose uptake by the cells.

Because normal basal levels of growth hormone are low, it is sometimes necessary to stimulate the secretion of the hormone to rule out hyposecretion. Various substances can be used in these provocative tests, including arginine, insulin, arginine-insulin, levodopa, and, less frequently, vasopressin, glucagon, exercise, or tolbutamide. Careful medical evaluation of the patient is necessary before insulin is used as a provocative agent so that a hypoglycemic crisis can be prevented.

### Purpose of the Test

Growth hormone levels are evaluated to diagnose growth disorders and possible pituitary tumors. Abnormal linear growth may be a result of several factors: genetics, chronic disease, malnutrition, and so forth. Growth hormone levels will assist in determining the cause of the growth disorder and thereby influence therapy and prognosis.

| | |
|---|---|
| **Procedure** | Serum growth hormone levels are measured by RIA. Five milliliters of venous blood is drawn into a red-topped tube and is sent to the laboratory. |

**Findings**

**Elevated Values**

Pituitary tumor      Acromegaly
Hypothalamic tumor    Gigantism

**Decreased Values**

Dwarfism
Metastatic or anoxic
  pituitary destruc-
  tion

**Interfering Factors**

- Failure to fast for 8 to 12 hours before the test
- Administration of radioactive scan within 7 days
- Medications such as amphetamines, arginine, beta blockers, chlorpromazine, corticosteroids, dopamine, glucagon, insulin, levodopa, and oral contraceptives

**Nursing Implementation**

■

*Critical Thinking 20–10*
A neighbor's child is the shortest child in his class. His parents ask you if he should be tested. What initial assessments should you make in helping the parents come to a decision?

**Pretest**

Instruct the patient to limit activity and not eat or drink for 8 to 12 hours before the specimen is collected.
Obtain a drug history to determine if any interfering medication is being taken.
Inquire if the patient has undergone any recent radioactive scans.

**During the Test**

The nurse takes actions similar to those for other venipuncture procedures.

**Posttest**

The patient can resume diet and the medications that were withheld.
Send the specimen to the laboratory on ice.
Normal activity may be resumed.

## Growth Hormone Stimulation Test

**(Serum)**      Synonyms: Arginine test, insulin tolerance test (ITT)

**Normal Values**

With arginine: >7 ng/mL *or* SI >7 µg/L
With insulin (with serum glucose of <40 mg/dL): >20 ng/mL *or* SI >20 µg/L
With propranolol and glucagon: >10 ng/mL *or* SI >10 µg/L

## Background Information

Review the preceding section on growth hormone.

| | |
|---|---|
| **Purpose of the Test** | The growth hormone stimulation test is usually performed to evaluate children and infants with retarded growth. It is also used to support the diagnosis of pituitary tumor. A variety of stimulants can be used to stimulate the secretion of the growth hormone, including arginine, glucagon, propranolol, insulin, levodopa, exercise, and corticotropin-releasing hormone (CRH). Arginine and insulin are the most frequently used stimulants.

The insulin tolerance test may be used to distinguish primary versus secondary adrenocorticoid insufficiency by measuring ACTH levels instead of growth hormone levels. |
| **Procedure** | Depending on the substance used, slight variations exist in the method. With arginine, a baseline sample of 5 mL of venous blood is obtained in a red-topped tube. A venous infusion of arginine is then administered. After the arginine infusion is completed (in approximately 30 minutes), 30 minutes are allowed to pass. Three venous samples are then obtained at 30-minute intervals. Ion exchange chromatography is used to analyze the blood samples.

If insulin is used, a baseline venous sample is taken, after which 100 units of regular insulin is given intravenously over 2 to 3 minutes. Venous samples are taken at 15, 30, 45, 60, 90, and 120 minutes after the administration of insulin. Blood glucose levels must fall to below 40 mg/dL within 1 hour after the insulin is given for an accurate evaluation. |
| **Findings** | **Elevated Values**

No growth hormone deficiency

**Decreased Values**

Pituitary dwarfism
Pituitary tumors |
| **Interfering Factors** | • Failure to comply with fasting or activity restrictions
• Alcohol
• Medications such as amphetamines, beta blockers, calcium gluconate, estrogen, spironolactone, and steroids |
| **Nursing Implementation** | **Pretest**

Assess patients at risk if a growth hormone stimulation test with insulin is planned. This includes patients with cardiovascular disease, epilepsy, a history of a cerebrovascular accident, or adrenal insufficiency. |

Instruct the patient to limit physical activity and not to eat or drink for 12 hours before the test.

Instruct the patient not to drink alcohol for 24 hours before the blood is drawn.

Obtain a medication history to determine if any interfering drug is being taken. Check with the prescriber about withholding any interfering medication.

Instruct the patient to lie down quietly for 90 minutes before the blood is drawn.

### During the Test

An intravenous catheter (heparin lock) is inserted to prevent multiple venous punctures.

A baseline venous sample is taken.

If arginine is used, an infusion is given over 30 minutes in the arm opposite the heparin lock used for blood sampling. Thirty minutes after the arginine infusion is completed, three additional blood specimens are obtained at 30-minute intervals.

If insulin is used, 100 units of regular insulin is given over 2 to 3 minutes. Blood specimens are drawn at 15, 30, 45, 60, 90, and 120 minutes.

Observe the patient carefully. Stop the test if serious signs of hypoglycemia occur (e.g., vertigo, chest pain).

### Posttest

The patient can resume medication schedule, diet, and physical activities.

Ensure that the patient who received insulin as a stimulant has adequate food intake.

## Growth Hormone Suppression Test

**(Serum)**                                   Synonym: Glucose loading test

| Normal Values | Growth hormone levels decrease to undetectable to <3 ng/mL *or* SI <3 μg/L in 30–120 minutes |
| --- | --- |

### Background Information

The growth hormone suppression test is performed after high levels of growth hormone are found. Normally, the ingestion of glucose causes a decrease in the secretion of growth hormone. In patients with hypersecretion of growth hormone, however, a significant decrease does not occur.

### Purpose of the Test

This test is usually performed to assess an increase in growth hormone levels and to confirm the diagnoses of gigantism in children and acromegaly in adults.

### Procedure

A baseline venous blood sample, 5 mL, is drawn into a red-topped tube. The patient ingests a glucose solution. After 1 to 2 hours, another blood sample is drawn. RIA is used to assess the samples.

| | |
|---|---|
| **Findings** | **Maintenance of High Growth Hormone Levels** |
| | Acromegaly |
| | Gigantism |

| | |
|---|---|
| **Interfering Factors** | • Noncompliance with activity restrictions and fasting |
| | • Radioactive scans within the previous week |
| | • Medications such as amphetamines, arginine, beta blockers, chlorpromazine, dopamine, glucagon, histamine, insulin, levodopa, nicotinic acid, and steroids |

**Nursing Implementation**

■

*Critical Thinking 20–11*
Your adult patient with a potential diagnosis of acromegaly is withdrawn, keeps the curtain drawn around her bed, and never leaves the room. What possible nursing diagnosis is appropriate?

**Pretest**

Instruct the patient about the need to avoid physical activity for 10 to 12 hours before the test and to lie quietly for 30 minutes before the blood is drawn.
Instruct the patient not to eat or drink for 12 hours before the sample is taken.
Obtain a medication history to ensure that an interfering drug has not been taken.
Question the patient or check the patient's chart for any recent radioactive scans.

**During the Test**

Explain the purpose of the two venipunctures.
After the first specimen is obtained in the early morning, instruct the patient to drink the glucose solution *slowly* to minimize nausea.
Ensure that the second specimen is obtained 1 to 2 hours after the ingestion of glucose.

**Posttest**

The patient resumes normal diet and activity.

## 2-Hour Postprandial Glucose

**(Plasma)**    Synonym: 2-hour postprandial blood sugar

| | |
|---|---|
| **Normal Values** | Fasting blood glucose: <126 mg/dL *or* SI <6.993 mmol/L |
| | Values may be slightly elevated in elderly patients. |

### Background Information

In healthy individuals, the ingestion of food raises the blood glucose level, which is a potent stimulant for insulin release. The insulin level peaks in less than an hour. Normally, within 1½ to 2 hours, the glucose level will return to baseline. It may take slightly longer in older individuals for the value to return to a baseline level. The 2-hour postprandial glucose test evaluates whether the individual has an adequate insulin response to intake. A diabetic is considered in good control if the 2-hour postprandial glucose level is less than 130 mg/dL. In an undiagnosed case, a 2-hour postprandial glucose level greater than 140 mg/dL indicates that an oral glucose tolerance test (OGTT) should be performed, because this test has more controlled variables.

---

**Purpose of the Test**

The 2-hour postprandial glucose test is performed to support the diagnosis of diabetes mellitus and to evaluate the management of a patient with diabetes mellitus.

---

**Procedure**

Two hours after a meal is ingested, venipuncture is performed to obtain 5 mL of blood in a red-topped tube for a plasma or serum glucose level determination.

---

**Findings**

A 2-hour postprandial glucose determination greater than 126 mg/dL is consistent with the diagnosis of diabetes mellitus. Diagnosis is not made with a 2-hour postprandial glucose test; an elevation indicates a need for a fasting blood sugar or oral glucose tolerance test.

---

**Interfering Factors**

- Noncompliance with dietary requirements
- Cushing's disease or Cushing's syndrome
- Infection
- Malabsorption syndrome
- Malnutrition
- Severe stress
- Medications such as arginine, beta-adrenergic blockers, epinephrine, glucocorticoids, glucose administered intravenously, hypoglycemic agents, insulin, lithium, phenothiazines, and phenytoin

---

**Nursing Implementation**

**Pretest**

Instruct the patient to eat normally before the test.

**During the Test**

The patient ingests a meal containing at least 100 g of carbohydrate.
Instruct the patient not to eat or drink for 2 hours after the meal is ingested.
Venipuncture is performed to obtain a blood glucose level 2 hours after the meal.

**Posttest**

The patient resumes a normal diet.

---

## Insulin, Blood
**(Serum, Plasma)**          Synonyms: None

---

**Normal Values**

**Fasting**
Adult: 5–25 µU/mL *or* SI 34–172 pmol/L
Newborn: 3–20 µU/mL *or* SI 21–138 pmol/L

*Continued on following page*

*Continued*

> 1 hour after eating: 50–130 µU/mL *or* SI 347.3–902.8 pmol/L
> 2 hours after eating: <30 µU/mL *or* SI <208.4 pmol/L

## Background Information

Insulin is a protein hormone produced and secreted by the pancreas. It has a short half-life (3 to 5 minutes) and is broken down by the liver and kidneys. Insulin is secreted in response to food intake. It increases in concentration within 10 minutes of eating, peaks in 30 to 45 minutes, and returns to baseline levels within 90 to 120 minutes. Normally, insulin levels increase as blood glucose levels increase.

Without insulin, carbohydrate, protein, and fat metabolism are affected, resulting in hyperglycemia and metabolic acidosis.

## Purpose of the Test

Insulin levels are determined to assess for insulin-producing tumors, to confirm suspected insulin-resistant states, and as part of the evaluation of glucocorticoid insufficiency.

## Procedure

Insulin levels may be assessed by random venous sampling or during a glucose tolerance test. A specimen is obtained by venipuncture and collected in an anticoagulated tube. The specimen is assessed by RIA.

## Findings

**Elevated Values**

| | | |
|---|---|---|
| Acromegaly | Insulinoma | Vagal stimulation |
| Cushing's syndrome | Liver disease | |
| Hyperinsulinism | Pancreatic lesions | |

**Decreased Values**

Insulin-dependent
    diabetes mellitus
Hypopituitarism

## Interfering Factors

- Noncompliance with test protocol
- Insulin antibodies
- Medications such as ACTH, catecholamines, colchicine, diazoxide, oral contraceptives, phenytoin, steroids, sulfonylureas, thyroid hormones, vinblastine, and radioisotopes

## Nursing Implementation

Care varies according to whether a fasting sample is used or the insulin level is being obtained as part of the OGTT (see pp. 000–000 for discussion of this test).

### Pretest

Take a medication history to determine if any interfering drugs are being taken. Check to determine if these drugs are to be withheld. If the patient is receiving insulin therapy, the insulin is withheld until the test is performed.

Assess the patient's stress level, which may increase endogenous glucocorticoid secretion.

If a fasting insulin sample is to be drawn, instruct the patient not to eat or drink for 7 hours before the blood is drawn.

### During the Test

Observe the patient for hyperglycemia if the insulin is withheld and for hypoglycemia because of the fasting state.

If performed with an OGTT, a blood sample for insulin is obtained each time a glucose level specimen is drawn.

### Quality Control

Send the specimen to the laboratory immediately, because it must be centrifuged within 30 minutes and frozen until the assay can be performed.

### Posttest

The patient resumes normal medication schedule and diet therapies.

## Ketones, Serum
(Serum, Plasma)   Synonyms: Acetoacetate, acetones

| Normal Values | Negative: <2 mg/dL *or* SI <0.34 nmol/L |
|---|---|

### Background Information

Without adequate insulin, three major ketone bodies accumulate in the blood: acetone, acetoacetate acid, and beta-hydroxybutyric acid.

### Purpose of the Test

Serum ketone levels are measured to distinguish between diabetic ketoacidosis and hyperosmolar coma. With diabetic ketoacidosis, incomplete fatty acid metabolism leads to increasing ketones in the blood. Patients with hyperosmolar coma produce minimal or no ketosis in the presence of extremely high levels of serum glucose. The mechanism of maintaining nearly normal ketone levels in hyperosmolar coma is not known. It is theorized that these patients have sufficient insulin to break down fatty acids or are glucagon resistant.

The severity of the ketosis will influence the therapy for uncontrolled diabetes.

| | |
|---|---|
| **Procedure** | Venipuncture is performed to obtain 2 mL of blood in a red-topped tube, if a serum ketone level is desired. If a plasma level is ordered, a gray-topped tube is needed. |

**Findings**

**Elevated Values**

| | | |
|---|---|---|
| Alcoholism | Isopropanol | Starvation |
| Decreased caloric | poisoning | Uncontrolled diabetes |
| intake (dieting) | Propranolol | mellitus |
| Eclampsia | poisoning | Gierke's disease |

**Interfering Factors**

- Hemolysis of specimen

**Nursing Implementation**

The nurse's duties are similar to those performed in other venipuncture procedures.

## Ketones, Urinary

**(Urine)**   Synonyms: Acetoacetate, acetones

| | |
|---|---|
| **Normal Values** | Negative |

## Background Information

Without adequate insulin, three major ketone bodies accumulate in the blood and are excreted in the urine. These ketone bodies are acetone, acetoacetic acid, and beta-hydroxybutyric acid. Ketones form as fats, and fatty acids are broken down.

A variety of commercial products are available to test for ketones in the urine. The most popular products are Acetest tablets, Ketostix, and Keto-Diastix. These products measure acetone and acetoacetate acid levels but not beta-hydroxybutyric acid, which may be the dominant ketone in patients with poorly controlled diabetes mellitus.

Urinary ketone testing is usually performed in conjunction with urinary glucose testing. It may be carried out randomly to evaluate a suspected diagnosis of uncontrolled diabetes mellitus or four times a day to regulate insulin coverage.

**Purpose of the Test**

Urine is tested for ketone bodies to evaluate the patient with diabetes mellitus and to diagnose carbohydrate deprivation. The concentration of urine ketones can be used to adjust insulin requirements in diabetic patients and to monitor patients on low-carbohydrate diets.

**Procedure**

With the Acetest tablet, one drop of urine is placed on a tablet. With the Ketostix or Keto-Diastix, the reagent strip is dipped in the urine. The color change of the tablet or on the strip is compared to the chart provided by the manufacturer to determine the presence and concentration of ketones.

| **Findings** | **Elevated Values** | | |
|---|---|---|---|
| | Alcoholic keto-<br>    acidosis<br>Fever | High-fat diet<br>Hypermetabolic states<br>Starvation | Uncontrolled diabetes<br>    mellitus |

**Interfering Factors**

- Using products that have been exposed to light or are outdated
- Bacteria in the urine

**Nursing Implementation**

**Pretest**

Instruct the patient about the double-void technique.

**During the Test**

Instruct the patient to void, discard this urine, wait 30 minutes, and void into a clean, dry container.
Check voided urine within 60 minutes.
The method of checking for ketones varies with the product. Follow the manufacturer's guidelines.

**Posttest**

Document the results, usually on a flow chart.
Adjust insulin dosage as ordered based on the results.

## Long-Acting Thyroid Stimulator

**(Serum)**    Synonym: LATS

| **Normal Values** | Negative |
|---|---|

### Background Information

Long-acting thyroid stimulator is a globulin that binds to thyroid receptor sites and stimulates thyroid activity. It helps to differentiate between Graves' disease and nodular toxic goiter or other disorders.

### Purpose of the Test

The determination of long-acting thyroid stimulator levels is performed to support the diagnosis of Graves' disease.

### Procedure

Venipuncture is performed and blood is collected in a heparinized tube. The specimen is assessed by mouse bioassay.

| | |
|---|---|
| **Findings** | **Elevated Values** |
| | Graves' disease |
| | Nodular toxic goiter |
| | (rare) |

| | |
|---|---|
| **Interfering Factors** | • Radioactive iodine |

| | |
|---|---|
| **Nursing Implementation** | The nursing actions are similar to those in other venipuncture procedures. |
| | **Pretest** |
| | Schedule any test requiring radioactive iodine for after blood for long-acting thyroid stimulator levels is drawn. |

## Metyrapone Testing

| | |
|---|---|
| **(Serum)** | Synonym: Metyrapone stimulation test |

| | |
|---|---|
| **Normal Values** | 11-deoxycortisol level >7 µg/dL *or* SI >202 nmol/L |

### Background Information

Review the section on plasma ACTH (pp. 552–554). Metyrapone is given to block cortisol synthesis. A decrease in cortisol will normally stimulate ACTH secretion, which, in turn, will increase the secretion of 11-deoxycortisol. If an increase occurs after the metyrapone is given, ACTH and adrenal function are normal. If an abnormal result occurs, that is, no increase in 11-deoxycortisol occurs, the diagnosis of adrenal insufficiency is established; however, it is not known whether it is primary or secondary adrenal failure.

The *insulin-induced hypoglycemia test* is similar to the metyrapone test. The hypoglycemia causes a stress response normally resulting in the secretion of CRH, which causes an increase in ACTH secretion. This test allows the assessment of the hypothalamic-pituitary axis.

| | |
|---|---|
| **Purpose of the Test** | Metyrapone testing is performed to diagnose adrenal insufficiency and to assess pituitary-adrenal reserves. |

| | |
|---|---|
| **Procedure** | Metyrapone is given in the evening. The next morning, a venipuncture is performed to obtain 7 to 10 mL of blood in a red- or green-topped tube. |

| | | |
|---|---|---|
| **Findings** | Adrenal hyperplasia | Ectopic ACTH |
| | Adrenal tumor | syndrome |

| | |
|---|---|
| **Interfering Factors** | • Recent radioisotope therapy or testing<br>• Medication such as chlorpromazine |
| **Nursing Implementation** | The nursing actions are similar to those carried out in the determination of cortisol levels (see pp. 564–566). |
| **Complications** | For a patient with adrenocorticoid insufficiency, the administration of metyrapone, which inhibits cortisol production, may precipitate an addisonian crisis (Table 20–3). |

## Oral Glucose Tolerance Test

**(Plasma)**    Synonyms: OGTT, GTT

| | |
|---|---|
| **Normal Values** | Baseline fasting blood glucose level: 70–105 mg/dL *or* SI 3.9–5.8 mmol/L<br>30-minute blood glucose level: 110–170 mg/dL *or* SI 6.1–9.4 mmol/L<br>60-minute blood glucose level: 120–170 mg/dL *or* SI 6.7–9.4 mmol/L<br>90-minute blood glucose level: 100–140 mg/dL *or* SI 5.6–7.8 mmol/L<br>120-minute blood glucose level: 70–120 mg/dL *or* SI 3.9–6.7 mmol/L |

### Background Information

Fasting blood glucose level determinations, if repeated, are usually adequate to diagnose diabetes mellitus if the plasma glucose level is greater than 126 mg/dL. However, if the fasting blood glucose levels are questionable, and clinical indications make diabetes mellitus likely, an oral glucose tolerance test (OGTT) or an intravenous glucose tolerance test (IVGTT) may be performed. The American Diabetes Association recommends that pregnant women at the 24th to 28th week of gestation have a OGTT done using 50 g of glucose. If any abnormality results, a repeat OGTT is done with 100 g of glucose. Many recommend that any pregnant woman at risk for gestational diabetes have the OGTT done in the 16th to 18th week of pregnancy and repeat the test at the 24th to 28th week. Other indications include delivery of an infant weighing more than 9 lb (4.1 kg), frequent vaginal yeast infections, and impotence in males.

The *intravenous glucose tolerance test* is similar to the OGTT. It is usually ordered when the patient has a problem with gastrointestinal absorption. It is not preferable to the OGTT because it bypasses normal glucose absorption and, therefore, normal changes in gastrointestinal hormones.

| Table 20–3 | Complications of Metyrapone Testing | |
|---|---|
| **Complication** | **Nursing Assessment** |
| Addisonian crisis | Hypotension<br>Hyponatremia<br>Hyperkalemia<br>Muscle weakness<br>Shock |

Patient preparation for the IVGTT is the same as that for the OGTT, except that the glucose load (0.5 g/kg of ideal body weight) is given intravenously over 2 to 3 minutes. The fasting blood glucose levels after the IVGTT are similar to those after an OGTT, except that the 30-minute ingestion fasting blood glucose level tends to be higher.

| | |
|---|---|
| **Purpose of the Test** | The OGTT is performed to confirm the diagnosis of diabetes mellitus. |
| **Procedure** | After the ingestion of a glucose load, venous blood samplings for plasma glucose are obtained at the time of ingestion and then at 30, 60, 90, and 120 minutes after the glucose load is given. |
| **Findings** | The OGTT confirms the diagnosis of diabetes mellitus if the 2-hour blood glucose level is greater than 200 mg/dL and at least one other blood glucose determination is greater than 200 mg/dL. Blood glucose levels between the diagnostic criteria and normal values are called *impaired glucose tolerance*. |

**Interfering Factors**

- Noncompliance with dietary and fasting requirements
- Alcohol ingestion
- Being bedridden
- Cushing's syndrome or Cushing's disease
- Infection
- Malabsorption syndrome
- Malnutrition
- Pregnancy
- Severe stress
- Smoking
- Medications such as amphetamines, arginine, beta-adrenergic blockers, diuretics, epinephrine, glucocorticoids, glucose administered intravenously, insulin, lithium, oral contraceptives, oral hypoglycemic agents, phenothiazines, phenytoin, and salicylates

**Nursing Implementation** **Pretest**

Instruct the patient to take in at least 150 to 250 g of carbohydrates per day for 3 days before the test to optimize insulin secretion.

Instruct the patient not to drink or eat for 8 hours before the test begins. The patient is also instructed to avoid stimulants and not to smoke or perform any unusual activity for 8 hours before the test.

Take a medication history to determine if any interfering drugs are being taken. Check with the prescriber to determine if medications should be withheld. Oral hypoglycemic agents are withheld for 2 weeks before an OGTT is performed.

Question the patient regarding any recent acute illnesses. The OGTT should be delayed for at least 2 weeks after an acute illness.

### During the Test

A fasting blood glucose determination is performed (usually in the early morning between 7 and 9 AM).

Within 5 minutes of obtaining the baseline fasting blood glucose level, the patient drinks 75 g of glucose in 300 mL of water. Children are given 1.5 g of glucose per kilogram of ideal body weight. The glucose solution should be ingested within 5 minutes.

Venipunctures are performed to obtain blood glucose readings at 30, 60, 90, and 120 minutes after the glucose solution is ingested. If a hypoglycemic reaction is suspected, a 3-hour blood specimen is obtained.

Observe the patient for a hyper- or hypoglycemic reaction.

The patient may drink water during the collection period.

### Posttest

The patient resumes taking medications that were withheld.

A normal diet and activity level are resumed.

■
*Critical Thinking 20–12*
Following a OGTT, three newly diagnosed diabetics have been identified. They are 4, 13, and 27 years old. Will the age of the patient influence the nurse's teaching plan?

---

## Osmolality, Plasma

**(Plasma, Serum)**        Synonyms: None

---

**Normal Values**

Adults: 285–300 mOsm/kg $H_2O$ *or* SI 280–300 mmol/kg
Children: 270–290 mOsm/kg $H_2O$ *or* SI 270–290 mmol/kg

---

### Background Information

Osmolality is a measure of the number of particles dissolved in a solution. In the blood, the osmolality is created by sodium, chloride, bicarbonate, proteins, glucose, and urea dissolved in the plasma.

Osmolality is affected by an increase or decrease in fluid volume or by an increase or decrease in blood particles.

---

**Purpose of the Test**

Plasma osmolality is determined to assess the person's fluid status and identify ADH abnormalities.

---

**Procedure**

Venipuncture is performed to obtain 1 mL of blood in a red-topped tube. Osmolality is measured by the freezing point depression of solution using an osmometer or cryoscope or by the vapor pressure or dew point osmometer.

---

**Findings**

**Increased Values**

| | | |
|---|---|---|
| Alcoholism | Diabetes insipidus | Hyperglycemia |
| Aldosteronism | High-protein diet | Hypernatremia |
| Dehydration | Hypercalcemia | Hyperkalemia |

**Decreased Values**

Addison's disease
Fluid overload
Hyponatremia
Liver failure with
  ascites

Syndrome of inappro-
  priate antidiuretic
  hormone

---

**Interfering Factors**

- Hemolysis of specimen
- Medications
- Diuretics
- Mineralocorticoids

---

**Nursing Implementation**

The nursing actions are similar to those of other venipuncture procedures.

---

**Critical Values**

**<265 mOsm/kg H$_2$O (SI <265 mmol/kg H$_2$O) and >320 mOsm/kg H$_2$O (SI >320 mmol/kg H$_2$O)**

Assess patient fluid status. Notify the physician, especially if the patient is increasingly stuporous. Initiate seizure precautions for high osmolality levels.

---

## Osmolality, Urine

**(Urine)**

Synonyms: None

---

**Normal Values**

24-hour urine specimen (with normal diet and fluid intake): 500–800 mOsm/kg H$_2$O or SI 500–800 mmol/kg H$_2$O

Random urine specimen: 50–1,200 mOsm/kg H$_2$O or SI 50–1,200 mmol/kg H$_2$O

---

### Background Information

Osmolality is a measure of the number of particles that are dissolved in a solution. Thus, urine osmolality varies based on the person's fluid status and the metabolic waste products being excreted. If the patient is overhydrated, the urinary osmolality decreases as output increases. If the person is dehydrated, the urine osmolality increases as the output decreases. Urine osmolality is based on the concentration ability of the kidneys and the serum levels of sodium, chloride, bicarbonate, proteins, glucose, and urea.

---

### Purpose of the Test

Urine osmolality is determined to assess the ability of the kidneys to concentrate or dilute urine and to identify antidiuretic hormone (ADH) abnormalities.

| | |
|---|---|
| **Procedure** | Ten milliliters of urine is collected in a sterile container and is sent to the laboratory if a random urine specimen is desired. For a 24-hour specimen, all urine voided in a 24-hour period is sent to the laboratory. |

**Findings**

**Increased Values**

Addison's disease
Azotemia
Cirrhosis of the liver
Dehydration

Diabetes mellitus
Diarrhea
Hyperglycemia
Hypernatremia

Syndrome of inappropriate antidiuretic hormone

**Decreased Values**

Aldosteronism
Diabetes insipidus
Glomerulonephritis

Hypocalcemia
Hyponatremia
Overhydration

Sickle cell anemia

**Interfering Factors**

- Noncompliance with nothing-by-mouth status
- Glucosuria
- Recent scans requiring radiopaque dyes
- Medications
- Antibiotics
- Diuretics
- Volume expanders

**Nursing Implementation**

Nursing care is similar to that for other 24-hour urine collection procedures. Or, for a random specimen, perform the following.

**Pretest**

Instruct the patient not to eat or drink overnight before the urine is collected for a random specimen.

**During the Test**

Obtain 10 mL of urine in a sterile container.

**Posttest**

Send the specimen to the laboratory immediately.

## Parathyroid Hormone

(Serum)    Synonyms: Parathormone, PTH

**Normal Values**

(Interpreted in relation to serum calcium levels)
Intact parathyroid hormone: 210–310 pg/mL *or* SI 210–310 ng/L
N-terminal fraction: 230–630 pg/mL *or* SI 230–630 ng/L
C-terminal fraction: 410–1,760 pg/mL *or* SI 410–1,760 ng/L

## Background Information

Parathyroid hormone is produced and secreted by the parathyroid glands. Its role in the body is the regulation of calcium. Its secretion is based on a negative feedback mechanism with calcium (Fig. 20–5).

Parathyroid hormone affects calcium levels by stimulating osteoclast activity in the bone and inhibiting osteoblast activity. This causes bone reabsorption, which shifts calcium and phosphate out of the bone into the blood. Parathyroid hormone also causes increased reabsorption of calcium at the kidney's distal tubules and decreased reabsorption of phosphate at the proximal tubules. The result of parathyroid hormone activity is an increase in calcium in the blood with a decrease in plasma phosphate levels.

**Purpose of the Test**

A parathyroid hormone determination is performed to diagnose suspected parathyroid disorders. It may be performed to differentiate among clinical diagnoses that result in calcium and phosphate abnormalities.

**Procedure**

Parathyroid hormone is measured by RIA, which can measure biologically active intact parathyroid hormone. This fraction represents only a small portion of the total parathyroid hormone. Alternatively, RIA can measure C-terminal or N-terminal portions of the hormone. Two venous samples, 3 mL each in red-topped tubes, are needed.

**Findings**

**Elevated Values**

Hyperparathyroidism

**Decreased Values**

Hypoparathyroidism
Lung, kidney,
    pancreatic, or
    ovarian cancer

**Interfering Factors**

- Noncompliance with fasting requirements
- Elevated lipid levels

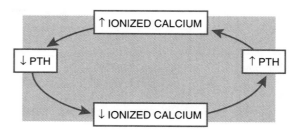

**Figure 20–5**
Regulation of parathyroid hormone (PTH) secretion.

**Nursing Implementation**     The actions of the nurse are similar to those carried out in other venipuncture procedures.

### Pretest

Instruct the patient not to eat or drink for 12 hours before the test.

### Posttest

The patient may resume a normal diet.
Send the specimen to the laboratory on ice.

## Renin, Plasma

**(Plasma)**     Synonyms: Plasma renin activity, PRA

**Normal Values**

> **Adult**
> Recumbent position: 0.2–1.6 ng/mL/hr *or* SI 0.2–1.6 µg X hr$^{-1}$ X L$^{-1}$
> Upright position: 0.7–3.33 ng/mL/hr *or* SI 0.7–3.33 µg X hr$^{-1}$ X L$^{-1}$
> **Infant:** 2.4–37.0 ng/mL/hr *or* SI 2.4–37 µg X hr$^{-1}$ X L$^{-1}$
> **Young child:** 1.0–11.2 ng/mL/hr *or* SI 1.0–11.2 µg X hr$^{-1}$ X L$^{-1}$
> **Child:** 0.5–5.9 ng/mL/hr *or* SI 0.5–5.9 µg X hr$^{-1}$ X L$^{-1}$

### Background Information

Renin is a proteolytic enzyme produced and secreted by the juxtaglomerular cells of the kidneys. Renin is secreted whenever a reduction of blood pressure to the kidneys occurs. Renin in the circulation acts on angiotensinogen to form angiotensin I, which is converted to angiotensin II—a powerful vasoconstrictor and stimulant for aldosterone secretion. This action is called the renin-angiotensin-aldosterone system or axis (see Fig. 20–2).

Because renin is a powerful vasoconstrictor, its role in hypertension has been studied. Most patients with hypertension have normal renin levels. Some hypertensive patients with excessive fluid retention have low renin levels, and other hypertensive patients have high renin levels.

It has been difficult to correlate renin levels with clinical states, because renin levels vary between individuals and because laboratory techniques vary in the measurement of these levels. In addition, many factors will influence secretion rates of renin, including dietary ingestion of sodium. For this reason, some clinicians correlate renin levels with the sodium content of the patient's diet. The sodium content of the diet is measured by a 24-hour urine sodium level test.

Another method to evaluate renin is to perform a *sodium-depleted renin test,* during which a diuretic (usually furosemide) is given.

**Purpose of the Test**     Plasma renin levels are determined as part of hypertension screening and to diagnose primary aldosteronism.

**Procedure**     Procedures vary. A random renin test simply requires a venipuncture to obtain 10 mL of blood in a lavender-topped tube containing EDTA. The specimen is placed on ice and immediately sent to the laboratory. If the renin level is to be correlated with sodium intake, a 24-hour urine specimen is required.

If a renin determination from a renal vein is planned, it is carried out under fluoroscopy; a catheter is inserted into the renal vein via the femoral vein. The specimen is assayed by RIA.

| Findings | | | |
|---|---|---|---|
| | **Elevated Values** | | |
| | Hypertension | Hypovolemia | Addison's disease |
| | Cirrhosis | Hypokalemia | Chronic renal failure |
| | **Decreased Values** | | |
| | Fluid retention with high-sodium diet | Excessive licorice intake | Cushing's syndrome |
| | Primary aldoster-onism | Hypertension with fluid retention | |

**Interfering Factors**

- Noncompliance with dietary and medication restrictions
- Improper positioning during the test
- Medications such as antihypertensives, clonidine, diuretics, estrogen, minoxidil, nitroprusside, propranolol, reserpine, and vasodilators

**Nursing Implementation**

■

*Critical Thinking 20–13*
A random renin level is ordered for a young child. The physician orders it done after the patient has been in the upright position for 2 hours. How can a busy nurse ensure this positioning?

The actions of the nurse vary depending on the technique used.

**Pretest**

Instruct the patient on the technique.

If a random sampling is ordered, instruct the patient to maintain a prone position or an upright position for 2 hours before the test. The position is based on physician preference.

If a renal vein level determination is ordered, explain the need to go to the radiology department for fluroscopy. Explain equipment, groin preparation, and local anesthesia.

If a sodium depletion renin test is ordered, assess the patient's cardiovascular status before a diuretic is given. Instruct the patient to maintain a low-sodium diet for 3 days before the test.

**Table 20–4  Complications of Adrenal Vein Renin Level Assay**

| Complication | Nursing Assessment |
|---|---|
| Bleeding | Observe puncture site and area under patient for blood |
| | Restlessness |
| | Tachycardia |
| | Decreased urinary output |
| | Hypotension |
| Hematoma | Observe site for swelling |
| | Check distal pulses |
| | Check extremity for color and temperature |

### Posttest

If the femoral approach to the renal vein is used, assess the site for hematoma and bleeding.

---

**Complications**

The only complications expected with renin evaluation are those associated with femoral vein access: bleeding and hematoma formation (Table 20–4).

---

## Resin Triiodothyronine Uptake

**(Serum)**     Synonyms: $T_3$ resin uptake test, $RT_3U$, $T_3$ uptake ratio, triiodothyronine resin uptake test

---

**Normal Values**     25%–35% *or* SI 0.25–0.35

---

### Background Information

The resin triiodothyronine uptake test is determined to estimate the *free triiodothyronine index* (FT$_3$I). In many institutions, the assay of free triiodothyronine has replaced the index, because the index is an estimate of the free hormone levels.

The resin triiodothyronine uptake test assesses the capacity of the blood proteins to bind with thyroid hormones. It does not measure the hormones themselves.

---

**Purpose of the Test**

The resin triiodothyronine uptake test is performed to diagnose hyper- and hypothyroidism.

---

**Procedure**

Venipuncture is performed to obtain a serum specimen to which radioactive triiodothyronine is added. Radioactive triiodothyronine is used instead of thyroxine because more triiodothyronine is bound to the resin, which has a lower affinity to endogenous protein-binding sites. After the resin is mixed with the radioactive triiodothyronine in serum, it is removed, and the amount of radioactivity absorbed is measured.

The measurement of the free triiodothyronine index is obtained by multiplying the resin uptake and the total thyroid hormone concentration. The index is not a direct measurement of the free thyroid hormone, but a estimate.

The normal free triiodothyronine index is 24 to 67.

---

**Findings**

**Elevated Values**

Hyperthyroidism

**Decreased Values**

Hypothyroidism

| | |
|---|---|
| **Interfering Factors** | • Renal failure |
| | • Malnutrition |
| | • Metastatic disease |
| | • Liver dysfunction |
| | • Critical illness |
| | • Medications such as ACTH, androgens, barbiturates, chlorpromazine, estrogen, furosemide, glucocorticoids, heroin, lithium, methadone, phenylbutazone, propylthiouracil, and thyroid replacement |
| **Nursing Implementation** | The nurse takes actions similar to those taken in other venipuncture procedures. |

## 17-Hydroxycorticosteroids

**(Urine)**                                                    Synonym: 17-OHCS

| | |
|---|---|
| **Normal Values** | **Adult male:** 4.5–12 mg/24 hr *or* SI 12.4–33.1 μmol/24 hr |
| | **Adult female:** 2.5–10 mg/24 hr *or* SI 6.9–27.6 μmol/24 hr |
| | **Children** |
| | 8–12 years: <4.5 mg/24 hr *or* SI <12.4 μmol/24 hr |
| | <8 years: <1.5 mg/24 hr *or* SI <4.14 μmol/24 hr |

### Background Information

17-Hydroxycorticosteroids (17-OHCS) are urinary steroids (cortisol and cortisone metabolites) used to assess adrenal function. An increase in 17-OHCS in the urine reflects an increase in plasma cortisol. With the direct measurement of plasma cortisol and free cortisol, the frequency of 17-OHCS determinations has significantly decreased.

When assessing 17-OHCS values, it is necessary to consider the patient's body type. Obese or muscular individuals will have higher 17-OHCS levels than will those with normal body types because of an increase in cortisol metabolism. To adjust to body type, some clinicians correlate the 17-OHCS to the creatinine clearance.

| | |
|---|---|
| **Purpose of the Test** | 17-OHCS levels are obtained to assess adrenal function. |
| **Procedure** | A 24-hour urine specimen is obtained. The urine is assessed by colorimetric reaction. |
| **Findings** | **Elevated Values** |

| | | |
|---|---|---|
| Adrenal cancer | Hyperthyroidism | Severe hypertension |
| Cushing's syndrome | Pituitary tumor | Acromegaly |
| Extreme stress | Obesity | |

**Decreased Values**

| | | |
|---|---|---|
| Addison's disease | Liver failure | Congenital adrenal |
| Hypothyroidism | Renal failure | hyperplasia |
| Starvation | Pregnancy | Hypotension |

**Interfering Factors**

- Failure to collect all the urine during the 24-hour collection period
- Failure to keep specimen on ice or refrigerated
- Medications such as chloral hydrate, chlorpromazine, colchicine, erythromycin, estrogens, oral contraceptives, paraldehyde, quinidine, quinine, reserpine, and spironolactone

**Nursing Implementation**

**Pretest**

Take the patient's medication history to assess for interfering factors.

Explain the collection procedure to the patient, especially the need to collect *all* the urine for 24 hours.

Instruct the patient to avoid excessive physical activity during the testing period.

**During the Test**

At the start of the test, instruct the patient to void at 8 AM and discard this urine. The collection period begins at this time, and all the urine is collected for 24 hours, including the 8 AM specimen of the following morning.

On the requisition slip and specimen label, write the patient's name and the time and date of the start and finish of the test period.

Keep the urine and collection container refrigerated or on ice during the collection period.

**Posttest**

Arrange for prompt transport of the cooled specimen to the laboratory.

## 17-Ketogenic Steroids

**(Urine)**                    Synonym: 17-KGS

**Normal Values**

**Adult male:** 4–14 mg/24 hr *or* SI 13–49 µmol/24 hr
**Adult female:** 2–12 mg/24 hr *or* SI 7–42 µmol/24 hr
**Children**
    11–14 years: 2–9 mg/24 hr *or* SI 7–31 µmol/24 hr
    <11 years: 0.1–4 mg/24 hr *or* SI 0.3–14 µmol/24 hr

## Background Information

17-Ketogenic steroids (17-KGS) include the metabolites of cortisol and other steroids. 17-KGS determination is not performed often because direct measurement of plasma cortisol and free cortisol has become more common.

| | |
|---|---|
| **Purpose of the Test** | Determination of 17-KGS levels is performed to assess adrenal function and support the diagnosis of Cushing's syndrome or Addison's disease. |

| | |
|---|---|
| **Procedure** | A 24-hour urine specimen is collected. The urine is assessed colorimetrically. |

**Findings**

**Elevated Values**

Adrenal cancer

Adenoma

Adrenogenital
   syndrome

Cushing's syndrome

Extreme stress

Ectopic ACTH-
   producing tumors

**Decreased Values**

Addison's disease

Cretinism

Hypopituitarism

Generalized wasting
   disease

**Interfering Factors**

- Failure to collect all the urine during the 24-hour collection period
- Failure to keep the specimen cool during the collection period
- Physical exercise
- Physical or emotional stress, or both
- Medications such as estrogens, hydralazine, penicillin, phenothiazines, quinine, reserpine, steroids, and thiazides

**Nursing Implementation**

**Pretest**

Take the patient's medication history to assess for interfering factors.

Explain to the patient the need to collect *all* the urine for 24 hours.

Instruct the patient to avoid excessive physical activity during the collection period.

**During the Test**

At the start of the test, instruct the patient to void at 8 AM and discard this urine. The collection period begins at this time, and all the urine is collected for 24 hours, including the 8 AM specimen of the following morning.

On the requisition slip and specimen label, write the patient's name and the time and date of the start and finish of the test period.

Keep the urine and collection container refrigerated or on ice throughout the test period.

Arrange for prompt transport of the cooled specimen to the laboratory.

## 17-Ketosteroids, Urinary

(Urine)         Synonym: 17-KS

| Normal Values | **Adult male:** 10–25 mg/24 hr *or* SI 35–87 µmol/24 hr |
|---|---|
| | **Adult female:** 6–14 mg/24 hr *or* SI 21–49 µmol/24 hr |
| | **Children** |
| | 10–14 years: 1–6 mg/24 hr *or* SI 2–21 µmol/24 hr |
| | <10 years: <3 mg/24 hr *or* SI <10 µmol/24 hr |

## Background Information

Urinary 17-ketosteroids measure the metabolites of androgens. Determination of 17-ketosteroids is rarely carried out because (1) plasma levels of the androgens are available, (2) it requires a 24-hour urine specimen, and (3) multiple drugs interfere with an accurate measurement.

## Purpose of the Test

Determination of 17-ketosteroids is performed to assess adrenal and gonadal function.

## Procedure

A 24-hour urine specimen is collected and assessed by colorimetric analysis.

## Findings

**Elevated Values**

Adrenal carcinoma
Adenoma

Cushing's syndrome
Extreme stress

**Decreased Values**

Addison's disease       Cretinism       Hypopituitarism

## Interfering Factors

- Failure to collect all the urine in the 24-hour period
- Failure to keep the specimen on ice or refrigerated during the collection period
- Hematuria
- Contrast dyes
- Increased exercise
- Stress
- Medications such as ACTH, estrogens, glucocorticoids, hydralazine, morphine, oral contraceptives, penicillin, phenothiazines, quinine, reserpine, and thiazides

## Nursing Implementation

**Pretest**

Instruct the patient to avoid excessive physical activity and stressful situations. Take a medication history to determine if interfering drugs are being taken. Explain to the patient the need to obtain *all* the urine during the collection time.

### During the Test

At the start of the test, instruct the patient to void at 8 AM and discard this urine. The collection period starts at this time, and all urine is collected for 24 hours, including the 8 AM specimen of the following morning.

On the requisition slip and specimen label, write the patient's name and the time and date of the start and finish of the collection period.

Keep the urine and collection container refrigerated or on ice throughout the collection period.

### Posttest

Arrange for prompt transport of the cooled specimen to the laboratory.

## Thyroglobulin Autoantibodies

**(Serum)**                    Synonym: Antithyroid antibodies

| Normal Values | Titer less than 1:100 by immunofluorescence; negative by hemagglutination method |
|---|---|

### Background Information

Some thyroid disorders may be autoimmune in origin. To evaluate this potential cause, antithyroid antibodies are measured. One of these antibodies is thyroglobulin autoantibody. The thyroglobulin autoantibodies act on the antigen *thyroglobulin*, the storage form of thyroid hormones. Although the presence of these antibodies helps confirm the diagnosis of autoimmune disease, their absence does not rule out the potential diagnosis.

### Purpose of the Test

Thyroglobulin antibodies are evaluated to detect autoimmune-based thyroid disease.

### Procedure

Venipuncture is performed to obtain 7 mL of blood in a red-topped tube. The specimen is assessed by immunofluorescence or hemagglutination technique.

### Findings

**Elevated Values**

| | | |
|---|---|---|
| Graves' disease | Hypothyroidism | Rheumatoid arthritis |
| Hashimoto's thyroiditis | Nontoxic nodular goiter | Systemic lupus erythematosus |
| Hyperthyroidism | Pernicious anemia | Thyroid cancer |

### Interfering Factors

- Oral contraceptives

### Nursing Implementation

The nursing actions are similar to those of other venipuncture techniques.

## Thyroid Microsomal Autoantibodies

**(Serum)** Synonym: Antithyroid antibodies

**Normal Values**   Titer less than 1:100 by immunofluorescence method; negative by hemagglutination method

### Background Information

Antithyroid antibodies are present in autoimmune diseases of the thyroid gland. Thyroid microsomal antibodies act against the lipoprotein microsomal antigen found in the thyroid gland. Evaluation of the antibody formation provides help in diagnosing autoimmune-based disorders of the thyroid gland. Although the presence of the antibody helps confirm the cause of the disorder, its absence does not usually rule out the potential cause.

### Purpose, Procedure, Findings, and Nursing Implementation

The purpose, the procedure, the findings, and the nursing implementation of the thyroid microsomal autoantibodies test are as for the thyroglobulin autoantibodies test.

## Thyrotropin

**(Serum)** Synonyms: Thyroid-stimulating hormone, TSH

**Normal Values**   Adult: 0.4–8.9 U/mL *or* SI 0.4–8.9 mU/L
Newborn, whole blood: <20 U/mL *or* SI <20 mU/L

### Background Information

Thyrotropin (TSH) is secreted by the anterior pituitary gland via a negative feedback mechanism (see Fig. 20–6). Thyrotropin causes the thyroid gland to increase its production and secretion of thyroid hormones.

Because of thyrotropin's regulatory mechanism with the thyroid hormones, its level will be affected by primary thyroid abnormalities. If the patient has hyperthyroidism, thyrotropin will be suppressed. If the patient has primary hypothyroidism, thyrotropin secretion will become markedly elevated. This elevation may create a compensatory euthyroid state. Exogenous thyroid hormones will also suppress thyrotropin secretion. TSH varies very little with age. The American College of Obstetricians and Gynecologists recommend that all women older than 65 years have the TSH level evaluated every 3 to 5 years. Although the TSH level is normally stable throughout life, even after menopause, the TSH level is used to assess thyroid function.

**Purpose of the Test**   Thyrotropin levels are obtained to (1) diagnose hypothyroidism, (2) distinguish between primary and secondary hypothyroidism, and (3) monitor patient response to thyroid replacement therapy.

| | |
|---|---|
| **Procedure** | Venipuncture is performed to obtain 7 mL of blood in a red-topped tube. If the test is required on a newborn, a heelstick is performed and the blood is collected on filter paper. |

**Findings**

**Elevated Values**

| | | |
|---|---|---|
| Addison's disease | Pituitary adenoma | Thyroid cancer |
| Goiter (some forms) | Primary hypo- | |
| Hyperpituitarism | thyroidism | |

**Decreased Values**

| | | |
|---|---|---|
| Hyperthyroidism | Secondary hypothy- | Thyroiditis |
| Overdose of exoge- | roidism | |
| nous thyroid | Tertiary hypothy- | |
| replacement | roidism | |

**Interfering Factors**

- Radioisotope administration within 1 week
- Extreme stress
- Medications such as aspirin, corticosteroids, dopamine, heparin, lithium, potassium iodide, and thyroid replacement therapy

**Nursing Implementation**

Nursing actions resemble those of other venipuncture procedures.

**Pretest**

Assess for and report any clinical states that would increase the patient's endogenous glucocorticoid levels.
Check with the prescriber regarding withholding medications that may interfere with test results.

## Thyrotropin-Releasing Hormone Test

(Serum)       Synonyms: TSH test, TSH-releasing hormone, TSH stimulation test

**Normal Values**

After TSH is given, TSH increases.
Male: 14–24 µU/mL *or* SI 14–24 mU/L
Female: 16–26 µU/mL *or* SI 16–26 mU/L

## Background Information

Thyrotropin-releasing hormone (TRH) is produced and secreted by the hypothalamus. It acts as moderator of the thyroid hormone-thyrotropin negative feedback mechanism. In response to synthetic TRH being given intravenously, the anterior pituitary gland will normally increase its secretion of thyrotropin within 5 minutes. The thyrotropin levels peak in 20 to 30 minutes and will return to baseline within 2 to 4 hours.

| | |
|---|---|
| **Purpose of the Test** | TRH determinations are rarely performed today, because the thyrotropin (TSH) test is usually adequate to support the diagnosis. TRH testing is performed when clinical manifestations of thyroid dysfunction are evident, but other tests are not clear. |

| | |
|---|---|
| **Procedure** | TRH determinations may be performed in a number of ways, with the dose and route of the TRH varying. The most common method is the bolus intravenous administration of 200 to 500 µg of synthetic TRH after blood is drawn for a baseline thyrotropin level. After 30 minutes (and sometimes again after 60 minutes), when the thyrotropin response is normally peaking, a second specimen is drawn for a thyrotropin determination. |

**Findings**

**Elevated Values**

Normal response
Hypothyroidism

**Decreased Values**

| | | |
|---|---|---|
| Cushing's syndrome | Hyperthyroidism | Pituitary lesions |
| Depression | Multinodular goiter | Renal failure |

**Interfering Factors**

- Corticosteroids
- Levodopa
- Salicylates (high dose)

**Nursing Implementation**

The nursing implementation for this test is similar to that for thyrotropin testing (see pp. 605–606).

**Pretest**

Explain to the patient the need for multiple venipuncture procedures.

## Thyroxine, Total

**(Serum)**     Synonyms: $T_4$, total $T_4$

**Normal Values**

**Adult:** 5–12 µg/dL *or* SI 64.4–154.4 nmol/L
**Children**
    10–20 years: 4.2–11.8 µg/dL *or* SI 54.11–151.9 nmol/L
    1–10 years: 6.4–15 µg/dL *or* SI 82.41–93.1 nmol/L
    2–10 months: 7.8–16.5 µg/dL *or* SI 100.4–212.4 nmol/L
**Newborn:** 6.4–23.2 µg/dL *or* SI 82.4–298.6 nmol/L

## Background Information

The thyroid gland produces and secretes the hormones thyroxine and triiodothyronine. This gland takes up iodide from the extracellular fluid and uses the iodide to produce thyroglobulin, the precursor of all thyroid hormones. The thyroglobulin is stored in the thyroid gland until thyroxine and triiodothyronine are processed before secretion from the gland. Secretion of triiodothyronine and thyroxine is primarily regulated by a negative feedback mechanism with thyrotropin. Thyrotropin is secreted by the anterior pituitary gland (Fig. 20–6).

Once secreted by the thyroid gland, triiodothyronine and thyroxine are bound primarily to thyroid-binding globulin and to a lesser degree to albumin and prealbumin. The small amount of the hormones not bound to protein is called *free thyroxine* and *free triiodothyronine*. It is the free hormones that are biologically active. The bound hormones are released from the protein as the hormones are needed. In the peripheral circulation, thyroxine will lose one of its iodide molecules and become triiodothyronine, the more potent of the thyroid hormones.

Because the majority of the thyroid hormones are bound to protein, the evaluation of thyroid hormone levels should include the person's protein levels. If the patient has decreased proteins to carry the hormone, a greater amount of the hormone will be in the free state or active form. RIA measures both bound and unbound thyroxine.

When needed, thyroxine converts to triiodothyronine to bind with its target cells. Its action is to increase the basal metabolic rate; therefore, its effect is widespread. By increasing the basal metabolic rate, thyroid hormones increase oxygen consumption and produce heat. Triiodothyronine and thyroxine are needed for conversion of carotene to vitamin A in the liver, are essential for normal growth and development, stimulate secretion of growth hormone, and increase the affinity of beta-adrenergic receptors to catecholamines.

| | |
|---|---|
| **Purpose of the Test** | Thyroxine levels are obtained to evaluate thyroid function, confirm the diagnosis of hyper- or hypothyroidism, and evaluate therapy for hyper- or hypothyroidism. |
| **Procedure** | Venipuncture is performed to obtain 5 mL of blood in a red-topped tube. RIA is used to assess the hormone level.<br><br>If a thyroxine determination is ordered on a newborn, umbilical cord blood may be used or a heelstick can be performed. With the heelstick method, special filter paper is used to blot the blood, and the filter paper is sent to the laboratory in a container that protects against light. |

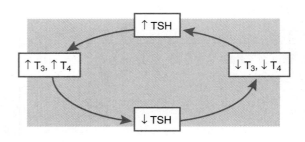

**Figure 20–6**
Thyroid hormone regulation. Thyroid hormone production and secretion are based on a negative feedback mechanism, with thyroid-stimulating hormone (TSH) secreted by the anterior pituitary gland. $T_3$ = triiodothyronine; $T_4$ = thyroxine.

| | |
|---|---|
| **Findings** | **Elevated Values** |

Hyperthyroidism
Acute or subacute
   thyroiditis

**Decreased Values**

Hypothyroidism        Myxedema
Chronic or subacute   Cretinism
   thyroiditis

**Interfering Factors**

- Liver disorders, which affect blood protein levels
- Protein-wasting diseases such as chronic renal failure
- Medications such as androgens, aspirin, chlorpropamide, chlorpromazine, estrogen, heparin, iodides, thyroid replacement medications, lithium, methadone, phenothiazines, phenytoin, reserpine, steroids, sulfonamides, sulfonylureas, and tolbutamide

**Nursing Implementation**

■

*Critical Thinking 20–14*
After a heelstick is performed on an infant to obtain a thyroxine level, the mother begins to sob uncontrollably. How can the nurse best help the mother? What nursing diagnosis should be validated by nursing assessments?

Nursing actions are similar to those used in other venipuncture procedures.

**During the Test**

If a heelstick is performed, the heel is first cleansed with antiseptic and the skin is pierced with a sterile lancet. Completely saturate the circles on the filter paper.

Because pregnancy will normally cause an increase in thyroxine levels, indicate on the requisition slip if the patient is pregnant.

**Posttest**

Send the filter paper to the laboratory in a container that protects against light.

**Critical Values**

**<2.0 µg/dL (SI <26 nmol/L) and >20 µg/dL (SI >257 nmol/L)**

For low thyroxine levels, assess the patient for myxedema coma. For high thyroxine levels, assess the patient for thyroid storm. Assessments for both extremes of thyroxine levels include careful evaluation of the patient's mental status. Report decreased mentation to the physician immediately.

## Thyroxine-Binding Globulin

(Serum)            Synonym: TBG

**Normal Values**

Adult: 1.2–3.0 mg/dL *or* SI 12–30 mg/L
Child: 2.9–5.0 mg/dL *or* SI 29–50 mg/L
Infant: 1.6–4.2 mg/dL *or* SI 16–42 mg/L

## Background Information

Thyroxine-binding globulin (TBG) is the primary protein carrier of thyroxine and triiodothyronine. The thyroid hormones bound to TBG provide a storehouse of the hormones, which are released from the protein as needed. Since TBG carries approximately 70% of the total amount of thyroid hormones in the circulation, TBG levels significantly affect total hormone concentrations. In addition to increased or decreased levels of TBG affecting hormone levels, factors may exist that affect the binding capacity of triiodothyronine and thyroxine to TBG. These factors may interfere with test results.

| | |
|---|---|
| **Purpose of the Test** | TBG is evaluated when clinical manifestations of thyroid dysfunction and thyroid hormone levels do not correlate. |

| | |
|---|---|
| **Procedure** | Venipuncture is performed to collect 7 mL of blood in a red-topped tube. TBG levels are assessed by RIA or electrophoresis. |

**Findings**

**Elevated Values**

| | | |
|---|---|---|
| Congenital abnormality | Estrogen therapy Hepatitis, acute | Hypothyroidism Pregnancy |

**Decreased Values**

| | | |
|---|---|---|
| Androgens Cirrhosis of the liver Congenital abnormality | Glucocorticoids Hyperthyroidism Recent surgery Renal failure | Starvation |

**Interfering Factors**

- Heparin
- Phenylbutazone
- Phenytoin
- Salicylates

**Nursing Implementation**

The nurse takes actions similar to those taken in other venipuncture procedures.

**Pretest**

Obtain a medication history to determine if any drug is being taken that affects normal thyroid binding.

## Tolbutamide Stimulation Test

**(Serum)**          Synonyms: None

| | |
|---|---|
| **Normal Values** | Serum insulin level: <195 µU/mL *or* SI <1,354 pmol/L |

### Background Information

Tolbutamide (Orinase) is an oral hypoglycemic agent. Its duration of action is short, being rapidly inactivated by the liver. For this reason, tolbutamide is used in stimulation tests to evaluate exaggerated and prolonged insulin secretion. This condition may occur with insulinoma, which is an insulin-secreting tumor of the pancreatic islets of Langerhans. It presents with spontaneous fasting hypoglycemia.

The goal in giving tolbutamide is to create a hypoglycemic state and see the insulin response to the induced hypoglycemia. If the insulin secretion stays at high levels and is prolonged, the test result is positive.

| | |
|---|---|
| **Purpose of the Test** | The tolbutamide stimulation test is performed to identify insulin-producing tumors of the pancreas. |
| **Procedure** | The tolbutamide stimulation test is performed by administering tolbutamide intravenously over a 2-minute period. Serum insulin levels are obtained every 5 minutes for 15 minutes. |
| **Findings** | If the insulin level is maintained or prolonged, the test confirms the diagnosis of insulinoma. |
| **Interfering Factors** | • Liver disorders<br>• Renal failure<br>• Medications such as chloramphenicol, dicumarol, MAO inhibitors, phenylbutazone, salicylates, and sulfonamides |

**Nursing Implementation**

See section on serum insulin (pp. 585–587).

**Pretest**

Explain to the patient the need for several venipuncture procedures.

**During the Test**

Observe the patient for a reaction to tolbutamide, which is most commonly a skin rash.

**Posttest**

Observe the patient for prolonged hypoglycemia, especially in elderly individuals.

| | |
|---|---|
| **Complications** | Prolonged hypoglycemia may occur with the administration of tolbutamide (Table 20–5). |

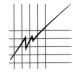

| Table 20–5 | Complications of Tolbutamide Stimulation Test | |
|---|---|---|
| | **Complication** | **Nursing Assessment** |
| | Hypoglycemia | Anxiety |
| | | Diaphoresis |
| | | Hunger |
| | | Palpitations |
| | | Tachycardia |
| | | Tremulousness |
| | | Vagueness |
| | | Ataxia |
| | | Convulsions |
| | | Coma |

## Triiodothyronine

**(Serum)**  Synonym: $T_3$

### Normal Values

**Adult:** 40–204 ng/dL *or* SI 0.6–3.1 nmol/L
**Children**
 10–20 years: 80–213 ng/dL *or* SI 1.2–3.3 nmol/L
 1–10 years: 105–269 ng/dL *or* SI 1.6–4.1 nmol/L
 1–12 months: 105–245 ng/dL *or* SI 1.6–3.7 nmol/L
**Newborn:** 100–740 ng/dL *or* SI 1.5–11.4 nmol/L

### Background Information

See discussion on thyroxine (pp. 607–609).

### Purpose of the Test

Triiodothyronine levels are obtained as part of the diagnostic process to determine hyper- or hypothyroidism and to diagnose triiodothyronine toxicosis.

### Procedure

Venipuncture is performed to obtain 3 mL of blood in a red-topped tube.

### Findings

**Elevated Values**

| | | |
|---|---|---|
| Hyperthyroidism | Toxic adenoma of the | Toxic nodular goiter |
| Pregnancy | thyroid gland | |

**Decreased Values**

| | | |
|---|---|---|
| Hypothyroidism | Recent surgery | Sick euthyroid |
| Liver disease | Renal disease | syndrome |

| **Interfering Factors** | • Significant increase or decrease in thyroxine-binding globulins<br>• Medications such as estrogen, heparin, iodides, triiodothyronine replacement therapy, lithium, methadone, methimazole, methylthiouracil, phenylbutazone, phenytoin, progestins, propranolol, propylthiouracil, reserpine, salicylates, steroids, and sulfonamides |
| --- | --- |

| **Nursing Implementation** | Nursing actions are similar to those for other venipuncture procedures. |
| --- | --- |

## Vasopressin

**(Plasma)**    Synonyms: ADH, antidiuretic hormone

| **Normal Values** | If serum osmolality is >290 mOsm/kg: 2–12 pg/mL *or* SI 1.85–11.1 pmol/L<br>If serum osmolality is <290 mOsm/kg: <2 pg/mL *or* SI <1.85 pmol/L |
| --- | --- |

### Background Information

Vasopressin (ADH) is produced by the hypothalamus and stored in the posterior pituitary gland. Its major function in the body is to act on the cells in the collecting ducts of the kidney, making them more permeable to water. The result is an increased reabsorption of water. This action is independent of electrolyte levels, and electrolytes are *not* reabsorbed with the water. The purpose of this action is to maintain normal plasma osmolality. ADH also has a vasopressor effect. It causes arteriole smooth muscles to constrict, thus elevating the blood pressure.

ADH is released from the posterior pituitary gland in response to several stimuli. The major stimulus is an increase in plasma osmolality. Whenever the osmoreceptors in the anterior hypothalamus sense even minor changes in plasma osmolality, neural stimulation of the pituitary gland will result in an increased secretion of ADH, which will result in an increased reabsorption of water at the renal collecting ducts. With the increase in water in the extracellular fluid, blood tonicity will decrease and urine osmolality will increase. Because the increase in water results in decreased blood osmolality, the osmoreceptors will cease the neural stimulation necessary for ADH secretion (Fig. 20–7).

Another stimulant for ADH release is the extracellular fluid volume. A drop in blood volume is sensed by stretcher receptors primarily in the vena cava and right atrium. By way of the brain stem, these receptors tell the hypothalamus to stimulate

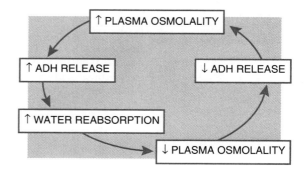

**Figure 20–7**

Vasopressin (ADH) regulation. ADH is secreted by the posterior pituitary gland primarily in response to an increase in plasma osmolality.

the release of ADH from the posterior pituitary gland. The resultant increase in fluid volume from water retention results in a decrease in stretcher receptor stimulation. In addition, as arterial blood pressure drops, pressor receptors found in the aorta and coronary sinuses will stimulate the release of ADH to increase extracellular fluid volume and thus the patient's blood pressure.

ADH secretion may be increased by drugs (e.g., nicotine, opiates, barbiturates, chlorpropamide) and severe pain, stress, and hyperthermia. Decreased sensitivity of the kidneys to ADH occurs with the intake of lithium carbonate and deme-clocycline.

| | |
|---|---|
| **Purpose of the Test** | A serum ADH determination is obtained to diagnose diabetes insipidus and syndrome of inappropriate antidiuretic hormone. |

| | |
|---|---|
| **Procedure** | Venipuncture is performed to obtain 5 mL of blood in a red-topped tube. |

**Findings**

**Elevated Values**

Syndrome of inappro-
priate antidiuretic
hormone

**Decreased Values**

Diabetes insipidus

**Interfering Factors**

- Noncompliance with diet, activity, and medication restrictions
- Pain
- Stress
- Mechanical ventilation
- Alcohol
- Medications such as anesthetics, carbamazepine, chlorothiazide, cyclophosphamide, estrogen, oxytocin, and vincristine

**Nursing Implementation**

**Pretest**

Instruct the patient not to eat or drink for 12 hours before the test.
Instruct the patient not to drink alcohol for 24 hours before the test.
Instruct the patient to limit physical activity for 12 hours before the test. The patient should lie down and rest for 30 minutes before the blood is drawn.
Obtain a medication history to determine if any interfering drugs are being taken. Check with the prescriber to determine if these drugs are to be withheld or continued.
Assess the patient for pain and stress, which may interfere with results.

**During the Test**

Perform venipuncture.

**Posttest**

Instruct the patient to resume normal activity and diet. Administer prescribed medications that were withheld for the test.

## Vitamin D, Activated

**(Serum, Plasma)**              Synonym: 1,25-dihydroxycholecalciferol

| Normal Values | 25–45 pg/mL *or* SI 60–108 nmol/L |
| --- | --- |

### Background Information

Activated vitamin D is produced from vitamin D by the liver and kidneys. Vitamin D is derived from the action of ultraviolet light on a group of provitamins in the skin. Levels of vitamin D usually decrease in the winter months. Vitamin D is also derived from vitamin D enriched foods. Vitamin D is first converted in the liver to 25-hydroxycholecalciferol and then to 1,25-dehydroxycholecalciferol in the kidney. Activated vitamin D elevates plasma calcium and phosphate levels by increasing intestinal absorption of calcium and phosphate and increasing the release of calcium from bone into blood.

### Purpose of the Test

Activated vitamin D levels are assessed to evaluate causes of hypocalcemia. They are usually obtained with parathyroid hormone levels.

### Procedure

A fasting venous specimen is needed. If a serum level test is ordered, 5 mL of blood is collected in a red-topped tube. If a plasma level is desired, 5 mL of blood is collected in a green-topped tube.

### Findings

**Elevated Values**

Hyperparathyroidism
Overdose of vita-
   min D
Sarcoidosis

**Decreased Values**

| | | |
| --- | --- | --- |
| Anticonvulsants | Malabsorption | Pseudohypoparathy- |
| Hepatic failure | syndrome | roidism |
| Hypoparathyroidism | Osteomalacia | Renal failure |
| Isoniazid | | |

### Interfering Factors

- Phosphorus deficiency
- Prolonged lack of exposure to sunlight

| | |
|---|---|
| **Nursing Implementation** | The nurse performs actions similar to those in other venipuncture procedures. |
| | **Pretest** |
| | Instruct the patient not to eat or drink for 8 hours before the test. |

## Water Deprivation Test

(Urine)                              Synonyms: Dehydration test, concentration test

| | |
|---|---|
| **Normal Values** | Specific gravity: 1.025–1.032 |
| | Osmolality: >800 mOsm/kg *or* SI >800 mmol/kg |

### Background Information

Normally, as fluid intake is withheld, blood osmolality increases, urine output decreases, and urinary osmolality increases. The increase in serum osmolality causes an increase in ADH secretion. In patients with diabetes insipidus (DI), a normal response to increased plasma osmolality does not occur; instead, little or no increase in ADH occurs, resulting in little or no change in urinary output or osmolality.

DI may be caused by a defect in production, release, or utilization of ADH. If DI is a result of a problem in production (hypothalamic) or release (pituitary) of ADH, it is called *neurogenic* or *central* DI. If DI is caused by a failure of the kidney to respond to ADH, it is called *nephrogenic* DI. The water deprivation test supports the diagnosis of DI.

As part of the water deprivation test, a *vasopressin stimulation test* or *ADH stimulation test* may be performed to distinguish between neurogenic and nephrogenic DI. This distinction is important in determining appropriate treatment plans.

| | |
|---|---|
| **Purpose of the Test** | The water deprivation test is performed to diagnose DI and to assess the kidney's ability to concentrate urine based on extracellular fluid load. |

| | |
|---|---|
| **Procedure** | During the test, the patient is deprived of fluid intake, and periodic urine specimens are obtained for osmolality and specific gravity determinations. The urine is collected in separate clean containers and placed on ice or refrigerated. Strict urinary output measurements are maintained. |
| | If a vasopressin stimulation test is included, hypertonic saline or nicotine is given to stimulate ADH release. If complete neurogenic DI is present, no change is noted in urinary output or osmolality. If partial neurogenic DI is present, only minor changes occur. If desired, a vasopressin test may be performed. After vasopressin is given, no change will occur in urinary output or osmolality if nephrogenic DI is present. With central DI, the urine osmolality will increase and the urinary output will decrease. |

| | |
|---|---|
| **Findings** | If no change in urine osmolality exists, the diagnosis of DI is supported. |

| **Interfering Factors** | • Noncompliance with fluid restrictions<br>• Inability to complete test because of hypovolemia<br>• Glucosuria<br>• Administration of radiopaque dyes within 7 days |
|---|---|

**Nursing Implementation**

### Pretest

Assess the patient's hemodynamic status. If a vasopressin test is planned, check for a history of coronary artery disease, because vasopressin may cause coronary artery spasm.

Obtain baseline serum and urine specimens for osmolality determinations.

Baseline weight is obtained before the evening meal on the day before testing.

### During the Test

Assess the patient for hypovolemia (tachycardia, orthostatic hypotension).

Observe the patient to ensure compliance with nothing-by-mouth status.

Obtain a urine specimen every 2 hours. Label each specimen with the time and the amount obtained. Document urinary output.

Weigh patient every 2 to 4 hours. Maintain the patient on nothing-by mouth status until 2% to 5% of the patient's weight is lost (this takes approximately 6 to 12 hours).

After 2% to 5% of patient body weight is lost and urinary output continues with urinary osmolality plateauing, an ADH stimulation test may be performed by administering hypertonic saline (3% sodium chloride) or nicotine as ordered.

If a vasopressin test is to be performed, check the patient's blood pressure and document it; notify the physician if the patient is hypertensive. Aqueous vasopressin is given subcutaneously or intravenously. Collect the urine specimen for amount and osmolality 1 hour after vasopressin administration. Another method is to give long-acting vasopressin in oil intramuscularly the night before the test. Urine is collected in the morning three times at hourly intervals. This method cannot be performed in conjunction with the water deprivation test.

*Critical Thinking 20–15*
When a water deprivation test is being done, how does a nurse assess for psychogenic polydipsia? If psychogenic polydipsia is suspected, what should the nurse do?

**Complications**

Hypovolemia may occur with the water deprivation test (Table 20–6). Patients with DI will continue to put out urine even though they have no intake. If a vasopressin test is performed, the administration of vasopressin may produce

### Table 20–6 Complications of the Water Deprivation Test

| Complication | Nursing Assessment |
|---|---|
| Hypovolemia | Tachycardia and orthostatic hypotension (early signs) |

the complications of high blood pressure or coronary artery spasms, or both (Table 20–7).

## Water-Loading Test

**(Plasma, Urine)** Synonyms: None

| **Normal Values** | Urinary output increases, and plasma and urine osmolality decrease. |
| --- | --- |

### Background Information

Review the discussion of plasma ADH (pp. 555–558). Normally, with an increase in fluid intake, urinary output will increase to maintain a normal plasma osmolality. As the urine volume increases, its osmo- lality decreases. However, patients with syndrome of inappropriate antidiuretic hormone (SIADH) will not respond to increasing fluid intake.

| **Purpose of the Test** | The water-loading test is performed to diagnose SIADH. |
| --- | --- |

| **Procedure** | With the water-loading test, the patient orally ingests a water load of 20 to 25 mL/kg of body weight. Hourly serum and urine osmolality and urine outputs are recorded for 4 hours. |
| --- | --- |

| **Findings** | Little or no change in urinary output or plasma and urine osmolality readings supports the diagnosis of SIADH. |
| --- | --- |

| **Interfering Factors** | • Patient is unable to drink the required volume of fluid<br>• Medications such as demeclocycline, diuretics, and lithium carbonate |
| --- | --- |

| **Nursing Implementation** | **Pretest**<br><br>Assess the patient for hyponatremia.<br>Obtain a cardiac history of the patient, the results of which may require that the test be canceled.<br>Weigh the patient. |
| --- | --- |

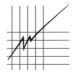

**Table 20–7  Complications of the Vasopressin Test**

| Complication | Nursing Assessment |
| --- | --- |
| Coronary spasms | Angina<br>ST changes on monitor |

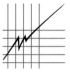

### Table 20–8  Complications of the Water-Loading Test

| Complication | Nursing Assessment |
|---|---|
| Water intoxication | Hyponatremia |
| | Lethargy |
| | Confusion |
| | Stupor |
| | Muscular twitching |
| | Convulsions |
| | Coma |

### During the Test

Instruct the patient to drink the required fluid.

Obtain hourly output measurements and send blood and urine to the laboratory for osmolality determination. On the requisition slip, indicate the hour of the specimen, with zero hour being the time the patient ingested the fluid. See discussion of plasma and urine osmolality for the nursing procedures associated with the collection of these samples. Observe the patient for water intoxication.

### Posttest

Weigh the patient.

**Complications**

When patients with SIADH undergo the water-loading test, their output is not increased. The increased fluid load in the extracellular fluid can cause dilutional hyponatremia, also called *water intoxication* (Table 20–8).

## Diagnostic Procedures

## Computed Tomography of the Adrenal Glands

**(Imaging)**     Synonyms: CT scan of the adrenal glands, adrenal scan

**Normal Values**     Negative; no tumor or enlargement

## Background Information

A CT scan of the abdomen is performed to visualize the adrenal glands. Its purpose is to identify adrenal tumors (adrenal carcinomas and adenomas) and to differentiate tumors from hyperplasia. CT scanning has almost completely replaced adrenal arteriography.

An adrenal CT scan is performed using iodocholesterol iodine 131 as the contrast agent, which is given intravenously.

**Nursing Implementation**    **Pretest**

Check for allergy to iodine. (Review Chapter 12 for discussion of CT scanning and the other nursing responsibilities for this procedure.)

## Computed Tomography of the Pancreas

**(Imaging)**                    Synonym: CT scan of the pancreas

| **Normal Values** | Negative; no tumor or inflammation |
|---|---|

## Background Information

CT scanning of the pancreas is performed to diagnose tumors (benign or malignant) and pancreatitis (acute or chronic) and to localize abscesses. The scan may be carried out with or without contrast medium, usually depending on whether the person is allergic to the dye. (Review Chapter 12 for a discussion of CT scanning and the nursing responsibilities for this diagnostic procedure.)

## Pancreatic Ultrasonography

**(Ultrasound)**                Synonym: Pancreatic sonogram

| **Normal Values** | Normal size and morphologic features |
|---|---|

## Background Information

The pancreas is both an exocrine organ and an endocrine organ. The exocrine function consists of the production and excretion of digestive enzymes required for the absorption of ingested food. The endocrine function consists of the production and secretion of hormones necessary for cellular nutrition.

A pancreatic sonogram assesses the size, shape, and positioning of the organ. Inflammation of the pancreas, as well as calculi, cysts, pseudocysts, and tumors, can be identified by ultrasound.

| **Purpose of the Test** | An ultrasound of the pancreas is performed to support the diagnosis and progression of pancreatitis and to identify tumors, cysts, and pseudocysts. Ultrasound may be used as a guide for fine needle biopsy of the pancreas. |
|---|---|

| **Procedure** | See Chapter 8 on ultrasound. |
|---|---|

**Findings**

| Abscess | Cancer | Pseudocyst |
|---|---|---|
| Acute or chronic pancreatitis | Cyst | |

**Interfering Factors**

- Barium or gas in the bowel
- Dehydration
- Noncompliance with fasting
- Obesity

**Nursing Implementation**

Review Chapter 8.

### Pretest

Instruct the patient not to eat or drink for 12 hours before the test.
Schedule any barium studies for after the sonogram.
Explain to the patient the need to distend the stomach to visualize the entire pancreas.

### During the Test

Encourage the patient to drink the prescribed fluid (500 to 1,000 mL of juice).
Place the patient in the supine position. The patient is usually repositioned during the procedure to a sitting position.

### Posttest

The patient resumes a normal diet.

## Pituitary Magnetic Resonance Imaging

(Imaging)                Synonyms: None

| **Normal Values** | Normal pituitary size and configuration |
|---|---|

## Background Information

MRI has significantly affected endocrine diagnoses because of its ability to identify small lesions of the pituitary gland. In most cases, it has eliminated the need for angiography in patients with suspected aneurysms or vascular malformations. With MRI, the pituitary stalk and gland as well as the optic chiasm and the intercavernous portion of the carotid artery are visualized.

| **Purpose of the Test** | MRI of the pituitary gland is performed to identify suspected hypothalamic-pituitary tumors and vascular abnormalities, including aneurysms, infarctions, and malformations. |
| --- | --- |

| **Procedure** | MRI of the pituitary gland is usually performed once without contrast dye and then again with a contrast agent. Usually, gadolinium diethylenetriamine-pentaacetic acid is given intravenously as the contrast medium. |
| --- | --- |

| **Findings** | Adenomas | Craniopharyngiomas | Gliomas |
| --- | --- | --- | --- |
| | Aneurysm | Hemochromatosis | Vascular malforma- |
| | Arachnoid cysts | Germinomas | tions |

| **Interfering Factors** | • Patient has claustrophobia |
| --- | --- |

| **Nursing Implementation** | See Chapter 12 for the nursing responsibilities associated with this diagnostic procedure. |
| --- | --- |

## Radioactive Iodine Uptake Study

(Imaging)    Synonym: RAIU

| **Normal Values** | After 6 hours: 3%–13% |
| --- | --- |
| | After 24 hours: 8%–29% |

## Background Information

Radioactive iodine uptake can be a helpful index of thyroid function, because the thyroid gland takes up from the extracellular fluid only the amount of iodide it needs for the synthesis of the thyroid hormones. The iodide not used is excreted in the urine. The thyroid gland does not distinguish between radioactive and nonradioactive iodine.

The thyroid uptake of radioactive iodine will be influenced by dietary iodine, which will be taken up at the same time as the radioisotope. Generally, the greater the amount of thyroid hormone produced, the greater the need for iodide and the higher the radioactive iodine uptake. Usually, radioactive iodine uptake increases with hyperthyroidism and decreases with hypothyroidism.

| **Purpose of the Test** | The radioactive iodine uptake test assesses thyroid function to confirm the diagnosis of hyper- or hypothyroidism. |
| --- | --- |

| **Procedure** | Sodium iodide 123 is given to the patient orally. After 6 hours and again after 24 hours, a gamma scintillation counter is used to measure the radioactivity over the thyroid gland. |
| --- | --- |

**Findings**

**Elevated Values**

| | | |
|---|---|---|
| Hashimoto's thyroiditis | Hypoalbuminemia | Lithium ingestion |
| Hyperthyroidism | Iodine-deficient goiter | |

**Decreased Values**

Excessive iodide
    intake
Hypothyroidism
Thyrotoxicosis as a
    result of ectopic
    thyroid metastasis,
    spontaneously
    resolving hyperthy-
    roidism, subacute
    thyroiditis, or
    thyrotoxicosis
    factitia

**Interfering Factors**

- Dietary intake of iodized foods (e.g., salt, bread)
- Iodine-deficient diet
- Previous radiographic studies with iodine-based dye
- Severe diarrhea
- Renal failure
- Noncompliance with dietary restrictions
- Medications such as anticoagulants, antihistamines, antithyroid medications, corticosteroids, lithium, multivitamins, penicillin, phenothiazides, phenylbutazone, salicylates, and thyroid hormones

**Nursing Implementation**

**Pretest**

Instruct the patient not to eat or drink for 12 hours before the test.

Obtain a medication history to determine if any interfering drugs were taken.

Schedule any x-ray studies requiring dyes for after the radioactive iodine uptake study.

Describe the scanning equipment to the patient. The probe is placed over the anterior portion of the neck. Emphasize that no discomfort is involved but that the patient must lie absolutely still while the scan is performed.

Ensure that a signed consent form has been obtained.

Tell the patient that the oral radioactive iodine must be ingested. It has little or no taste. It comes in capsule or liquid form.

Explain to the patient the need for two scans, because the uptake of the radioactive iodine is usually maximized at 24 hours but some thyroid conditions may cause the peak uptake to occur earlier.

### During the Test

Two hours after ingestion of the radioactive iodine, a light meal may be consumed.

Transport the patient to the nuclear medicine laboratory when scheduled.

### Posttest

The patient resumes a normal diet.

Observe for allergic response to the dye.

Wear gloves for 24 hours after the test when handling the patient's bedpan or urinal. Wash hands with soap and water after removing gloves.

Instruct the patient to wash hands with soap and water after voiding for 24 hours.

## Radionuclide Thyroid Scanning

(Imaging)                                        Synonyms: None

| Normal Values | Normal anatomic position and size |
|---|---|

### Background Information

To produce its hormones, the thyroid gland must extract iodide from the extracellular fluid. Once it has taken up enough iodide to meet its needs, the iodide left in the extracellular fluid is excreted in the urine. The thyroid gland cannot distinguish between dietary iodine and radioactive iodine. Thus, it will take up the radioactive iodide, which can be scanned by a gamma camera. The functioning of the thyroid gland can be evaluated by the amount of radioactive iodide it takes up. In thyrotoxic states, more iodide is needed and the uptake is increased, whereas in hypothyroid states, less than normal amounts of iodide are needed and thus less is taken up by the thyroid gland.

| Findings | **Increased Uptake** |
|---|---|
| | Hyperthyroidism |

**Decreased Uptake**

Hypothyroidism
Cretinism

In addition to an increase or decrease in uptake by the thyroid gland, scanning may also identify "hot" or "cold" spots. Cold nodules are areas of the gland that take up less or no radioactive iodine. Hot nodules are areas that take up more radioactive iodine than does the surrounding tissue. Cold spots may indicate cancer, whereas hot spots are usually not malignant. An echogram (sonogram) may be obtained to distinguish if the cold spot is a solid or semicystic lesion or a pure cyst. Pure cysts are rarely cancerous.

| **Interfering Factors** | • Ingestion of foods and medications containing iodine |
| | • Recent studies using iodine-based dyes |

**Nursing Implementation**

**Pretest**

Inquire if the patient is allergic to iodine or seafood.

Ask women if they are pregnant or breastfeeding.

Ask if any x-ray studies requiring contrast media have been performed within the past 2 months.

Instruct the patient to avoid iodized salt or iodinated salt substitutes and seafood for a week before the test.

Instruct the patient not to eat or drink for 12 hours before the test.

Check with the prescriber to determine if interfering medications are to be withheld.

Ensure that an informed consent form is signed.

Warn the patient that when the intravenous radioactive iodine is given, he or she may feel warm, flushed, and nauseous. Deep breathing may relieve the nausea.

Inform the patient that the procedure takes approximately 20 minutes.

**During the Test**

Transport the patient to the nuclear medicine laboratory.

Iodine 123 is given orally or intravenously.

**Posttest**

Iodine 123 is excreted in the urine within 24 hours. The patient resumes a normal diet.

## Thyroid Biopsy

**(Pathology)**    Synonyms: None

**Normal Values**    Normal cells

### Background Information

A thyroid biopsy is usually performed by fine needle aspiration (FNA). FNA has replaced surgical removal as a diagnostic technique because it avoids surgical risk and is less traumatic for the patient.

### Purpose of the Test

A biopsy is performed to differentiate the cause of thyroid nodules or lumps. Thyroid nodules are more common in women and occur at any age.

Thyroid cancer is rare; most nodules are benign. The biopsy will identify malignant thyroid nodules, follicular neoplasms, and benign lesions.

**Procedure**

FNA is usually carried out in the operating room to maintain sterile technique. It usually requires a local anesthetic only, which permits it to be performed on an outpatient basis. A 23- or 25-gauge biopsy needle is used to aspirate tissue from the nodule. Another method is called the capillary method, in which the needle is inserted into the nodule; with an up-and-down motion, tissue accumulates in the needle until blood is seen in the hub of the needle. The tissue is assessed by cytologic examination.

**Findings**

Benign thyroid nodules
Cancer of the thyroid gland

Follicular neoplasm (cancerous or benign)

**Interfering Factors**

- Noncompliance with dietary restrictions
- Failure to place specimen in preservative immediately after aspiration
- Inadequate amount of tissue obtained

**Nursing Implementation**

**Pretest**

Assess the patient's level of anxiety, because fear of cancer may be significant or may interfere with the patient's ability to understand explanations.
Instruct the patient not to eat or drink for 12 hours before the test.
Prepare the patient for the operating room according to hospital protocol.
Ensure that a signed informed consent form has been obtained.
Administer preprocedure medication as prescribed.

**During the Test**

The patient is positioned on the back with a small pillow under the shoulders.

**Table 20–9  Complications of Thyroid Biopsy**

| Complication | Nursing Assessment |
|---|---|
| Bleeding | Overt bleeding<br>With hematoma<br>  Swelling<br>  Stridor<br>  Dyspnea |
| Edema | Swelling<br>Stridor<br>Dyspnea |
| Infection | Malaise<br>Fever<br>Tenderness<br>Redness |

A local anesthetic may or may not be given. General anesthesia may be required in some cases.

Encourage the patient not to move or swallow as the local anesthetic is given.

Support the patient, who will feel pressure as the procedure is performed.

Direct pressure is maintained on the site after the needle is removed for 10 to 15 minutes.

### Posttest

Reassure the patient that tenderness at the biopsy site is normal.

Position the patient in a semi-Fowler's position with a small pillow under the head to remove stress from the site.

An ice pack may be ordered.

Instruct the patient to support the head when changing position.

Keep site clean and dry.

---

**Complications**

Complications of a thyroid biopsy are rare. Most patients complain only of some tenderness, but the nurse should observe for bleeding, edema, and infection (Table 20–9).

---

## References

Alzaid, A. A. (1996). Microalbuminuria in patients with NIDDM: An overview. *Diabetes Care, 19,* 79–86.

Barrett-Conner, E., Schrott, H. G., Greendale, G., Kritz-Silverstein, D., Espeland, M. A., Stern, M. P., Bush, T., & Perlman, J. A. (1996). Factors associated with glucose and insulin levels in healthy postmenopausal women. *Diabetes Care, 19,* 333–340.

Brown, S. A., & Hanis, C. L. (1995). A community-based, culturally sensitive education and group-support intervention for Mexican Americans with NIDDM: A pilot study of efficacy. *Diabetes Educator, 21,* 203–209.

Cate, J. C., & Papadea, C. (1995). Parathyroid hormone part I: Measurement and clinical use. *Laboratory Medicine, 26,* 599–602.

Chaisson, K. M. (1995). Comparison of arterial and capillary blood glucose with the use of the Accu-Chek III. *Clinical Practice Issues, 10,* 27–30.

Chang, H., Anderson, G. C., & Wood, C. E. (1995). Feasible and valid saliva collection for cortisol in transitional newborn infants. *Nursing Research, 44,* 117–119.

Curtis, P., & Dworkin, H. (1995). Nuclear medicine and the thyroid gland: A retrospective review. *Journal of Nuclear Medicine Technology, 23,* 8S–15S.

Daniels, G. H. (1995). Thyroid function tests: How to use the new assays in hypothyroidism and euthyroid sick syndrome. *Consultant, 35,* 714–723.

Dawson-Hughes, B., Harris, S. S., & Dallal, G. E. (1997). Plasma calcidol, season, and serum parathyroid hormone concentrations in healthy elderly men and women. *American Journal of Clinical Nutrition, 65,* 67–71.

Frati, A. C., Iniestra, F., & Ariza, C. R. (1996). Acute effect of cigarette smoking on glucose tolerance and other cardiovascular risk factors. *Diabetes Care, 19,* 112–117.

Fraynor, S. M. (1997). Clinical pathology rounds: Glycosylated hemoglobin electrophoresis. *Laboratory Medicine, 28,* 370–373.

Gibson, R. G., Fineberg, S. E., & Bridges, J. M. (1996). Accuracy of a rapid quantitative bedside beta-hydroxbutyrate test system. *Clinical Laboratory Science, 9,* 282–287.

Goff, J., & Rogers, B. P. (1995). Selecting a bedside glucose monitor for outpatient clinics. *Clinical Nurse Research, 4,* 105–113.

Greendyke, R. M., & Gifford, F. R. (1997). Testing blood glucose at the bedside in a chronic care hospital. *Laboratory Medicine, 28,* 63–67.

Haugen, B. R. (1996). Thyroid cancer: When to suspect, what to do. *Consultant, 36,* 419–430.

Hawes, A. S., Richardson, R. P., Antonacci, A. C., & Calvano, S. E. (1995). Chronic pathophysiologic elevation of corticosterone after thermal injury or thermal injury and burn wound infection adversely affects body mass, lymphocyte numbers, and outcome. *Journal of Burn Care and Rehabilitation, 16,* 1–15.

Hudak, C. H., Gallo, B. M., & Morton, P. G. (1998). *Critical care nursing* (7th ed.). Philadelphia: J. B. Lippincott.

Lehmann, C. A. (1998). *Saunders manual of clinical laboratory science.* Philadelphia: W. B. Saunders.

Li, K., & Huang, H. (1997). Comparing urinary reagent strips for detecting glycosuria in patients with diabetes mellitus. *Laboratory Medicine, 28,* 397–401.

Koistinen, P., Martikkala, V., Karpakka, J., Vuolteenaho, O., & Leppaluoto, J. (1996). The effects of moderate altitude on circulating thyroid hormones and thyrotropin in training athletes. *Journal of Sports Medicine and Physical Fitness, 36,* 108–111.

Mitchell, D. H., & Owens, B. (1996). Replacement therapy: Arginine vasopressin (AVP), growth hormone (GH), cortisol, thyroxine, testosterone and estrogen. *Journal of Neuroscience Nursing, 28,* 140–152.

Papadea, C., & Cate, J. C. (1995). Intact parathyroid hormone immunoradiometric assays. *Laboratory Medicine, 26,* 671–676.

Rusterholtz, A. (1996). Interpretation of diagnostic laboratory tests in selected endocrine disorders. *Nursing Clinics of North America, 31,* 715–720.

Schilling, J. S. (1997). Hyperthyroidism: Diagnosis and management of Graves' disease. *Nurse Practitioner, 22,* 72–90.

Speicher, C. E. (1998). *The right test* (3rd ed.). Philadelphia: W. B. Saunders.

Stepp, C. A., & Woods, M. (1998). *Laboratory procedures for medical office personnel.* Philadelphia: W. B. Saunders.

Thelan, L. A., Urden, L. D., Lough, M. E., & Stacy, K. M. (1998). *Critical care nursing diagnosis and management.* St. Louis: Mosby–Year Book.

Wang, D. H., Koehler, S. M., & Mariash, C. N. (1996). Detecting Graves' disease. *Physicians and Sports Medicine, 24,* 35–40.

Westphal, S. A., & Palumbo, P. J. (1995). The trouble with glycosylated hemoglobin. *Patient Care, 29,* 95–96.

# CHAPTER 21

# Renal and Urinary Tract Function

The kidneys perform the processes of regulation, excretion, and hormonal production. Under normal anatomic and physiologic conditions, the kidneys help maintain body tone, fluid volume, acid-base balance, and the chemical balance of extracellular fluids.

The ureters, bladder, and urethra are the other components of the urologic system that guide the flow of urine in excretory functions. The prostate gland surrounds part of the bladder neck and urethra in the male. Alterations in the anatomy or physiology of these parts can result in urinary obstruction.

The laboratory tests presented in this chapter evaluate renal function based on changes in blood chemistry test results and urine analyses. Blood test results can also indicate the presence of prostate cancer markers. Additional laboratory tests are appropriate for the evaluation of renal function and other functions throughout the body; these multisystem laboratory tests are presented in Chapter 5.

The diagnostic procedures presented in this chapter are used to identify abnormalities of structure and function of the renal and urologic system. The tests evaluate sources of obstruction, abnormalities in renal blood flow, and changes in the cells. The structural abnormalities can also alter renal function, as measured by the blood and urine laboratory tests.

## Laboratory Tests

## Albumin, Urinary

**(Urine)**     Synonyms: None

| Normal Values | Microalbumin: Less than 2 mg/dL<br>Reagent strip: Negative |
| --- | --- |

## Background Information

Evaluation of protein in the urine is done as part of urinalysis. Normally in the healthy adult, the excretion of protein is so small that it is undetectable by routine methods of analysis. Of the protein excreted, approximately 40% is albumin (Speicher, 1998). Because albumin can be tested by the use of reagent strips, urinary albumin testing is frequently used in the management of urinary disorders. Studies have shown that albumin in urine can be used as a predictor of complications associated with diabetes mellitus.

Various methods are available for assessing urinary excretion of albumin, including radioimmunoassay (RIA), turbidimetric, and chemical methods and reagent strips. Reagent strips are sensitive to albumin, but not at very low levels. To evaluate microalbuminuria, laboratory analysis is necessary.

## Purpose of the Test

Urinary excretion of albumin is evaluated to assess renal function, determine effectiveness of therapy, and differentiate renal disorders. It is being increasingly used to screen for the complications associated with diabetes mellitus.

## Procedure

For a reagent strip analysis of albumin, a random urine specimen is collected in a clean container. A first voided urine specimen is preferred. For microalbuminuria, the procedure varies with the method of analysis. With the turbidimetric method, a 24-hour specimen of urine is used with no preservative in the collection container.

## Findings

■

*Critical Thinking 21–1*
Your patient has a chronic renal disorder. The urinalysis indicates protein in the patient's urine, but when you check the urine with a dipstick, the result is negative for protein. Is the dipstick unreliable?

**Elevated Values**

| | | |
|---|---|---|
| Amyloidosis | Heavy metal poison- | Renal transplant |
| Cystic kidney | ings | rejection |
| Cystitis | Multiple myeloma | Urinary tract malig- |
| Diabetes mellitus | Nephritis | nancies |
| (complications of) | Nephropathies | |
| Glomerulonephritis | Pyelonephritis | |

## Interfering Factors

• With reagent strips: Highly concentrated urine; highly alkaline urine; specimen contaminated with bacteria, blood, ammonia compounds, or chlorhexidine
• With turbidimetric method: Ingestion of cephalosporin, penicillin, sulfonamides, or tolbutamide; recent administration of radiocontrast dyes

## Nursing Implementation

Care is dependent on the method of analysis. Check with the laboratory regarding the method and specimen required.

### Home Testing for Urinary Albumin

Assess the patient's understanding of the purpose of home testing and the need to notify the physician if albumin is spilled or if its concentration increases. Instruct the patient to use the first voided urine in the morning. Warn the patient that any vigorous exercise will increase the excretion of albumin in the urine. Teach the patient how to follow the manufacturer's instructions for using the dipstick. Timing varies by manufacturer. Instruct the patient to keep the top on the reagent strip container. Warn the patient that abnormal results must be checked by laboratory analysis of urinary albumin, because changes in specific gravity may affect results.

## Calculus Analysis

**(Qualitative Chemical Analysis)**

Synonyms: Kidney stone analysis, renal calculus analysis, nephrolithiasis analysis

**Normal Values**

No kidney stones are present in the urine.

### Background Information

A renal calculus is commonly called a *stone*. It forms in the renal pelvis; descends through the ureter, bladder, and urethra; and exits from the body in the urine. Calculi are of various sizes, textures, colors, and chemical compositions.

**Calcium Stones.**   The most common type of renal calculi are calcium stones. They are caused by excess calcium in the urine and consist of calcium phosphate, calcium oxalate, or a combination of the two chemical salts. These dark-colored stones are usually hard and have a rough surface. The underlying causes of calcium stone formation are thought to be increased intestinal absorption of dietary calcium, poor renal tubular resorption of calcium, a loss of calcium from bone, or any combination of these factors. Calcium stones make up 75% of all urinary stones (Baer, 1996).

**Struvite Stones.**   This type of stone is sometimes called an *infection stone* because of its association with chronic urinary tract infection. It is not known whether the stone causes the infection to occur or the infection causes the stone to form. This pale stone is usually large and soft. It is also called a *staghorn calculus* because of its characteristic shape as it forms within the renal pelvis. The chemical composition is magnesium ammonium phosphate and carbonate apatite. This calculus is sometimes called a *phosphate stone* based on its chemical composition.

**Uric Acid Stones.**   These stones consist of uric acid and urate crystals. They are yellow-brown and moderately hard. They form in the presence of excess uric acid and concentrated acidic urine. Underlying causes include primary gout, dehydration, and some medications, including thiazide diuretics and salicylates.

**Cystine Stones.**   These stones occur infrequently. They are dark yellow-brown and greasy. Their formation is caused by an autosomal recessive inborn error in metabolism that impairs the absorption of amino acids. Because of this deficit in metabolism, cystine and other amino acids are excreted in urine. The precipitate forms both crystals and stones.

**Purpose of the Test**

The analysis of urinary calculi is used in the work-up for nephrolithiasis. It determines the chemical composition of the stone and provides data regarding the metabolic factors that result in stone formation.

**Procedure**

All urine is strained through a gauze strainer or a fine mesh sieve. Any stones that are recovered are placed in a glass bottle or plastic container and sent to the laboratory for qualitative analysis.

**Findings**

**Abnormal Values**

| | | |
|---|---|---|
| Urolithiasis | Gout | Urinary tract |
| Hypercalciuria | Primary cystinuria | infection |
| Hyperparathyroidism | Dehydration | Other infection |

**Nursing Implementation**

**Pretest**

Teach the patient to use a clean container to collect the urine every time he or she voids. The first voided specimen of the morning is particularly important, because the stone may pass during the night.

Each collected specimen is to be poured through the strainer or sieve. The gauze or mesh is examined to see if a stone is present. Teach the patient to look carefully, because the stone can be as small as the head of a pin.

If a stone is recovered, it is placed in a clean, lidded container. Label the container with the patient's name, other identifying data, and the date, time, and source of the stone.

**Posttest**

Send the stone to the laboratory in the labeled container. If the stone is enmeshed in the gauze, place both the stone and the gauze in the container.

Specify on the requisition form that the source of the stone is urinary, and include the date and time that the stone was passed.

**Quality Control**

Do not wrap or place the stone on adhesive tape to secure it. The adhesive interferes with the infrared spectroscopy examination that is used to analyze the stone.

## Creatinine

**(Serum)**

Synonyms: Plasma creatinine, pCR

**Normal Values**

Adult male: 0.7–1.3 mg/dL *or* SI 62–115 µmol/L
Adult female: 0.6–1.1 mg/dL *or* SI 53–97 µmol/L
Adolescent: 0.5–1 mg/dL *or* SI 44–88 µmol/L
Child: 0.3–0.7 mg/dL *or* SI 27–62 µmol/L
Infant: 0.2–0.4 mg/mL *or* SI 18–35 µmol/L
Newborn: 0.3–1 mg/dL *or* SI 27–88 µmol/L

## Background Information

Creatinine is an amino acid and waste product of protein metabolism. It is derived from creatine, which is synthesized in the liver, kidneys, and pancreas and stored in muscle tissue. As creatine is metabolized in the muscle, creatinine is produced. Creatinine is released into the extracellular fluid and excreted through the kidneys.

In the kidneys, creatinine is filtered by the glomeruli and is usually not resorbed. Additional creatinine is secreted by the renal tubules. When the kidneys are functional, they maintain the serum creatinine level at a minimal low level. When renal function is impaired, the creatinine level increases.

When glomerular filtration decreases to half its normal rate and only about half the nephrons are functioning, the serum creatinine level rises to about double the normal value. As renal failure progressively worsens, the serum creatinine level continues to rise. Effectiveness of treatment can be evaluated by the serum creatinine level's decreasing.

The serum levels of creatinine decrease in conditions that cause decrease in muscle mass, in muscle-wasting diseases, and in liver disease. In these disorders, less creatine synthesis and storage, and therefore less creatinine production, occur.

## Purpose of the Test

Serum creatinine determination is the most common laboratory test used to evaluate renal function and to estimate the effectiveness of glomerular filtration.

## Procedure

A red-topped tube is used to collect 10 mL of venous blood. For infants and small children, a heelstick puncture is used to fill a capillary pipette.

### Quality Control

Venipuncture technique must be smooth, with a blood flow that fills the vacuum tube readily. If the blood has excessive turbulence because of flawed technique, the hemolysis of the erythrocytes will alter the results.

## Findings

### Elevated Values

Acute or chronic
 renal failure
Uremia or azotemia
Renal artery stenosis

Congestive heart
 failure
Shock
Dehydration

Rhabdomyolysis
Acromegaly

### Decreased Values

Advanced liver
 disease
Long-term corticoste-
 roid therapy

Hyperthyroidism
Muscular dystrophy
Paralysis
Dermatomyositis

Polymyositis

## Interfering Factors

- Hemolysis
- Warming of the specimen

## Nursing Implementation

Care of the venipuncture site is included in the plan. In addition, perform the following.

*Critical Thinking 21–2*
Normally, the urea-to-creatinine ratio is 10:1. Your patient's ratio is 20:1. What does this mean?

### Pretest

Instruct the patient to fast from food and fluids for 8 hours before the test, when indicated by the laboratory protocol. In some methods of analysis, lipemia and the recent ingestion of meat can cause a false elevation in the test results.

### Posttest

Arrange for prompt transport of the specimen to the laboratory. Prolonged delay causes ammonia to form in the specimen. Warming will cause a falsely elevated test result.

## Creatinine Clearance, 24-Hour Urine

(Urine)        Synonyms: Ccre, Ccr, urine creatinine

**Normal Values**

**Mean Creatinine Clearance**
Adult male: 1–2 g/day *or* SI 8.8–17.7 mmol/day; 90–139 mL/min/1.73 m² *or* SI 0.87–1.34 mL/sec/m²
Adult female: 0.8–1.8 g/day *or* SI 7.1–15.9 mmol/day; 80–125 mL/min/1.73 m² *or* SI 0.77–1.2 mL/sec/m²
Child: 70–140 mL/min/1.73 m² *or* SI 1.17–2.33 mL/sec/m²

## Background Information

Creatinine is an amino acid waste product that is derived from muscle creatinine, a product of protein metabolism. It is distributed throughout body fluids and is excreted by the kidneys. In the process of urinary elimination, creatinine is freely filtered by the glomeruli, usually without resorption by the tubules. Additional creatinine is secreted by the proximal renal tubules. The total amount of creatinine excreted in urine is called *creatinine clearance.*

In the course of renal failure, diminished glomerular filtration occurs. Once the glomerular filtration rate is reduced by half, the renal tubules compensate by increasing their secretion of creatinine. As chronic renal failure or uremia becomes severe, an eventual reduction occurs in the excretion of creatinine by both the glomeruli and the tubules. Age affects creatinine clearance.

The amount of urinary creatinine is increased significantly by muscle necrosis and muscle atrophy because of protein catabolism. It is decreased significantly in acute and advanced chronic renal failure because of the kidneys' inability to filter and secrete this waste product. Creatinine clearance decreases by 10% per decade after age 40 years, whereas serum creatinine shows little variation.

The urinary creatinine clearance test is usually accompanied by a serum creatinine test. The blood test may be performed at the midpoint in urinary collection or at the start or completion of the urine collection, depending on laboratory protocol.

## Purpose of the Test

The urine creatinine clearance test is performed to help assess renal function and creatinine excretion. It is also used to monitor the progress of renal disease.

## Procedure

The test usually requires urine collection for 24 hours, but collection periods of 4 or 12 hours are sometimes prescribed.

## Findings

**Elevated Values**

| | | |
|---|---|---|
| Muscular dystrophy | Muscular inflammatory disease | Anemia |
| Polymyositis | Hyperthyroidism | Leukemia |
| Paralysis | | |

**Decreased Values**

Glomerulonephritis
Congestive heart
  failure
Acute tubular
  necrosis

Advanced pyelone-
  phritis
Shock
Polycystic kidney
  disease

Renal malignancy
Dehydration
Bilateral ureteral
  obstruction
Nephrosclerosis

**Interfering Factors**

- Excessive exercise in the test period
- Failure to collect all the urine
- Failure to time the test accurately
- Warming of the urine specimen
- High protein intake before the test

**Nursing Implementation**

### Pretest

Instruct the patient to avoid excessive intake of meat on the day before the test.
Instruct the patient to collect all urine for the 24-hour period of the test,
  storing the container in the refrigerator or on ice.
Encourage adequate hydration before and during the test, and omit coffee and
  tea during the test.

### During the Test

At 8 AM, instruct the patient to void and discard the urine. The test begins at
  this time, and all subsequent urine specimens are collected for 24 hours,
  including the 8 AM specimen of the next morning.
Advise the patient to avoid vigorous exercise during the test period.
Ensure that the patient's name and the time and date of the start and finish of
  the test are written on the label and requisition slip.

### Posttest

Arrange for prompt transportation of the refrigerated specimen to the laboratory.

## Electrolytes, 24-Hour Urine

(Urine)

Synonyms: Sodium, urine; chloride, urine; potassium, urine; calcium, urine; magnesium, urine

**Normal Values**

**Sodium**
  Adult: 40–220 mEq/24 hr *or* SI 40–220 mmol/24 hr
  Male child (6–10 years): 41–115 mEq/24 hr *or* SI 41–115 mmol/24 hr
  Female child (6–10 years): 20–69 mEq/24 hr *or* SI 20–69 mmol/24 hr
  Male child (10–14 years): 63–117 mEq/24 hr *or* SI 63–117 mmol/24 hr
  Female child (10–14 years): 48–168 mEq/24 hr *or* SI 48–168 mmol/24 hr
**Chloride**
  Adult (≤60 years): 110–250 mEq/24 hr *or* SI 110–250 mmol/24 hr
  Adult (>60 years): 95–195 mEq/24 hr *or* SI 95–195 mmol/24 hr
  Child (<6 years): 15–40 mEq/24 hr *or* SI 15–40 mmol/24 hr

*Continued on following page*

*Continued*

> Male child (6–10 years): 36–110 mEq/24 hr *or* SI 36–110 mmol/24 hr
> Female child (6–10 years): 18–74 mEq/24 hr *or* SI 18–74 mmol/24 hr
> Male child (10–14 years): 64–176 mEq/24 hr *or* SI 64–176 mmol/24 hr
> Female child (10–14 years): 36–173 mEq/24 hr *or* SI 36–173 mmol/24 hr
> Infant: 2–10 mEq/24 hr *or* SI 2–10 mmol/24 hr
>
> **Potassium**
> Adult: 25–125 mEq/24 hr *or* SI 25–125 mmol/24 hr
> Male child (6–10 years): 17–54 mEq/24 hr *or* SI 17–54 mmol/24 hr value
> Female child (6–10 years): 8–37 mEq/24 hr *or* SI 8–37 mmol/24 hr
> Male child (10–14 years): 22–57 mEq/24 hr *or* SI 22–57 mmol/24 hr
> Female child (10–14 years): 18–58 mEq/24 hr *or* SI 18–58 mmol/24 hr
> Infant: 4.1–5.3 mEq/24 hr *or* SI 4.1–5.3 mmol/24 hr
>
> **Calcium**
> Adult (normal calcium intake): 100–300 mg/day *or* SI 2.5–7.5 mmol/day
> Adult (low calcium intake): 50–100 mg/day *or* SI 1.25–3.75 mmol/day
> Adult (calcium-free diet): 5–40 mg/day *or* SI 0.13–1 mmol/day
> Infant and child: <6 mg/kg/day *or* SI <0.15 mmol/kg/day
> **Magnesium:** 7.3–12.2 mg/dL *or* SI 3–5 mmol/day

## Background Information

Electrolytes are ions that are present in body fluids. Sodium, chloride, potassium, and bicarbonate are important determinants of osmolarity, pH, and hydration in both intracellular and extracellular fluid. The concentrations of intracellular and extracellular electrolytes also regulate membrane potentials and the functions of nerve, heart, and muscle tissue.

In normal physiology, the daily intake of foods includes a renewing supply of electrolytes. The glomeruli filter the electrolytes from the blood, and the renal tubules resorb most of them for recirculation and redistribution as needed. Electrolyte excesses are not resorbed and are excreted in the urine.

The normal urinary excretion of electrolytes is dependent on the amount of intake, the serum level, and the state of hydration of the body. The equilibrium of water and electrolytes is controlled by renal, adrenal, posterior pituitary, and hypothalamic functions.

**Sodium and Chloride.**   In patients with endocrine deficiency, an excess amount of diuretic medication, or renal disease that affects the renal tubules, the kidneys cannot conserve the sodium and chloride through renal tubular resorption.

Thus, the urinary electrolyte levels rise as the electrolytes are lost from the body.

Nonrenal causes of low levels of sodium and chloride in the urine include intestinal problems that affect the digestion or absorption of the electrolytes and losses of these electrolytes via other mechanisms of excretion. Additionally, problems that cause water retention dilute the concentration of electrolytes in body fluids. The kidneys respond by greater resorption and conservation of the sodium and chloride, and a lower amount of these electrolytes is excreted in the urine. Aldosterone and other adrenocorticoid hormones promote the resorption of sodium and chloride, with reduced loss of electrolytes in the urine.

When renal conditions cause low levels of sodium and chloride in the urine, conditions that cause prerenal azotemia or acute oliguria prevent glomerular filtration of blood. Depending on the severity of the condition, fewer electrolytes are removed from the blood, and urinary excretion of electrolytes is minimal.

**Potassium.**   Nonrenal conditions that result in excess potassium in the urine include excessive potassium intake in food or medication. Excess aldosterone and adrenocortical hyperfunction both promote potassium excretion in the urine. Catabolism and lysis of cells cause the release of potassium into extracellular fluid and ultimately into the urine. Renal conditions that cause excess potassium in the urine include metabolic acidosis and renal tubular disease that prevents resorption of the potassium.

Nonrenal causes of decreased urinary potassium include conditions that either prevent intestinal absorption of this electrolyte or cause a loss of the electrolyte via another route. When the serum level is low, the kidneys will compensate and resorb more potassium, allowing less to be lost in the urine. Additionally, adrenocortical hypofunction and a deficiency of aldosterone promote potassium resorption by the renal tubules, with less potassium to be excreted in the urine.

Renal causes of low levels of potassium in the urine are acute or advanced chronic renal disease. When diminished renal circulation and diminished glomerular filtration occur, less urine is produced and less excess serum potassium is eliminated.

**Calcium.**    Calcium is maintained in homeostatic balance in the blood by the functions of the intestine, bones, and kidneys. This balance is regulated by the interplay of parathyroid hormone, calcitonin, and vitamin $D_1$, the active form of vitamin D. The daily intake of calcium in food provides a continual renewal of the supply of calcium that is available for the body. In daily excretion of excess supply, the glomeruli of the kidneys filter calcium out of the blood and the renal tubules resorb the amount needed to maintain a normal serum value. Excess calcium is removed from the body in urine, feces, and sweat.

Parathyroid hormone prevents hypocalcemia by increasing the resorption of calcium by the bones and renal tubules. When the renal tubules resorb calcium, less calcium is present in the urine. Calcitonin works in the opposite way; it prevents hypercalcemia by decreasing the resorption of calcium by the bones and renal tubules. When the renal tubules resorb less calcium, more calcium is present in the urine. Vitamin $D_1$ acts on the mucosa of the small intestine to allow the absorption of dietary calcium.

The normal excretion of urinary calcium varies with dietary intake. The average calcium intake for adults is 600 to 800 mg/day (SI 15 to 20 mmol/day). Patients who follow a calcium-restricted diet

or who consume less than the average amount of daily calcium have a lower normal value of calcium in the urine.

An excessive calcium level in the urine is called *hypercalciuria*. It is identified as a calcium value in the urine of more than 350 mg/day (SI 8.75 mmol/day). The excess urinary calcium can result from increased intestinal absorption, increased bone resorption, or impaired renal tubular resorption. Increased intestinal absorption can result from low serum phosphorus levels, excessive loss of phosphorus from the kidneys, or excessive vitamin D intake. Increased bone resorption means that excess calcium is released from bone. The excess calcium enters the serum and ultimately is released in the urine. This can occur with immobility; bone diseases, including malignancy; and endocrine disorders, including hyperparathyroidism, thyrotoxicosis, and Cushing's disease. Excess calcium in the urine can cause the formation of urinary calculi. The most common calcium stones are composed of calcium oxalate, and a few are composed of calcium phosphate.

A diminished amount of calcium in the urine is called *hypocalciuria*. It can result from a deficiency of parathyroid hormone, vitamin D disorders, renal diseases that limit glomerular filtration or cause loss of serum proteins, bone diseases that increase the skeletal uptake of calcium, and digestive disorders that inhibit the intestinal absorption of calcium.

**Magnesium.**    The magnesium cation is derived from the intake of food. Most of the magnesium cation is stored in soft and hard tissues, and a small amount is maintained in homeostatic balance in the serum and extracellular fluid. The excess dietary intake is not absorbed and is eliminated in feces. The kidneys maintain major control of the serum level by conserving magnesium in tubular resorption processes or by eliminating the excess in the urine.

In normal physiologic function, an excess of serum magnesium causes the renal tubules to resorb less, resulting in a greater amount of magnesium in the urine. A low level of serum magnesium causes the renal tubules to resorb more magnesium, resulting in less of the cation in the urine.

In pathophysiologic processes, an excess of magnesium in the urine can be caused by damage to the renal tubules, with a failure to resorb the magnesium. As a result of the renal loss, the serum value can become low. A low level of magnesium in the urine can be caused by advanced renal failure with an inability of the glomeruli to filter out the magnesium from the blood. If the magnesium does not enter the nephrons, it does not appear in the urine. Other diverse causes of excess or reduced magnesium in the urine also exist.

The physiology of magnesium is not fully understood, and its measurement by laboratory analysis is not standardized. Little of this cation is present in the serum because so much of it is stored in the soft tissue, muscle, and bone. When the serum value is abnormal, the urine is usually tested to obtain additional data. One of the problems of urine testing is that little agreement exists regarding the normal range of urine values. Because the normal values vary among laboratories and geographic regions, the reference value of a particular laboratory may vary from the value listed in this text.

## Purpose of the Test

Urine electrolytes are used to help monitor renal function, fluid and electrolyte balance, and acid-base balance. The urinary calcium level is used to evaluate bone disease, parathyroid disorders, nephrolithiasis, calcium metabolism, and idiopathic hypercalciuria.

## Procedure

A 24-hour urine specimen is collected in a large, clean urine collection container. Alternative methods include a 12-hour urine collection or a single random urine sample for electrolyte testing. If a 24-hour urine test for protein or creatinine clearance is also ordered, these tests can be performed simultaneously with the urine electrolyte test, using the same specimen.

## Findings

**Elevated Values**

SODIUM AND CHLORIDE

| | | |
|---|---|---|
| Increased sodium chloride intake | Renal tubular acidosis | Acute or chronic renal failure |
| Adrenal failure | Syndrome of inappropriate antidiuretic hormone | |
| Addison's disease | | |
| Nephritis (salt-wasting) | Alkalosis | |
| | Diuretic therapy | |

POTASSIUM

| | | |
|---|---|---|
| Increased potassium intake | Metabolic acidosis | |
| Cushing's syndrome | Adrenocorticotropic hormone or cortisone treatment | |
| Aldosteronism | | |
| Renal tubular disease | Salicylate poisoning | |

CALCIUM

| | | |
|---|---|---|
| Hyperparathyroidism | Multiple myeloma | Skeletal immobility |
| Vitamin D toxicity | Thyrotoxicosis | Degenerative liver disease |
| Malignancy of bone | Paget's disease | |
| Renal tubular acidosis | Sarcoidosis | Cushing's disease |
| Sarcoma | Osteoporosis | Diabetes mellitus |
| Nephrolithiasis | Schistosomiasis | |

MAGNESIUM

| | | |
|---|---|---|
| Chronic renal disease | Bartter's syndrome | Cisplatin therapy |
| Addison's disease | Ingestion of excess | Diuretic therapy |
| Chronic alcoholism | magnesium | |

**Decreased Values**

SODIUM AND CHLORIDE

| | | |
|---|---|---|
| Decreased sodium chloride intake | Congestive heart failure | Intestinal fistula |
| Cushing's syndrome | Nephrotic syndrome | Severe burns |
| Cirrhosis (with ascites) | Prerenal azotemia | Excessive sweating |
| | Vomiting, diarrhea | Metabolic acidosis |

POTASSIUM

| | |
|---|---|
| Addison's disease | Nephrosclerosis |
| Acute glomerulone-phritis | Malabsorption syndrome |
| Pyelonephritis | Metabolic alkalosis |

CALCIUM

| | | |
|---|---|---|
| Hypoparathyroidism | Nephrosis | Renal osteodystrophy |
| Hypothyroidism | Steatorrhea | Vitamin D-resistant rickets |
| Pseudohypoparathy-roidism | Acute nephritis | Vitamin D deficiency |
| Celiac disease | Hypocalciuric hypercalcemia | |

MAGNESIUM

| | | |
|---|---|---|
| Advanced kidney failure | Diabetic acidosis | Primary aldoste-ronism |
| Acute or chronic diarrhea | Starvation | Malabsorption |
| | Pancreatitis | |
| | Dehydration | |

**Interfering Factors**

- Failure to collect all the urine during the 24-hour collection period
- Failure to refrigerate the specimen
- For magnesium testing: Contact with a metal bedpan or urinal

**Nursing Implementation**

**Pretest**

Obtain a urine collection container from the laboratory for the collection of all urine in the 24-hour test period.

If the test is used to evaluate nephrolithiasis, instruct the patient to eat the usual diet for 3 days before the test. If the patient is already receiving a calcium-restricted diet as part of the calcium stone prevention treatment, instruct the patient to maintain the dietary restriction before and during the test period.

When thiazide diuretics are used to prevent formation of calcium stones, instruct the patient to continue the medication before and during the test. Thiazides are effective in lowering the urine calcium levels, and the benefits of the medication can be evaluated.

### During the Test

Instruct the patient to void at 8 AM and discard the specimen. The test begins immediately thereafter, and all urine is collected for the next 24 hours, including the 8 AM specimen of the next morning.

Keep the urine in the refrigerator or on ice throughout the collection period.

Ensure that the patient's name and the date and time of the start and finish of the test are written on the label and the requisition slip.

Instruct the patient to use the special laboratory container to collect the urine. If a bedpan or urinal is used for voiding, it must be made of plastic, not metal.

### Posttest

Arrange for prompt transport of the chilled specimen to the laboratory.

## Erythropoietin

**(Serum)**  Synonym: EP

**Normal Values**  5–36 µU/mL *or* SI 5–35 IU/L

### Background Information

Erythropoietin is a hormone manufactured primarily by the kidneys. Its action is to regulate erythropoiesis, meaning that it stimulates or promotes the proliferation, differentiation, and maturation of erythrocyte precursor cells of the bone marrow. In normal kidneys, the stimuli to produce erythropoietin are hypoxia and decreased renal oxygenation.

In the anemia of renal disease, the erythropoietin level is low. In cases of end-stage renal disease or after bilateral nephrectomy, the ability to produce erythropoietin is greatly reduced, and erythropoiesis by the bone marrow is limited.

In chronic iron deficiency anemia and other types of anemia and after a moderate blood loss, the erythropoietin level is elevated as the kidneys respond to the need for more red blood cells and oxygen. The erythropoietin level rises dramatically in pregnancy and with erythropoietin-producing tumors.

### Purpose of the Test

Measurement of erythropoietin is performed to investigate some anemias and the anemia of end-stage renal disease. It also may be used to differentiate between primary and secondary polycythemia vera or to detect the recurrence of an erythropoietin-producing tumor.

### Procedure

A red-topped tube is used to collect 7 mL of venous blood.

| Findings | **Elevated Values** | | |
|---|---|---|---|
| | Anemias<br>Secondary polycythemia (pulmonary fibrosis, chronic obstructive pulmonary disease) | Erythropoietin-producing tumor (cerebellar hemangioblastoma, renal tumor, hepatoma, pheochromocytoma) | Polycystic kidney disease<br>Early renal transplant rejection |

**Decreased Values**

End-stage renal failure
Primary polycythemia (polycythemia vera)

---

**Interfering Factors**     • Pregnancy

---

**Nursing Implementation**     No specific patient instruction or intervention is needed.

---

## Phenylalanine, Blood

**(Blood)**          Synonyms: Phe, PKU test, phenylalanine screening test, Guthrie screening test

---

**Normal Values**

**Guthrie test:** <2 mg/day/L *or* SI 121 µmol/L
**Fluorometry Method**
 Full-term newborn: 1.2–3.4 mg/dL *or* SI 73–206 µmol/L
 Premature newborn: 2–7.5 mg/dL *or* SI 121–454 µmol/L
 Adult: 0.8–1.8 mg/dL *or* SI 48–109 µmol/L

---

### Background Information

In normal amino acid metabolism, the enzyme phenylhydroxylase is needed to convert phenylalanine to tyrosine. When this enzyme or its cofactor $BH_4$ is absent, the levels of phenylalanine and phenylpyruvic acid, a phenylalanine metabolite, rise in the blood and urine.

Phenylketonuria (PKU) is an inherited disorder of amino acid metabolism that is characterized by elevated levels of phenylalanine and phenylpyruvic acid. Unless early detection and proper dietary intervention occur, the elevated blood level of phenylala-

nine will cause central nervous system damage and mental retardation. The possible panic range of the Guthrie test is 4 mg/dL or higher (SI 242 µmol/L). Within 10 days of birth, a newborn with undetected and untreated hyperphenylalaninemia may have a serum level of 15 to 30 mg/dL (SI 907–1,815 µmol/L).

The phenylalanine level is not elevated at birth because no dietary intake of protein has occurred. In the infant who has a defect in amino acid metabolism, the serum level begins to rise within 24 hours after starting to feed with milk or formula. The ideal time to screen the blood for phenylalanine is 48 to 72 hours after birth or 2 days after the newborn begins to feed.

State laws require PKU testing of all newborns within a specified period. If the blood phenylalanine test is performed in the first 24 hours of life, the test should be repeated after feeding has begun. The repeat test greatly reduces the chance of a false-negative result.

The blood phenylalanine test is a screening tool that identifies only hyperphenylalaninemia. Further testing is needed to verify the cause of the elevated blood level. If an elevated result occurs, the test is repeated in 24 hours to ensure accuracy.

Premature or low-birth-weight infants have higher serum values than do full-term infants of normal weight. This false-positive serum elevation is caused by immaturity of the liver. Antibiotics also interfere with the Guthrie method of analysis and cause a false-positive result.

---

### Purpose of the Test

The blood phenylalanine test is performed to detect PKU and other causes of hyperphenylalaninemia. It is also used to monitor patients who have PKU and are being maintained on a phenylalanine-restricted diet.

---

### Procedure

A heelstick puncture is used to obtain 2 to 3 drops of blood. The blood sample is collected by capillary tube or PKU card or filter paper. The circles are filled by blotting the blood onto the paper.

**Quality Control**

With the filter paper or card, only one side of the paper is blotted to fill the circles. The paper should not be turned over to soak the other side. Cord blood cannot be used for this test.

---

### Findings

**Elevated Values**

| | |
|---|---|
| Phenylketonuria | Liver disease |
| Severe burns | Sepsis |
| Hyperphenylalanin-emia | Galactosemia |

---

### Interfering Factors

- Little to no ingestion of milk
- Insufficient quantity of blood
- Antibiotics
- Recent exchange transfusion

---

### Nursing Implementation

■

*Critical Thinking 21–3*
After drinking chocolate milk at school, a 7-year-old child with PKU has a slightly elevated blood phenylalanine level. This is not the first time that she has eaten prohibited foods. How can the nurse help the child follow her diet?

**Pretest**

Ensure that the laboratory requisition slip includes the name, date, time of the test, date of birth, and time of the first milk feeding. Note the administration of antibiotics or blood transfusion.

**Posttest**

Arrange for prompt transport of the specimen to the laboratory.

# Phenylalanine, Urine

(Urine)                              Synonym: PKU urine test

**Normal Values**

> Ferric chloride method: Green color is positive for phenylpyruvic acid.
> Phenastix method (urine reagent dip strip): Persistent blue-gray to green-gray color is positive for phenylpyruvic acid.

## Background Information

In normal amino acid metabolism, phenylalanine is converted to tyrosine. The enzyme phenylalanine hydroxylase and other cofactors must be present for this conversion to take place. Normal renal function provides for glomerular filtration of the amino acids, with tubular resorption of the filtrate.

When the enzyme or its cofactors are absent and an intake of protein exists as the source of amino acids, the levels of phenylalanine and phenylpyruvic acid (the phenylalanine metabolite) rise in the blood. The increase of amino acids in the plasma concentration results in an increase in glomerular filtration, but the renal tubules cannot resorb all the excess. Thus, the overflow of phenylalanine and phenylpyruvic acid is excreted in the urine.

PKU is one type of aminoaciduria. It is an inherited disorder of amino acid metabolism caused by the absence of phenylalanine hydroxylase. If the condition remains undetected or uncontrolled by dietary therapy, damage to the central nervous system and mental retardation will occur.

Phenylpyruvic acid is not present in the urine at birth because an intake of protein from breast milk or infant formula must first occur. If the amino acid metabolism is impaired, a rapid rise of phenylalanine in the blood will occur. This can be detected readily by the serum phenylalanine test, which is the primary screening test for PKU.

In hyperphenylalaninemia, the presence of phenylpyruvic acid is not detectable in the urine for 2 to 6 weeks after birth. Once the serum level of phenylpyruvic acid rises to 10 to 20 mg/dL, the metabolite appears in the urine. Because of the time delay, the phenylalanine urine test is not used as an initial screening test for PKU.

**Purpose of the Test**

The urine phenylalanine test is used to assist in the detection of hyperphenylalaninemia, including PKU. The test is also used to monitor the effect of dietary treatment for patients who have a defect in amino acid metabolism.

**Procedure**

A freshly voided specimen of urine is collected in a plastic urine collection container.

**Findings**

**Abnormal Values**

Phenylketonuria
Non-PKU hyperphenylalaninemia

**Interfering Factors**

- Inadequate labeling

- Improper collection procedure
- Diluted urine

| **Nursing Implementation** | **Pretest** |

For testing infants and small children, teach the parent to apply the urine collection bag and transfer the urine to a collection container.

**Posttest**

Ensure that the time and date of voiding are written on the label and requisition slip.
Arrange for the transport of the urine to the laboratory within 1 hour.

## Prostate-Specific Antigen

**(Serum)**                          Synonym: PSA

| **Normal Values** | 40–49 years old: Less than 1.5 ng/mL *or* SI 1.5 µg/L<br>50–59 years old: Less than 2.5 ng/mL *or* SI 2.5 µg/L<br>60–69 years old: Less than 4.5 ng/L *or* SI 4.5 µg/L<br>70–80 years old: Less than 7.5 ng/L *or* SI 7.5 µg/L (Statland, 1996) |

### Background Information

Prostate-specific antigen (PSA) is a tumor marker for adenocarcinoma of the prostate gland. This antigen is an enzyme that is manufactured exclusively by the prostate gland, establishing its specificity and usefulness in detecting abnormal prostatic tissue growth. Prostate-specific antigen is produced by the epithelial cells of the gland in normal, benign hypertrophy and malignant prostate conditions, but the amount of the enzyme varies with each type of condition (Table 21–1).

**Benefits.**   The best use of the prostate-specific antigen test is to monitor patients after treatment for adenocarcinoma of the prostate gland. The test is highly predictive of residual or recurrent disease after treatment by radical prostatectomy, radiation therapy, or antiandrogen treatment. Following treatment, the patient is monitored by the prostate-specific antigen test for a number of years. The test will detect renewed malignant growth in localized or distant metastatic sites long before the recurrence can be detected by other diagnostic methods.

In 1994, the U.S. Food and Drug Administration (FDA) approved the use of prostate-specific antigen as a screening tool for prostate cancer when

**Table 21–1   Abnormal Values of Prostate-Specific Antigen**

| Condition | Laboratory Values |
|---|---|
| Male with benign prostate hypertropy | $10.2 \pm 8.97$ ng/mL *or* SI $10.2 \pm 8.97$ µg/L |
| Prostate cancer | |
|    Stage A | $9.39 \pm 8.09$ ng/mL *or* SI $9.39 \pm 8.09$ µg/L |
|    Stage B | $17.45 \pm 16.83$ ng/mL *or* SI $17.45 \pm 16.83$ µg/L |
|    Stage C | $55.14 \pm 51.65$ ng/mL *or* SI $55.14 \pm 51.65$ µg/L |
|    Stage D | $118.92 \pm 50$ ng/mL *or* SI $118.92 \pm 50$ µg/L |

the prostate-specific antigen test is used with the digital rectal examination. In combination, the abnormal results are valid indicators for a biopsy of the prostatic tissue. Research (Diefenbach, Ganz, Pawlow, & Gutrie, 1996) indicates that men are unaware of the PSA test as a method of screening for cancer. Public education is needed.

**Limitations.** Although this is the first and only organ-specific tumor marker and it is a valuable test in specific situations, the test has some problems of reliability and specificity. By itself, prostate-specific antigen cannot be used as a cancer screening tool for the healthy male population, because it is not specific enough to consistently distinguish between benign and malignant conditions.

The recent FDA decision regarding the prostate-specific antigen test and digital rectal examination as an approved screening tool raises concerns about the cost of testing (and follow-up biopsy) when the PSA test, even in combination with the digital rectal examination, still has a high false-positive rate.

The prostate-specific antigen test lacks specificity to distinguish between benign prostatic hypertrophy and an early stage of prostatic malignancy. As seen in Table 21–1, the elevated value for benign prostatic hypertrophy may be in the same range as the value for stage A of malignant growth.

Prostate-specific antigen testing cannot be used by itself to stage the malignancy. As seen in Table 21–1, the abnormal values often rise proportionately with the severity or extent of the malignancy. This correlation, however, is not always consistent or reliable, particularly in the early stages of malignancy.

---

## Purpose of the Test

*Critical Thinking 21–4*
A male friend says his doctor told him not to bother having a PSA test done. He asks you if his doctor's advice is reliable. How do you respond?

As a tumor marker for adenocarcinoma of the prostate gland, the test is used to monitor the postsurgical patient who has had a radical prostatectomy. It is used to evaluate for recurrence or residual tumor and helps identify the need for additional treatment. In combination with the digital rectal examination, it is recommended as a screening tool for all men older than 50 years and for men older than 40 years who have additional risk factors, including African-American men and men who have a positive family history of prostate cancer.

---

## Procedure

A red-topped tube is used to collect 7 to 10 mL of venous blood.

---

## Findings

**Elevated Values**

Adenocarcinoma of the prostate
Benign prostatic hypertrophy

Prostatitis
Urinary retention
Prostatic infarct

---

## Interfering Factors

• Recent urethral instrumentation

---

## Nursing Implementation

**Pretest**

Collect the specimen before any prostate manipulation.
Schedule the test for at least 2 weeks after any urethral instrumentation procedure such as a transurethral resection, prostatic biopsy, or cystoscopy, because these procedures will cause a release of the prostate-specific antigen.
Because a fasting specimen is preferred, instruct the patient to cease food intake for 8 hours before the test.

### Posttest

Arrange for prompt transport of the specimen to the laboratory.

**Quality Control**

Once the blood is centrifuged and the serum extracted, the serum is stable at room temperature for 24 hours. Thereafter, it must be stored at −20°C or lower.

## Prostatic Acid Phosphatase

**(Serum, Vaginal Secretions)**    Synonyms: PAP, acid phosphatase

**Normal Values**

**Serum**
4-Nitrophenyl phosphate method at 37°C (male): 0.13–0.63 U/L
Tartrate resistance fraction (male): 0.2–3.5 U/L *or* SI 2.2–10.5 U/L
Thymolphthalein monophosphate method at 37°C: <1.9 U/L
**Vaginal secretions:** <2 U/L

### Background Information

Acid phosphatase is an enzyme that is present in high concentrations in the prostate gland and its secretions. In serum, although its value is elevated in association with metastatic cancer of the prostate, it is likely to remain in a normal range during the early stage of the disease. The normal value varies with the method of analysis used.

Other acid phosphatase isoenzymes are present in body tissues, including platelets, erythrocytes, liver, spleen, and bone marrow. These tissue sources can also release small amounts of prostatic acid phosphatase into the serum.

**Serum.**    For many years, prostatic acid phosphatase was used as a tumor marker to diagnose and help stage adenocarcinoma of the prostate gland. Today, the prostate-specific antigen test has surpassed the prostatic acid phosphatase test in the diagnosis and evaluation of carcinoma of the prostate gland. The prostatic acid phosphatase test is still used with the prostate-specific antigen test in the evaluation and staging of metastatic prostate cancer. The tartrate-resistant method of analysis remains an important diagnostic test for hairy cell leukemia.

**Vaginal Secretions.**    Prostatic acid phosphatase is present in prostatic secretions and therefore in semen. In cases of alleged rape, the vaginal secretions are tested for acid phosphatase.

### Purpose of the Test

Acid phosphatase is used to assist with the staging of metastatic adenocarcinoma of the prostate gland. After treatment for the malignancy, it assists in the evaluation for recurrence of the disease.

### Procedure

A red- or purple-topped tube with ethylenediaminetetraacetic acid or acid phosphatase anticoagulant is used to collect 7 mL of venous blood.

### Quality Control

Venipuncture technique must be smooth, with a blood flow that fills the vacuum tube readily. If the blood has excessive turbulence because of flawed venipuncture technique, the hemolysis of the erythrocytes will alter the results.

---

**Findings**

### Elevated Values

| | | |
|---|---|---|
| Metastatic cancer of the prostate | Niemann-Pick disease | Prostatitis |
| Hairy cell leukemia | Advanced Paget's disease | Metastatic cancer of bone |
| Gaucher's disease | Benign prostatic hypertrophy | Prostatic infarct |
| Hemolytic diseases | | |

---

**Interfering Factors**

- Hemolysis
- Warming of the specimen
- Failure to maintain nothing-by-mouth status
- Lipemia

---

**Nursing Implementation**

### Pretest

To avoid a false-positive elevation, schedule this test for several days after any diagnostic test that manipulates the prostate gland (transurethral resection, bladder catheterization, digital examination).

Collect the specimen before any prostate manipulation is done.

Instruct the patient to discontinue all food and fluids for 8 hours before the test, because lipemia interferes with the laboratory analysis.

### Posttest

Arrange for prompt transport of the specimen to the laboratory.

### Quality Control

The blood must be centrifuged promptly and the serum tested or put on ice for rapid cooling. If the specimen is warmed, within 1 hour the serum value will be lowered falsely. If testing is delayed, the specimen is acidified with acetic acid or citrate buffer.

---

## Protein Electrophoresis, 24-Hour Urine

**(Urine)**     Synonym: Urine protein electrophoresis

---

**Normal Values**

40–150 ng/24 hr *or* SI 40–150 mg/24 hr
No monoclonal gammopathy (M protein) noted

## Background Information

Normally, a small amount of protein exists in the urine. About one third of it is albumin, and the remainder consists of plasma proteins, including many small globulins.

When excessive protein appears in the urine, the causes can be broadly categorized as glomerular disorders, tubular disorders, or overflow proteinuria. In the first two categories, the problems are related to renal damage. The third category is characterized by excessive protein produced by nonrenal disease. The proteins are filtered by the glomeruli, but the large amount prevents effective resorption by the tubules. Thus, an "overflow" of protein into the urine occurs.

Protein electrophoresis is a laboratory method used to identify the predominant proteins in the urine. In abnormal glomerular permeability, albumin, $alpha_1$-proteins, and transferrin are predominant. In tubular proteinemia, $alpha_2$- and $beta_2$-microglobins are predominant.

The Bence Jones protein is one of the proteins of overflow proteinuria. Its presence in the urine is associated with multiple myeloma, macroglobulinemia, and malignant lymphoma. Protein electrophoresis analyzes for the presence of monoclonal gammopathy (M protein). On the electrophoresis pattern, the M protein is demonstrated by a sharp spike in the globulin region.

---

**Purpose of the Test**

Protein electrophoresis of the urine is used to identify the different types of protein loss in the urine and to evaluate patients with known or suspected multiple myeloma.

---

**Procedure**

A single voided specimen of urine is placed in a clean urine container.

---

**Findings**

**Abnormal Values**

GLOMERULAR-PATTERN PROTEINURIA

Glomerular diseases
Nephrotic syndrome

OVERFLOW-PATTERN PROTEINURIA

Multiple myeloma          Lymphoma
Waldenström's             Amyloidosis
  macroglobulinemia

TUBULAR-PATTERN PROTEINURIA

Fanconi's syndrome     Wilson's disease      Renal transplant
Cystinosis             Pyelonephritis          rejection

---

**Interfering Factors**

- Hematuria

---

**Nursing Implementation**

**Pretest**

Instruct the patient to collect a routine urine specimen.
Instruct female patients to collect the urine at a time when no menstrual flow occurs.

### Posttest

Refrigerate the urine until it is transported to the laboratory.

## Specific Gravity

**(Urine)**      Synonyms: None

| **Normal Values** | 1.003–1.029 |
| --- | --- |

### Background Information

The specific gravity of urine is the ratio of the weight of a given volume of urine to the weight of the same volume of distilled water at a constant temperature. The urine specific gravity will vary within the individual based on his or her diet and fluid status. Increased fluid intake normally decreases the specific gravity of urine. Decreased fluid intake normally increases the urine specific gravity.

**Purpose of the Test**      Specific gravity reflects the ability of the kidneys to concentrate and dilute urine. It assesses renal function and the hormonal regulation of fluid balance, specifically the antidiuretic hormone.

**Procedure**      Urine specific gravity is measured as part of urinalysis (see Chapter 3), by hydrometer or by a reagent strip.

**Findings**      See Chapter 3.

**Interfering Factors**
- Excessive protein in the urine
- Alkaline urine

**Nursing Implementation**      The actions of the nurse are dependent on the method used to measure the specific gravity. See Chapter 3 for the urinalysis method.

     If a hydrometer (urinometer) is used, perform the following.

### Pretest

Obtain a urinometer calibrated to measure urine specific gravity at room temperature.

### Quality Control

Accuracy of the urinometer can be assessed by using distilled water, which has a specific gravity of 1.000.

### During the Test

Instruct patient to void into a clean container.

Allow the urine to reach room temperature.

Wearing gloves, pour fresh urine into the urinometer's cylinder until it is three-fourths full.

Remove any foam with filter paper.

Gently insert the hydrometer into the cylinder using a gentle spinning motion.

Read the specific gravity at eye level (Fig. 21–1).

### Posttest

Disinfect the urinometer.

Remove gloves and wash hands.

Document the specific gravity.

Reagent strips are replacing the use of hydrometers in measuring specific gravity. The reagent strip pad will change color according to the concentration of ions in the urine.

### Quality Control

Check the vial of reagent strips for product dating. Do not use them after the manufacturer's expiration date. Always store strips in the manufacturer's darkened container. Do not expose the container to direct sunlight or extreme heat.

### During the Test

Instruct the patient to void into a clean container.

Dip the reagent strip into the urine.

Wait the time specified by the manufacturer.

Compare the resultant color with the chart provided.

### Posttest

Document the specific gravity.

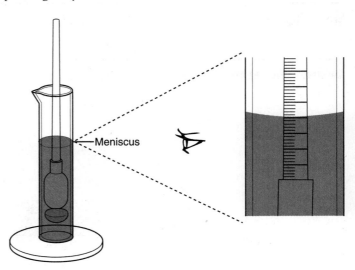

**Figure 21–1**
Hydrometer. (Reproduced with permission from Stepp, C. A., & Woods, M. [1998]. *Laboratory procedures for medical office personnel.* Philadelphia: W. B. Saunders.)

# Urea Nitrogen

**(Serum)**          Synonyms: Blood urea nitrogen, BUN

| | |
|---|---|
| **Normal Values** | Older adult (>60 years): 8–23 mg/dL *or* SI 2.9–8.2 mmol/L<br>Child to adult (1–60 years): 5–20 mg/dL *or* SI 1.8–7.1 mmol/L<br>Infant (birth–1 year): 4–19 mg/dL *or* SI 1.4–6.8 mmol/L |

## Background Information

Blood urea nitrogen (BUN) is the major nitrogenous end product of protein and amino acid catabolism. It is produced in the liver and distributed throughout intracellular and extracellular fluid. Urea nitrogen is excreted from the body primarily by the kidneys; lesser amounts are excreted in sweat or degraded by intestinal bacteria.

In the kidneys, almost all urea is filtered out of the blood by glomerular function. Some urea is resorbed with water in the renal tubules, but most is removed from the body in urine. The amount of urea excreted is dependent on the state of hydration and renal perfusion. If the patient is dehydrated, low tubular flow of urinary filtrate occurs, and more urea is absorbed. If overhydration and a high tubular flow rate exist, less urea is resorbed, resulting in a lower serum level.

In addition to dehydration, the urea nitrogen level can rise from renal and nonrenal factors. Nonrenal factors include increased urea production associated with increased dietary protein intake and increased catabolism, such as occurs with corticosteroid therapy or muscle-wasting diseases. When excess urea is produced, the serum level rarely rises above 40 mg/dL (SI >14.2 mmol/L). Some medications will cause a *slight* increase in the BUN level.

In renal causes of an elevated BUN level, the problem can be prerenal, intrarenal, or postrenal. Prerenal disease includes poor renal blood flow, as in shock or renal artery stenosis. The impaired perfusion slows the glomerular filtration rate. Intrarenal disease includes damage to the renal parenchyma. Renal causes of azotemia result in a dramatic rise in the BUN level. Generally, the urea nitrogen level does not begin to rise until a loss of at least 50% of glomerular function occurs (Henry, 1996). Postrenal problems are related to obstruction in the kidney or in the urinary tract. This causes an increase in tubular resorption of the urea.

| | |
|---|---|
| **Purpose of the Test** | The BUN level is used to evaluate renal function. With the serum creatinine level, it is used to monitor patients in renal failure or those receiving dialysis therapy. |
| **Procedure** | A red-topped tube is used to obtain 10 mL of venous blood. |

| | | | |
|---|---|---|---|
| **Findings** | **Elevated Values** | | |
| | Acute or chronic renal failure | Stress | Dehydration |
| | Shock | Congestive heart failure | Hyperalimentation |
| | Renal artery stenosis | Burns | Ketoacidosis |
| | Hemorrhage | Increased protein intake | Long-term steroid therapy |
| | Postrenal syndrome | | Diabetes mellitus |

**Decreased Values**

| | | |
|---|---|---|
| Overhydration | Intravenous therapy | Acromegaly |
| Starvation | Low-protein diet | Severe liver damage |

---

**Interfering Factors**  • None

---

**Nursing Implementation**  Care of the patient is similar to that for other venipunctures.

---

**Critical Value**

**100 mg/dL or higher (SI 35.7 mmol/L or higher)**

This value is extremely elevated and defines the condition of uremia. The patient will be stuporous or comatose. Generally, renal failure is identified at much lower levels.

---

## Uric Acid, Urine

(Urine)  Synonyms: None

**Normal Values**

Average diet (adult): 250–750 mg/24 hr *or* SI 1.48–4.43 mmol/24 hr
Low purine diet (male): <420 mg/24 hr *or* SI <2.83 mmol/24 hr
Low purine diet (female): <400 mg/24 hr *or* SI <2.36 mmol/24 hr
High purine diet (adult): <1,000 mg/24 hr *or* SI <5.9 mmol/24 hr

## Background Information

As an end product of protein metabolism, uric acid and urate crystals are excreted by the kidneys and bowel. Hyperuricosuria, a high level of uric acid in the urine, may be caused by excess secretion or excess production of uric acid.

**Uric Acid Excretion.**   The excretion of uric acid is influenced by a number of normal variables. A high intake of purine foods results in a high level of uric acid excretion in the urine. Normal urine has a saturated level of uric acid, with urate crystals in the sediment of the urine. If the urine is acidic and concentrated, uric acid becomes insoluble and produces greater quantities of urate crystals. Abundant crystals form a thick sludge that can block renal tubules or cause uric acid stone formation.

**Uric Acid Production.**   Some pathologic conditions cause increased uric acid production and ultimately excess uric acid excretion. These condi-

tions include metabolic abnormalities such as gout and glycogen storage diseases. Intestinal changes such as ileostomy or other intestinal diversions cause the urine to become acidic. The acidity increases the urinary precipitation of urate crystals.

When leukemia is treated with cytotoxic drugs or when malignant tumors are irradiated, tumor necrosis and a metabolic breakdown of nucleoprotein occur. The massive amount of uric acid and urate crystal production can cause an acute or dangerous elevation of the urine uric acid level. The urate crystals can block the renal tubules and ureters, resulting in renal failure.

If mild to severe renal failure or other kidney disease that inhibits renal function occurs, the urinary excretion of uric acid will be low, even though normal to excessive uric acid production and a high serum uric acid level exist.

**Purpose of the Test**

The urinary uric acid test measures the urinary excretion of uric acid in patients with renal calculi or in those at risk for the development of a calculus. The test is also used to assess the effect of enzyme deficiency or metabolic abnormality that results in the overproduction of uric acid.

**Procedure**

A 24-hour urine collection is used to measure the amount of daily uric acid that is excreted. The laboratory will provide a collection container with sodium hydroxide, which keeps the pH of the urine in an alkaline state. This prevents precipitation of urate crystals.

**Findings**

**Elevated Values**

| | | |
|---|---|---|
| Uric acid nephrolithiasis | Acute leukemia of childhood | Surgical jejunoileal bypass |
| Viral hepatitis | Radiation therapy | Sickle cell anemia |
| Gout | Lymphatic leukemia | Polycythemia vera |
| Glycogen storage disease | Crohn's disease | Tumor lysis syndrome |
| Leukemia, chronic myeloid | Lymphosarcoma | |
| Lesch-Nyhan syndrome | Ulcerative colitis | |
| | Wilson's disease | |
| | Ileostomy | |
| | Cystinosis | |

**Decreased Values**

| | | |
|---|---|---|
| Chronic glomerulonephritis | Diabetic glomerulosclerosis | Folic acid deficiency |
| Collagen disease | Lead toxicity | Xanthinuria |

**Interfering Factors**

- Failure to collect all urine during the test period
- Failure to store the specimen properly
- High- or low-purine diet
- Many medications (including aspirin, antiinflammatory drugs, diuretics, vitamin C, and x-ray contrast medium)

**Nursing Implementation**

**Pretest**

Instruct the patient to collect all urine of the test period and store it in a large container. Some laboratories require the specimen to be refrigerated or stored on ice during the test period. Other laboratories do not require refrigeration.

**During the Test**

Discard the 8 AM specimen. All urine is collected for 24 hours, including the 8 AM specimen of the following morning.

Ensure that the label and requisition slip contain the patient's name and the time and date of the start and finish of the test.

■

*Critical Thinking 21–5*
The patient's 24-hour urine collection is under way when you notice that no written documentation exists about the time the test started. How can you resolve this problem?

### Posttest

List all medications taken by the patient on the requisition slip.
Arrange for transport of the specimen to the laboratory.

## Urine Protein, 24-Hour

**(Urine)**                                    Synonyms: None

| **Normal Values** | 40–150 mg/24 hr *or* SI 40–150 mg/24 hr |
|---|---|

### Background Information

Protein is minimally present in the urine of individuals with normal renal function. The urinary proteins consist of albumin and many small globulins. In normal renal anatomy and physiology, the albumin molecules are quite large, and most cannot be filtered through the glomerular membrane. The smaller globulins are filtered by the glomeruli, but most are resorbed by the proximal tubules. Additional glycoproteins are secreted by cells in the distal tubules and the ascending Henle's loop. These minimal losses of protein into the urine are considered normal.

Urinary protein levels can increase after strenuous exercise, with salt depletion, or during a period of dehydration or febrile illness. These events cause a higher level of proteinuria but are not considered indications of renal or urinary tract disease.

| **Purpose of the Test** | The urine protein test is used to help confirm the presence of renal disease. |
|---|---|

| **Procedure** | A 24-hour urine specimen is collected in a large, clear, glass or plastic container. |
|---|---|

### Findings

**Elevated Values**

Glomerulonephritis
Renal transplant
    rejection
Tubular necrosis
Chronic pyelone-
    phritis

Nephrotic syndrome
Diabetic glomerulo-
    sclerosis
Renal failure
Urinary tract infec-
    tion

Toxemia of pregnancy
Multiple myeloma
Congestive heart
    failure
Malignant hyperten-
    sion

### Interfering Factors

- Contamination of the specimen with mucus, vaginal or prostatic secretions, or white blood cells
- Dilute urine from excessive fluid intake
- Failure to collect all urine
- Warming of the specimen

**Nursing Implementation**

### Pretest

Instruct the patient to collect all urine for a 24-hour period. The specimen must be refrigerated or kept on ice throughout the test period.

Advise the patient to drink a regular amount of fluids during the test period.

### Quality Control

Excessive fluid intake will dilute the urine and give a false-negative value.

### During the Test

Have the patient void at 8 AM and discard the urine.

The test period starts at this time, and all urine is collected for 24 hours, including the 8 AM specimen of the following morning.

Ensure that the patient's name and the time and date of the start and finish of the test are written on the label and requisition slip.

### Posttest

Keep the specimen refrigerated until it is transported to the laboratory.

---

## Diagnostic Procedures

## Angiography, Renal

**(Radiography)**

Synonyms: None

The arterial circulation to the kidneys and within the kidneys is visualized using an iodinated contrast medium and radiography. The contrast material is administered via a femoral or brachial artery. An arterial catheter is passed from the aorta into the right and left renal arteries. As the dye is injected via the catheter, rapid, timed x-ray films are taken to visualize the arterial circulation and tissue perfusion.

Arterial circulatory impairment includes aneurysm, arteriosclerosis, renal artery stenosis, and renal artery infarction. Abnormalities of renal tissue include chronic pyelonephritis, renal abscess, tumor, cyst, pseudotumor, and hematoma.

A complete discussion of angiography is presented in Chapter 11.

## Biopsy, Prostate

**(Tissue Biopsy)**

Synonyms: Core biopsy of the prostate gland, fine needle aspiration biopsy of the prostate gland, FNB of the prostate

| **Normal Values** | Normal prostate tissue with no evidence of tumor or infection |

## Background Information

Prostate cancer usually consists of multiple tumors that originate in the peripheral area of the prostate gland. The majority of these cases are adenocarcinomas.

A biopsy of the prostate gland is indicated when a palpable nodule exists; when alteration in size, shape, or texture of prostate tissue occurs; when abnormal findings occur on ultrasound of the prostate; or when elevated blood levels of the tumor markers prostatic acid phosphatase and prostate-specific antigen exist.

The microscopic study of the biopsy tissue confirms the diagnosis. If the tissue sample is malignant, it provides identification of the tumor type, including the tumor grading and local staging of the cancer.

A number of methods can be used to obtain the biopsy sample. An open biopsy means that the peritoneal area is incised and a wedge of prostate tissue is removed surgically. The tissue sample may also be obtained during a transurethral resection procedure. Each of these methods requires general or spinal anesthesia.

Needle aspiration biopsy is performed via a transrectal or perineal approach. Ultrasound may be used during the procedure to guide the placement of the needle and confirm the presence of the needle in the tumor tissue (Fig. 21–2). A core biopsy procedure uses a larger needle (14 to 18 gauge) that may be attached to an automated core biopsy gun. The core biopsy needle has a higher accuracy rate in establishing the diagnosis. A fine needle aspiration biopsy uses a narrow, flexible prostatic aspiration needle.

## Purpose of the Test

A prostate biopsy is used to determine the cause of an enlarged prostate gland and to diagnose prostate cancer.

## Procedure

The procedure varies dependent on whether an open or needle biopsy is done. If an open biopsy is performed, care is similar to the pre- and postoperative

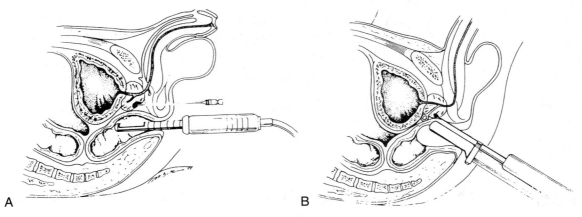

A                                                                    B

**Figure 21–2**

Ultrasound-guided prostate biopsy. A, Transperineal approach. B, Transrectal approach. (Reproduced with permission from Muldoon, L., & Resnick, M. I. [1989]. Results of ultrasonography of the prostate. *Urologic Clinics of North America, 16,* 699.)

care of a patient with prostatic surgery. With a needle biopsy, a local anesthetic is given to the perineum. Using sterile technique, a needle is inserted into the prostate. Several samples of tissue are aspirated.

| Findings | Abnormal Values | | |
|---|---|---|---|
| | Cancer of the prostate gland | Benign prostatic hypertrophy | Lymphoma Prostatitis |

**Interfering Factors**

- Failure to maintain nothing-by-mouth status
- Acute prostatitis

**Nursing Implementation**

### Pretest

Instruct the patient regarding the procedure, and obtain written consent from the patient or the person legally designated to make the patient's health care decisions.

Instruct the patient to take a disposable phosphate (Fleet) enema on the night before or in the early morning before the procedure. No food or fluids are permitted for 12 hours before the test in preparation for possible anesthesia.

Assist the patient in removing all clothes and putting on a hospital gown.

Have the patient void to empty the bladder.

Place the patient in the lithotomy position.

Administer sedation as ordered.

### During the Test

For the transperineal approach, assist with the preparation of the local anesthetic. It will be injected by the physician into the perineal area between the scrotum and the rectum.

Provide comfort and reassurance to the patient who may be anxious and afraid. Momentary pain is felt as the anesthetic is injected. Additionally, the patient may worry about the possible diagnosis.

Place the biopsy specimen in a sterile container with a preservative such as formalin or Zenker's fluid. In some cases, cultures or tissue slides are prepared immediately. Label all specimens with the patient's name and the tissue source.

Send the specimens to the laboratory without delay.

Apply an adhesive bandage to the perineal biopsy site. No dressing is used for the transrectal approach.

### Posttest

Take vital signs, and record the results. If general anesthesia was used or if the patient is unstable, continue monitoring the vital signs at regular intervals.

Assess for pain, and offer pain medication as needed.

Observe the biopsy site for signs of bleeding into the dressing or into local tissue.

Assess for difficulty in voiding or hematuria.

Instruct the patient to take the prescribed antibiotic for 2 days to prevent infection.

**Complications**     The most common complication of this procedure is infection, particularly in patients who have unknown prostatitis. It is also possible for the biopsy needle to penetrate the bladder or prostatic urethra or for bleeding to occur.

The complications of prostate biopsy are presented in Table 21–2.

## Biopsy, Renal

**(Tissue Biopsy)**     Synonyms: Kidney biopsy, fine needle aspiration biopsy of the kidney, FNB of the kidney

### Background Information

Biopsy of the kidney provides specific information regarding the pathophysiologic changes in the tissue. Other laboratory tests and noninvasive procedures are performed first to obtain as much diagnostic information as possible. The broad categories of pathophysiologic conditions that require renal biopsy include acute renal failure, renal tumor, renal transplant rejection, asymptomatic hematuria, proteinuria of unknown origin, or questions regarding drug toxicity and untoward reaction to medication.

A renal biopsy may be done as a surgical procedure or by fine needle biopsy. Needle biopsy may be performed to diagnose renal cancer. It is used when computed tomography (CT) or magnetic resonance imaging (MRI) findings are inconclusive, to investigate metastatic disease or recurrence of cancer, and to diagnose type of renal tumor in the patient who is a poor surgical risk.

In renal transplant patients, the donor kidney can show signs of transplant rejection. Without biopsy, early accurate diagnosis of rejection is difficult because of other possible causes of renal dysfunction that produce the same symptoms. Fine needle aspiration biopsy is minimally invasive and can be used repeatedly on the same patient.

**Purpose of the Test**     Renal biopsy is used to determine the exact pathologic state and diagnosis of the renal disorder, monitor the progression of the renal disease, evaluate the response to treatment, and assess for rejection of the renal transplant.

**Table 21–2     Complications of Biopsy of the Prostate**

| Complication | Nursing Assessment |
| --- | --- |
| Sepsis | Redness |
| | Localized swelling |
| | Fever |
| | Pain |
| | Purulence |
| Bladder or urethral puncture | Hematuria |
| | Frequency |
| | Urinary retention |
| Bleeding | Ecchymosis |
| | Hematoma |
| | Swelling |
| | Pain |
| | Hematuria |

| | |
|---|---|
| **Procedure** | After administration of local anesthesia, a biopsy needle is inserted percutaneously or through a small incision. While the needle is advanced into the kidney, ultrasound or x-ray films are used to guide the exact placement and location. A syringe is used to aspirate a small core of tissue from the renal cortex. The total time needed to obtain the specimen is about 15 minutes. |

**Findings**

**Abnormal Values**

| | | |
|---|---|---|
| Acute or chronic glomerulonephritis | Amyloid infiltration of the kidney | Renal transplant rejection or failure |
| Goodpasture's syndrome | Systemic lupus erythematosus | Renal cell carcinoma |
| | | Wilms' tumor |

**Interfering Factors**

- Failure to maintain nothing-by-mouth status
- Coagulation disorder
- Urinary tract infection
- Nonfunction of one kidney

**Nursing Implementation**

**Pretest**

Ensure that written informed consent has been obtained from the patient or the person legally responsible for the patient's health care decisions.

Check that all screening tests are completed and that the results are posted in the patient's chart. Coagulation studies, including prothrombin time testing, activated partial thromboplastin time testing, platelet level determination, and hematocrit testing, are performed to verify clotting ability. Urinalysis identifies the presence of any infection.

Take baseline vital signs and record the results.

Administer sedation as ordered.

**During the Test**

Cleanse the skin of the lower back with antiseptic.

Provide reassurance to the patient to help alleviate anxiety.

When the needle is to be inserted, instruct the patient to take a deep breath and hold it. Assist the patient in remaining still. A brief sensation of pain may occur, but it is mild.

After the needle is removed, apply pressure to the puncture site for 20 minutes to help promote clotting.

Apply a sterile dressing and adhesive bandage to the puncture site.

Place the biopsy specimen in a sterile container with normal saline.

Ensure that the container is labeled with the patient's name and the tissue source of the specimen.

Arrange for immediate transport of the specimen to the laboratory.

**Quality Control**

On arrival at the laboratory, the specimen must be fresh and moist to ensure accurate analysis.

### Posttest

Monitor vital signs every 15 minutes for 1 hour, every 30 minutes for the next hour, and at regular intervals thereafter.

At frequent intervals, observe the dressing and surrounding tissue for signs of bleeding.

For 8 hours, monitor each voided specimen for hematuria. Initially, a small amount of blood may be present, but it should disappear within the 8-hour period. In some institutions, the protocol is to collect every urine specimen separately, with a notation of the time and date of voiding written on the container. Over time, progressively less blood should be present, and the urine should return to its normal color.

Encourage the patient to drink extra fluids, if not contraindicated, to help promote urination.

Eight hours after the test, ensure that a specimen for hemoglobin and hematocrit determinations is drawn. When bleeding is excessive, different time intervals and repeat testing may be necessary.

Instruct the patient to lie flat for 12 to 24 hours. A sandbag in the flank area may be used to help promote compression of the tissue. After this period of immobility, bedrest or limited activity is maintained for 24 hours to prevent the onset of fresh bleeding.

Instruct the patient to avoid physical exertion, heavy lifting, and trauma to the lower back for several days.

---

**Complications**

Although renal biopsy is considered safe, with a low complication rate, the procedure has some risks. These complications include retroperitoneal and urinary tract hemorrhage, pneumothorax, biopsy of other abdominal viscera, and infection. A summary of the complications of renal biopsy appears in Table 21–3.

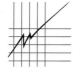

**Table 21–3   Complications of Renal Biopsy**

| Complication | Nursing Assessment |
| --- | --- |
| Bleeding | Hematuria (microscopic or gross) |
| | Dizziness, weakness |
| | Pallor |
| | Falling hematocrit value |
| | Falling hemoglobin value |
| | Tachycardia |
| | Hypotension |
| | Pain (dorsal, flank, or shoulder) |
| Infection | Fever |
| | Burning on urination |
| | Urinary frequency |
| Pneumothorax | Dyspnea |
| | Cyanosis |
| | Hypotension |
| | Restlessness, apprehension |

## Computed Tomography, Kidney

**(Tomography)**

Synonyms: CT, CAT, CT scan

Computed tomography (CT) of the kidney produces many axial slices for imaging renal tissue. Tumors, cysts, and other lesions are clearly demonstrated. The scan can also be used to detect or evaluate calculi, obstruction, congenital abnormalities, infections, and polycystic disease. An iodine-based contrast medium is used.

    A complete discussion of CT is presented in Chapter 12.

## Cystoscopy

**(Endoscopy)**

Synonyms: None

**Normal Values**

No anatomic or structural abnormalities are present.

### Background Information

Cystoscopy provides direct visualization of the urinary bladder. When the urethra also is examined, the procedure is called *cystourethroscopy.*

    The examination is performed with a cystoscope—a thin, lighted tube with a telescopic lens. The procedure may be performed in the urologist's office or in the operating room with local, spinal, or general anesthesia. Following the diagnostic component, treatment may include dilation of stricture, cauterization of bleeding spots, removal of superficial tissue, implantation of radium seeds, and placement of a ureteral stent or catheter.

    Cystoscopy is used to investigate the cause of painless hematuria, particularly when cancer of the epithelial lining is suspected. It also is part of the investigation into the cause of urinary incontinence or retention. The examiner is able to visualize the location, extent, and exact nature of the problem.

### Purpose of the Test

Cystoscopy is used to diagnose and evaluate structural and functional changes of the urinary bladder.

### Procedure

With the patient under local anesthesia, the cystoscope is inserted through the urethra into the urinary bladder. Once the bladder is filled with saline for irrigation, all aspects of the bladder walls are examined. Biopsy samples for tissue examination and cell washings for cytologic analysis may be carried out. Urine samples may be collected from the bladder or from each ureter. The procedure takes 30 to 45 minutes.

### Findings

**Abnormal Values**

Cancer of the bladder
Polyps
Diverticulum of the
    bladder

Bladder fistula
Bladder stones
Bladder neck stricture
Congenital anomaly

Benign prostatic
    hypertrophy
Cancer of the prostate
    gland

| | |
|---|---|
| **Interfering Factors** | • Failure to maintain nothing-by-mouth-status<br>• Acute infection of the bladder, urethra, or prostate gland |

**Nursing Implementation**

### Pretest

Ensure that written informed consent is obtained from the patient or the person legally designated to make health care decisions for the patient.

When bowel emptying is part of the protocol, instruct the patient to administer an enema the night before or the morning of the test.

For general or spinal anesthesia preparation, instruct the patient to fast from food and fluids for 8 hours before the procedure. For local anesthesia, fasting from food is required, but clear liquids on the morning of the test are permitted.

Take baseline vital signs and record the results.

Administer preoperative sedatives or antispasmodics as prescribed.

### During the Test

Provide reassurance to the patient who is awake during the procedure. The instillation of the local anesthetic into the urethra is mildly painful until the tissue becomes numb. When the bladder is filled with saline, discomfort and the urge to void are normal sensations.

Assist with the collection of specimens.

The biopsy tissue is placed in a sterile glass container with formalin preservative. For the cytologic study, 50 to 75 mL of bladder irrigation fluid is placed in a sterile jar with 50% alcohol as a preservative.

Assist with the collection of urine specimens and mark their source (bladder, right ureter, left ureter).

### Posttest

Take vital signs and record the results. For patients who have undergone general anesthesia, continue monitoring the vital signs every 15 to 30 minutes until the patient is stable.

Assess for pain or bladder spasms and medicate as needed.

Encourage extra oral fluids to promote adequate hydration and the voiding of urine.

Instruct the patient to void within 8 hours after the test. Notify the physician if the patient is unable to void within this time.

Reassure the patient that it is normal to have a burning sensation on voiding and to see a small amount of blood or pink-tinged urine. These problems usually disappear after the third voiding.

At home, warm tub baths can help alleviate the discomfort or pain of bladder spasms. Instruct the patient to avoid alcohol for 48 hours because of its irritant effect on the bladder mucosa.

To prevent infection, instruct the patient to take the prescribed antibiotic as ordered.

**Complications**

The more common complications of cystoscopy are persistent bleeding, infection, and urinary retention. Because the patient usually goes home soon after the test, a review of abnormal problems should be provided, and the patient should be advised to notify the urologist when these problems occur. The complications of cystoscopy are presented in Table 21–4.

## Intravenous Pyelogram

**(Radiography)**  Synonyms: IVP, excretory urogram, EUG, intravenous urography, IVU, IUG

| Normal Values | No anatomic or physiologic abnormalities are noted in the kidneys, ureters, or bladder. |
| --- | --- |

### Background Information

The intravenous pyelogram is a basic urologic procedure that uses contrast medium and radiography to visualize the anatomy and function of the urinary tract. The intravenous contrast material is filtered from the blood by the kidneys. The x-ray films demonstrate the contrast medium entering the renal pelvis of each kidney and then flowing through the ureters and into the bladder (Fig. 21–3).

When a time delay occurs before the injected contrast medium reaches the renal pelvis, the delay is an indication of prerenal vascular obstruction or poor renal function. The x-ray films also demonstrate abnormalities of position, shape, size, or structure of the organs of the urinary tract. Clear detail and precise location of a stricture, dilation, calculus, obstruction, tumor, or filling defect can be seen.

The intravenous pyelogram is being replaced by CT, ultrasound, and digital subtraction angiography. The contrast medium used in an intravenous pyelogram can be toxic to the kidneys or can cause an allergic type of reaction that can be severe, so alternative methods are replacing this procedure.

### Purpose of the Test

The intravenous pyelogram is used to evaluate the structure and function of the kidneys, ureters, and bladder. It assesses the cause of nontraumatic hematuria, locates the precise site of obstruction, and investigates the cause of flank pain or renal colic.

### Table 21–4   Complications of Cystoscopy

| Complication | Nursing Assessment |
| --- | --- |
| Bleeding | Persistent, painless hematuria<br>Bright red urine<br>Passage of blood clots |
| Urinary obstruction | Inability to urinate within 8 hr despite a full bladder and desire to void |
| Infection | Flank or abdominal pain<br>Chills<br>Fever<br>Pyuria |

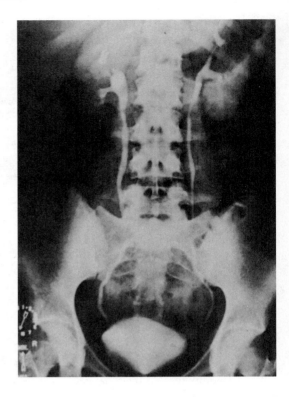

**Figure 21–3**
Intravenous pyelogram (IVP). The calices of the kidneys, ureters, and bladder appear white because of the use of contrast medium. (Reproduced with permission from Thompson, M. A. [1994]. *Principles of imaging science and protection* [Vol. 2, Slide 291A]. Philadelphia: W. B. Saunders.)

| | |
|---|---|
| **Procedure** | A initial x-ray film is taken to provide baseline information. After an intravenous injection of contrast material, timed radiographs are taken of the urinary tract. Films at 1 minute visualize the kidneys; at 3 to 5 minutes, the renal collecting system is visualized; at 10 minutes, the ureters are seen; and at 20 to 30 minutes, filling of the bladder is seen. A postvoiding film demonstrates the ability of the bladder to empty. The test requires 1 to 1½ hours to complete. |

**Findings**

**Abnormal Values**

| | | |
|---|---|---|
| Hydronephrosis | Tumor | Nonfunctioning |
| Renal or ureteral calculi | Pyelonephritis | kidney |
| Hydroureter | Renal tuberculosis | |
| Polycystic kidney disease | Absent kidney | |
| | Congenital anomalies | |

**Interfering Factors**

- Renal failure
- Feces, gas, or barium in the colon
- Recent gallbladder series
- Failure to maintain nothing-by-mouth status

**Nursing Implementation**

### Pretest

Ask the patient about any history of allergy to shellfish or iodine or of a previous reaction to an x-ray study that used contrast medium.

Schedule the intravenous pyelogram for before any barium test or gallbladder series that also uses iodinated contrast material.

Ensure that a signed informed consent form has been obtained from the patient or the person legally designated to make health care decisions for the patient.

Instruct the patient regarding the pretest bowel cleansing procedure that removes gas and fecal matter. This includes taking the prescribed laxative or cathartic the night before the test and an enema or suppository on the morning of the test.

Instruct the patient to discontinue food intake for 8 hours before the test. Fluids are permitted.

### Quality Control

> Patients who are dehydrated are at high risk for the development of renal failure as a result of the toxic effect of the contrast medium on the kidney tissues. Assess and report indications of fluid deprivation.

Ensure that recent blood urea nitrogen and creatinine test results are posted in the chart. These tests help identify patients who are at risk and help determine a safe dose of contrast medium.

Record baseline vital signs.

### During the Test

Assist the patient as the contrast medium is administered. It is common for the patient to experience a brief burning sensation or a metallic taste in the mouth, or both.

Have an emesis basin within reach, because nausea and vomiting may occur.

### Posttest

Take the vital signs and record the results.

Continue the intravenous fluid replacement and encourage the patient to take oral fluids.

**Complications**

During the test, a small number of patients have a vasovagal response to the contrast material. Atropine is kept on hand to overcome this side effect. An allergic or anaphylactic response can occur immediately or hours later. This response varies from a rash and hives to acute respiratory distress. A mild reaction is treated with antihistamines or steroids. A severe reaction is treated with intravenous epinephrine and oxygen, with additional measures taken as needed. An emergency cart is maintained in the radiology suite at all times.

Patients with diabetes and preexisting renal disease may develop impaired renal function, which can occur from 1 to 4 days after the study is completed. Usually it is a transitory problem and the kidneys return to their baseline level of function. A summary of the complications of intravenous pyelography is presented in Table 21–5.

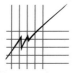

### Table 21–5 Complications of Intravenous Pyelography

| Complication | Nursing Assessment |
|---|---|
| Vasovagal response | Flushing |
| | Hypotension |
| | Bradycardia |
| Allergic-type reaction | Hives, rash |
| | Urticaria |
| | Flushing |
| | Hypotension |
| | Tachycardia |
| | Dyspnea |
| | Stridor |
| | Laryngospasm |
| Nephrotoxicity | Elevated blood urea nitrogen level |
| | Elevated creatinine |
| | Oliguria |

## Magnetic Resonance Imaging, Urinary Tract

**(Tomography)**      Synonym: MRI

Magnetic resonance imaging (MRI) produces a sharp image of the kidneys and can distinguish the renal cortex from the renal medulla. The vascular system can be imaged without the use of contrast material, and the staging of renal cell carcinoma is effective. Bladder tumors and their malignant extension into perivesicular fat or lymph nodes are shown clearly. MRI can distinguish benign from malignant growth in the prostate and can detect cancer invasion into seminal vesicles and pelvic lymph nodes.

A complete discussion of MRI is presented in Chapter 12.

## Plain X-Ray Film, Renal Tract

**(Radiography)**      Synonyms: KUB; kidney, ureter, bladder

The plain x-ray film of the renal tract is a basic radiologic film that demonstrates the size, shape, and position of the organs of the renal tract. It can identify enlargement of the kidneys, as in hydronephrosis or tumor growth, and shrinkage of the kidney from chronic pyelonephritis or renal ischemia. Visible calcifications include calculi of the kidney, ureter, or bladder; renal tuberculosis; renal tubular acidosis; and calcifications in the bladder wall and ureters from the *Schistosoma* parasite.

A complete discussion of radiography is presented in Chapter 9.

## Renal Scan

**(Radionuclide Imaging)**      Synonyms: None

The renal scan uses radionuclides to investigate renal failure and evaluate the function of the renal vascular system, the kidneys, and the ureters. The renal scan assesses the kidneys or the renal transplant for adequacy of renal blood flow, tissue perfusion, glomerular filtration, tubular excretion, and ureteral function.

The scan can demonstrate the prerenal disorders of renal artery stenosis or occlusion. Within the kidney, renal perfusion, glomerular filtration rates, and tubular transport rates can be semiquantified. Intrarenal disorders identified by the renal scan include acute tubular necrosis, glomerulonephritis, vasculitis, and acute interstitial nephritis. The scan also demonstrates postrenal problems, including obstruction of the ureter or ureters or ureterovesicular reflux.

A complete discussion of nuclear diagnostic tests is presented in Chapter 10.

## Retrograde Pyelography
**(Radiography)**                Synonyms: None

The retrograde pyelogram provides radiographic visualization of the bladder, ureters, and renal pelvis following the retrograde instillation of sterile contrast medium into the renal collecting system. Generally, this procedure is used during or after cystoscopy or to evaluate the placement of a ureteral stent or catheter.

In the past, the procedure was used to diagnose postrenal obstruction. It was also an alternative imaging procedure for when intravenous pyelography was not possible or when the intravenous pyelogram results were not clear. As a result of improvements in the contrast medium used in intravenous pyelography and the use of ultrasound, retrograde pyelography is used much less frequently. Retrograde pyelography carries the risk of urinary tract infection and sepsis.

## Ultrasound, Renal
**(Ultrasound)**                Synonyms: None

Renal ultrasound clearly defines the kidneys—their size, shape, position, collecting systems, and surrounding tissues. Renal masses greater than 2 cm are readily detected. Renal cysts are a frequent finding. The procedure also identifies the location and severity of obstruction. In addition to its diagnostic uses, renal ultrasound may be used as a guide for needle placement in renal biopsy, for drainage of a renal abscess, or for placement of a nephrostomy tube.

A complete discussion of ultrasound is presented in Chapter 8.

## Ultrasound, Transrectal
**(Ultrasound)**                Synonym: TRUS

Transrectal ultrasound is a procedure that positions the ultrasound instrument and its high-frequency transducer in the rectum. The sound wave echoes are converted into images of the prostate gland. One use of ultrasound is to differentiate malignant from benign prostatic disease.

Other uses of transrectal ultrasound include monitoring the size of the gland, staging prostate cancer, evaluating treatment, evaluating urodynamics, and providing a visual guide to the prostate gland during a prostate biopsy procedure.

A complete discussion of ultrasound is presented in Chapter 8.

## Uroflowmetry

**(Manometry)**                    Synonyms: None

| Normal Values | No anatomic or physiologic abnormalities are noted in the kidneys, ureters, or bladder. |
|---|---|

**Urine Volume**
66–80 years: ≥200 mL
46–65 years: ≥200 mL
14–45 years: ≥200 mL
8–13 years: ≥100 mL
4–7 years: ≥100 mL

**Flow Rate**
Male (66–80 years): 9 mL/sec
Female (66–80 years): 10 mL/sec
Male (46–65 years): 12 mL/sec
Female (46–65 years): 15 mL/sec
Male (14–45 years): 21 mL/sec
Female (14–45 years): 18 mL/sec
Male (8–13 years): 12 mL/sec
Female (8–13 years): 15 mL/sec
Male (4–7 years): 10 mL/sec
Female (4–7 years): 10 mL/sec

## Background Information

The broad category of urodynamic studies consists of several tests that evaluate voiding and lower urinary tract function. Uroflowmetry is the initial test that is performed to assess bladder and sphincter function. This test is generally ordered for patients with incontinence or retention of urine.

Urinary incontinence is the involuntary leakage of urine through the urethral meatus. When incontinence is defined by its symptomatology, the problem is called urge incontinence, stress incontinence, or total incontinence. When the incontinence is defined by its cause, the problem is one of bladder storage, bladder emptying, or urinary sphincter dysfunction. Urinary retention or obstruction may be classified as bladder or urethral dysfunction.

Determination of the urinary flow rate is a non-invasive procedure that provides measurable baseline data about the patient's ability to void. The data measure the volume of urine voided, the pattern of micturition, and the time and rate of voiding. The patient's data are compared with normal micturition patterns and numeric values of the flow rate. When the patient's values are higher than normal, the problem is one of incontinence. When the patient's values are lower than normal, the problem is one of impaired urinary flow.

In any person, the urinary flow rate varies with the volume of urine that is voided. The patient's results are compared with normal values based on the volume voided. The flow rate of any individual also varies from one voiding episode to another. The uroflowmetry test is repeated several times to obtain reliable data. Additionally, normal voiding rates vary between males and females and among different age groups across the life span. The interpretation of the patient's values is age specific and gender specific.

| | |
|---|---|
| **Purpose of the Test** | Uroflowmetry is used to help evaluate lower urinary tract dysfunction. |

**Procedure**

The patient urinates into a toilet that is equipped with a funnel and uroflowmeter. As voiding activates the uroflowmeter and its transducer, electronic data are received, transmitted, analyzed, and recorded. Specific variations in the procedure are based on differences in manufacturers' equipment and laboratory protocol. The total time for completion of the test is 10 to 15 minutes.

**Findings**

**Elevated Values**

Conditions that cause reduced urethral resistance

Incontinence (stress, urge, or total)

**Decreased Values**

Urethral or bladder neck obstruction
Poor muscular contraction of the bladder

**Interfering Factors**

- Body movement during voiding
- Toilet tissue in the apparatus
- Straining during urination

**Nursing Implementation**

■

*Critical Thinking 21–6*
Twice your adult patient having a uroflowmetric test done has discarded the toilet paper into the collection container. You explained the procedure twice to the patient. What should you do?

**Pretest**

Instruct the patient to drink fluids and refrain from voiding for several hours before the test.
Ensure the patient's privacy for the test. The bathroom contains a toilet with the uroflowmeter installed in it.
Instruct the patient to void into the urometer funnel without straining or body movement. No toilet tissue should be discarded into the funnel or collection container.

**Posttest**

No specific patient instruction or intervention is needed.

**References**

Agrawal, B., Berger, A., Wolf, K., & Luft F. C. (1996). Microalbuminuria screening by reagent strip predicts cardiovascular risk in hypertension. *Journal of Hypertension, 14,* 223–228.
Albin, R. J. (1996). New PSA test eliminates biopsy for BPH patients. *Medical Laboratory Observer, 28,* 10, 12.
Alzaid, A. A. (1996). Microalbuminuria in patients with NIDDM: An overview. *Diabetes Care, 19,* 79–86.

Anderson, J. R., Strickland, D., Corbin, D., Byrnes, J. A., & Zweiback, E. (1995). Age-specific reference ranges for serum prostate-specific antigen. *Urology, 46,* 54–57.
Arroyo, A. J., Burns, J. B., & Patel, Y. P. (1996). Derived GFR (dGFR) values from Technetium-99m-MAG3 data: A comparison with the 24-hour creatinine clearance. *Journal of Nuclear Medicine Technology, 24,* 223–226.

Baer, D. M. (1996). Urinary calculi. *Medical Laboratory Observer, 28,* 15–16.

Bowe, K. (1995). Phenylketonia: An update for pediatric community health nurses. *Pediatric Nursing, 21,* 191–194.

Brunzel, N. A. (1994). *Fundamentals of urine and body fluid analysis.* Philadelphia: W. B. Saunders.

Clochesy, J. M., Breu, C., Cardin, S., Whittaker, A. A., & Rudy, E. B. (1996). *Critical care nursing* (2nd ed.). Philadelphia: W. B. Saunders.

Cronan, J. J. (1996). Percutaneous biopsy. *Radiologic Clinics of North America, 34,* 1207–1223.

Diefenbach, P. N., Ganz, P. A., Pawlow, A. J., & Gutrie, D. (1996). Screening by the prostate-specific antigen test: What do the patients know? *Journal of Cancer Education, 11,* 39–44.

Fastbom, J., Wills, P., Cornelius, C., Viitanen, M., & Winblad, B., (1996). Levels of serum creatine and estimated creatinine clearance over the age of 75: A study of an elderly Swedish population. *Archives of Gerontology and Genetics, 23,* 179–188.

Feinfeld, D. A., Guzik, H., Carvounis, C. P., Lynn, R. I., Somer, B., Aronson, M. K., & Frishman, W. H. (1995). Sequential changes in renal function test in the old old: Results from the Bronx longitudinal aging study. *Journal of the American Geriatrics Society, 43,* 412–414.

Fleming, M. (1996). Automated microalbumin assay using the Abbott Spectrum. *Laboratory Medicine, 27,* 339–341.

Frizzell, J. (1998). Avoiding lab test pitfalls. *American Journal of Nursing, 98,* 34–37.

Hadeed, V., & Trump, D. J. (1996). Prostate cancer: Update on the why, when, and how of screening. *Consultant, 36,* 2036–2047.

Henry, J. B. (1996). *Clinical diagnosis and management by laboratory methods* (20th ed.). Philadelphia: W. B. Saunders.

Lehmann, C. A. (Ed.) (1998). *Saunders manual of clinical laboratory science.* Philadelphia: W. B. Saunders.

McLeary, R. D. (1995). Transrectal ultrasound of the prostate. *Applied Radiology, 24,* 13–18.

Mercader, V. P., Gatenby, R. A., & Curtis, B. R. (1996). Radiographic assessment of genitourinary trauma. *Trauma Quarterly, 13,* 129–151.

Middleton, M. L., & Blaufox, M. D. (1996). Renal scintigraphy: Practical applications. *Applied Radiology, 25,* 6–17.

Morton, K. A., Pisani, D. E., Whiting, J. H., Cheung, A. K., Arias, J. M., & Valdivia, S. (1997). Determination of glomerular filtration rate using technetium-99m-DTPA with differing degrees of renal function. *Journal of Nuclear Medicine Technology, 25,* 110–114.

Newman, J. (1996). Epidemiology, diagnosis and treatment of prostate cancer. *Radiographic Technology, 68,* 39–68.

Niskanen, L. K., Penttila, K., Parviainen, M., & Uusitupa, M. J. (1996). Evolution, risk factors, and prognostic implications of albuminuria in NIDDM. *Diabetes Care, 19,* 486–492.

Ouslander, J. G., Schapirs, M., & Schnelle, J. F. (1995). Urine specimen collection from incontinent female nursing home residents. *Journal of the American Geriatrics Society, 43,* 279–281.

Riley, M. D., & Dwyer, T. (1998). Microalbuminuria is positively associated with usual dietary saturated fat intake and negatively associated with usual dietary protein intake in people with insulin-dependent diabetes mellitus. *American Journal of Clinical Nutrition, 67,* 50–57.

Savage, S., Estacio, R., Jeffers, B., & Schrier, R. W. (1996). Urinary albumin excretion as a predictor of diabetic retinopathy, neuropathy, and cardiovascular disease in NIDDM. *Diabetes Care, 19,* 1243–1247.

Speicher, C. E. (1998). *The right test* (3rd ed.). Philadelphia: W. B. Saunders.

Statland, E. (1996). PSA reference values. *Medical Laboratory Observer, 28,* 16–17.

Thelan, L. A., Urden, L. D., Lough, M. E., & Stacy, K. M. (1998). *Critical care nursing diagnosis and management.* St. Louis: Mosby.

Tietz, N. W. (Ed.) (1995). *Clinical guide to laboratory tests.* Philadelphia: W. B. Saunders.

Waldman, A. R., & Osborne, D. M. (1994). Screening for prostate cancer. *Oncology Nursing Forum, 21,* 1512–1517.

Zauderer, B. (1996). Age-related changes in renal function. *Critical Care Nursing Quarterly, 19,* 34–40.

# CHAPTER 22

# Reproductive Function

This chapter addresses the tests that are related to reproduction and childbearing. The span of diagnostic tests is extensive. Some are measurements of sexual maturation, and others are assessments that are performed before conception, during pregnancy, during labor, or after delivery. Also included are diagnostic tests and procedures that investigate infertility, genetic alteration, hormonal imbalance, the effects of aging, and malignancy of the reproductive organs.

Patients who undergo tests that are related to reproduction represent the entire spectrum of the human life span. Because of new prenatal technology in diagnostic testing and treatment, the embryo and fetus can also be tested.

The development of new diagnostic technologies and the expanded understanding of genetics have increased our knowledge and ability to identify causes of prenatal risk. Laboratory tests that are performed on cord blood provide direct diagnostic data about the fetus itself. This allows intervention and treatment at a much earlier stage of gestation than was possible in the past.

A number of the diagnostic tests and procedures include genetic analysis of the parents and family. The analyses may be performed before or after conception. The blood of the developing fetus also may be examined to detect an inherited or acquired genetic abnormality that could adversely affect growth and development. The results of genetic testing provide knowledge, but they do not always provide certainty about the eventual outcome and health status of the offspring.

Knowledge about the future can be a blessing for the prospective parents, but it can also create a painful burden or a serious dilemma for them. Prenatal diagnostic technology promotes pregnancy outcomes based on "choice, rather than chance." The diagnostic knowledge forces the prospective parents to make conscious, rational decisions and influences the path of life of the fetus (Satish, 1992).

The rapid advances in diagnostic testing also create ethical and legal dilemmas. Some of the advances are powerful enough to create eventual changes within society itself. In nursing, these advances also create changes in professional practice. The need for the nurse's knowledge of the new diagnostic technologies to grow is ongoing. The nurse must also understand the implications of the findings for the patient.

During the period of diagnostic testing, the patient can experience anxiety. The fears are often related to the possible results of the tests and may also be related to the risk of the tests, such as potential harm to the pregnancy or to the fetus.

The patient may express feelings of depression, irritability, invasion of privacy, personal inadequacy, or even failure. The tests are often expensive and multiple, causing varying degrees of financial strain. The interaction between the nurse and the patient can help alleviate the stress, correct misconceptions, and provide empathetic support as the patient makes decisions about treatment, the continuation or termination of the pregnancy, or the future health care needs of the child.

## Laboratory Tests

## Alpha$_1$-Fetoprotein, Serum

**(Serum)**                    Synonyms: Maternal serum alpha-fetoprotein, MSAFP

**Normal Values**

**Pregnancy (Median Values)**
14th week: 25.6 ng/mL *or* 25.6 µg/L
15th week: 29.9 ng/mL *or* 29.9 µg/L
16th week: 34.8 ng/mL *or* 34.8 µg/L
17th week: 40.6 ng/mL *or* 40.6 µg/L
18th week: 47.3 ng/mL *or* 47.3 µg/L
19th week: 55.1 ng/mL *or* 55.1 µg/L
20th week: 64.3 ng/mL *or* 64.3 µg/L
21st week: 74.9 ng/mL *or* 74.9 µg/L

## Background Information

In the pregnant female, alpha$_1$-fetoprotein (AFP) testing is used for intrauterine screening, optimally in the 16th to 18th weeks of pregnancy. Abnormally elevated serum and amniotic fluid values are often present in cases of open neural tube defects, which include spina bifida, myelomeningocele, omphalocele, esophageal atresia, duodenal atresia, and anencephaly. Other abnormalities of the fetus may also cause an elevation of AFP. The causes of abnormally decreased values during pregnancy include Down syndrome, trisomy 18, fetal death, spontaneous abortion, and molar pregnancy.

When the serum value is greater than two times the median value, the patient is considered to have additional risk. Additional testing by ultrasound is done to verify fetal malformation, multiple gestation, or an incorrect estimation of gestational age (Rose & Mennuti, 1993). The elevated serum test value can be a false-positive result, particularly if an incorrect maternal weight or gestational age is factored into the interpretation of the result. A

follow-up amniocentesis is recommended for patients who have an ultrasound result that does not explain the abnormal AFP value.

In addition to the high rate of false-positive results, the maternal serum alpha$_1$-fetoprotein test cannot detect closed types of neural tube defects, such as hydrocephalus. Despite these limitations, the test is used for screening of pregnancies because it is an early indicator of open neural tube defects, Down syndrome, and other conditions caused by chromosomal disorder in the fetus (Green & Statham, 1993).

A borderline or abnormal maternal serum alpha$_1$-fetoprotein test result creates strong feelings of anxiety and worry for the expectant parents. They may have to face the issue of termination of the pregnancy. Doubt, uncertainty, grief, anxiety, fear for their baby, or consideration of an abortion can all be sources of stress or conflict. In addition, the meaning of this pregnancy can be altered for the couple, and worry about the development of the fetus can continue even after follow-up testing reveals normal results (Santalahti, Latikka, Ryynanen, et al., 1996).

Once the abnormal test result is known and the mother or parents consider follow-up testing, the nurse can provide psychological support and serve as a family educator and advo-cate. The nurse can also help the family understand the meaning of the results, including the benefits and limitations of this screening test (Coving-ton, Gieleghem, Madison, et al., 1996).

A complete discussion of this test is presented in Chapter 19.

## Androstenedione

**(Serum)**    Synonyms: None

**Normal Values**

**Adult**
   Male: 75–205 ng/dL *or* SI 2.6–7.2 nmol/L
   Female: 85–275 ng/dL *or* SI 3–9.6 nmol/L
**Child**
   10–17 years: 8–240 ng/dL *or* SI 0.3–8.4 nmol/L
   1–10 years: 8–50 ng/dL *or* SI 0.3–1.7 nmol/L
   1–12 months: 6–68 ng/dL *or* SI 0.2–2.4 nmol/L
**Newborn:** 20–290 ng/dL *or* SI 0.7–10.1 nmol/L

## Background Information

Androstenedione is an androgen precursor hormone that converts to testosterone in the male and to estrogens in the female. It is synthesized by the adrenal cortex in males and females and is also synthesized in the ovaries of females. In normal physiology, the level of the hormone rises sharply after puberty and peaks in the young adult. After menopause, the level decreases abruptly in women. The hormone has a diurnal pattern and peaks in the blood level at about 7 AM, with the lowest blood level occurring at 4 PM each day.

The hirsute female experiences excessive growth of body hair, similar to the hair distribution of the male. An elevated level of androstenedione may be the cause of this virilization.

## Purpose of the Test

This test may be used to evaluate androgen production in the hirsute female. It also may be used to identify the cause of gonadal impairment, menstrual irregularity, and premature sexual development.

## Procedure

A red-topped tube is used to collect 10 mL of venous blood.

## Findings

**Elevated Values**

| | | |
|---|---|---|
| Cushing's syndrome | Gynecomastia (in males) | Premature sexual development |
| Congenital adrenal hyperplasia | Ovarian hyperplasia | Osteoporosis |
| Adrenal tumor | Stein-Leventhal syndrome | Hirsutism |
| Ovarian tumor | Endometriosis | Testicular tumor |
| Polycystic ovaries | | |

### Decreased Values

| | | |
|---|---|---|
| Sickle cell anemia | Ovarian failure | Adrenal failure |

---

**Interfering Factors**

- Menstruation
- Recent radioactive isotope scan

---

**Nursing Implementation**　Nursing care includes care of the venipuncture site.

### Pretest

For the menstruating female, schedule the test for at least 1 week before or 1 week after menstruation. For all patients, schedule this test for before a nuclear scan, because the radioisotopes of the scan would interfere with the method of laboratory analysis.

Instruct the patient that it is preferable to fast from food and fluids for 8 hours before the test (Jacobs et al., 1996).

The blood should be drawn early in the morning (7 AM) because of the diurnal rhythm of the hormone.

### Posttest

Place the specimen on ice and arrange for prompt transport to the laboratory.

The laboratory analysis should be performed within 1 hour. If a delay occurs in the laboratory, the serum must be frozen.

---

**Critical Value**

>1,000 ng/dL *or* SI >34.9 nmol/L

This extreme level suggests diagnosis of a virilizing tumor. Notify the physician of this elevated result.

---

## Cancer Antigen 125
**(Serum, Body Fluids)**　Synonym: CA 125

---

**Normal Values**

<35 U/mL *or* SI <35 kU/L

---

## Background Information

Cancer antigen 125 (CA 125) is a tumor marker for ovarian cancer. The serum antigen is produced by the genes of malignant cells and normal endometrial and uterine tissue. The antigen has a minimal presence in the blood and body fluids unless these tissues are destroyed and the antigen is released from the cells. The antigen can be detected by laboratory radioimmunoassay methodology.

A variety of different malignant and benign disorders cause a rise in cancer antigen 125. The level rises in the first trimester of pregnancy, during menstruation, and in some nonmalignant disorders. It also rises in gynecologic malignancy and in metastatic disease of a nongynecologic origin. Also, cancer antigen 125 testing may not detect ovarian cancer at an early stage of growth (Held, 1996).

Because of the variables that can result in false-positive results and a failure to detect the onset of the tumor, cancer antigen 125 testing cannot be used to screen for ovarian cancer (Carlson, Skates, & Singer, 1994).

Despite the problems with sensitivity and reliability that prevent its use for screening, cancer antigen 125 testing is valuable in selected situations. A serum value greater than 35 kU/mL (SI >35 kU/L) is positive and correlates with malignancy. Further diagnostic testing is needed. A persistently rising cancer antigen 125 value may be associated with advancing malignancy, particularly advanced ovarian cancer. Conversely, in the patient with known ovarian cancer, a decline in the cancer antigen 125 value indicates a good response to treatment.

In cases of suspected malignancy in the abdominal or pleural cavity, the body fluid obtained during paracentesis or thoracentesis may be analyzed for cancer antigen 125. The malignant cells of cancers of the pancreas and lung release this antigen into the fluid of the body cavity.

## Purpose of the Test

The serum cancer antigen 125 level determination is used to monitor the progress of disease in patients with ovarian cancer after the surgical removal of a tumor. The analysis of body fluids for cancer antigen 125 helps diagnose metastasis to an organ in the body cavity.

## Procedure

**Serum.**  A red-topped tube with a serum separator is used to collect 10 mL of venous blood.

**Body Fluid.**  During the aspiration procedure, some of the body fluid is collected in three sterile tubes (with red, green, and lavender tops). Because a series of tests will be performed on the specimens, sufficient fluid must be available. Two of the tubes contain anticoagulant to prevent clotting by fibrinogen.

## Findings

**Elevated Values**

| | | |
|---|---|---|
| Ovarian cancer | Adenocarcinoma of | Pregnancy |
| Adenocarcinoma of | the lung, colon, | Endometriosis |
| the cervix, endo- | pancreas, or breast | Menstruation |
| metrium, or | Acute pelvic inflam- | Ovarian-tubal abscess |
| fallopian tubes | matory disease | |

## Interfering Factors

- Inadequate specimen identification
- Recent radioactive isotope scan

## Nursing Implementation

For the serum test, nursing care includes care of the venipuncture site.

### Pretest

Schedule this test for before or at least 7 days after any radioimmunoassay scan. The radioisotopes of the scan would interfere with the radioimmunoassay method of analysis.

If this test is to be performed on a body fluid sample obtained by thoracentesis or paracentesis, follow the nursing care procedures described in Chapters 14 and 19 of this text.

For the patient with a history of cancer, provide empathetic support. Her anxiety level is likely to be high because of the implications of a potentially elevated test result.

### Posttest

Before leaving the patient's bedside or the treatment table, ensure that the specimen tubes are correctly identified. When the specimen is a body fluid, ensure that the source of the fluid (thoracentesis or paracentesis fluid) is written on the requisition slip.

Arrange for prompt transport of the specimen to the laboratory.

When the patient with a known history of ovarian cancer has a rising or elevated level of cancer antigen 125, a high probability exists that the cause is progression or recurrence of the malignancy. Before new treatment is instituted, additional diagnostic testing (including surgery or biopsy, or both) to examine abnormal tissue is indicated (Jacobs et al., 1996). Provide additional emotional support to help the patient cope during the stress of additional testing and in the decision making that is part of the overall treatment plan.

| **Critical Value** | **>65 kU/mL *or* SI >65 kU/L** |
| --- | --- |
| | Ninety percent of patients with a pelvic mass and a serum value at this level have a pelvic malignancy (Jacobs et al., 1996). Alert the physician of this extreme elevation. |

## Estradiol, Serum

**(Serum)**                    Synonym: $E_2$

| **Normal Values** | **Adult** |
| --- | --- |
| | Premenopausal female: 30–400 pg/mL *or* SI 110–1,468 pmol/L |
| | Postmenopausal female: 0–30 pg/mL *or* SI 0–110 pmol/L |
| | Male: 10–50 pg/mL *or* SI 37–184 pmol/L |

### Background Information

The ovaries, testes, and placenta are capable of the biosynthesis of all steroids, including the sex hormones. Estradiol is the most potent of the estrogen hormones. Estradiol is secreted by the ovaries in the female, and it is produced by the testes in the male. The estradiol level is sharply decreased or absent in postmenopausal women.

### Purpose of the Test

The measurement of serum estradiol aids in the analysis and evaluation of female infertility, menstrual irregularity, amenorrhea, or sexual precocity in the child. In the male, this test may be used to help evaluate a feminizing condition.

| **Procedure** | A red-topped tube is used to collect 10 mL of venous blood. |
|---|---|

| **Findings** | **Elevated Values** |
|---|---|

Polycystic ovary            Gynecomastia
Adrenal tumor               Hepatic cirrhosis
Ovarian neoplasm or         Hyperthyroidism
  tumor

**Decreased Values**

Anorexia nervosa            Ovarian hypo-
Amenorrhea                    function
Ovarian dysfunction

| **Interfering Factors** | • Recent radioactive isotope scan |
|---|---|

| **Nursing Implementation** | Nursing care includes care of the venipuncture site. |
|---|---|

**Pretest**

■
*Critical Thinking 22–1*
Your patient has started her infertility work-up. She expresses
feelings of sadness because of
the inability to conceive. What
assessment findings would validate a nursing diagnosis of situational low self-esteem?

Schedule this test for before or at least 7 days after a radioimmunoassay scan. The radioisotopes of the scan would interfere with the radioimmunoassay method of analysis.

**Posttest**

To assist in the correct interpretation of the results, include the patient's age, the phase of menstrual cycle, and the time that the test specimen was obtained.

Arrange for prompt transport of the specimen to the laboratory.

## Estriol, Pregnancy
**(Serum, Urine)**

Synonyms: $E_3$; total serum estriol, pregnancy; total urine estriol, pregnancy

| **Normal Values** | **Serum** (Tietz, 1995) |
|---|---|

28–30 weeks of gestation: 38–140 ng/mL *or* SI 132–486 nmol/L
32–34 weeks of gestation: 35–260 ng/mL *or* SI 121–902 nmol/L
36–38 weeks of gestation: 48–570 ng/mL *or* SI 167–1,978 nmol/L
40 weeks of gestation: 95–460 ng/mL *or* SI 330–1,596 nmol/L
**Urine** (Tietz, 1995)
First trimester of pregnancy: 0–800 μg/24 hr *or* SI 0–2,776 nmol/24 hr
Second trimester of pregnancy: 800–12,000 μg/24 hr *or* SI 2,776–41,640 nmol/24 hr
Third trimester of pregnancy: 5,000–50,000 μg/24 hr *or* SI 17,350–173,500 nmol/24 hr

## Background Information

During pregnancy, estriol is the predominant estrogen present in the serum and urine. Because this hormone is synthesized by the placenta, the serum and urine values are considered a measure of the integrity and well-being of the fetal-placental-maternal unit. Because the normal serum values vary greatly according to the test methodology used, the nurse uses the reference values provided by the laboratory that performed the test.

Because serum levels rise progressively during a normal pregnancy, the number of weeks of gestation is a necessary consideration in the interpretation of the test result. The serum level of estriol also fluctuates in a diurnal rhythm, with the highest value occurring at midday. To increase

the reliability of the test results, each test specimen is drawn at the same time of day. Because of the fluctuations in values, no single test specimen is used for interpretation. Instead, a series of test values are used to calculate the average test result.

When the serial test results are declining or are at a lower-than-normal level, the fetus is considered to be in danger. Immediate further investigation of the status of fetal health is indicated. This is particularly true in the high-risk pregnancy. Because alternative tests and technologic procedures are available that are better able to visualize the fetus or monitor for fetal distress, this test may not be used in most facilities.

| | |
|---|---|
| **Purpose of the Test** | In the later stages of pregnancy, the results of the serial estriol test are used to evaluate fetal well-being and placental function, especially in the high-risk pregnancy. |

| | |
|---|---|
| **Procedure** | **Serum.**   A red- or green-topped tube is used to obtain 5 to 7 mL of venous blood from the pregnant female.<br>**Urine.**   A special laboratory container is used to collect a 24-hour specimen. |

**Findings**

**Decreased Values**

| | | |
|---|---|---|
| Diabetes mellitus | Preeclampsia | Hemoglobinopathy |
| Fetal growth retardation | Fetal adrenal aplasia | |
| Postmaturity | Erythroblastosis fetalis | |
| Fetal encephalopathy | Intrauterine death | |

**Interfering Factors**

- Recent radioisotope scan
- Improper urine collection procedure
- Failure to collect all the urine of the test period
- Failure to refrigerate the urine specimen
- Improper labeling

**Nursing Implementation**   For the serum test, nursing care includes care of the venipuncture site.

### Pretest

#### Urine Collection

Provide both written and verbal instructions regarding the collection of the urine. These instructions must include the specific times for the collection period.

### During the Test

The first voided specimen of the morning is discarded, and the urine collection period begins at 8 AM.

The patient places all urine for 24 hours into the container. This includes the first voided specimen of the next morning.

Keep the specimen and container on ice or refrigerated during the collection period. This prevents deterioration of the urine.

During the collection period, all urine is added to the container. If any urine spills or if a specimen is discarded accidentally, the test is invalidated. The stored specimen is discarded, and a new collection period is started on the following day.

### Posttest

#### Serum and Urine

Label the urine container (not the lid) with the patient's name and other appropriate identifying data. Include the time and date of the start and completion of the urine collection period.

Include the weeks of gestation on the requisition slip of each test.

Arrange for prompt delivery of the specimen to the laboratory.

#### Quality Control

> For the serum specimen, the cells must be separated from the serum and the serum frozen immediately. The urine specimen must be refrigerated continuously until the urine is analyzed.

---

**Critical Values (Urine)**

**<4 mg/24 hr or 40% below the average result of the last three values**

Fetal well-being is at risk. Immediate evaluation of the status of the mother and the fetus is indicated.

---

## Estrogen-Progesterone Receptor Assay

**(Tissue Biopsy)**     Synonym: ER-PgR

---

**Normal Values**

Negative: <3 fmol/mg of cytosol protein *or* SI <3 nmol/kg of cytosol protein
Borderline: 3–10 fmol/mg of cytosol protein *or* SI 3–10 nmol/kg of cytosol protein
Positive: >10 fmol/mg of cytosol protein *or* SI >10 nmol/kg of cytosol protein

## Background Information

The biopsy specimen of malignant breast tissue is tested to identify the presence of estrogen receptor sites and progesterone receptor sites. Although the name of the assay is written as a single entity, the tests are actually two different assays. One is for estrogen, and the other is for progesterone. Generally, both tests are performed on the tissue sample to provide the most complete information regarding the potential effectiveness of hormonal therapy on the malignant tumor.

When the results of the estrogen receptor assay or of both the estrogen and the progesterone assays are positive, the tumor is likely to respond to androgen therapy or tamoxifen as a supplemental or palliative method of treatment. In each test, a value greater than 100 fmol/mg of cytosol protein (SI >100 nmol/kg of cytosol protein) is considered strongly positive and has the best potential for an effective treatment result. The laboratory term *fmol/mg of cytosol protein* or its SI equivalent is the measurement of the binding capacity of the protein that is present at the receptor sites. The test results are usually available 1 week after the biopsy is performed.

| | |
|---|---|
| **Purpose of the Test** | The assay is used to identify primary or metastatic tumors of the breast that would respond favorably to hormonal therapy. |
| **Procedure** | A biopsy specimen of abnormal breast tissue is obtained and placed in a jar or waxed cardboard container. This jar or container is placed immediately in a larger container with ice. |
| **Findings** | **Positive Values** <br><br> Breast cancer that may respond to hormonal therapy |
| **Interfering Factors** | • Use of a fixative on the tissue specimen <br> • Delay in transport of the specimen <br> • Inadequate tissue specimen <br> • Warming of the specimen |
| **Nursing Implementation** | **Pretest** <br><br> The pretest preparation of the patient is presented in the section on breast biopsy in this chapter. <br> If the patient receives hormonal therapy for contraception, menopausal therapy, or antiestrogen therapy, these hormones should be discontinued before the breast biopsy is performed. <br> On the requisition slip, identify the source and site of the tissue (left or right breast). <br><br> **During the Test** <br><br> Ensure that no preservative is used on the specimen. Place the container with the specimen on ice. |

Deliver the specimen to the pathologist present in the operating suite, or have the specimen sent to the laboratory. The specimen is sent as soon as it is obtained, without waiting for closure of the incision or completion of the biopsy procedure.

### Quality Control

> The specimen must be prepared for frozen section within 15 to 30 minutes to prevent deterioration of the proteins at the receptor sites.

### Posttest

The posttest nursing care consists of postoperative care for the patient with a breast biopsy.

## Estrogens, 24-Hour Urine

(Urine)  Synonym: Total urinary estrogens

**Normal Values**

Postmenopausal female: <20 µg/24 hr *or* SI 69 µmol/24 hr
Premenopausal female: 15–80 µg/24 hr *or* SI 52–277 µmol/24 hr
Male: 15–40 µg/24 hr *or* SI 52–139 µmol/24 hr
Child: <10 µg/24 hr *or* SI <35 µmol/24 hr

### Background Information

The ovaries, placenta, testes, and adrenal glands are capable of the biosynthesis of all steroids, including the sex hormones. The liver and many other organs metabolize and conjugate estrogen. Ultimately, the conjugated forms of estrogen are excreted in the urine or feces. Estradiol, estrone, and estriol are three estrogen hormones measured in the total urinary estrogen test. The amount and composition of the estrogens varies between the sexes and among age groups, based on differences in physiologic function.

In the nonpregnant female, estradiol is the most potent estrogen, and it is secreted from the follicular fluid of the ovaries. Most estrone is produced by conversion of the adrenal steroidal hormone, but some is secreted from the ovaries or is converted from estriol. The amount of estrogen fluctuates during the menstrual cycle. The highest level occurs during the ovulation cycle. In pregnancy, estriol is produced by the fetal-placental unit.

The postmenopausal woman produces a lower amount of total estrogen because of the decreased estrogen secretion from the ovaries. The primary source of this woman's estrogen is the conversion of adrenal hormone to estrone. The testes of the male also produce some estrogen in the form of estradiol and some estrone.

### Purpose of the Test

The measurement of urinary estrogen is used to evaluate ovarian function, predict ovulation, determine the cause of amenorrhea, evaluate excess or decreased estrogen conditions, and help diagnose a testicular tumor.

### Procedure

A special plastic collection bottle with a boric acid preservative is used to collect all urine for a 24-hour period.

| **Findings** | **Elevated Values** | | |
|---|---|---|---|
| | NONPREGNANT FEMALE | | |
| | Ovarian tumor<br>Adrenocortical tumor | Adrenocortical<br>hyperplasia | |
| | MALE | | |
| | Testicular tumor | | |
| | **Decreased Values** | | |
| | Ovarian dysfunction<br>Pituitary gland<br>hypofunction | Ovarian insufficiency<br>Adrenal gland<br>hypofunction | Menopause<br>Anorexia nervosa |

| **Interfering Factors** | • Improper storage of the specimen<br>• Incomplete collection of the urine |
|---|---|

**Nursing Implementation**

**Pretest**

Provide both written and verbal instructions regarding the collection of urine. These instructions must include the specific times for the collection period.

**During the Test**

The first voided specimen of the morning is discarded, and the urine collection period begins at 8 AM.

All urine for a 24-hour period is placed in the container. This includes the first voided specimen of the next morning.

To prevent deterioration, maintain the specimen and container on ice or refrigerated during the collection period.

During the time period, all urine is added to the collection container. If any urine spills, or if a specimen is discarded accidentally, the test is invalidated.

**Posttest**

Label the urine container (not the lid) with the patient's name and other appropriate identifying data. Include the time and date of the start and completion of the urine collection period.

For the pregnant woman, include the weeks of gestation on the requisition slip. For all patients, include the patient's sex and age on the requisition slip.

Arrange for prompt delivery of the specimen to the laboratory.

## Follicle-Stimulating Hormone

(Serum, Urine)                 Synonyms: FSH, follitropin

**Normal Values**

**Serum (adult male):** 1.42–15.4 mLU/mL *or* SI 1.42–15.4 IU/L
**Serum (Adult Female)**
Follicular phase: 1.37–9.9 mLU/mL *or* SI 1.37–9.9 IU/L

Ovulatory peak: 6.17–17.2 mLU/mL *or* SI 6.17–17.2 IU/L
Luteal phase: 1.09–9.2 mLU/mL *or* 1.09–9.2 IU/L
Postmenopausal phase: 19.3–100.6 mLU/mL *or* SI 19.3–100.6 IU/L
**Serum (Child 1–10 Years)**
Male: 0.3–4.6 mLU/mL *or* SI 0.3–4.6 IU/L
Female: 0.68–6.7 mLU/mL *or* SI 0.68–4.6 IU/L
**Urine**
Adult male: 3–11 U/24 hr *or* SI 3–11 IU/24 hr
Female (non-midcycle): 2–15 U/24 hr *or* SI 2–15 IU/24 hr
Prepubertal child (male or female): <1.0–3.4 U/24 hr *or* SI <1.0–3.4 IU/24 hr

## Background Information

Follicle-stimulating hormone (FSH), like luteinizing hormone, is a gonadotropin manufactured by the anterior pituitary gland. The target organs of FSH are the ovaries and testes. Often, the determination of the FSH level is carried out at the same time as the luteinizing hormone (LH) level determination because of the common source of tissue synthesis and action on target organs.

In the ovulating female, the FSH level is somewhat high in the preovulatory phase. Just before midcycle, it surges to a peak level. Thereafter, a sharp decline followed by maintenance of the lower level of FSH occurs during the luteal phase. In both the male and the female, as the FSH and LH levels suddenly rise, their combined function is to stimulate the granulosa cells of the ovaries or Leydig's cells of the testes. This assists with the maturation of the oocyte and spermatozoa.

The flow of FSH is described as pulsatile or intermittent throughout the day and night. For the female patient, some laboratories require three separate blood samples at 15- to 30-minute intervals. This provides control for the problem of episodic secretion. For the adult male, the secretion of FSH is somewhat episodic, but not as much as in the female. In the young child, the FSH level is low and rises gradually with the onset of puberty. By midpuberty, the FSH level is equivalent to that of the adult.

Urinary collection may be used, because the 24-hour collection period is not affected by the pulsatile, episodic variations that can alter the results of the blood test.

## Purpose of the Test

The measurement of FSH is used to differentiate between primary and secondary gonadal failure of pituitary or hypothalamic origin. It is used to help diagnose gonadal dysfunction or failure, including delayed sexual maturation, menstrual disturbance, or amenorrhea. It is also used to evaluate infertility in the female and testicular dysfunction in the male.

The urinary values are most useful for children with precocious puberty. The urine study is also used to identify the time of ovulation when in vitro fertilization is planned.

## Procedure

**Serum.** A red- or green-topped tube is used to collect 7 to 10 mL of venous blood.

**Quality Control**

Venipuncture technique must be smooth, with a blood flow that fills the vacuum tube readily. If the blood has excessive turbulence because of flawed venipuncture technique, the hemolysis of the erythrocytes will alter the test results.

**Urine.**   A large plastic urine container is used to collect all urine for 24 hours. Some laboratories recommend boric acid preservative, but others do not.

| | |
|---|---|
| **Findings** | **Elevated Values** |

| | |
|---|---|
| Primary testicular failure | Idiopathic precocious puberty |
| Ovarian agenesis | Menopause |
| Klinefelter's syndrome | Central nervous system lesion |
| Castration | Orchitis |

**Decreased Values**

| | |
|---|---|
| Polycystic disease of the ovary | Hypothalamic disorder |
| Pregnancy | Adrenal tumor |
| Anterior pituitary hypofunction | Congenital adrenal hypoplasia |
| Anorexia nervosa | Sickle cell disease |

**Interfering Factors**

- Recent radioactive isotope scan
- Incomplete urine collection
- Inadequate preservation of the urine
- Hemolysis

**Nursing Implementation**

For the blood test, nursing care includes care of the venipuncture site, as presented in Chapter 2.

### Pretest

Schedule this test for before any nuclear scan examination, because the radioactive isotopes of the scan would interfere with the radioimmunoassay examination used in this test.

### Urine Collection

Provide both written and verbal instructions regarding the collection of the urine. These instructions must include the specific times of the collection period.

### During the Test

The first voided specimen of the morning is discarded, and the urine collection period begins at 8 AM.

All urine is collected for 24 hours and placed in the container. This includes the first voided specimen of the next morning.

Maintain the specimen and container on ice or refrigerated during the collection period. This prevents deterioration.

All urine is added to the collection container during the 24 hours. If any urine spills, or if a specimen is discarded accidentally, the test is invalidated.

## Posttest

On the urine requisition slip, write the time and date of the start and completion of the test.

For both tests, write the date of the last menstrual period on the requisition slip.

For both the blood and the urine test, the specimen must be delivered to the laboratory without delay. The urine must be kept chilled or refrigerated until it is prepared for analysis.

## Human Chorionic Gonadotropin, Serum

**(Serum)**                    Synonyms: hCG

| | |
|---|---|
| **Normal Values** | **Qualitative measurement:** Negative<br>**Quantitative Measurement**<br>Male and nonpregnant female: <5 mIU/mL *or* SI <5 IU/L<br>Pregnant female (1 week of gestation): 5–50 mIU/mL *or* SI 5–50 IU/L<br>Pregnant female (4 weeks of gestation): 1,000–30,000 mIU/mL *or* SI 1,000–30,000 IU/L<br>Pregnant female (6–8 weeks of gestation): 12,000–270,000 mIU/mL *or* SI 12,000–270,000 IU/L<br>Pregnant female (12 weeks of gestation): 15,000–220,000 mIU/mL *or* SI 15,000–220,000 IU/L |

## Background Information

Human chorionic gonadotropin (hCG) is a hormone normally produced by the developing placenta. In the normal, nonpregnant person, only a trace amount of this hormone is found in the blood. In abnormal conditions, the hormone is produced by some germ cell malignancies and malignancy of other organs. This glycoprotein hormone consists of two subunits called alpha- and beta-hCG. The serum assay usually measures the beta subunit (Tietz, 1995).

The measurement of the beta subunit detects a normal pregnancy within 6 to 10 days after the fertilized egg is implanted. During the early part of a normal pregnancy, the amount of hCG shows a dramatic rise in the blood. The level generally peaks in the 7th to 10th week of gestation. Very high values suggest a multiple pregnancy. In ectopic pregnancy, however, the secretion of hCG is much lower and does not progress in the same pattern.

Benign or malignant trophoblastic disease is usually associated with very high levels of hCG.

The trophoblastic abnormalities include hydatidiform mole, invasive mole, and choriocarcinoma. After surgical removal of a hydatidiform mole or chorionic cancer, the serum level recedes and returns to normal within 8 to 12 weeks. Once the serum level is normal for several consecutive weeks, the patient is considered free of disease. Because it is a tumor marker, the serum level continues to be monitored monthly for 1 year. A persistent elevation or a slow rate of decline of the serum value indicates an invasive malignancy with the need for chemotherapy (Aziz, 1996).

Germ cell tumors of the testes or ovaries also cause a rise in the serum value of human chorionic gonadotropin. As a tumor marker, postoperative serial testing for hCG can reveal the presence of recurrence and metastasis of ovarian or testicular cancer. For postoperative surveillance, this test is combined with other diagnostic tests to increase the accuracy in detection of recurrence (Aziz, 1996).

**Purpose of the Test**

The serum measurement of hCG is used to detect an early pregnancy, to help confirm the diagnosis of a trophoblastic or germ cell tumor, and to monitor the patient after the surgical removal of a tumor. In postsurgical removal of a trophoblastic or germ cell tumor, the follow-up testing helps evaluate the need for additional treatment.

**Procedure**

A red-topped tube is used to obtain 10 mL of venous blood.

**Quality Control**

> Venipuncture technique must be smooth, with a blood flow that fills the vacuum tube readily. If the blood has excessive turbulence because of flawed venipuncture technique, the hemolysis of the erythrocytes will alter the test results.

**Findings**

■

*Critical Thinking 22–2*
In the third month of pregnancy, the patient's serum hCG value declines sharply. Until the viability of the fetus can be determined, how can the nurse provide support to the patient?

**Elevated Values**

| | | |
|---|---|---|
| Pregnancy | Choriocarcinoma | Cancer of the lung, |
| Hydatidiform mole | Ovarian-testicular | stomach, liver, or |
| Islet cell neoplasm of | teratoma | colon |
| the pancreas | | |

**Decreased Values**

Ectopic pregnancy
Threatened abortion

**Interfering Factors**

• Recent radioactive isotope scan
• Hemolysis

**Nursing Implementation**

**Pretest**

It is preferable to schedule this test for before or at least 7 days after a nuclear scan.

**Quality Control**

> Some laboratories use a radioimmunoassay method of analysis. If this method is used, the radioisotopes of a nuclear scan interfere with the analysis and results.

**Posttest**

On the requisition slip, include the date of the patient's last menstrual period. This information is used to help determine whether the results are within normal limits. Arrange for prompt transport of the specimen to the laboratory.

| **Critical Value** | **>100,000 mIU/mL (SI >100,000 IU/L)** |
|---|---|
| | In the nonpregnant patient, a severely elevated level indicates choriocarcinoma. In the postsurgical patient with this diagnosis, the elevated value identifies a recurrence and the need for chemotherapy (Aziz, 1996; Jacobs et al., 1996). The nurse notifies the physician of the abnormally elevated test result. |

## Human Chorionic Gonadotropin, Urine

(Urine)    Synonyms: Pregnancy test, hCG

| **Normal Values** | Male, nonpregnant female: Negative |
|---|---|
| | Pregnant female: Positive |
| | Home testing: Negative; not pregnant |

### Background Information

Almost immediately after the fertilized ovum is implanted, hCG production and secretion begin. During the early phase of the pregnancy, the serum hCG rises rapidly and reaches a peak about 60 to 80 days after the last menstrual period. Thereafter, it tapers off a bit but is sustained at an elevated level throughout the pregnancy.

The urinary level of this hormone is also elevated in the same pattern as the serum level is elevated. Once the pregnancy is completed or terminated, the urinary value converts to negative within 2 weeks.

In addition to pregnancy, some malignancies produce hCG. The serum and urine levels are elevated in these conditions.

### Purpose of the Test

This urine test confirms pregnancy within 6 days of conception. If a teratogenic medication or treatment such as x-ray, chemotherapy, or radiotherapy must be given to a young, sexually active female, the test can screen for an unknown pregnancy before treatment begins. The test is also used on an emergency basis to determine if pregnancy is the cause of pelvic pain.

### Procedure

A clean plastic container is used to collect a first voided morning specimen of urine.

#### Home Testing

The test stick is dipped in the urine for 10 to 20 seconds so that the absorbent area is covered. Some manufacturers recommend placing the test stick on a level surface and pouring a small amount of urine into the absorbent area. Wait 3 minutes to read the result.

**Findings**

**Positive Values**

Pregnancy
Choriocarcinoma
Lung, colon, pancre-
    atic, or stomach
    cancer

Ovarian tumor
Testicular tumor
Melanoma
Multiple myeloma

**Negative Values**

Threatened abortion
Ectopic pregnancy

**Interfering Factors**

- Hematuria
- Bacteriuria
- Proteinuria
- Detergent or soap in the specimen container

**Nursing Implementation**

**Pretest**

Instruct the patient to collect a single specimen of urine in the laboratory col-
    lection container. The urine should be from the first voided morning
    specimen, collected on arising from sleep. This urine sample is more concen-
    trated and produces the most accurate result.

**Posttest**

Ensure that the container has a lid in place and that a label with correct identi-
    fication is on the container.
Arrange for prompt delivery of the urine to the laboratory.

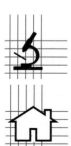

**Quality Control**

The urine is stable for 4 hours at room temperature. If a delay occurs before analysis is performed, the specimen must be refrigerated.

**Home Testing**

Teach the patient to follow the manufacturer's instructions exactly. The test is accurate as early as the first day of a missed period. A positive result is shown by the emergence of two colored lines in the test well. The control (C) line means that the test is valid. The test (T) line means that the test result is positive. Instruct the patient to seek professional advice as a follow-up to the positive test result.

   Warn the patient that false-negative results can occur because of failure to follow the instructions (Davidaud et al., 1993; Hicks, 1993), testing too soon after conception, diluted urine, or taking the drug carbamazepine (Tegretol). Testing can be repeated in 2 weeks, but if amenorrhea persists, the patient should see her physician (Cunningham et al., 1997). False-positive results can occur because of protein or blood in the urine (Stepp & Woods, 1998) and because of the drugs methadone (Dolophine), chlordiazepoxide (Librium), and promethazine (Phenergan) (Hicks, 1993).

## Luteinizing Hormone

**(Serum, Urine)**          Synonyms: LH, lutropin

**Normal Values**

**Serum**
Adult male: 1–8 mU/mL *or* SI 1–8 U/L
Adult female (follicular phase): 1–12 mU/mL *or* SI 1–12 U/L
Adult female (midcycle peak): 16–104 mU/mL *or* SI 16–104 U/L
Adult female (luteal phase): 1–12 mU/mL *or* SI 1–12 U/L
Adult female (post menopause): 16–66 mU/mL *or* SI 16–66 U/L
Child (6 months–10 years): 1–5 mU/mL *or* SI 1–5 U/L
**Urine**
Adult male: 9–23 U/24 hr
Adult female: 4–30 U/24 hr
Male child (1–10 years): <1–5.6 U/24 hr
Female child (1–10 years): 1.4–4.9 U/24 hr
**Home test:** Negative

### Background Information

Luteinizing hormone (LH) is a gonadotropin synthesized and secreted by the anterior pituitary gland. The regulation of the flow of the hormone is carried out by the hypothalamus and the pituitary glands. The target organs of LH are the ovaries of the female and the testes of the male (Mahon, Smith, & Burns, 1998).

In the course of the menstrual cycle, the serum level of LH is low in the follicular phase. It surges to a peak at midcycle and then sharply decreases to a low level during the luteal phase. The LH preovulatory stimulus initiates ovarian activity, including progesterone production and the maturation of the oocyte. All these activities must occur before a mature oocyte is released in ovulation. In the male, LH secretion is more episodic, with smaller surges throughout each day. LH is needed for the maturation of spermatozoa.

In the early years of childhood, the serum level of LH remains low. The LH concentration increases during puberty, and by the end of puberty it is equivalent to that of the adult.

The urine measurement of LH is used to detect the day of the LH surge in the preovulatory phase of the menstrual cycle. The urine test becomes positive when the LH level rises, about 24 to 48 hours before ovulation occurs.

The LH test may be performed with the follicle-stimulating hormone (FSH) test. These hormones have similar structure and secretion patterns, and they are both manufactured by cells of the anterior pituitary gland.

### Purpose of the Test

The measurement of LH is used to help diagnose gonadal dysfunction or failure, including delayed sexual development, amenorrhea, and menstrual irregularity. It also is used as part of infertility evaluation in the female and testicular dysfunction evaluation in the male. In home testing, the test is used to detect the LH surge as an early predictor of ovulation.

### Procedure

**Serum.**  A red-topped or green-topped tube is used to collect 10 mL of venous blood.

**Urine.** A large bottle is used to collect urine for 24 hours. Some laboratories require the addition of boric, acetic, or hydrochloric acid. Other laboratories require no preservative in the bottle.

**Home Testing.** A single midafternoon or early-evening specimen of urine is collected in a plastic container. The test stick is dipped in the urine for 10 to 20 seconds so that the absorbent area is covered. Some manufacturers recommend placing the test stick on a level surface and pouring a small amount of urine into the absorbent area. Wait 3 minutes to read the result. When the result is positive, the test line changes color (often to deep pink, purple, or blue).

---

## Findings

### Elevated Values

Primary gonadal
  dysfunction
Polycystic ovary
  syndrome

Post menopause
Pituitary adenoma
Castration
Ovarian failure

### Decreased Values

Pituitary or hypotha-
  lamic syndrome
Severe stress
Malnutrition
Anorexia nervosa

Isolated gonadotropic
  deficiencies
Congenital adrenal
  hyperplasia
Delayed puberty

Adrenal tumor

---

## Interfering Factors

• Recent radioactive isotope scan

---

## Nursing Implementation

### Pretest

Schedule this test for before or at least 7 days after a nuclear scan.

### Quality Control

> The measurement of LH is carried out by radioimmunoassay. The radioisotopes of a nuclear scan would interfere with the analysis and results.

### Urine Collection

Provide both written and verbal instructions regarding collection of urine.
  These instructions must include the specific times for the collection period.

### During the Test

For the 24-hour collection, the first voided specimen of the morning is discarded, and the urine collection period begins at 8 AM.
All urine collected in the 24-hour period is placed in the container. This includes the first voided specimen of the next morning.
Keep the specimen and container on ice or refrigerated during the collection period. This prevents the specimen's deterioration.

All urine collected during this period is added to the collection container. If any urine spills, or if a specimen is discarded accidentally, the test is invalidated.

## Posttest

On the urine requisition slip, write the time and date of the start and completion of the test.

For serum and 24-hour urine tests, write the date of the last menstrual period on the requisition slip.

For both these tests, the specimen must be delivered to the laboratory without delay.

### Quality Control

The 24-hour urine specimen must be kept chilled or refrigerated until it is prepared for analysis.

### Home Testing

Teach the patient to follow the manufacturer's instructions exactly. The elevated level of LH appears in the urine (the test result turns positive) about 32 hours before ovulation occurs (Hammond & Steinkamph, 1992). A positive result is shown by the emergence of two colored lines in the test well. The control (C) line means the test is valid. The test (T) line means the test result is positive. If the patient has intercourse on the first or second day after the LH surge (after a positive test result), she is more likely to conceive.

Advise the patient that despite manufacturers' claims of very high accuracy rates, home ovulation test kits have only a 72% to 75% accuracy rate. In detection of the LH surge as a predictor of ovulation, the home test kits may not help in becoming pregnant, and they should not be used as a method to avoid pregnancy. Additionally, the home test kits are expensive, and some patients require additional assistance although written instructions are provided (Anderson, Eccles, & Irvine, 1996; Fehring, 1992).

# Pregnanetriol

**(Urine)**  Synonyms: None

**Normal Values**

**Adult male:** 0.4–2.5 mg/day *or* SI 1.2–7.5 µmol/day
**Adult Female**
  Follicular phase: 0.1–1.8 mg/day *or* SI 0.3–5.3 µmol/day
  Luteal phase: 0.9–2.2 mg/day *or* SI 2.7–6.5 µmol/day
**Child**
  0–5 years: <0.1 mg/day *or* SI <0.3 µmol/day
  6–9 years: <0.3 mg/day *or* SI <0.9 µmol/day

## Background Information

17-Hydroxyprogesterone is a substrate needed to produce cortisol, an adrenocortical steroid. Pregnanetriol, a ketogenic steroid, is a metabolite of 17-hydroxyprogesterone. When adrenal function is normal, minute amounts of pregnanetriol are present in the urine. If adrenal insufficiency prevents or limits the synthesis of cortisol, an increase in adrenocorticotropic hormone production, increased release of adrenal androgens, and increased release of 17-hydroxyprogesterone into the serum occur. The increase of serum 17- hydroxy-progesterone causes an increase in pregnanetriol in the urine.

The increase in adrenal androgens results in virilization of the female. The infant female may show masculinization of the external genitals at birth, and female secondary sex characteristics may fail to develop in the older female child. The increase in adrenal androgens may cause precocious development in the male child.

## Purpose of the Test

The measurement of this urinary metabolite helps confirm the diagnosis of adrenal hyperplasia. It also is used to monitor cortisol replacement.

## Procedure

A large, clean collection bottle is used to collect urine for 24 hours.

**Quality Control**

Some laboratories require a boric acid preservative to be added to the container. To preserve the urine, the specimen is refrigerated or cooled throughout the collection period.

## Findings

**Elevated Values**

Congenital adrenal
   hyperplasia
Adrenal tumor
Insufficient cortisol
   replacement

Stein-Leventhal
   syndrome
21-Hydroxylase
   deficiency
Ovarian tumor

## Interfering Factors

- Muscular exercise
- Warming of the specimen
- Failure to collect the entire specimen

## Nursing Implementation

**Pretest**

Instruct the patient or the parent of the small child that no physical exertion must occur before or during the test period. This is because physical activity increases the urinary metabolic output and causes a falsely elevated test result.

Provide both written and verbal instructions regarding the collection of urine. These instructions must include the specific times for the collection period.

For the infant or small child, the pediatric collection bag is to be taped to the clean perineal area. A diaper is applied over the bag to help maintain its position and to prevent removal of the bag by the child.

**During the Test**

The first voided specimen of the morning is discarded, and the urine collection period begins at 8 AM.

All urine is collected for 24 hours and placed in the container. This includes the first voided specimen of the next morning.

Maintain the specimen and container on ice or keep them refrigerated during the collection period. The chilling temperature prevents deterioration.

During the period of collection, all urine is added to the collection container. If any urine spills, or if a specimen is discarded accidentally, the test is invalidated.

## Posttest

On the urine requisition slip, write the time and date of the start and completion of the test.

The specimen must be delivered to the laboratory without delay. The urine must be kept chilled or refrigerated. In the laboratory, the urine can be frozen until the analysis is performed.

# Progesterone

**(Serum)**    Synonym: $P_4$

| Normal Values | |
|---|---|
| | **Adult male:** 13–97 ng/dL *or* SI 0.4–3.1 nmol/L |
| | **Menstruating Female** |
| | Follicular phase: 15–70 ng/dL *or* SI 0.5–2.2 nmol/L |
| | Luteal phase: 200–2,500 ng/dL *or* SI 6.4–79.5 nmol/L |
| | **Pregnant Female** |
| | First trimester: 1,025–4,400 ng/dL *or* SI 32.6–139.9 nmol/L |
| | Second trimester: 1,950–8,250 ng/dL *or* SI 62.0–262.4 nmol/L |
| | Third trimester: 6,500–22,900 ng/dL *or* SI 206.7–728.2 nmol/L |

## Background Information

The androgenic sex hormone progesterone is synthesized in various body tissues. In the male and the nonmenstruating female, the source is the adrenal gland and the conversion of pregnenolone and pregnenolone sulfate. In the menstruating female, it is produced by the ovaries. During pregnancy, progesterone is synthesized in great quantity by the placenta, and the serum level rises progressively throughout the term of the pregnancy.

In the menstruating female, the corpus luteum of the ovary produces a small but steady supply during the preovulatory or follicular phase of the menstrual cycle. After ovulation, the progesterone level rises over a 4- to 5-day period in the luteal phase of the menstrual cycle. The serum level reaches and maintains its peak for about 1 week and then falls rapidly before the start of menstruation. A normal value in the luteal phase indicates that the patient is ovulating normally.

Progesterone functions to help prepare the endometrium of the uterus for the implantation of the fertilized ovum. To determine the day of ovulation, serial blood samples are obtained during the menstrual cycle. Serial testing may also be done throughout a pregnancy to monitor for abnormal gestational development of the fetus, such as inevitable abortion. To determine the serum value in the luteal phase, the blood sample is drawn on the eighth day after a urinary luteal hormone surge.

## Purpose of the Test

Serum progesterone levels are used to determine ovulation and to assess the function of the corpus luteum, particularly in cases of habitual abortion or infertility.

| | |
|---|---|
| **Procedure** | A red-topped tube is used to obtain 10 mL of venous blood. |

**Findings**

**Elevated Values**

| | |
|---|---|
| Congenital adrenal hyperplasia | Molar pregnancy |
| | Ovarian tumor |

**Decreased Values**

Threatened abortion
Short luteal phase syndrome
Ectopic pregnancy

**Interfering Factors**

• Recent radioactive isotope scan

**Nursing Implementation**

Nursing care includes care of the venipuncture site.

**Pretest**

Schedule this test for before or at least 7 days after a nuclear scan.

**Quality Control**

The measurement of progesterone is performed by the radioimmunoassay method of analysis. The radioisotopes of a nuclear scan would interfere with the analysis and results.

When a series of blood tests throughout the menstrual cycle is required, make sure that the patient understands the testing plan and schedule of test dates.

**Posttest**

On the requisition slip, write the pertinent data, including the patient's sex, the date of the patient's last menstrual period, and the trimester of pregnancy. These data are used to help determine whether the results are within normal limits. Arrange for prompt transport of the specimen to the laboratory.

**Quality Control**

As soon as the cells have been separated out, the serum must be refrigerated or frozen.

**Critical Value**

**<5–10 ng/dL (SI <15.9–31.8 mmol/L)**

In the pregnant female, this severely low level indicates a possible pathologic pregnancy. If the level is 5 ng/dL or lower (SI 15.9 mmol/L or lower), the low value indicates nonviability of the pregnancy. The condition may be a failing intrauterine pregnancy or an ectopic pregnancy. The nurse alerts the physician of the very low result.

# Prolactin

**(Serum)** Synonyms: PRL, lactogenic hormone

## Normal Values

Adult: 0–20 ng/mL *or* SI 0–20 µg/L
Pregnancy (third trimester): 95–473 ng/mL *or* SI 95–473 µg/L
Newborn: <30–495 ng/mL *or* SI 30–495 µg/L

## Background Information

Prolactin is a hormone produced by the anterior pituitary gland that is needed for lactation. Its production and release into the blood are controlled by the inhibiting and releasing factors of the hypothalamus and a number of other internal and external variables.

Prolactin has a diurnal rhythm; the serum level rises during sleep and is at its highest level several hours after waking. It rises progressively during pregnancy, and after delivery it returns to a baseline value in the woman who does not breast-feed. The hormone is usually mildly elevated in the breast-feeding mother. The hormone prolactin is at an elevated level in the fetus and neonate but declines to a normal level a few weeks after birth. Serum levels also can rise after stress or exercise and during venipuncture procedures.

The serum prolactin level can be lower than normal because of damage to the pituitary gland. The low level prevents lactation in the postpartum mother. In the male or female with excess flow of this hormone, the cause may be a problem in the hypothalamus, pituitary gland, or adrenal gland. The elevated level affects gonadal function and can cause galactorrhea (inappropriate lactation), anovulation, hirsutism, or infertility. A prolactin-secreting tumor causes a dramatic rise in the serum.

## Purpose of the Test

The measurement of serum prolactin is used to evaluate oligorrhea, amenorrhea, or galactorrhea. It may assist in the diagnosis of pituitary gland or hypothalamus dysfunction.

## Procedure

A chilled, red-topped tube is used to collect 10 mL of venous blood 3 to 4 hours after arising from sleep.

### Quality Control

Venipuncture technique must be smooth, with a blood flow that fills the vacuum tube readily. If the blood has excessive turbulence because of flawed venipuncture technique, the hemolysis of the erythrocytes will alter the test results.

## Findings

### Elevated Values

| | | |
|---|---|---|
| Hypothalamus-pituitary disease (sarcoidosis, metastatic cancer) | Prolactin-secreting pituitary tumor | Renal failure |
| | Hypothyroidism | Anorexia nervosa |
| | Acromegaly | Cirrhosis of the liver |
| | | Adrenal insufficiency |

**Decreased Values**

Pituitary infarction or
necrosis

---

**Interfering Factors**

- Alcohol intake
- Failure to fast in the pretest period
- Recent radioactive isotope scan
- Warming of the specimen
- Hemolysis
- Sleep disturbance

---

**Nursing Implementation**

For care of the venipuncture site, see Chapter 2.

**Pretest**

Schedule this test for before or at least 7 days after a nuclear scan.

**Quality Control**

The measurement of progesterone is carried out by radioimmunoassay. The radioisotopes of a nuclear scan would interfere with the analysis and the results.

Instruct the patient to abstain from alcohol in the 24 hours before the blood is drawn and to fast from food for 8 hours before the test.
Schedule the blood to be drawn between 8 and 10 AM or 3 to 4 hours after arising from sleep. This helps control for diurnal fluctuations.

**Posttest**

Ensure that the blood is placed on ice immediately.
Arrange for prompt transport of the specimen to the laboratory.

**Quality Control**

The cells must be separated from the serum by refrigerated centrifuge. The serum can be maintained for 24 hours at a temperature of 4°C. If additional delay occurs before analysis, the serum must be frozen.

---

**Critical Values**

**>200 ng/mL (SI >200 µg/L)**

In the nonpregnant or nonlactating patient, a severe elevation indicates a prolactin-secreting tumor. The nurse should alert the physician of the abnormal test result.

---

## Semen Analysis

(Ejaculate)                    Synonyms: Sperm analysis, sperm count, seminal cytology

**Normal Values**

**Physical Analysis**
Appearance: Opalescent gray-white color
Volume: 2–5 mL
Coagulation-liquefaction: Coagulates rapidly; forms water droplets in 10 to 60 minutes
pH: 7.2–7.8
**Chemical Analysis**
Acid phosphatase: >200 U per ejaculate
Citric acid: >52 µmol per ejaculate
Fructose: >13 µmol per ejaculate
Zinc: >2.4 µmol per ejaculate
**Microscopic Analysis**
Motility: >50% sperm with moderate to rapid linear (forward) motion
Concentration: 20–250 × 10⁶ spermatozoa per milliliter of ejaculate
Morphology: >50% of spermatozoa have normal structure and shape
Viability: >50% of spermatozoa are alive
Leukocytes: <1 × 10⁶/mL of ejaculate
Antisperm antibodies: Negative

## Background Information

Semen consists of secretions from the testes, epididymis, seminal vesicles, and prostate gland. The spermatozoa are produced in the testes and released into the semen. The semen serves as the transport medium for the mature spermatozoa.

In cases of infertility, the analysis of the semen is usually the first test to be performed on the male. Infertility may result from a decreased amount of sperm, called *oligospermia*. Sterility results from nonviable sperm, called *azoospermia*. The semen specimen is examined for physical and chemical characteristics and then for microscopic visualization of the sperm and a leukocyte count. Because the concentrations of sperm can vary significantly, two to three samples are examined in a 2- to 3-month period.

**Physical Analysis.** Semen is a liquid having a characteristic gray-white, opalescent color. Abnormal color changes can include red, often caused by blood, or yellow, as associated with certain drugs. Clear semen is often indicative of a low sperm count. The semen is usually somewhat viscous. It usually coagulates after ejaculation but then liquefies in about 30 minutes. The failure to liquefy after 60 minutes is abnormal.

**Chemical Analysis.** The elements of chemical analysis provide information about factors that influence sperm motility, fertilization ability, and

sperm health (Yablonsky, 1996). The pH of fresh semen is in the range of 7.2 to 7.8. A lower-than-normal pH is associated with a problem in the epididymis, vas deferens, or seminal vesicles. A higher-than-normal pH is associated with infection. Seminal fluid fructose determination is a common clinical test in the analysis of semen. A normal value verifies the secretory ability of the seminal vesicles and the integrity of the ejaculatory ducts and vas deferens. A low fructose level is associated with a low sperm count. The levels of zinc, citric acid, and acid phosphatase are measures of the secretory ability of the prostate gland.

**Microscopic Examination.** The mobility of the sperm and the quality of the movement are important characteristics, because mobile sperm are able to reach the ovum. Both speed and linear (forward) progression are evaluated.

The sperm count, or *concentration*, is a measure of the quantity of sperm. Sperm counts of fewer than 20 million per milliliter or more than 250 million per milliliter are abnormal and are associated with infertility. Sperm morphologic features or the measurements of the head, midpiece, and tail are part of the analysis for defects. Some of the common abnormal morphologic conditions are presented in Figure 22–1. When more than 50% of the sperm have a normal

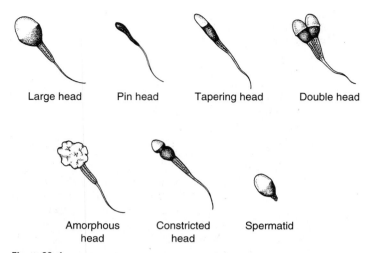

Large head   Pin head   Tapering head   Double head

Amorphous
head

Constricted
head

Spermatid

**Figure 22–1**

Abnormal sperm morphologic features. (Reproduced with permission from Brunzel, N. A. [1994].
*Fundamentals of urine and body fluid analysis.* Philadelphia: W. B. Saunders.)

structure, the sperm morphologic state is called
normal.

The semen is also examined microscopically
for viable sperm. In a fresh normal specimen, at
least 50% of the sperm are alive. Immature sperm
may be present in great numbers, and they are
indicative of infertility. The ejaculate is examined
for cells, particulate matter, and debris. When more
than 1 million leukocytes are present, the results
indicate inflammation that probably originates
in the prostate gland or seminal vesicles.

Under the microscope, the sperm may also
agglutinate, or clump together. This occurs in
the presence of immunoglobulin G (IgG), immunoglobulin A (IgA), or immunoglobulin M (IgM)
antisperm antibodies, and the clumping is associated with infertility. Either the male or the female
may produce the antibodies, but once agglutination
occurs, the sperm cannot penetrate or progress
through the cervical mucus to reach the ovum
(Brunzel, 1994).

Using the immunobead binding method
and light microscopy, the amount of antisperm antibodies can be quantified. The sperm and
immunobeads are incubated together. If antisperm
antibodies are present on the surface of the
sperm, the immunobeads will attach to the antibodies. A weakly positive response occurs when
20% to 49% of the sperm are bound to the immunobeads. An intermediate response occurs when
50% to 89% of the sperm are bound to the immunobeads. A high response is present with 90% to
100% binding of the sperm with the immunobeads
(Nakamura, 1996). For infertility testing, antisperm antibodies may be detected by serum testing
of the male and the female.

The semen specimen is a potential biohazard
that may contain an infectious organism, such as
the human immunodeficiency virus, hepatitis virus,
or herpesvirus. To prevent accidental transmission, universal precautions must be used when
handling the semen specimen.

## Purpose of the Test

Semen analysis is used to investigate infertility in the male. It is also used to
evaluate the effectiveness of vasectomy. In special situations, it may be part of
medicolegal testing, such as in cases of alleged rape or sexual abuse.

## Procedure

A special wide-mouthed, clean, plastic or glass container is used to collect ejaculate, which is usually produced by masturbation. Two to three specimens

are usually required. They are collected at least 7 days apart and within a 3-month period.

### Quality Control

> Some plastic containers are toxic to spermatozoa. The correct container should be provided by the laboratory.

If the patient cannot produce the sperm by masturbation, special nonspermicidal condoms can be provided by the laboratory. Regular condoms are not acceptable because of the lubricant and spermicidal preparation that is on or in them.

---

**Findings**

### Abnormal Values

| Testicular failure | Genital infection | Prostatic dysfunction |
| Obstruction of the ejaculatory ducts | Cryptorchidism Hyperpyrexia | Postvasectomy azoospermia |

---

**Interfering Factors**

- Exposure of the ejaculate to intense sunlight or chilling temperatures
- Delay in the analysis of the specimen
- Use of lubricant or over-the-counter condom
- Incomplete collection of the ejaculate

---

**Nursing Implementation**

### Pretest

Instruct the patient regarding the method of specimen collection. The instructions are given verbally in a professional and sensitive manner. A written copy of the instructions is also given to the patient. These instructions include the following.

Use the sterile container that is provided by the laboratory.

Collect the specimen by masturbation. If this is not possible or acceptable, a special condom provided by the laboratory can be used. Coitus interruptus is also acceptable, but the amount of ejaculate will be less (Spear & Niederberger, 1996).

Instruct the patient to practice sexual abstinence for at least 2 days but not more than 7 days before the specimen is collected.

Provide a clean, comfortable room for the patient. It should be in or near the laboratory because of the short time before liquefaction occurs. If these arrangements are not possible, the specimen can be obtained at home.

Special transport instructions are provided regarding avoidance of sunlight, cooling, spillage, and delay in delivery of the specimen to the laboratory.

### During the Test

To protect the spermatozoa from cold shock, the collection container should be at room temperature or warmed before the ejaculate is produced. The container can be warmed under the patient's arm or next to his body (Brunzel, 1994).

The complete ejaculate must be placed in the specimen container.

## Posttest

If the nurse handles the container, gloves must be worn to protect from possible exposure to acquired immunodeficiency syndrome (AIDS). If the nurse has an open cut or wound on the skin, he or she must not handle the specimen container (Jacobs et al., 1996).

Ensure that the container and the requisition slip are labeled, including the patient's name, the date, and the time of specimen collection. The period of sexual abstinence is included in the documentation.

Ensure that the specimen is delivered to the laboratory within 1 hour. The specimen must be analyzed within 2 hours, or it must be rejected by the laboratory.

To protect the specimen from deterioration during transport, instruct the patient to perform the following: Place the lid securely on the container, and protect the specimen from chilling and sunlight by placing it next to the body, in an inside coat pocket, or under the arm.

### Quality Control

> The specimen must not be exposed to chilling or sunlight, because these negative conditions reduce the motility of the sperm.

## Testosterone, Total, Free

**(Serum)**                    Synonyms: None

**Normal Values**

**Total Testosterone**
Adult male: 280–1,100 ng/dL *or* SI 9.72–38.17 nmol/L
Adult female: 15–70 ng/dL *or* SI 0.52–2.43 nmol/L
Male child (1–5 years): 0.3–30.0 ng/dL *or* SI 0.10–1.04 nmol/L
Female child (1–5 years): 2–20 ng/dL *or* 0.07–0.69 nmol/L

**Free Testosterone**
Adult male: 50–210 pg/mL *or* SI 174–729 pmol/L
Adult female: 1.0–8.5 pg/mL *or* SI 3.5–29.5 pmol/L
Male child (6–9 years): 0.1–3.2 pg/mL *or* SI 0.3–11.1 pmol/L
Female child (6–9 years): 0.1–0.9 pg/mL *or* SI 0.3–3.1 pmol/L

## Background Information

Total testosterone consists of the measurement of testosterone that is free, loosely bound to albumin, and strongly bound to sex-hormone–binding globulin. Free testosterone is the amount of the total hormone that is unbound in the serum. Because free testosterone is the active form of the hormone, its determination is the more significant test.

In the male, almost all the testosterone is synthesized by the testes. In the female, small amounts are synthesized by the ovaries and adrenal glands, and additional amounts are converted from androstenedione. Testosterone is the dominant androgen and in the male is responsible for spermatogenesis (Mahon, Smith, & Burns, 1998). Androgens affect many other organs and tissues, resulting in increased total body mass and *hirsutism*, the distribution of body hair. When hirsutism is excessive, it is due to excessive testosterone or its hormonal precursor, androstenedione.

## Purpose of the Test

The measurement of serum testosterone is used to diagnose precocious sexual development in the boy who is younger than 10 years. It helps diagnose deficient activity of the testes or ovaries. It is part of the testing that determines the cause of male infertility or sexual dysfunction. In the female, it helps determine the cause of hirsutism or virilization.

## Procedure

A red-topped tube is used to collect 10 mL of venous blood.

## Findings

**Elevated Values**

Ovarian tumor
Adrenal tumor
Hyperthyroidism
Congenital adrenal
  hyperplasia

Testicular tumor
Idiopathic precocious
  puberty
Central nervous
  system lesion

**Decreased Values**

Cirrhosis of the liver
Excessive alcohol
  intake
Hypopituitarism

Estrogen therapy
Severe obesity
Renal failure
Malnutrition

Down syndrome
Cryptorchidism

## Interfering Factors

- Recent radioactive isotope scan

## Nursing Implementation

For care of the venipuncture site, see Chapter 2.

**Pretest**

Schedule this test for before or at least 7 days after a nuclear scan.

**Quality Control**

The measurement of testosterone is carried out by radioimmunoassay. The radioisotopes of a nuclear scan would interfere with the analysis and the results.

**Posttest**

Arrange for prompt transport of the specimen to the laboratory.

**Quality Control**

Once the cells have been separated out, the serum must be refrigerated.

## Diagnostic Procedures

## Amniocentesis and Amniotic Fluid Analysis

**(Amniotic Fluid)**   Synonyms: None

**Normal Values**

Chromosome analysis: Normal karyotype
Alpha$_1$-fetoprotein: <2.5 multiple of median value (MOM)
Acetylcholinesterase: Negative
Rh Incompatibility
  Freda classification: Negative or 1+
  Optical density at 450 nm (delta 450): 0–0.2
  Bilirubin: 0.01–0.03 mg/dL $or$ SI 0.02–0.06 µmol/L
Creatinine
  36 weeks of gestation: 1.6–1.8 mg/dL $or$ SI 141–159 µmol/L
  37–38 weeks of gestation: >2 mg/dL $or$ SI >177 µmol/L
Lecithin-to-sphingomyelin ratio: >2
Phosphatidylglycerol: Present
Pulmonary surfactant: Positive; foam stability index: >0.48
Meconium: Absent

## Background Information

Amniotic fluid is the fluid that surrounds the fetus in the uterus. During pregnancy, it provides the medium for water, electrolyte, and other solute exchange with the fetus. The fetus swallows the amniotic fluid for hydration and urinates into the fluid to eliminate metabolic wastes. Throughout the pregnancy, the amniotic fluid bathes the fetal lungs. The amniotic fluid is also in continuous exchange with maternal plasma, so complete cleansing and change of the fluid occur every 2 to 3 hours.

**Amniocentesis.**   This is the percutaneous needle aspiration of a sample of amniotic fluid for the purpose of laboratory analysis. As seen in Table 22–1, several reasons exist to perform amniocentesis. The biochemical and cytologic analyses provide data regarding the fetus and the pregnancy.

When the purpose of the amniocentesis is to screen for fetal abnormality, it is performed early in the second trimester. By that time, fetal cell samples are available for chromosomal study, and sufficient amniotic fluid is available to obtain the fluid and cell samples. Usually, the procedure is performed in the 15th to 17th weeks of gestation, when the risk to the fetus is lower and sufficient time is available to provide the appropriate counseling and discuss treatment alternatives. If an early amniocentesis is performed (in the 11th to 12th weeks of gestation), the risk is greater for fetal loss or development of talipes equinovarus in the infant (Wilson, Johnson, Dansereau, 1998; Whittle, 1998).

When the purpose of the amniocentesis is to

### Table 22–1   Amniocentesis: Timing, Purposes, and Potential Findings

| Gestation | Indications | Potential Abnormalities |
|-----------|-------------|-------------------------|
| 15–17 wk | Maternal age >35 yr | Trisomy 21 (Down syndrome) Neural tube defect (spina bifida, anencephaly) |
| | Sex determination of the fetus | Sex-linked recessive disorders (hemophilia, Duchenne's muscular dystrophy) |
| | Family history of chromosomal abnormality | |
| | Family history of metabolic disorder | Inborn errors of metabolism (Tay-Sachs disease, Gaucher's disease, Niemann-Pick disease; galactosuria, maple syrup disease, homocystinuria) |
| | Family history of hemoglobinopathy | Hemoglobin disease (thalassemia, sickle cell anemia) |
| 20–42 wk | Management of a problem pregnancy | Maternal heart disease, diabetes, endocrine disorder; analysis of amniotic fluid for fetal thyroid hormone, glucose, estriol, L/S ratio* |
| | Assessment of fetal distress | Rh incompatibility, infection, fetal pulmonary immaturity |

*L/S ratio = lecithin-sphingomyelin ratio.

evaluate a problem pregnancy or to identify a change in the health status of the fetus, the procedure is performed in the late part of the second trimester or during the third trimester. In high-risk pregnancy, it may be advisable to terminate the pregnancy by delivery of the preterm infant. Severe maternal illness or a maternal condition can adversely affect the fetus. The status of fetal health and fetal maturity are considerations that influence the decision making and timing of the delivery.

**Amniotic Fluid Analysis.**   Normal amniotic fluid is colorless to pale yellow. When the fluid is a darker yellow or amber, the cause is excessive bilirubin and biliverdin. A dark green color is caused by meconium. Blood colors the fluid pink to red. The specimen should contain no blood. If the specimen contains blood, the source can be a maternal vein, the placenta, the fetus, or the cord. Another possibility is that it is caused by the insertion of the needle during the procedure.

**Chromosomal Analysis.**   A *karyotype* is the complement of chromosomes. In humans, the normal karyotype consists of 46 chromosomes aligned in a standard sequence, with defined location, size, structure, and banding patterns.

Chromosomal abnormalities are detected by analysis of fetal cells that are present in the amniotic fluid. Trisomy 21 and other trisomy conditions caused by the translocation of genes have the highest incidence in women older than 35 years. Chromosome analysis can also detect neural tube defects that include anencephaly, myelomeningocele, and spina bifida. The analysis can also detect genetic abnormalities that cause more than 80 different types of inborn errors of metabolism. They include disorders of lipid, carbohydrate, glycoprotein, mucopolysaccharide, amino acid, and organic acid metabolism. The use of gene probe technology can also identify other genetic disorders, including cystic fibrosis, muscular dystrophy, sickle cell anemia, and hemophilia. Additional information about genetic testing is presented in Chapter 13.

When a genetic abnormality is encountered, the parents need comprehensive information about the health status of the fetus. They need to make an informed decision about the pregnancy, and the choices are painful. The alternatives include termination of the pregnancy or completion of the pregnancy with preparation for the special health care needs of the newborn. Genetic counseling precedes the amniocentesis and is also provided when a genetic abnormality is encountered.

**Alpha₁-Fetoprotein.** $Alpha_1$-fetoprotein is a glycoprotein that is made in the yolk sac, fetal intestinal tract, and liver. It is present in the fetal serum and in the amniotic fluid. The amount increases steadily during fetal growth, with a maximal level at about 12 weeks of gestation. Thereafter, the concentration decreases as a greater proportion of amniotic fluid is produced.

Amniotic fluid $alpha_1$-fetoprotein is used to detect neural defects, such as spina bifida or anencephaly, and nonneural defects, such as congenital nephrosis or atresia in the upper gastrointestinal tract.

**Acetylcholinesterase.** This enzyme is present in high concentrations in cerebrospinal fluid. It is not present in the amniotic fluid with a normal fetus, but if a neural tube defect exists, such as anencephaly or spina bifida (open or closed), the cerebrospinal fluid leaks into the amniotic fluid. If the fetus has a ventral wall defect such as an omphalocele, acetylcholinesterase also leaks into the amniotic fluid, and the test result is positive.

**Rh Incompatibility.** Amniocentesis can usually detect Rh incompatibility after 30 weeks of gestation. The analysis is based on the amount of free bilirubin in the fluid. Higher values indicate the degree of hemolysis that is occurring in the fetus.

**Bilirubin.** Unconjugated bilirubin is produced by the fetus during normal erythrocyte destruction. The amount of bilirubin is minimal and is removed by the placenta and maternal circulation. With hemolytic disease, however, a continual and excessive destruction of the fetal erythrocytes occurs. The amount of unconjugated bilirubin rises dramatically in the amniotic fluid in direct correlation with the severity of the disease.

The most common cause of hemolytic disease

of the newborn is incompatibility of the maternal antibodies with the fetal erythrocyte antigen. The problem is usually a result of the mix of the Rh-negative antibodies of the mother with the $Rh_oD$ antigen of the fetus, but other Rh antibodies can also cause hemolysis of fetal erythrocytes.

**Creatinine.** This test measures renal function and renal maturity of the fetus. These values are also a measure of fetal lung maturity, because the development of the lungs is dependent on the normal development of the kidneys. The critical value is a creatinine level of less than 1.6 mg/dL (SI <141 μmol/L). This lower-than-normal value implies that the fetus is immature or premature. If it is delivered at this stage of development, the fetus is likely to experience respiratory distress syndrome.

**Lecithin-to-Sphingomyelin Ratio.** The lecithin-to-sphingomyelin (L/S) ratio is a major indicator of fetal pulmonary maturity. Lecithin is the major compound of pulmonary surfactant, the phospholipid substance needed for alveolar function. Sphingomyelin is produced in cell membranes, but its function is unknown. In the early stages of gestation, these two substances are produced in approximately equivalent amounts (a ratio of 1:1 or 1).

As the fetus matures beyond 34 to 36 weeks of gestation, the concentration of lecithin increases and the sphingomyelin remains stable. Thus, an L/S ratio of greater than 2 means that about twice as much lecithin as sphingomyelin is present; this indicates fetal lung maturity. In a normal pregnancy, this value usually occurs at about the 36th week of gestation and thereafter. A ratio of less than 1.5 to 2 is the indicator of fetal lung immaturity, with the increased likelihood that the newborn infant will experience respiratory distress syndrome (McGee, 1997). In diabetic mothers, an L/S ratio of greater than 3.5 is the normal value for fetal lung maturity. This higher value is due to increased surfactant production in the fetus of the diabetic mother.

**Phosphatidylglycerol.** This is a lipid component of pulmonary surfactant that normally appears in the amniotic fluid after the 35th week of gestation. It is an indicator of fetal pulmonary maturity. Once it appears, little risk exists that the fetus will experience respiratory distress syndrome. Generally, this test is used with the L/S ratio determination to assess fetal lung maturity. Phosphatidylglycerol is also useful as a criterion for delivery in the high-risk pregnancy that is complicated by type I diabetes mellitus.

**Pulmonary Surfactant.** The lungs are one of the late-maturing organs of the fetus. Surfactant is a lipid and protein substance produced by the mature epithelial cells of the alveoli. Surfactant enables the walls of the alveoli to expand and contract in the function of respiration. Because amniotic fluid bathes the lungs of the fetus, a certain amount of the surfactant produced appears in the fluid. The amount of surfactant is one of the predictors of fetal maturity and viability.

Pulmonary surfactant is measured by the *shake test*, also known as the *foam stability index* (FSI). In the laboratory, amniotic fluid samples are mixed with different amounts of ethanol in test tubes. The tubes are shaken to produce foam and bubbles that indicate that surfactant is present. The FSI represents the highest concentration of the mixture that produces a foam that does not dissolve. FSI values greater than 0.48 indicate fetal pulmonary maturity (Brunzel, 1994).

**Meconium.** The staining is caused by the release of mucuslike fetal intestinal secretions into the amniotic fluid. It is an abnormal sign that indicates fetal distress and the need for immediate delivery of the fetus.

| | |
|---|---|
| **Purpose of the Test** | Amniocentesis is used to detect genetic or chromosomal abnormalities in the fetus. It is also used to assess fetal maturity or fetal distress in the management of a problem pregnancy. |

| | |
|---|---|
| **Procedure** | Ultrasound is used to locate the position of the fetus, the placenta, and the pool of amniotic fluid, and it guides the insertion of the needle. Using sterile technique, several syringes and a long needle are used to aspirate 12 to 20 mL of amniotic fluid from the uterus (Fig. 22–2). The fluid is placed in sterile brown plastic containers for transport to the laboratory. |

**Quality Control**

Glass containers cannot be used, because cells adhere to the surface of the glass. A brown container is used to protect the solution and bilirubin from the sunlight. If such a container is not available, a clear container can be used. It is covered immediately with aluminum foil to prevent oxidation from sunlight.

| | |
|---|---|
| **Findings** | **Elevated Values**<br><br>ALPHA₁-FETOPROTEIN |

ALPHA$_1$-FETOPROTEIN

Neural tube defects: anencephaly, spina bifida, myelocele, hydrocephaly

Nonneural tube defects: congenital nephrosis, esophageal atresia, duodenal atresia

ACETYLCHOLINESTERASE

Neural tube defect
Fetal thyroid disease

RH INCOMPATIBILITY

Fetal hemolysis of erythrocytes (erythroblastosis fetalis)

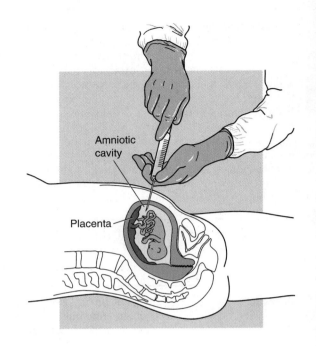

**Figure 22–2**
Amniocentesis. Once the needle is inserted through the skin and the uterine wall, a sample of amniotic fluid is aspirated with a syringe.

BILIRUBIN

Rh incompatibility

L/S RATIO

Maternal diabetes

PULMONARY SURFACTANT

Maternal diabetes          Premature rupture of          Hemoglobinopathy
Placenta previa              membranes                    Malnutrition
Intrauterine growth        Toxemia                        Drug addiction
   retardation             Hypertension

MECONIUM

Fetal distress

**Decreased Values**

BILIRUBIN

Fetal immaturity

CREATININE

Fetal immaturity

L/S RATIO

Fetal pulmonary
   immaturity

PHOSPHATIDYLGLYCEROL

Fetal pulmonary
immaturity

PULMONARY SURFACTANT

| | | |
|---|---|---|
| Polyhydramnios | Anemia | Advanced maternal |
| Hypothyroidism | Renal disease | age |
| Liver disease | Syphilis | Toxoplasmosis |

---

**Interfering Factors**

- Exposure of specimen to sunlight
- Contamination of specimen (blood, meconium)
- Recent radioactive isotope scan
- Position of the placenta
- Delay in delivery of specimen to laboratory

---

**Nursing Implementation**

### Pretest

After the patient receives a complete explanation of the amniocentesis procedure from the physician, obtain written consent from the patient or the
person who is legally responsible for the patient's health care decisions.

Provide instructions regarding pretest preparation. These instructions vary,
depending on the gestation of the pregnancy.

For a pregnancy that is less than 20 weeks of gestation, instruct the woman to
drink extra fluids 1 hour before the test and not to urinate until the test is
completed. A full bladder raises the uterus up and out of the pelvis so
that the uterine contents can be visualized.

For a pregnancy that is greater than 20 weeks of gestation, no requirements
exist for fluid intake. Instruct the woman to void before the procedure
begins. With the larger size of the uterus, an empty bladder is less likely to
be punctured during the procedure.

Assist the patient in removing her clothes, putting on a hospital gown, and
lying supine on the examining table.

Obtain and record vital signs, including the blood pressure, temperature, pulse,
respirations, and fetal heart rate. This establishes the baseline values that are
needed for comparison in the posttest period.

Provide emotional support for the patient. Anxiety about the procedure and the
status of the fetus' health is common.

### During the Test

Position the patient with her hands behind her head to help prevent contamination of the sterile field.

After ultrasound has located the fetus' position, the placenta, and the pool of
amniotic fluid, wash the abdomen with povidone-iodine solution and
drape the sterile field.

Comfort the patient during the administration of the local anesthetic in the
intended area of the abdomen. Some stinging may be felt during the
injection.

After the fluid sample is withdrawn, assist with its placement in the specimen
containers.

Once the needle is withdrawn, place a small adhesive bandage over the site of the needle puncture.

### Posttest

Monitor and record the blood pressure, pulse, respirations, and fetal heart rate every 15 minutes for 30 to 60 minutes. They should remain within normal limits and be comparable to the pretest data.

Ensure that the specimen is correctly labeled. The requisition slip should state the source of the fluid and the period of gestation of the pregnancy.

Arrange for prompt transport of the specimen to the laboratory.

### Quality Control

In the laboratory, the specimen used for cellular analysis is kept at room temperature. The specimen used for biochemical analysis is centrifuged and refrigerated or placed on ice. Phospholipid is metabolized when kept uncentrifuged at room temperature. This specimen is also kept in a dark place to prevent photo-oxidation of the bilirubin.

If the patient feels faintness, nausea, or cramps, place her on her right side to relieve the uterine pressure.

At the time of discharge, instruct the patient to rest at home until the cramping subsides. Light activity can then resume. Posttest activity restrictions for the next several days include no bending at the waist, no lifting of anything heavier than 20 pounds, and avoidance of strenuous exercise (Wright, 1994).

Provide the patient with written instructions to notify the physician immediately about any symptoms of itching, fever, leakage of fluid, severe abdominal pain, or unusual (increased or decreased) fetal activity.

### Critical Values

**RH incompatibility: Delta 450 spectral analysis 0.3–0.7; Freda classification 3+ or higher**
**Bilirubin: >0.47 mg/dL (SI >8 μmol/L)**

These values indicate severe fetal distress, and the higher values indicate impending fetal death. The nurse should notify the physician of these very abnormal results.

### Complications

The overall incidence of complications from amniocentesis is less than 0.5% (Satish, 1992; Wright, 1994). The complications include spontaneous rupture of the membranes, premature labor, spontaneous abortion, stillbirth, bleeding from a traumatic tap, and infection.

The nursing assessment of complications of amniocentesis is presented in Table 22–2.

## Breast Biopsy

**(Tissue Biopsy)**

Synonyms: None

### Normal Values

No malignant cells are seen.

**Table 22–2  Complications of Amniocentesis**

| Complication | Nursing Assessment |
|---|---|
| Premature labor | Leakage of fluid from the vagina<br>Severe, persistent uterine cramping<br>Uterine contractions |
| Bleeding | Blood in the amniotic fluid (port-wine–colored fluid)<br>Fetal lethargy or hyperactivity |
| Infection | Chills, fever<br>Purulent drainage at the puncture site<br>Uterine cramping<br>Fetal lethargy |

## Background Information

A suspicious palpable or nonpalpable lesion of the breast requires a biopsy to determine the cause and differentiate between benign and malignant tissue. A mammogram is often performed before the biopsy to visualize the size and location of the growth. Several methods can be used to obtain the tissue specimen.

**Surgical Biopsy.**   Using mammogram visualization, a localizing needle and a wire with a hook are implanted in the tumor. This helps to locate the abnormal tissue that is to be biopsied. After the patient is transferred to the operating room with the wire in place, the biopsy is performed under local or general anesthesia.

A surgical incision is made near the area of the wire and the abnormal breast tissue. In an *excisional biopsy,* the cyst, fibroadenoma, or calcified area is removed. In an *incisional biopsy,* a wedge of tissue is removed from the larger tumor mass. Sutures or surgical clips are used to close the incision (Buyske, MacKarem, Ulmer, & Hughes, 1996).

Disadvantages to the incisional biopsy procedure exist. Many nonpalpable lesions are benign. The external scar may be disfiguring, and the internal scarring impairs visualization in future mammography examinations. Also, because of bleeding or slippage of the localizing wire, the abnormal tissue might not be removed. In this case, the biopsy must be repeated.

**Fine Needle Aspiration Biopsy.**   This procedure is performed by inserting a thin, hollow needle into the lump or cyst. Aspiration removes the fluid of the cyst or a sample of tissue from a solid tumor.

Needle aspiration has advantages that include the ability to drain or collapse a benign cyst, to remove a small lesion by aspiration, and to obtain a tissue sample without disfigurement. The disadvantage is that without direct visualization, it is difficult to locate the abnormal tissue with pinpoint accuracy.

**Core Biopsy.**   This procedure uses a bigger-gauge needle and an automated biopsy gun to obtain a larger tissue sample. The needle is advanced to the appropriate depth, and then the gun is fired to advance the needle and extract a core of tissue. A local anesthetic is used to perform either the fine needle aspiration biopsy or the core biopsy.

**Localization Methods.**   It is sometimes difficult to locate the abnormal tissue because it is small and the breast is moveable. In addition, the mammogram provides a two-dimensional image without measurement of the depth of the tissue where the lesion is located. The localization may be done by palpation and clinical examination or by the use of grid coordinates to help with freehand needle placement. Ultrasound can be used to visualize and guide the placement of the needle.

Increasingly, stereotactic guidance is used to provide three-dimensional imaging for either surgical or needle biopsy measures. In this procedure, automated mammography and computers provide a three-dimensional view for precise localization of the abnormal tissue. Based on imaging, computer control, and the alignment of needle holders and guides, the needle is inserted and guided to the precise location and depth of the lesion. The radiologist can then insert dye or a wire hook to identify the location for the surgeon. Alternatively, the radiologist can perform a core needle biopsy with a biopsy gun (Newman, 1996). The average time to do the stereotactic needle placement and obtain the biopsy is 1 hour, but some procedures take up to 4 hours.

**Psychosocial Concerns.**    Women who must undergo breast biopsy experience varying degrees of distress, depression, anxiety, and heightened emo-

tion. The anxiety can be very high, particularly in women who have limited social support, less life satisfaction, higher feelings of hopelessness, or concurrent stress from other causes. The emotions experienced include fear of a possible malignancy, fear of the unknown, concerns about family health, fear of the biopsy procedure, and fear of the pain from the procedure (Kelly & Winslow, 1996; Northouse, Jeffs, Cracchiolo-Caraway, Lampman, & Dorris, 1995; Poole, 1997).

---

**Purpose of the Test**    The biopsy distinguishes benign from malignant breast disease.

---

**Procedure**    Fluid or tissue is removed from the breast lesion. The fluid aspiration sample will be used to make slides for microscopic analysis. Microscopic examination of permanent slides of the tissue will be performed. Frozen section examination may be done when the size of the tissue sample is sufficient. An estrogen-progesterone assay may be performed.

---

**Findings**    **Abnormal Values**

| | | |
|---|---|---|
| Fibroadenoma | Duct papilloma | Calcification |
| Fat necrosis | Mastitis | Cystosarcoma |
| Carcinoma | Fibroplasia | Granular cell tumor |
| Abscess | Lipoma | |

---

**Interfering Factors**    • Inadequate tissue sample

---

**Nursing Implementation**    **Pretest**

After the patient has been informed of the procedure and the reason for it, obtain written consent from the patient or the person legally responsible for the patient's health care decisions. Provide supplemental information, and answer the patient's questions in layperson language, as needed (Northouse, Tocco, & West, 1997).

If surgical biopsy and general anesthesia are planned, instruct the patient to fast from food and fluids for 8 hours before the surgery.

Assist the patient in removing all clothes and putting on a hospital gown.

Assess and record the vital signs, including temperature, blood pressure, pulse, and respirations.

Provide emotional support through the personalization of care. Assist the patient in reducing her stress by listening, providing explanations, affirming feelings, or using diversions, as indicated (Northouse et al., 1997).

For needle aspiration or incisional biopsy, place the patient in a supine position. For stereotactic needle biopsy, the patient sits erect in a chair with the breast compressed between the module and the compression plate, similar to the compression used in mammography.

### During the Test

Clean the breast tissue with povidone-iodine.

With the surgical or fine needle biopsy approach, apply the sterile drapes over the correct breast.

Assist with the preparation of the local anesthetic.

Provide support to the patient during the procedure. The patient can feel the injection of the anesthetic and the compression of the plates that squeeze the breast and hold the tissue immobile. Some patients can feel the push and pull of the needle, some pain, and other sensations such as stinging and the coldness of the compression plates. They are also uncomfortable because of positioning, with the head and neck turned to the side.

Assess the patient for early signs of fainting, such as lightheadedness, dizziness, pallor, and diaphoresis.

Some patients will faint during the procedure. The nurse or technician must be prepared to help the patient to prevent an injury from a fall. The compression plates must be released and the patient assisted to a Trendelenburg position in the examining chair.

Once the tissue is obtained, place the specimen in a sterile, dry, labeled container. Place the container on ice, and arrange for immediate transport of the specimen to the laboratory. If a frozen section can be done, the specimen may be given directly to the pathologist or technician who is waiting in the room.

When microscopic slides are prepared, the aspirated material is used to prepare two to four slides. The smears are fixed immediately with 95% alcohol or a spray-on cytologic fixative. The slides are then transported to the laboratory immediately.

Apply a dry, sterile dressing to the incision or puncture site.

### Posttest

Take vital signs and record the results. When a general anesthetic is used, monitor the vital signs every 15 to 30 minutes until the patient is reactive, alert, and stable.

To help the patient cope with postoperative depression or anxiety, encourage the patient to return to normal activity as soon as possible. After a surgical procedure, however, vigorous exercise must be avoided for 2 weeks.

To relieve surgical pain, instruct the patient to use warm, moist compresses or a heating pad and to wear a supportive bra.

Instruct the patient to shower or bathe as usual, using unscented soap for the needle puncture site. Cleansing of the surgical incision is prescribed by the surgeon.

The surgical dressing is changed once a day.

Advise the patient to inform the surgeon of inflammation, infection, or excessive pain in the incision.

Until the biopsy results are known, it is common for the patient to continue to experience anxiety and uncertainty in the postprocedure period.

**Complications**

The complications of incisional biopsy are cellulitis and hematoma. The needle aspiration methods can produce bruising, particularly when multiple needle insertions and aspirations occur during the procedure. The nursing assessment of complications of breast biopsy is presented in Table 22–3.

**Table 22–3    Complications of Breast Biopsy**

| Complication | Nursing Assessment |
| --- | --- |
| Cellulitis, infection | Fever<br>Headache<br>Malaise<br>Pain in the breast<br>Redness<br>Swelling |
| Hematoma | Swelling in the breast<br>Pain<br>Ecchymosis<br>Leakage of blood from the incision |

## Colposcopy

**(Endoscopy, Biopsy)**        Synonyms: None

**Normal Values**        No abnormalities of the vagina or cervix are noted.

## Background Information

The colposcope is a microscope with a bright light that is inserted into the vagina. In the examination of the vagina and cervix, it provides 10 to 40 times the magnification of the surface epithelium and underlying connective tissue. The goal is to identify precursor changes in cervical tissue before the changes advance from benign or atypical cells to cervical cancer. The location of the changes is often at or near the squamocolumnar junction.

The colposcopy procedure is done because the results of the Papanicolaou (Pap) smear were abnormal. As a follow-up examination, colposcopy allows for more precise examination of the cervix and vagina for cellular and vascular changes. Endocervical curettage is used to scrape the tissue and obtain cell samples of the endocervical canal, and a biopsy forceps is used to nip small samples of tissue from the cervix. After a biopsy, bleeding is controlled with an application of silver nitrate, pressure, or sutures.

Significantly abnormal tissue that may be invasive carcinoma appears as a large lesion, one that is dull gray-white or has visible dilated blood vessels. A low-grade lesion that has tiny red dots or a mosaic pattern from the connection of capillaries is also suspicious. The colposcopy examination takes 10 to 15 minutes to perform.

**Psychological Considerations.**   The patient is likely to become concerned when told that the Pap smear is abnormal and that follow-up colposcopy is needed. Fear, nervousness, and anxiety are common responses. During the waiting period before colposcopy is scheduled, the woman may experience sleep disturbances or crying episodes. Fear of cancer is prevalent (Nugent & Clark, 1996).

Some women do not know what a colposcopy is, why it is needed, and what the implications of the findings are. Because of fear and anxiety, some may fail to keep their appointment for the colposcopy. For some, a total lack of information exists, and for others, fear of the possibility of tumor or cancer already exists. Most are nervous and frightened. Before the examination, they desire more information about the test and its implications (Tomaino-Brunner, Freda, & Runowicz, 1996).

| | |
|---|---|
| **Purpose of the Test** | Colposcopy is performed to further evaluate an abnormal Pap smear, to monitor for precancerous abnormalities, or to evaluate a lesion of the vagina or cervix. |

| | |
|---|---|
| **Procedure** | A colposcope is inserted into the vagina to provide magnification and illumination of vaginal and cervical tissue. A tissue biopsy is performed. |

**Findings**

**Abnormal Values**

| | | |
|---|---|---|
| Atrophic cellular changes | Papilloma | Cervical erosion |
| Cervical intraepithelial neoplasia | Condyloma | Invasive carcinoma |
| | Infection, inflammation | |

**Interfering Factors**

- Vaginal creams
- Menstruation

**Nursing Implementation**

### Pretest

Before the test, provide information and education about the test to all women who are scheduled for colposcopy. The information should include what the test is, why it is needed, and what the patient will feel as the test is performed. The anticipatory teaching can help reduce anxiety (Nugent & Clark, 1996).

Schedule the procedure for the early part of the menstrual cycle, preferably between days 8 and 12. In this period, the cervical mucus is clear and thin and allows maximum visibility.

Instruct the patient to refrain from the application of any creams or vaginal medications, because they obscure the view of the cervix.

After the patient has been informed about the procedure, obtain written consent from the patient or the person legally responsible for the patient's health care decisions.

Assist the patient in removing all clothes and putting on a hospital gown.

### During the Test

Place the patient in the lithotomy position with the legs supported in stirrups.

During the insertion of the speculum and colposcope, instruct the patient to breathe through the mouth to help relax the muscles.

As endocervical curettage is done to obtain the specimen, the patient can feel a "pinch" or a brief cramping sensation. Also, she can hear the snipping sound when the clamp closes as a small piece of biopsy tissue is obtained (Nugent & Clark, 1996).

Once the glass slides are prepared with cell scrapings, apply the fixative to prevent drying of the cells. If biopsy specimens are taken, place the tissue on hard brown paper or on a nonstick gauze (Telfa). Each sample is placed in a separate specimen jar that contains fixative.

## Posttest

Ensure that all specimens are labeled appropriately and that the requisition slip identifies the source of the tissue.

Arrange for prompt transport of the specimen to the laboratory.

When a cervical biopsy is performed, instruct the patient to refrain from sexual intercourse and to avoid the insertion of anything into the vagina until the lesion is healed. Arrange for a follow-up appointment to evaluate the healing process.

## Computed Tomography, Pelvis

**(Tomography)**                Synonyms: None

In the evaluation of the female pelvis, computed tomography (CT) with intravenous contrast material produces clear, cross-sectional images of the pelvic tissues and organs. The pelvic CT scan is often used to determine the extent of malignancy or the source of infection. For these purposes, the scan usually includes the abdomen and the pelvis so that nearby organs, structures, and blood vessels are visualized. Oral and rectal barium contrast material may be administered to opacify the bowel loops. If a pelvic tumor or abscess is located, the CT scan is used to guide the placement of a needle in a percutaneous aspiration biopsy or in a percutaneous needle drainage of the purulence.

The scout view of the CT scan may be used to perform CT pelvimetry on the pregnant woman, particularly when the fetus is in a breech position. When compared with radiography, the CT measurements are more accurate, and less radiation exposure occurs for the mother and the fetus.

More extensive discussion of the CT scan is presented in Chapter 12.

## Cordocentesis and Fetal Blood Analysis

**(Fetal Blood)**                Synonyms: Percutaneous umbilical cord sampling, PUBS

**Normal Values**

**Fetal Blood Analysis**
Chromosomal analysis: Normal karyotype
Hematologic evaluation: Within normal limits for gestational age
Biochemistry analysis: Within normal limits for gestational age
IgG antibodies: Within normal limits
IgM antibodies: Within normal limits
Coagulation factors: Factors II, V, VIII, and IX are present

## Background Information

Cordocentesis is a method of obtaining a fetal blood specimen during pregnancy by venipuncture of an umbilical vein. The cordocentesis procedure can be performed in the second or third trimester, but for the purpose of genetic studies, the procedure is performed around the 15th to 16th weeks of gestation. The normal values of fetal cord blood vary based on the gestational age of the fetus.

### Fetal Blood Analysis

**Prenatal Chromosomal Analysis.** This procedure is performed on fetal lymphocytes obtained in the blood sample. The karyotype results are available in 2 to 3 days. The karyotype consists of the characteristics of the chromosomes, their number, form, size, structure, and grouping in the cell nucleus. Chromosomal abnormality in the fetus is identified.

The documentation of serious or severe chromosomal abnormality causes great emotional distress for the parents. Genetic counseling is an essential component of care and helps the parents make an informed choice about the continuation of the pregnancy. In obstetric management, the alternatives include continuation or termination of the pregnancy. If the pregnancy is continued, plans are made for intensive antepartal monitoring, for possible cesarean section for fetal distress during labor, and for the special postdelivery needs of the newborn.

**Congenital Infection.**   Infection in the pregnant woman can cross the placental barrier and infect the fetus. Some of the infections are teratogenic and have a devastating effect on the health and development of the fetus. The fetal blood analysis for infection includes measurement of fetal antibodies, white blood cells, eosinophils, liver enzymes, and platelets. Viral culture of the fetal blood and the amniotic fluid may be performed to identify the infectious organism.

Because fetal antibodies do not develop until the 22nd week of gestation, fetal cord blood samples cannot verify the infection before this time. Because of the legal limits of pregnancy termina-tion, little time is left to perform the cordocentesis, verify the fetal infection, and inform the parents. If the woman decides to terminate the pregnancy, the abortion procedure must be scheduled quickly.

**Thrombocytopenia.**   This is a low platelet count, which can result in fetal intracranial bleeding during pregnancy, labor, or the neonatal period. In most cases, the mother has immune thrombocytopenia and passively transmits the maternal antiplatelet antibodies to the fetus. If the fetus is affected, the treatment depends on the cause of the disorder and the severity of the platelet deficit. Several cordocentesis procedures may be performed to monitor the problem, and the fetus can receive a platelet transfusion by cordocentesis.

**Red Cell Isoimmunization.**   This occurs when the fetus has Rh-positive red blood cell antigens and the mother has Rh-negative erythrocytes. The maternal antibodies are transmitted to the fetus and result in fetal hemolysis of erythrocytes. If the erythrocyte incompatibility is not prevented or controlled, the fetus experiences a hemolytic anemia called *erythroblastosis fetalis* or *Rh disease.*

If the maternal serum antibody titer is greater than 1:64, the fetal risk increases and cordocentesis is indicated. The fetal cord blood is tested for blood type, the presence of Rh antigens, the hematocrit level, and the reticulocyte count. The treatment is individualized, but repeated cordocentesis may be used to monitor the problem and administer a fetal intravascular transfusion in utero as needed.

---

### Purpose of the Test
■

*Critical Thinking 22–3*
Will the identification of a chromosomal abnormality and the right to abortion ultimately result in the procreation of "perfect children" only?

Cordocentesis is used to obtain fetal blood for the identification of chromosomal abnormality, the detection of fetal infection, and the assessment for fetal anemia or other hematologic abnormality. It is also used to monitor fetal growth and development and the state of fetal health during the gestational period.

---

### Procedure

Guided by ultrasound, a sterile 20- to 22-gauge spinal needle is inserted through the woman's abdomen and uterus. The needle is then advanced into the umbilical cord until it is placed in one of the umbilical veins (Fig. 22–3). Once the needle placement is verified, a syringe is used to aspirate 0.5 to 3 mL of venous blood. The blood is then transferred to microtubes for the specific laboratory analyses.

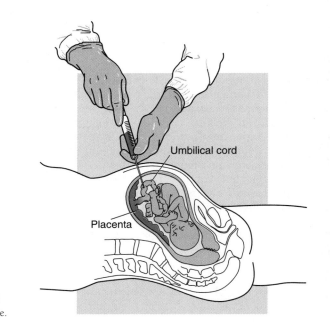

Umbilical cord

Placenta

**Figure 22–3**
Cordocentesis. The needle is advanced through the skin and into the uterus. Once the needle punctures the umbilical cord and one of the uterine veins, cord blood is aspirated by syringe.

| Findings | Abnormal Values | | |
|---|---|---|---|
| | CHROMOSOMAL DISORDER | | |
| | Trisomy<br>Fragile X syndrome<br>Sex chromosome<br>  mosaicism | Dysmorphic syn-<br>  dromes<br>Inborn errors of<br>  metabolism | |
| | INFECTION | | |
| | Toxoplasmosis<br>Rubella | Varicella<br>Cytomegalovirus | Human parvovirus<br>B19 |
| | COAGULOPATHY | | |
| | Hemophilia A<br>Hemophilia B | Von Willebrand's<br>  disease | |
| | ERYTHROCYTE DISORDERS | | |
| | Sickle cell anemia<br>Thalassemias<br>Spherocytosis | Enzyme deficiency<br>G-6-PD | |
| | HEMOLYTIC ANEMIA | | |
| | Rh disease<br>Minor antigen<br>  disorders | | |

PLATELET DISORDER

Thrombocytopenia

IMMUNODEFICIENCY

Severe combined immunodeficiency disorder
Chronic granulomatous disease

Wiskott-Aldrich syndrome
Ataxia telangiectasia
Homozygous C3 deficiency

Chédiak-Higashi syndrome

MISCELLANEOUS

Adrenoleukodystrophy
Familial hypercholesterolemia

Hyperphenylalaninemia

---

**Interfering Factors**

- Maternal obesity
- Uncooperative behavior
- Severe polyhydramnios
- Unfavorable fetal position
- Specimen contamination (amniotic fluid or blood)

---

**Nursing Implementation**

### Pretest

Once the woman has been informed of the procedure by her physician and has agreed to have the cordocentesis, obtain her written consent.

Assist the patient in removing all clothes and putting on a hospital gown.

Place the patient in a lateral position on the examining table.

Assess and record the mother's vital signs and the fetal heart rate.

Provide emotional support. The patient's anxiety level is often high because of concern for the safety of the fetus, fear of the procedure, or concern about the potential for abnormal test results.

### During the Test

Thoroughly cleanse the woman's abdomen with the appropriate povidone-iodine or surgical soap solution, and then place the surgical drape.

Assist with the preparation of the local anesthetic.

Reassure the patient when the injection causes a slight stinging sensation in the injection site on the abdomen.

Begin the frequent assessment and recording of the fetal heart rate. The fetal cardiac contractions can be counted during the imaging of the fetus on the ultrasound monitor.

Prepare any additional medications, as prescribed. If the fetus moves excessively, the mother may receive intravenous sedation to limit fetal movement. As an alternative, the fetus may receive an intravenous sedative or muscle relaxant via the umbilical vein.

Once the blood is obtained, assist with depositing it in the microtubes. Ensure that all blood samples and requisition forms are properly labeled. The data include the mother's name and age and the gestation of the pregnancy.

Each requisition slip clearly identifies the specimen as fetal blood (cord blood) obtained by cordocentesis.

### Posttest

Once the needle is removed, begin the monitoring of the fetal heart rate, and also assess and record the mother's vital signs.

In the recovery area, begin the external fetal monitoring of the fetal heart rate and uterine contractions. It is common for the mother to have mild uterine cramping for a short while. The fetal monitoring is discontinued when the fetal heart rate remains stable in a normal range and the uterine contractions cease.

At regular intervals, observe the abdomen for signs of bleeding. The small sterile dressing that covers the puncture site should remain dry and intact.

Administer prophylactic antibiotics, as prescribed.

In preparation for discharge, instruct the patient to rest for the remainder of the day. She should take her temperature at least two times per day. Fever greater than 100°F should be reported to her physician without delay. The patient is instructed to return to the physician for a follow-up evaluation and to learn the test results.

**Complications**

Although the cordocentesis procedure is a potential risk for the fetus, the overall complication rate of 1% to 2% or less is small (Mynaugh, 1996; Sonek & Nicolaides, 1994). Bleeding is the most common occurrence. Many pa-

**Table 22–4   Complications of Cordocentesis**

| Complication | Nursing Assessment |
| --- | --- |
| Fetal bradycardia | Fetal heart rate <120 beats/min<br>Fetal lethargy |
| Infection, fetal or maternal | **Maternal**<br><br>    Fever of 100°F or higher<br>    Chills<br>    Uterine cramping<br>    Possible redness, swelling, or purulence at the puncture site<br><br>**Fetal**<br><br>    Lethargy |
| Premature labor | Continual uterine contractions recorded on the fetal monitor<br>Sensations of uterine cramping, pain, or rhythmic contraction and relaxation of the uterus<br>Vaginal leakage of amniotic fluid |
| Bleeding, fetus, cord | Blood in the amniotic fluid<br>Fetal lethargy<br>Fetal hyperactivity<br>Continued staining or wetness of the dressing; pink drainage |

tients have minimal bleeding that ceases a few minutes after the needle is removed. If the bleeding from the cord is prolonged, the fetus may become anemic. Exsanguination can occur.

The more serious complications can have severe consequences. If prolonged fetal bradycardia or excessive bleeding occurs, an emergency cesarean section may be performed. With premature rupture of the membranes or ongoing preterm labor, the fetus may be delivered prematurely. Fetal death can occur as a result of these complications.

A summary of the complications of cordocentesis is presented in Table 22–4.

## Fetal Monitoring, External

**(Electric Monitoring)**    Synonym: External EFM

| **Normal Values** | Baseline fetal heart rate: 120–160 beats per minute<br>Variability: ±5–25 beats per minute |
|---|---|

## Background Information

The *fetal heart rate* is a reliable indicator of fetal well-being. It is also an indirect measurement of placental function. Placental blood flow provides oxygen to the fetal central nervous system and the reflexes that control fetal heart rate. The baseline fetal heart rate varies with the gestational age of the fetus. The normal rate is higher in the early months of gestation. It drops proportionally with advancing gestation, as the maturing fetal central nervous system exerts greater control over the fetal heart rate.

External monitoring is used to assess the fetus, particularly when a complication exists in the pregnancy. The fetal heart rate is monitored by a cardiotachometer, which amplifies the sounds and records the results on a graph. Simultaneously, a tokodynamometer measures and graphically records the pressure of uterine contractions (Fig. 22–4).

## Measurements

The normal baseline fetal heart rate is 120 to 160 beats per minute, with a variability of ±5 to 25 beats per minute. The fetal heart rate can change in response to uterine contractions, or the change in rate can be unrelated to contractions. In addition, the fluctuations of the fetal heart rate are assessed in terms of amplitude, lag time, and recovery time. The *amplitude* is the difference of beats per minute

between the baseline value and the maximum or minimum number of beats. The *lag time* is the difference between the peak of uterine contractions and the lowest point of deceleration. The *recovery time* is the difference between the end of the contraction and the return of the fetal heart rate to the baseline value.

**Antepartal Monitoring.**    The *nonstress test* assesses the fetal heart rate in response to fetal movement. The test monitors the fetal heart rate for 40 minutes during fetal rest or sleep as well as during fetal activity or movement. The fetal heart rate should increase in response to fetal movement. The normal nonstress test is also a good predictor of the health status of the fetus and a positive outcome of the pregnancy.

The *contraction stress test* identifies the fetus that already has diminished oxygenation to the central nervous system. The contraction is a source of stress because uterine and placental blood flow decreases during the contraction. When contractions occur, the healthy fetus sustains a normal baseline heart rate, with no decelerations. The fetus with compromised health or already-diminished blood flow responds to the contractions with late decelerations.

To obtain adequate data for the contraction stress test, the monitoring must evaluate the fetal

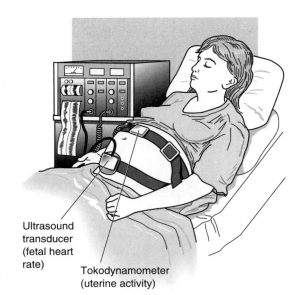

**Figure 22–4**
External fetal monitoring. The heart rate of the fetus is evaluated, particularly in response to uterine activity or contractions.

Ultrasound transducer (fetal heart rate)

Tokodynamometer (uterine activity)

response to at least three contractions in a 10-minute period. The contractions may occur naturally, or they may be stimulated. The stimulation can be carried out by having the patient rub one of her nipples to stimulate prolactin release and contractions, or it can be carried out by administering an intravenous dose of oxytocin.

**Intrapartum Monitoring.** External electronic fetal monitoring during labor provides a graphic recording of the fetal heart rate during contractions. Continual monitoring is not recommended for the patient who is at low risk and has had a normal pregnancy and normal labor. It is, however, highly informative in the moderate- to high-risk pregnancy or in cases of suspected or known problems with the fetus and its state of health.

---

**Purpose of the Test**

External fetal monitoring assesses fetal health and the fetal heart rate in non-stress situations during pregnancy or in stress situations that are provoked or occur during the contractions of labor.

---

**Procedure**

Using conductive gel on the skin, the cardiotachometer is placed on the woman's abdomen at the location at which the fetal heart tone is loudest. The tokodynamometer is placed over the fundus of the uterus to record the pressure of the contractions. Each transducer is attached with an abdominal belt or secured with an adhesive strip. The transducer is also connected by cable to the fetal monitor. After the recorder is set and adjusted, simultaneous linear graphic recordings occur.

| **Findings** | **Abnormal Values** | | |
|---|---|---|---|
| | MATERNAL PROBLEMS | | |
| | Fever<br>Tachycardia<br>Hypertension<br>Hypotension | Excess dosage of<br>narcotics, seda-<br>tives, or<br>tranquilizers | Ureteroplacental<br>insufficiency<br>Hyperthyroidism |
| | FETAL PROBLEMS | | |
| | Bradycardia<br>Arrhythmia<br>Central nervous<br>system depression<br>Hypoxia<br>Acidosis | Infection<br>Malposition<br>Temporary compres-<br>sion of fetal head<br>during contrac-<br>tions | Transitory umbilical<br>cord compression |

**Interfering Factors**

- Maternal obesity
- Excessive movement of the fetus or the mother
- Polyhydramnios

**Nursing Implementation**

**Pretest**

When monitoring is performed in the antepartum period, instruct the mother to eat a full meal before the test. This increases fetal activity. When the monitoring is performed during labor, the mother must remain without food and fluids. Assist the mother in removing all clothes and putting on a hospital gown.

Position her in a semi-Fowler's or left lateral position with the abdomen exposed.

As the equipment is prepared and applied, explain its purpose and show how the procedure benefits the mother and fetus. The woman should be reassured that the equipment cannot harm her or the fetus and that it does not interrupt the progress of labor.

**During the Test**

Once the monitoring begins, instruct the mother to avoid body movement for the first few minutes until the baseline recording is completed. Thereafter, she may move to change her position. During labor, she may move out of bed within the distance allowed by the monitoring cables to which she is attached.

Record any special events on the graph paper, including change in the patient's position, administration of medications, and procedures performed.

At intervals, check the positioning of the belts and transducers. They may fall off or slip out of position with the woman's activity.

Continuously evaluate the graphic recordings for abnormal results, and if they occur, notify the physician immediately. When the fetal heart rate indicates persistent fetal distress, cesarean section may be an urgent necessity.

### Posttest

Once the monitoring is completed, remove the belts and transducers. Cleanse the skin to remove the conductive gel.

When the woman has diabetes mellitus, hypertension, a pregnancy of more than 42 weeks of gestation, or preterm labor, or when fetal growth retardation occurs, the test is repeated on a weekly basis. Arrange the next appointment date.

## Fetal Monitoring, Internal

**(Electronic Monitoring)**   Synonyms: Internal EFM, direct fetal monitoring

**Normal Values**

Baseline fetal heart rate: 120–160 beats per minute
Variability: ±5–25 beats per minute

### Background Information

Internal electronic fetal monitoring provides an accurate recording of the fetal heart rate and uterine contractions during labor. It is an invasive procedure that poses some risk to the mother and the fetus, but the benefit is a more accurate assessment and monitoring of the fetus during labor. It is used in the high-risk pregnancy or when the fetal health is at risk or already compromised.

The fetal heart rate is monitored by a fetal electrode that is applied to the presenting part, often the scalp (Fig. 22–5). The electrode is connected by a wire to a metal plate on the mother's thigh. A cord goes from the plate to the monitor for a fetal heart rate graphic recording. The strength of

the uterine contractions is monitored by an intra-uterine pressure catheter. Within the tip of the catheter, the transducer or computer chip measures the pressures of the uterus during contraction and relaxation. The catheter is also connected by cable to the fetal monitor. The uterine pressure tracing is recorded simultaneously with the fetal heart rate.

To implant each monitor in the uterine cavity, the membranes must be ruptured. If they are still intact, amniotomy is performed. During implantation of the electrode, care is taken to avoid its placement in the eyes, fontanelle, face, or genitals of the fetus.

### Purpose of the Test

Internal fetal monitoring is used to assess the heart rate of the fetus who is at risk for uteroplacental insufficiency or fetal compromise. It is also used to monitor the strength of uterine contractions, particularly when oxytocin has been administered, when uterine dystocia is suspected, or when a trial of labor occurs after a previous delivery by cesarean section.

### Procedure

An electrode is inserted through a guide in the vagina and is implanted under the skin of the fetus. The monitoring device is connected to a metal plate on the mother's thigh and then to the fetal cardiac monitor. The internal pressure catheter is passed through the guide and advanced into the uterine cavity until its tip is located between the fetal head and the uterine cervix. This moni-

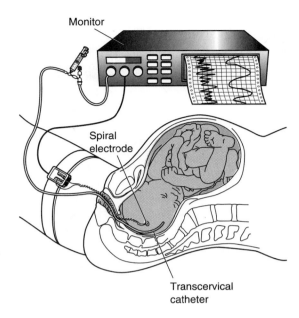

Monitor

Spiral
electrode

Transcervical
catheter

**Figure 22–5**
Internal fetal monitoring. The scalp of the fetus is punctured by
the implantation of the electrode. After delivery, the nurse
assesses the puncture site for signs of bleeding, hematoma,
tissue injury, and potential infection.

toring device is connected by a cord to a pressure reading device and then
by cable to the monitor.

| **Findings** | **Abnormal Values** | | |
|---|---|---|---|
| | MOTHER | | |
| | Infection, fever | Hyperthyroidism | Uterine dystocia |
| | Hypotension | Overmedication with | |
| | Tachycardia | a central nervous | |
| | Anemia | system depressant | |
| | FETUS | | |
| | Bradycardia | Congenital anomalies | Hypotension |
| | Malposition | (cardiac or | |
| | Hypoxia | cerebral) | |
| | Arrhythmia | Growth retardation | |

**Interfering Factors**
- Maternal obesity
- Excessive maternal or fetal activity
- Closed cervix
- Presenting part not fully descended or engaged

**Nursing Implementation**  **Pretest**

Once the woman receives a complete explanation of the procedure, obtain a
written consent.
Assist the woman into the lithotomy position with her legs in stirrups.

### During the Test

Assist the nurse-midwife or physician with the equipment needed for a sterile vaginal examination and placement of the monitors.

Apply conductive gel to the leg plate and use the strap to secure the plate to the mother's thigh. The uterine catheter is taped to the thigh. Connect the wires and cables correctly.

Turn on the recording device, run a test pattern, and begin the continuous monitoring. Observe for abnormal patterns.

If it helps the mother and her support person to relax, provide simple explanations about the variations in the recordings. Some individuals, however, are made more anxious by knowing every detail. Continue to provide encouragement to the mother as she progresses through labor.

On the paper recording strip, write the patient's name, identification number, weeks of gestation, and the time and date that the monitoring began. Whenever change in maternal or fetal activity, addition of medication, or change of equipment occurs, record the data on the electronic fetal monitor strip.

In the patient's chart, record the woman's vital signs, the time of the initiation of internal fetal monitoring, and any special procedures, such as amniotomy, that were performed.

### Posttest

Once the electrode and the catheter are removed and the infant is delivered, inspect the skin and puncture site for signs of laceration or infection. Record the results.

Apply an antiseptic or antibiotic solution to the site of skin puncture.

## Fetal Scalp Blood Sampling

**(Endoscopy, Capillary Blood)** Synonyms: None

| Normal Values | Fetal pH: 7.25–7.35 |
| --- | --- |

## Background Information

During labor, fetal distress and fetal hypoxia are indicated by a number of assessment findings (Saling, 1997). The fetal monitor may demonstrate late or variable deceleration, a change in heart rate (either bradycardia or tachycardia), or a loss of beat-to-beat variability. In addition, some meconium staining of the amniotic fluid may occur.

The pH of the capillary blood is similar to that of the arterial blood. The pH of fetal capillary blood is a direct assessment for fetal acidosis. In cases of fetal hypoxia, the pH of the fetal blood falls to less-than-normal levels. A borderline result is indicated by a pH of 7.2 to 7.25. When this slight decline occurs, additional blood specimens are obtained in 15 to 30 minutes. Acidosis is defined as a fetal pH of 7.2 or less, usually demonstrated in two consecutive blood samples. The acidosis confirms that the fetus is hypoxic and that fetal health is compromised. Immediate delivery by forceps or cesarean section is indicated.

To obtain the capillary blood sample, access to the scalp or skin of the fetus is necessary. The mother must be in active labor, with the membranes ruptured, the cervix partially dilated, and

the presenting part engaged. To obtain pertinent
and timely data, the blood must be analyzed within
10 to 15 minutes.

| | |
|---|---|
| **Purpose of the Test** | Fetal scalp blood sampling is carried out to determine the fetal capillary pH and to identify or confirm fetal acidosis. |
| **Procedure** | Under sterile conditions, an endoscope with a light is inserted through the vagina and up to the fetal scalp or presenting part (Fig. 22–6). After the fetal skin is cleansed, a scalpel blade is passed through the endoscope and is used to nick the fetal scalp or skin. Three long heparinized microtubes are used to collect the capillary blood specimen. Once the bleeding ceases, the endoscope is removed. |

**Findings**

**Decreased Values**

| | | |
|---|---|---|
| Fetal hypoxia | Fetal acidosis | Acute fetal distress |

**Interfering Factors**

- Intact membranes
- Undilated cervix
- Acute and ominous conditions that require immediate delivery (placenta previa, abruptio placentae)

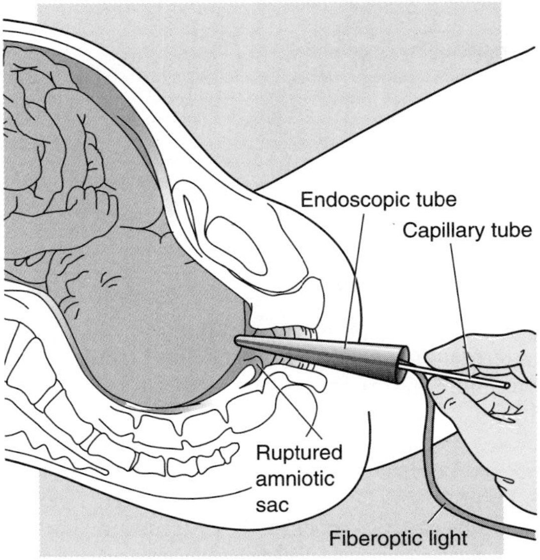

**Figure 22–6**

Fetal scalp blood sampling. During labor, the fetal scalp provides an excellent source of capillary blood, particularly useful for measuring pH. Once the infant is delivered, the nurse assesses the scalp for signs of bleeding, hematoma, tissue injury, and potential infection.

**Nursing Implementation**

### Pretest

Once the need for the test is explained to the mother, obtain her written consent to test the fetal blood.

Although the situation is urgent, provide appropriate support to the mother and her support person. Their anxiety level will be high.

Place the mother in the lithotomy or lateral position.

Notify the laboratory if the fetal blood sample requires immediate analysis.

### During the Test

Control the endoscopy light and pass the needed equipment to the individual obtaining the sample.

If the cervix is dilated manually, reassure the mother that it is normal to feel uterine cramping.

On receipt of the blood tubes, seal them with clay or wax.

Place the tubes on ice to minimize cellular respiration and alteration of the pH.

Label all specimens. Write the identification data, time, date, and source of the blood on the requisition slip.

Send the blood to the laboratory immediately.

### Posttest

Assist the mother to a lateral position.

As the mother and her support person await the test results, encourage them to support each other.

Document the procedure in the patient's chart.

If labor continues, assess the vaginal fluid for signs of additional blood that could come from the fetal puncture site. Continued fetal bleeding puts the fetus at greater risk.

After delivery, assess the puncture site and document its size and location. Cleanse the skin with an antiseptic, and apply antibiotic ointment.

## Hysterosalpingography

**(Radiography)**   Synonym: Hysterosalpingogram, HSG

**Normal Values**   Normal flow of dye through the uterus and fallopian tubes

## Background Information

As part of the infertility work-up in the female, the hysterosalpingogram is performed to identify anatomic abnormality of the uterus or occlusion of the fallopian tubes. The lumen of each of these structures is visualized. The tubes can be blocked because of external compression from an abdominal or pelvic abnormality, or internal blockage from scarring can exist. The uterus may have an anatomic abnormality, such as that caused by incomplete development of the uterus, or a congenital abnormality resulting from intrauterine exposure to diethylstilbestrol.

In normal anatomy, once the radiopaque dye is instilled into the uterine cavity, the effects of gravity and positional changes promote the flow of dye through the uterus and fallopian tubes and then into the abdominal cavity. If the contrast material does not enter the abdominal cavity, one or both tubes are blocked. The test requires 30 to 45 minutes to complete.

| | |
|---|---|
| **Purpose of the Test** | Hysterosalpingography is used to assess the patency of the fallopian tubes as part of infertility studies of the female. It also can identify abnormal development of the uterus and the presence of a uterine fistula. |
| **Procedure** | Radiopaque contrast medium is instilled through a catheter into the uterus. The patient's positional changes and a tilting of the table promote gravity flow of the contrast material. Fluoroscopic and x-ray films provide visualization of the interior surfaces of the uterus and fallopian tubes. |

**Findings**

**Abnormal Values**

Partial or complete
  obstruction of the
  fallopian tubes
Fibroid tumor of the
  uterus

Adhesions
Uterine fistula
Foreign body (e.g.,
  intrauterine device)
Uterine malformation

**Interfering Factors**

- Menstruation
- Pregnancy
- Active uterine bleeding
- Pelvic inflammatory disease
- Allergy to the contrast medium

**Nursing Implementation**

**Pretest**

Schedule this test during the early part of the menstrual cycle, before ovulation occurs. This prevents interference with ovulation, irradiation of the oocyte, or the possibility of an early phase of pregnancy.

Ensure that the patient has no current vaginal bleeding or gynecologic infection. When these conditions exist, the contrast material could be absorbed into the vasculature, or its flow could introduce microorganisms into the fallopian tubes.

Identify any patient with a history of allergy to iodine or shellfish or a reaction to a previous x-ray study that used iodinated contrast medium. If a positive allergic history exists, plans are made to premedicate the patient with steroids or an antihistamine, or both.

Once the patient is informed of the procedure, obtain written consent.

In the pretest preparation, instruct the patient to take the prescribed laxative on the night before the test. On the morning of the procedure, cleansing enemas are done until the returns are clear (Snopek, 1992).

Assist the patient in removing all clothes and putting on a hospital gown. Instruct the patient to void to empty the bladder. This prevents displacement of the uterus and fallopian tubes by an enlarged bladder.

Take the patient's vital signs and record the results.

**During the Test**

Place the patient in the lithotomy position.

Provide reassurance as the vaginal speculum is inserted, the cervix is cleansed with povidone-iodine, and the cannula is inserted. As the contrast material is instilled, the patient may experience temporary sensations of nausea, dizziness, bradycardia, or uterine cramping.

Between radiographic images, help the patient change position so that the contrast medium flows through the fallopian tubes.

### Posttest

Monitor and record the patient's vital signs.

Instruct the patient to gradually return to pretest activity levels.

---

**Complications**

An allergic reaction to the contrast medium can cause hives, urticaria, or hypotension.

---

## Laparoscopy, Pelvic

**(Endoscopy)**                     Synonym: Peritoneoscopy

---

**Normal Values**            No abnormalities of the ovaries, fallopian tubes, uterus, or peritoneal cavity are noted.

---

### Background Information

The laparoscope is a fiberoptic telescope that is used to visualize the peritoneal cavity, ovaries, uterus, and fallopian tubes. If a determination of tubal patency is to be included, hysterosalpingography is also performed. Additional surgical procedures such as tissue biopsy or tubal ligation may be part of the procedure.

Under general or local anesthesia, the peritoneal cavity is inflated with 2 to 3 L of carbon dioxide. The gas distends the abdomen wall so that the instruments can be inserted safely. The laparoscope is inserted through a small incision just below the umbilicus. If a surgical procedure is to be performed, a second incision is made in the lower abdomen for insertion of the additional instruments. To prevent trauma or injury, an indwelling catheter is used to keep the urinary bladder deflated.

---

**Purpose of the Test**

Laparoscopy is used to investigate the cause of pelvic pain, to detect endometriosis or an ectopic pregnancy, to identify a pelvic mass, or to determine if cancer is present or has metastasized.

---

**Procedure**

A laparoscope is used to visualize the size and shape of the uterus, ovaries, and fallopian tubes. The peritoneal cavity and peritoneum are observed for signs of infection, abscess, or adhesions. Biopsy of abnormal tissue may be performed.

---

**Findings**

**Abnormal Values**

| | |
|---|---|
| Ovarian cyst | Pelvic inflammatory |
| Endometriosis | disease |
| Ectopic pregnancy | Adhesions |
| Uterine fibroid | Abnormality of the |
| tumors | fallopian tubes |
| Pelvic abscess | Malignancy |

**Interfering Factors**

- Failure to maintain a nothing-by-mouth status
- Obesity
- Adhesions
- Advanced abdominal wall malignancy

**Nursing Implementation**

### Pretest

Instruct the patient to discontinue all food and fluids for 8 hours before the procedure is performed.

After the patient has been informed about the procedure, obtain written consent from the patient or the person legally responsible for the patient's health care decisions. Ensure that all preoperative laboratory work is completed and that the results are posted in the chart.

Assist the patient in removing all clothes and putting on a hospital gown.

Assess and record the vital signs, including temperature, blood pressure, pulse, and respirations.

Place the patient in the lithotomy position, with the legs supported in stirrups.

### During the Test

Insert the indwelling catheter into the bladder and connect it to the urinary collection system.

To help alleviate anxiety, provide reassurance or distraction, as indicated.

If a biopsy specimen is obtained, place the tissue in a glass container with preservative. Identify the tissue source on the requisition slip.

### Posttest

Monitor the vital signs every 30 minutes for 4 hours or until they are stable.

Ensure that the small dressing or dressings remain dry and intact.

Once the catheter is removed, monitor for voiding and urinary output.

Once the patient is alert, encourage ambulation and the oral intake of fluids. Carbonated beverages are avoided for 24 to 36 hours, because with the excess carbon dioxide in the abdomen, the intake of carbonated beverage can cause vomiting.

Provide pain medication as needed. Advise the patient that some pain in the abdomen and shoulder is to be expected for 24 to 36 hours. The cause is

**Table 22–5  Complications of Laparoscopy**

| Complication | Nursing Assessment |
| --- | --- |
| Hemorrhage | Hypotension<br>Tachycardia<br>Dizziness<br>Grossly bloody drainage from the incision |
| Infection | Fever<br>Malaise<br>Diaphoresis<br>Tachycardia<br>Abdominal pain |

the carbon dioxide gas, which will gradually be absorbed and exhaled from the lungs.

Instruct the patient to restrict physical activity for a few days until the incisions are healed. The patient must notify the physician of increasing abdominal pain, fever, or abnormal drainage.

## Complications

Laparoscopy can cause bleeding from the puncture of a blood vessel, infection from external contamination, or the accidental puncture of the intestine. Although these events can occur, they are quite rare. The complications of laparoscopy are presented in Table 22–5.

## Mammography

**(Radiography)**                    Synonym: Mammogram

## Normal Values

The breast tissue is within normal limits.

## Background Information

Mammography is used as a screening tool for breast cancer in asymptomatic women because it can identify tumors less than 5 mm in diameter (Peart, 1994). This small size is not palpable on physical examination. For the patient with an irregular area of tissue or a palpable growth, this x-ray method is used to obtain additional data about the abnormality.

The normal breast tissue of the younger woman is dense fibroglandular tissue. After childbearing and in older age, the glandular tissue atrophies and is replaced with fatty tissue. Because fatty tissue is radiolucent, lesions or masses are visible on mammography films. If a woman has silicone implants, however, mammography will be of little use. The prosthetic implants are radiopaque, and the early stages of breast malignancy cannot be visualized.

Malignancy of the breast appears as a dense mass with irregular margins or spiricules. The malignancy may also appear as numerous tiny clusters of calcification. The calcification can be caused by the secretion of calcium from tumor cells or tissue necrosis, or it can be caused by benign fibrocystic disease. Additional abnormalities that appear on mammography and may indicate malignancy include a newly developed area of density and asymmetry of the breast.

Benign growths are also visible, for example, fibroadenoma, cysts, and lymph glands. On mammography, these growths appear more rounded and have well-defined margins.

## Purpose of the Test

Mammography is used to screen for breast cancer, and it investigates a symptomatic change in the breast tissue. It also helps differentiate between benign and malignant diseases of the breast.

## Procedure

X-ray films of each breast are taken from different angles (Fig. 22–7).

## Findings

**Abnormal Values**

Benign cyst                    Malignancy of the
Microcalcifications            breast
Fibroadenoma

**Interfering Factors**
- Jewelry and clothing
- Scar tissue from previous surgery
- Body powders, creams, and deodorants
- Silicone breast implants

**Nursing Implementation**

**Pretest**

Instruct the patient to omit the use of body creams, powders, and deodorants

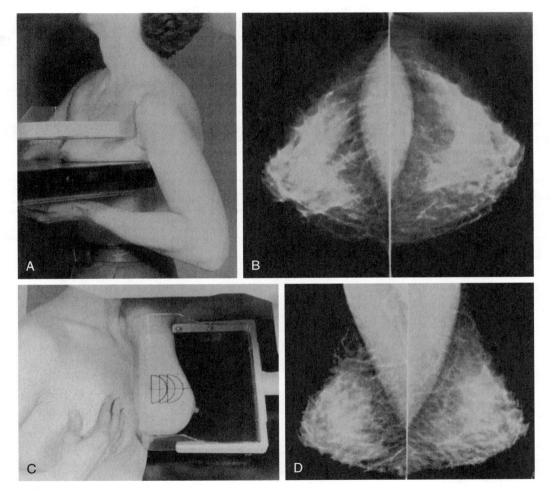

**Figure 22–7**

Mammography positioning and corresponding radiographic views. *A,* Positioning for craniocaudal view. *B,* Radiographs depicting properly positioned craniocaudal views. *C,* Positioning for mediolateral oblique view. *D,* Radiographs depicting properly positioned mediolateral oblique views. (Reproduced with permission from Prue, L. K. [1994]. *Atlas of mammographic positioning* [pp. 16, 17, 23, 24]. Philadelphia: W. B. Saunders.)

■
*Critical Thinking 22–4*
During a health teaching class at the senior center, the nurse discovers that only a few women have had a recent mammogram. Identify possible reasons for their omission of this health care screening test. How would you intervene?

on the day of the test. The metallic elements in these products interfere with visualization of the tissues.

Instruct the patient to remove all jewelry and clothing above the waist. The hospital gown is put on with the opening to the front.

### During the Test

Although the nurse does not perform the mammogram, he or she may be asked to describe the procedure.

The patient is positioned by seating her in front of the machine, with the breast placed on the platform over the x-ray cassette. The compressor is applied to the top of the tissue. The breast is squeezed between the two surfaces to hold the tissue firmly in place. The sensation is one of compression.

Each breast is radiographed separately.

### Posttest

Explain how the patient will learn of the results. Usually the report is sent to her personal physician.

No other posttest nursing measures are needed.

## Papanicolaou Smear

**(Cytologic Study)**          Synonyms: Pap smear, cervicovaginal cytology, cervical smear

| **Normal Values** | Bethesda system classification: Normal; within normal limits |
|---|---|

## Background Information

The Papanicolaou (Pap) smear is an inexpensive screening test to detect premalignant and malignant lesions of the cervix, vagina, and endometrium. The Papanicolaou smear test results use the Bethesda system as the accepted standard for reporting the cervical cytologic results.

The report informs about the adequacy of the specimen and the descriptive findings regarding infection or abnormal cell changes. In the Bethesda system, the descriptive categories include infections and reactive or reparative changes and epithelial or glandular cell abnormalities. With cell abnormality, the changes are graded in severity. The borderline lesion is defined as atypical squamous cells of undetermined significance (ASCUS). The squamous intraepithelial lesions (SIL) are graded from low grade to high grade. The low-grade squamous intraepithelial lesion (LSIL) consists of condyloma, mild dysplasia (CIN I)—a precancerous state—or both. A high-grade squamous intraepithelial lesion (HSIL) ranges from moderate dysplasia

(CIN II) to severe dysplasia (CIN III)—carcinoma in situ. Invasive carcinoma or adenocarcinoma is also included in the HSIL category (Prasad, 1995).

Abnormal Papanicolaou smear results, the patient's history of relevant risk factors, and the findings of the pelvic examination are the basis for an individualized treatment plan. This may include treatment for infection, repeat Papanicolaou smear testing at specific intervals, or colposcopy with possible biopsy.

**Psychosocial Concerns.**    When results of the Papanicolaou smear are abnormal, most women experience fear of cancer. They need information and support to clarify misconceptions and to encourage them to complete the follow-up testing (Mashburn & Scharbo-DeHaan, 1997). They may also fear the potential loss of sexual or reproductive function, or they may fear the follow-up test procedures. The anxiety may be expressed verbally, somatically (as with loss of sleep or weight gain), or emotionally with crying, anger, or irritation.

**Populations at Risk.**  Older, urban women with a low-income or poverty status and less education, who are of an ethnic minority, are at high risk for poor health and disease in general (Baldwin et al., 1996). In this population, the ethnic groups who are at higher risk for cancer of the cervix are women who are Hispanic, African-American, or Asian (Japanese, Filipino, and Vietnamese). This group of the population have a lower screening rate, a higher risk for cervical cancer, and a higher risk for a late diagnosis of this disorder. Following an abnormal Pap smear, they also have a low rate of follow-up diagnostic and treatment measures (Fox, Arnsberger, & Zhang, 1997).

| | |
|---|---|
| **Purpose of the Test** | The Papanicolaou smear is used to detect inflammation, premalignant changes, and malignancy or infection of the vagina and cervix. It is also used to evaluate the response of the cervix to chemotherapy or radiotherapy in the treatment of cancer. |

| | |
|---|---|
| **Procedure** | Using a vaginal speculum to enhance visibility, secretions and cells from the cervix and vagina are collected. The fluid and tissue scrapings are placed on glass slides and sprayed with or immersed in a fixative. |

**Quality Control**

> The speculum is not lubricated before insertion because the lubricant would interfere with the microscopic viewing of the slides. The fixative must be applied promptly to prevent drying of the cells.

| | |
|---|---|
| **Findings** | **Abnormal Values** |

| | | |
|---|---|---|
| Cervical dysplasia or cervical intraepithelial neoplasia | Cervicovaginal endometriosis | Lymphogranuloma venereum |
| Genital infection (viral, fungal, parasitic) | Condyloma | Carcinoma in situ |
| | Human papillomavirus | Adenocarcinoma |

| | |
|---|---|
| **Interfering Factors** | • Menstruation<br>• Recent douching<br>• Vaginal infection or medication<br>• Recent sexual intercourse<br>• Drying of the specimen<br>• Inadequate specimen |

| | |
|---|---|
| **Nursing Implementation** | **Pretest**<br>Schedule the test for when the patient is not menstruating.<br>Instruct the patient to refrain from sexual intercourse, douching, and vaginal medication for 48 hours before the test. Sexual intercourse can cause inflammation of the tissue. Douching can remove surface cells before the test sample is obtained. Medication obscures the microscopic examination of the |

cells. If vaginal infection is present, it will be treated and the Papanicolaou test postponed for 2 to 4 weeks.

Before the examination, instruct the patient to void.

### During the Test

Help the patient to lie on the table in the lithotomy position with the legs supported by stirrups. The elderly patient may need extra assistance in positioning because of stiffness and arthritis pain.

After the tissue and fluid samples are obtained, apply the fixative by spraying the samples or immersing them in solution. Identify each slide with the patient's name.

### Posttest

Help the patient get down from the table.

On the requisition slip, write the patient's name, age, date of last menstrual period, and the source of the specimen. The pertinent clinical data are also included, such as history of an abnormal Papanicolaou smear, carcinoma, radiation, chemotherapy, abnormal vaginal bleeding, exposure to diethylstilbestrol, a visible lesion, or recent pregnancy.

When the woman is informed of abnormal Papanicolaou test results, she often requires additional information about the meaning of the results and the follow-up measures. Recognize the patient's anxiety or confusion and intervene appropriately to help with the emotional stress. Additional information and repetition of the instructions may be needed.

To help promote Pap smear screening and follow-up care for underserved older women of ethnic minority groups, nurses can implement multiple interventions to provide a supportive climate. These measures include demonstrating concern for the patient as a person, making follow-up phone calls, speaking the patient's language, arranging convenient appointment times, and providing information about the test, the results, and the reason to have a repeat test or follow-up diagnostic measures, as appropriate (Baldwin et al., 1996; Fox et al., 1997; Mahon, 1996).

## Ultrasound, Pelvis

(Ultrasound)                               Synonyms: None

Gynecologic ultrasound can be performed transabdominally to scan multiple planes of the abdomen and pelvis. In a transvaginal approach, the ultrasound performs the scans in the coronal plane. In a comprehensive examination of the female, both the transabdominal and the transvaginal approach are used. Male pelvic ultrasonography usually uses an endorectal approach to examine the pelvic organs and structures (Fig. 22–8).

**Ultrasound in Pregnancy.**   In conditions related to pregnancy, ultrasound identifies an early ectopic pregnancy, a multiple pregnancy, fetal abnormality, and assessment of fetal growth. It is also used to guide aspiration procedures such as amniocentesis, cordocentesis, and the aspiration of multiple oocytes for in vitro fertilization.

**Female Pelvic Ultrasound.**   In the diagnosis of gynecologic problems, one use of ultrasound is to identify an ovarian malignancy at an early stage. In the case of abnormal uterine bleeding, it will identify submucous leiomyo-

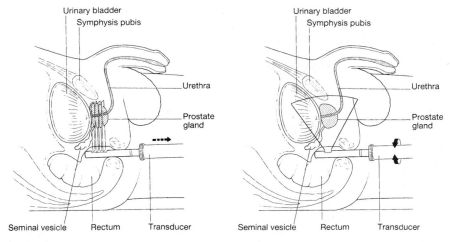

**Figure 22–8**
Ultrasound of the male pelvis. *Left,* Transverse plane—rectal approach. *Right,* Sagittal plane—rectal approach. (Reproduced with permission from Tempkin, B. B. [1993]. *Ultrasound scanning: Principles and protocols* [p. 197]. Philadelphia: W. B. Saunders.)

mas and evaluate the thickness of the uterine wall. Pelvic ultrasound often precedes any invasive gynecologic diagnostic test such as dilation and curettage. The procedure may also be used to monitor ovulation in the diagnosis and treatment of infertility and in the follow-up of treatment for pelvic inflammatory disease.

**Male Pelvic Ultrasound.** Ultrasonography in the male is used to assess the texture, size, and condition of the prostate gland, prostatic urethra, seminal vesicles, and vas deferens. It is also used to guide the placement of the needle during biopsy of the prostate gland. Ultrasound is part of the diagnostic work-up to detect and stage prostate cancer.

A complete discussion of ultrasound is presented in Chapter 8.

## References

Anderson, R. A., Eccles, S. M., & Irvine, D. S. (1996). Home ovulation testing in a donor insemination service. *Human Reproduction, 11*(8), 1674–1677.

Aziz, D. C. (1996). Tumor markers II. Clinical use of tumor markers based on outcome analysis. *Laboratory Medicine, 27*(12), 817–822.

Baldwin, D., Johnson, P., Cotanch, P., & Williams, J. (1996). *An afrocentric approach to breast and cervical cancer. Early detection and screening.* Washington, DC: American Nurses Publishing.

Brunzel, N. A. (1994). *Fundamentals of urine and body fluid analysis.* Philadelphia: W. B. Saunders.

Buyske, J., MacKarem, G., Ulmer, B. C., & Hughes, K. S. (1996). Breast cancer in the nineties. *AORN Journal, 64*(1), 64–65, 67–72.

Carlson, K. J., Skates, S. J., & Singer, D. E. (1994). Screening for ovarian cancer. *Annals of Internal Medicine, 121,* 2, 124–132.

Carpenter, V., & Colwell, B. (1995). Cancer knowledge, self-efficacy and cancer screening behaviors among Mexican-American women. *Journal of Cancer Education, 10*(4), 217–222.

Colodny, C. S. (1995). Procedures for your practice: Colposcopy and cervical biopsy. *Patient Care, 29*(11), 66–67.

Covington, C., Gieleghem, P., Board, F., Madison, K., Nedd, D., & Miller, L. (1996). Family care related to alpha-fetoprotein screening. *Journal of Obstetric, Gynecologic and Neonatal Nursing, 25,* 125–130.

Crum, C. P., & Newkirk, G. R. (1995). Abnormal Pap smears, cancer risk, and HPV. *Patient Care, 29*(11), 35–36, 38–40, 42.

Cunningham, F. G., MacDonald, P. C., & Gant, N. F. (1997). *Williams obstetrics* (20th ed.). Stamford, CT: Appleton & Lange.

Daily, C., Laurant, S. L., & Nunley, W. C. (1994). The prognostic value of serum progesterone and quantitative beta human chorionic gonadotropin in early human pregnancy. *American Journal of Obstetrics and Gynecology, 171*(2), 380–384.

Davidaud, J., Fournet, D., Ballongue, C., Guillem, G. P., Leblanc, A., Casellas, C., & Pau, B. (1993). Reliability and feasibility of pregnancy home-use tests: Validation and diagnostic evaluation by 638 volunteers. *Clinical Chemistry, 39*(1), 53–59.

Davidhizar, R., & Dowd, S. B. (1996). Fear in the patient with undiagnosed symptoms. *Journal of Nuclear Medicine Technology, 24*(4), 325–328.

Deane, K. A., & Degner, L. F. (1997). Determining the information needs of women after breast biopsy procedures. *AORN Journal, 65*(4), 767–768, 770–772, 775.

Depression follows miscarriage. (1997). *Journal of Psychosocial Nursing and Mental Health Services, 35*(6), 7.

Fehring, R. J. (1992). New technology in natural family planning. *Journal of Obstetric Gynecologic and Neonatal Nursing, 20*(3), 199–205.

Field, N. T., & Gilbert, W. M. (1997). Current states of amniotic fluid tests of fetal maturity. *Clinical Obstetrics and Gynecology, 40*(2), 366–386.

Fox, P., Arnsberger, P., & Zhang, X. (1997). An examination of differential follow-up rates in cervical cancer screening. *Journal of Community Health, 22*(3), 199–209.

Green, J., & Statham, H. (1993). Testing for fetal abnormality in routine antenatal care. *Midwifery, 9,* 124–135.

Hammond, K. R., & Steinkamph, M. P. (1992). Practical ways to monitor ovulation. *Patient Care, 26*(20), 123–125, 129–133, 137–138.

Held, J. L. (1996). Cancer care. Teaching your patients about PSA and CA 125 . . . tumor markers. *Nursing 96, 26*(2), 78.

Henry, J. B. (Ed.) (1996). *Clinical diagnosis and management by laboratory methods* (19th ed.). Philadelphia: W. B. Saunders.

Hicks, J. M. (1993). Home testing: To do or not to do? *Clinical Chemistry, 39*(1), 7–8.

Jacobs, D. S., Demott, W. R., Grady, H. J., Horvat, R. T., Huestis, D. W., & Kasten, B. L. (Eds.). (1996). *Laboratory test handbook* (4th ed.). Baltimore: Williams & Wilkins.

Jeffs, M., Cracchiolo-Caraway, A., Lampman, L., & Dorris, G. (1995). Emotional distress reported by women and husbands prior to a breast biopsy. *Nursing Research, 44*(4), 196–201.

Kadlec, J. V., & McPherson, R. A. (1995). Ethical issues in screening and testing for genetic diseases. *Clinics in Laboratory Medicine, 15*(4), 989–949.

Kelly, P., & Windslow, E. H. (1996). Needle wire localization for nonpalpable breast lesions: Sensations, anxiety levels, and informational needs. *Oncology Nursing Forum, 23*(4), 639–645.

Kottke, T. E., Trapp, M. A., Fores, M. M., Kelly, A. W., Jung, S. H., Novotny, P. J., & Panser, L. A. (1995). Cancer screening behaviors and attitudes of women in southeastern Minnesota. *Journal of the American Medical Association, 273*(14), 1099–1105.

Lauver, D., Nabholz, S., Scott, K., & Tak, Y. (1997). Testing theoretical explanations of mammography use. *Nursing Research, 46*(1), 32–39.

Mahon, C., Smith, L. A., & Burns, C. (1998). *An introduction to clinical laboratory science.* Philadelphia: W. B. Saunders.

Mahon, S. M. (1995). Prevention and early detection of cancer in women. *Seminars in Oncology Nursing, 11*(2), 88–102.

Mahon, S. M. (1996). Patient education. Educating women about early detection of gynecologic cancers using a brochure. *Oncology Nursing Forum, 23*(3), 529–535.

Mashburn, J., & Scharbo-DeHaan, M. (1997). A clinician's guide to Pap smear interpretation. *The Nurse Practitioner, 22*(4), 115–118, 124, 126–127, 130, 139, 143.

McGee, D. C. (1997). Lab values and diagnostics: Assessment of fetal lung maturity. *Neonatal Network: Journal of Neonatal Nursing, 16*(3), 59–63.

Mild cervical dysplasia: Repeat Pap smears vs. colposcopy. (1995). *Emergency Medicine, 27*(9), 67.

Mynaugh, P. A. (1996). Prenatal testing: Beyond the routine. *Office Nurse, 9*(6), 24–28.

Nakamura, R. M. (1996). Antisperm antibodies. *Medical Laboratory Observer, 28*(8), 14.

Newman, J. (1996). Role of stereotactic biopsy in diagnosing breast cancer. *Radiologic Technology, 68*(2), 131–152.

Northouse, L. L., Jeffs, M., Cracchiolo-Caraway, A., Lampman, L., & Dorris, G. (1995). Emotional distress reported by women and husbands prior to a breast biopsy. *Nursing Research, 44*(4), 196–201.

Northouse, L. L., Tocco, K. M., & West, P. (1997). Coping with a breast biopsy: How health care professionals can help women and their husbands. *Oncology Nursing Forum, 24*(3), 473–480.

Nugent, L. S., & Clark, C. R. (1996). Colposcopy: Sensory information for client education. *Journal of Obstetric Gynecologic and Neonatal Nursing, 25*(3), 225–231.

Peart, O. (1994). Helping patients overcome their fear of mammography. *Radiologic Technology, 66*(1), 34–40.

Pfeifer, D. J. (1995). The role of sonography in diagnosing and treating female infertility. *Journal of Diagnostic Medical Sonography, 11*(2), 61–66.

Poole, K. (1997). The emergence of the "waiting game": A critical examination of the psychosocial issues in diagnosing breast cancer. *Journal of Advanced Nursing, 25*(2), 273–281.

Prasad, C. J. (1995). Pathology of human papillomavirus. *Clinics in Laboratory Medicine, 15*(3), 685–704.

Rose, N. C., & Mennuti, M. T. (1993). Maternal serum screening for neural tube defects and fetal chromosome abnormalities. *The Western Journal of Medicine, 159*(3), 312–317.

Saling, E. (1997). Comments on the past and present situation of intensive monitoring of the fetus. *Neonatal Intensive Care, 10*(1), 40–44.

Santalahti, P., Latikka, A. M., Ryynänen, M., & Hemminki, E. (1996). Women's experiences of prenatal serum screening. *Birth, 23*(2), 101–107.

Satish, J. (1992). Prenatal genetics in laboratory medicine. *Clinics in Laboratory Medicine, 12,* 493–502.

Schapira, D. V., & Levine, R. B. (1996). Breast cancer screening, compliance and evaluation of lesions. *Medical Clinics of North America, 80*(1), 15–26.

Sharts-Hopko, N. C. (1997). STDs in women: What you need to know. *American Journal of Nursing, 97*(4), 46–55.

Slowey, K. B., Slowey, M. J., & Cato, J. (1996). Cardiac complications of laparoscopy: Anesthetic implications. *CRNA: The Clinical Forum for Nurse Anesthetists, 7*(1), 9–13.

Snopek, A. M. (1992). *Fundamentals of special radiographic procedures* (3rd ed.). Philadelphia: W. B. Saunders.

Sonek, J., & Nicolaides, K. (1994). The role of cordocentesis in the diagnosis of fetal well-being. *Clinics in Perinatology, 21*(4), 743–764.

Spear, K. A., & Niederberger, C. Ş. (1996). Male infertility: Evaluation and treatment. *Journal of Urologic Nursing, 15*(1), 1182–1193.

Stein, M. W. (1995). Ultrasound of pelvic inflammatory disease. *Applied Radiology, 24*(3), 21–25.

Stepp, C. A., & Woods, M. A. (1998). *Laboratory procedures for medical office personnel.* Philadelphia: W. B. Saunders.

Stringer, M., & Cohen, A. (1994). Fetal/maternal surveillance. *Journal of Perinatal Education, 3*(2), 29–34.

Sundaram, S. G., Goldstein, P. J., Manimekalai, S., & Wenk, R. E. (1992). Alpha-fetoprotein and screening markers of congenital disease. *Clinics of Laboratory Medicine, 18,* 481–492.

Tietz, N. W. (Ed.) (1995). *Clinical guide to laboratory tests* (3rd ed.). Philadelphia: W. B. Saunders.

Tomaino-Brunner, C., Freda, M. C., & Runowicz, C. D. (1996). "I hope I don't have cancer": Colposcopy and minority women. *Oncology Nursing Forum, 23*(1), 39–44.

Ungvarski, P. J. (1997). Update on HIV infection. *American Journal of Nursing, 97*(1, Nurse Practice Extra Edition), 44–52.

Urang, S., Davis, L., Elsberry, C. C., & Kozlowski, M. K. (1993). Fetal scalp blood sampling. *Journal of Nurse Midwifery, 38*(Suppl. 2), 2S–8S, 95S–99S.

Wallman, C. M., & Witt, C. L. (1997). Interpretation of fetal cord blood gases. *Neonatal Network: Journal of Neonatal Nursing, 16*(1), 72–75.

Whittle, M. J. (1998). Early amniocentesis: A time for a rethink. *The Lancet, 351*(9098), 226–227.

Wilson, R. D., Johnson, J. M., & Dansereau, J. (1998). Randomized trial to assess safety and fetal outcome of early and midtrimester amniocentesis. *The Lancet, 351*(9098), 242–247.

Wolfe, S. (1997). The great mammogram debate. *RN, 60*(8), 41, 44.

Woods, G. L. (1995). Update on laboratory diagnosis of sexually transmitted diseases. *Clinics in Laboratory Medicine, 15*(3), 665–684.

Wright, C. J., & Mueller, C. B. (1995). Screening mammography and public health policy: The need for perspective. *The Lancet, 346*(8966), 29–32.

Wright, L. (1994). Prenatal diagnosis in the 1990's. *Journal of Obstetric Gynecologic and Neonatal Nursing, 23*(6), 506–515.

Yablonsky, T. (1996). Male fertility testing. *Laboratory Medicine, 27*(6), 378–383.

# CHAPTER 23

# Neurologic Function

Neurologic laboratory tests and diagnostic procedures include both general and highly specific measures that provide data about the nervous system. The tests focus on the assessment of the skull, brain, spinal cord, central and peripheral nerves, and extracranial and intracranial circulation. The tests are used to confirm the presence and location of a lesion and to provide data about the cause of the problem. The tests are also used to gauge the progression of the disease or the patient's response to treatment.

Many of these tests provoke anxiety in the patient and the patient's family because of the fear of pain, the potential for a severe complication as a result of the procedure, and the threatening nature of the potential neurologic diagnosis.

Often, the patient who must undergo a neurologic diagnostic procedure already has abnormal assessment findings that result from disease or trauma. For example, he or she may be in a coma, mentally confused, paralyzed, or in severe pain. The patient's pretest condition and limitations are incorporated into the plan of care for each diagnostic test or procedure. The nurse's assistance provides accurate pretest preparation; patient safety; and measures to meet emotional, physical, and cognitive needs, with accurate assessment before, during, and after each test.

## Laboratory Tests

## Cerebrospinal Fluid Analysis and Lumbar Puncture

**(Cerebrospinal Fluid)**          Synonyms: CSF analysis, spinal tap, LP

**Normal Values**

**Cerebrospinal Fluid Analysis**
  Pressure: 80–180 mm $H_2O$ (lateral recumbent position)
  Appearance: Clear, colorless
**Microscopic Examination (Leukocyte Count)**
  Adult: 0–5 cells per µL *or* SI 0–5 × $10^6$/L
  Child (5–18 years): 0–10 cells per µL *or* SI 0–10 × $10^6$/L
  Neonate–1 year: 0–30 cells per µL *or* SI 0–30 × $10^6$/L
**Microscopic Examination (Differential Count)**
  Lymphocytes (adult): 40%–80% *or* SI 0.40–0.80 number fraction
  Monocytes (adult): 15%–45% *or* SI 0.15–0.45 number fraction
  Neutrophils (adult): 0%–6% *or* SI 0.00–0.06 number fraction
  Lymphocytes (neonate): 5%–35% *or* SI 0.05–0.35 number fraction
  Monocytes (neonate): 50%–90% *or* SI 0.50–0.90 number fraction
  Neutrophils (neonate): 0%–8% *or* SI 0.00–0.08 number fraction

*Continued on following page*

*Continued*

**Chemistry Analysis**
Lactate: 10–22 mg/dL *or* SI 1.1–2.4 mmol/L
Glucose: 50–80 mg/dL *or* SI 2.75–4.4 mmol/L
Total protein: 15–45 mg/dL *or* SI 150–450 mg/L
Albumin: 10–30 mg/dL *or* SI 100–300 mg/L
Immunoglobulin G: 1–4 mg/dL *or* SI 10–40 mg/L
**Protein Electrophoresis (Percentage of Total Protein)**
Prealbumin: 2%–7% *or* SI 0.02–0.07 number fraction
Albumin: 56%–76% *or* SI 0.56–0.76 number fraction
Alpha$_1$ globulin: 2%–7% *or* SI 0.02–0.07 number fraction
Alpha$_2$ globulin: 4%–12% *or* SI 0.04–0.12 number fraction
Beta globulin: 8%–18% *or* SI 0.08–0.18 number fraction
Gamma globulin: 3%–12% *or* SI 0.03–0.12 number fraction
**Myelin Basic Protein:** <2.5 ng/mL *or* SI <2.5 µg/L

## Background Information

About 70% of cerebrospinal fluid (CSF) is produced in the ventricles of the brain, with the remainder coming from the interstitial spaces of the cells of the brain and spinal cord. Continuous production, secretion, and reabsorption occur so that the volume of cerebrospinal fluid remains relatively constant. The total volume of cerebrospinal fluid for the adult ranges from 90 to 150 mL, and the total volume for the neonate is 10 to 60 mL. The fluid circulates throughout the subarachnoid space and continuously bathes the brain and spinal cord (Fig. 23–1).

The fluid protects and supports the central nervous system and provides the medium for the exchange of nutrients and metabolic wastes. Although the chemical composition of cerebrospi-

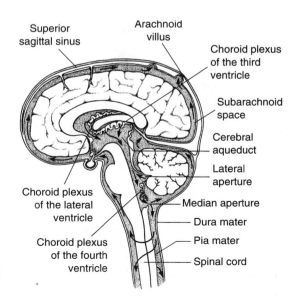

**Figure 23–1**
Circulation of the cerebrospinal fluid. A schematic representation of the brain and spinal cord, including the circulation of the cerebrospinal fluid. (Reproduced with permission from Brunzel, N. [1994]. *Fundamentals of urine and body fluid analysis* [p. 366]. Philadelphia: W. B. Saunders.)

nal fluid includes measurable electrolytes, ions, enzymes, and carbon dioxide, the significance of these values is not clearly understood (Brunzel, 1994). The chemistry values of protein, glucose, and lactate help in the diagnosis of neurologic disease, as does the presence of cells and microorganisms.

## Lumbar Puncture

This procedure is used to obtain the sample of cerebrospinal fluid for analysis. It involves the insertion of a sterile spinal needle between the lumbar vertebrae into the subarachnoid space. Because the spinal cord ends at L1 or L2 in adults, the spinal tap is performed below that level. The level of the tap is usually in the third or fourth lumbar interspace for adults and in the fourth or fifth interspace for children.

**Cerebrospinal Pressure.**   Once the needle is in the subarachnoid space, the pressure of the fluid is measured with a manometer attached to the needle. An elevated pressure reading is greater than 250 mm $H_2O$ (Bogousslavsky & Fisher, 1998). If the pressure is in the normal range, a specimen of up to 20 mL can be removed. After the removal of 10 to 20 mL of cerebrospinal fluid in a normal spinal tap, the closing pressure is usually 45 to 90 mm $H_2O$.

Because children have less total fluid in proportion to age and body size, the specimen sample must be considerably smaller. If the child's opening pressure is higher or lower than normal, a specimen of only 1 to 2 mL can be removed. This limitation is imposed because a risk exists of cerebellar herniation or spinal cord compression.

## Analysis of the Cerebrospinal Fluid

### Appearance

The normal cerebrospinal fluid is clear and colorless, with a viscosity similar to that of water. Cloudy fluid, called *pleocytosis,* is caused by an increased number of cells in the fluid. An increase in erythrocytes, leukocytes, microorganisms, or protein may occur. The cloudiness is sometimes measured on a scale of 0 to 4+ (from clear to cloudy).

Discoloration of the fluid, called *xanthochromia,* indicates that abnormal components are present in the fluid. The fluid may appear pink, orange, or yellow. The abnormal components include oxyhe-moglobin, carotene, bilirubin, and other substances. Gross blood may be present and is caused by a traumatic tap, a subarachnoid hemorrhage, or an intracerebral hemorrhage. The increased viscosity of the fluid may be caused by a metastatic mucin-secreting adenocarcinoma.

### Microscopic Examination

The normal total cell count is low in adults and in children of all ages. A slight increase in the number of monocytes occurs in the normal neonate. When a high elevation of leukocytes exists, the cause is often bacterial meningitis, but the count varies among infected patients. A cloudy specimen is associated with a white blood cell count of more than 200 cells per microliter, and a very high count may be greater than 50,000 cells per microliter. The erythrocyte count is of little diagnostic value, because the source of the red blood cells is usually the peripheral blood or a traumatic tap.

**Differential Cell Count.**   Normally, lymphocytes and monocytes are the predominant cells in cerebrospinal fluid. In bacterial meningitis, the neutrophil count is greatly elevated. In other causes of meningitis—including viral, tubercular, fungal, and syphilitic infection—an increased lymphocyte count exists. Other cells may be present and indicate abnormality. The presence of plasma cells can be a result of acute viral infection, a chronic inflammatory condition, or multiple sclerosis. A large increase in eosinophils is indicative of a parasitic or fungal infection but may also occur with a malfunctioning intracranial shunt or an intrathecal injection of medication or contrast medium. Malignant cells indicate a primary or metastatic tumor. Metastases are commonly from melanoma, leukemia, lymphoma, or cancer of the breast, lung, or gastrointestinal tract.

### Chemical Analysis

**Lactate.**   The lactate level increases in conditions of anaerobic metabolism, tissue hypoxia, and decreased oxygenation of the brain. The problem may be systemic and interfere with oxygen transport to the brain and central nervous system, or it may be a problem within the brain itself.

**Glucose.**   The glucose concentration is proportionate to the level of blood glucose. Within a period of 2 hours before the spinal tap, the glucose level in the cerebrospinal fluid is normally 60%

to 70% of the blood level. To interpret the glucose level of the cerebrospinal fluid correctly, a blood specimen must be drawn 30 to 60 minutes before the spinal tap is performed. Higher-than-normal values of glucose in the cerebrospinal fluid reflect hyperglycemia. Lower-than-normal values (<40 mg/dL) of glucose in the cerebrospinal fluid occur with many forms of meningitis, neoplasm, inflammatory disorder, and other conditions.

**Protein.** Some protein is normally present in the cerebrospinal fluid, but an excessive increase or decrease is indicative of a problem. The increased level may be the result of increased permeability of the blood-brain barrier, allowing protein to pass into the cerebrospinal fluid. It may also be the result of poor resorption of the protein or of an increase in immunoglobulin synthesis. Decreased protein values occur when an increase in water resorption occurs, such as with increased intracranial pressure or with leakage of the cerebrospinal fluid as the result of head trauma.

**Albumin.** Among the different proteins that compose the total protein value, albumin is the largest component. It enters the cerebrospinal fluid by crossing the blood-brain barrier. Therefore, the albumin level monitors its permeability.

**Immunoglobulin G.** Increased amounts of immunoglobulin G (IgG) may result from increased production of the antibody within the central nervous system or from an increase in the transport of the antibody across the blood-brain barrier. Elevated values are indicative of multiple sclerosis and other inflammatory disorders of the central nervous system.

**Protein Electrophoresis.** This test reveals the specific composition and distribution of the cerebrospinal fluid proteins. The primary purpose of this test is to identify *oligoclonal bands* in the gamma region. The presence of these bands is highly indicative of multiple sclerosis. Serum protein electrophoresis is performed on the patient's blood, which is drawn when the lumbar puncture is performed. In 90% of patients with multiple sclerosis, the oligoclonal bands are not present in the serum specimen, but they are present in the cerebrospinal fluid at some point during the course of the disease.

**Myelin Basic Protein.** Myelin basic protein is one of the proteins of the myelin sheath that surrounds axons of nerves. In multiple sclerosis and other demyelinating diseases, the myelin basic protein is released into the cerebrospinal fluid during an acute exacerbation of the disease and deterioration of the myelin sheaths. The test is used to monitor the disease and to identify patients who have multiple sclerosis but who do not demonstrate oligoclonal banding.

### Miscellaneous Tests

In addition to the standard tests, the cerebrospinal fluid may be cultured to identify the infectious agent. The common aerobic pathogens that cause meningitis are *Haemophilus influenzae, Neisseria meningitidis,* and *Streptococcus pneumoniae.* Other agents are fungal, parasitic, bacterial, tubercular, or viral in origin.

Immunologic examination may also be performed to detect the specific microbial antigen that is present in bacterial or fungal meningitis. Immunologic testing may include the testing performed to confirm neurosyphilis.

Cytologic examination may be performed to identify the cells of the primary or metastatic tumor. The malignant cells are shed from a malignant tumor that has extended into the ventricles or subarachnoid space.

---

**Purpose of the Test**

Lumbar puncture is performed to measure the pressure of the cerebrospinal fluid, to detect obstruction in the circulation of this fluid, and to obtain a sample of the cerebrospinal fluid for cellular, chemical, and microbiologic analysis.

Analysis of the cerebrospinal fluid is performed to confirm the diagnosis of infection in the central nervous system or to identify a tumor or hemorrhage in the brain, spinal cord, or surrounding lining of the tissues. It may be performed to confirm a chronic central nervous system infection such as neurosyphilis.

**Procedure**

**Lumbar Puncture.** Under sterile conditions and using local anesthesia, a spinal needle is inserted between the lower lumbar vertebrae and into the sub-arachnoid space (Fig. 23–2). After pressure measurements are determined, 15 to 20 mL of cerebrospinal fluid is collected in three or more sterile tubes.

**Findings**

**Elevated Values**

CELLS

Leukocytes: Bacterial meningitis
Neutrophils: Bacterial meningitis, encephalomyelitis, cerebral abscess, cerebral hemor-rhage, cerebral infarction, tumor
Lymphocytes: Meningitis, parasitic infection

Plasma cells: Multiple sclerosis, Guillain-Barré syndrome
Eosinophils: Parasitic infection, fungal infection, allergic reaction within the central nervous system

Malignant cells: Leukemia, lymphoma, medulloblastoma, metastatic carcinoma

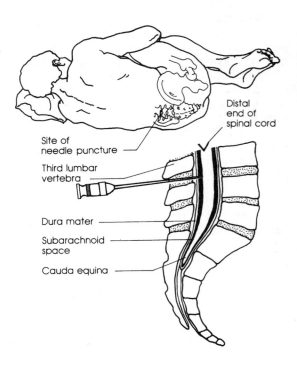

**Figure 23–2**
Patient position for lumbar puncture. The flexion of the lumbar spine widens the intervertebral spaces so that the needle can be inserted into the subarachnoid space more easily. (Repro-duced with permission from Dewit, S. C. [1992]. *Keane's essentials of medical surgical nursing* [3rd ed., p. 330]. Philadelphia: W. B. Saunders.)

CHEMISTRY

Lactate: Low arterial partial pressure of oxygen ($Po_2$), hypotension, stroke, hydrocephalus, brain trauma, cerebral edema, meningitis, cerebral arteriosclerosis

Glucose: Hyperglycemia

Total protein: Meningitis, stroke, extradural abscess, endocrine disorder, trauma, tumor, herniated disc, multiple sclerosis, neurosyphilis

Albumin: Viral meningitis, Guillain-Barré syndrome, collagen diseases

IgG: Multiple sclerosis, sclerosing panencephalitis, neurosyphilis

PROTEIN ELECTROPHORESIS

Alpha$_2$ globulin: Severe craniocerebral trauma

Myelin basic protein: Multiple sclerosis, head trauma, cerebrovascular accident, leukemia, neurosyphilis, systemic lupus erythematosus, Guillain-Barré syndrome

Gamma globulin: Multiple sclerosis

Oligoclonal bands: Multiple sclerosis, subacute sclerosing panencephalitis, Jakob-Creutzfeldt disease, encephalitis, Guillain-Barré syndrome, neurosyphilis, cerebrovascular accident, cerebral vasculitis, neoplasm

**Decreased Values**

Glucose: Acute or chronic meningitis, meningoencephalitis, systemic hypoglycemia, subarachnoid hemorrhage, neurosyphilis, sarcoidosis (meningeal), carcinomatous meningitis

Total protein: Trauma, dural tear; increased intracranial pressure

**Interfering Factors**

- Infection of skin or epidural abscess at the site of the proposed spinal tap
- Increased intracranial pressure
- Spinal block (incomplete or complete)
- Bleeding disorder

**Nursing Implementation**

### Pretest

After the physician explains the test to the patient, obtain written consent from the patient or the person legally responsible for the patient's health care decisions.

Ask the patient about any history of hemophilia, thrombocytopenia, other bleeding disorder, or anticoagulation therapy. Because these problems will result in prolonged bleeding into the tissues or cerebrospinal fluid, they are a relative contraindication to lumbar puncture.

Assist the patient in removing all clothing and putting on a hospital gown.

Monitor and record vital signs.

Place the patient in a lateral recumbent position with his or her back at the edge of the bed or examining table.

Flex the patient's neck and knees toward the chest (see Fig. 23–2). The flexion of the spine widens the intervertebral spaces.

### During the Test

Assist with the preparation of the equipment and sterile field, the antiseptic cleansing of the skin, and the preparation of the local anesthetic. Usually, 1 to 2 mL of lidocaine is administered subcutaneously by the physician.

Instruct the patient to remain absolutely still during the insertion of each needle. Hold the patient in position to help prevent movement.

Provide reassurance to the patient as the needles are inserted. The administration of the anesthetic causes a stinging sensation. Brief pain also occurs as the spinal needle penetrates the dura and enters the subarachnoid space.

Assist the patient in placing the legs in extension for the pressure reading.

Assist with the collection of the cerebrospinal fluid.

Mark the tubes "1," "2," "3," and so on, in the order in which they are collected.

■

*Critical Thinking 23–1*

As the patient is positioned for lumbar puncture, she tells you that she is very frightened. Before and during the procedure, what nursing interventions can you use to help her?

#### Quality Control

The first tube is used for chemical and immunologic analysis, because blood or tissue fluid will not alter these test results. The second tube is used for microbial analysis, and the third tube is used for microscopic examination of cells. If only a small amount of fluid is drawn, it is placed in a single tube, and the physician prioritizes the tests.

Arrange for immediate delivery of the specimen to the laboratory.

#### Quality Control

With delay, lysis of the white blood cells results in a false decrease in the cell count. Additionally, glycolysis causes a false rise in the lactate value, and the microbial organisms may be destroyed. If an unavoidable delay occurs in the laboratory, tube 1 (chemical and immunologic tests) is frozen. Tube 2 (microbiologic tests) is kept at room temperature, and tube 3 (cell counts and cytologic study) is refrigerated (Brunzel, 1994).

### Posttest

Monitor vital signs at regular and frequent intervals until they are stable. At the same time, assess the patient's level of consciousness and responsiveness.

Assess the puncture site for swelling, redness, or leakage of cerebrospinal fluid.

Instruct the patient to lie flat in a supine position for 1 to 6 hours. This helps prevent headache following lumbar puncture. If headache occurs, bedrest is extended to 12 hours.

Administer extra fluids to help the patient replace the volume of fluid in the subarachnoid space and to help prevent headache.

Administer the prescribed pain medication as needed.

At regular intervals, assess the patient's motor ability in the lower legs. If spinal blockage or severe compression of the cord occurs following the procedure, paresis can turn into paralysis. In addition, massive hematoma can occur within the subarachnoid space. This would compress the cauda equina and result in paralysis (Guberman, 1994).

| | |
|---|---|
| **Critical Value** | **A pressure measurement >300 mm H$_2$O** |
| | With a pressure reading at this very elevated level, the patient is in danger of a cerebellar herniation of the brain, with possible fatal consequences (Bogousslavsky & Fisher, 1998). The fluid sample removed should be very small. Treatment of the elevated pressure with urea or mannitol may be prescribed and another manometer testing done to ensure that the pressure has fallen (Adams, Victor, & Ropper, 1998). |

**Complications**

The most frequent complication of lumbar puncture is headache. Infection, hematoma, and bleeding can also occur. Although it is an infrequent complication, increased intracranial pressure can occur. The increase in the intracranial pressure may be caused by meningitis or brain tumor.

A summary of the complications of lumbar puncture is presented in Table 23–1.

## Diagnostic Procedures

Angiography, Brain, Head, and Neck   745

Computed Tomography, Cranial, Spinal   749

  Computed tomographic angiography   750

  Helical (spiral) computed tomography   750

Xenon computed tomography   750

Electroencephalography   750

Electromyography and Nerve Conduction Studies   753

Magnetic Resonance Imaging, Brain, Spinal Cord   756

  Magnetic resonance angiography   756

Myelography   757

Single Photon Emission Computed Tomography Scan, Brain   760

Single Photon Emission Computed Tomography Scan, Spine   762

Ultrasound, Cranial, Neck   763

X-Ray, Skull   764

X-Ray, Spine   764

## Angiography, Brain, Head, and Neck

**(Radiography)**   Synonym: Cerebral angiography

| | |
|---|---|
| **Normal Values** | No abnormalities of the tissue or vasculature are visualized. |

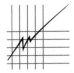

### Table 23–1  Complications of Lumbar Puncture

| Complication | Nursing Assessment |
|---|---|
| Spinal headache or post–lumbar puncture syndrome (PLPS) | Severe head pain on sitting up or standing<br>Nausea, vomiting<br>Dizziness, orthostatic hypotension |
| Increased intracranial pressure | Deteriorating level of consciousness (deepening stupor to coma)<br>Bradycardia<br>Elevated blood pressure<br>Slow or irregular respirations<br>Pupillary changes |
| Infection (meningitis) | High fever<br>Headache<br>Myalgia<br>Back pain<br>Photophobia<br>Deteriorating level of consciousness<br>Meningeal irritation (muscle stiffness or spasm in neck and other extensor muscles, positive, Kernig's sign, positive Brudzinski's sign)<br>Seizures |
| Complete spinal block | Paresis (weakness of the lower legs)<br>Paralysis of the lower legs<br>Signs of increased intracranial pressure |
| Bleeding, hematoma | Oozing of blood or cerebrospinal fluid from the puncture site<br>Localized swelling or edema near the puncture site<br>Bruising or ecchymosis near the puncture site |

## Background Information

Angiography of the brain, head, and neck provides clear imaging of intracranial and extracranial vascular abnormalities and their locations. Although the less invasive procedures of computed tomography (CT) and magnetic resonance imaging (MRI) have surpassed angiography for the imaging of tumors and trauma to the brain, angiography remains a mainstay in the investigation of the cerebral vasculature. Several different types of cerebral angiography can be performed.

**Cerebral and Arch Angiography.** In this type of angiography, a thin catheter is inserted via the femoral artery and passed up the aorta. At the aortic arch, the catheter is passed into the innominate, common carotid, or left subclavian artery, and then into the vertebral, internal, or external carotid artery. Once the catheter is in place, iodinated radiopaque contrast medium is injected under pressure, and rapid serial x-rays are taken. The contrast material provides visualization of the extracranial and intracranial circulation. In selected cases, a catheter is not passed through the arterial system. Instead, the contrast medium is introduced by a direct puncture of the common carotid artery or by a retrograde injection of contrast material into the brachial artery. The angiography procedure is sometimes called *plain film angiography* because of the use of simple x-ray or plain films for the imaging process.

**Digital Subtraction Angiography.** In this newer methodology, the visualization of the contrast medium and the vasculature is enhanced by computer resolution that subtracts out the images of bone and other overlying tissues that interfere with the visualization of the arteries. Digital subtraction angiography is particularly useful in the investigation of extracranial blood vessels. When the contrast material is injected into an artery, the procedure is called *intra-arterial digital subtraction angiography* (Fig. 23–3). The femoral artery is commonly used. With the assistance of computer resolution, the images are clearer and more magnified. When the contrast medium is injected into a vein, the procedure is called *intravenous subtraction angiography.* An antecubital vein is commonly used. Although the venous route is technically easier, and fewer complications or arterial emboli occur, the imaging is less clear. In addition, a greater number

of other complications are possible, including allergy or toxicity to the contrast medium (Snopek, 1992).

In addition to the visualization of the vasculature of the head, neck, and brain, cerebral angiography demonstrates the location and characteristic vascular patterns of different types of brain tumors. It locates and defines the source of a subarachnoid hemorrhage and also identifies vascular malformation. Thrombosis, embolic occlusion, or atheromatous stenosis can be seen when it occurs in a major extracranial or intracranial artery. Subdural hematoma is also visualized, because no contrast material is circulating in the space between the skull and the displaced brain tissue.

Some infrequent, but devastating, complications can occur with cerebral angiography. Many of the patients are elderly and in poor general health, with extensive arteriosclerotic disease or heart disease, or both. These problems make the patients more vulnerable to complications following the procedure.

---

**Purpose of the Test**

Cerebral angiography identifies abnormalities of the vasculature and the blood flow in the neck and brain. When intracranial or extracranial vascular surgery is indicated, it is used preoperatively to provide a precise image.

---

**Procedure**

Iodinated radiopaque contrast material is injected arterially or intravenously. Rapid serial x-ray films are taken to image the bolus of contrast medium as it moves through the circulation of the neck and the extracranial and intracranial blood vessels.

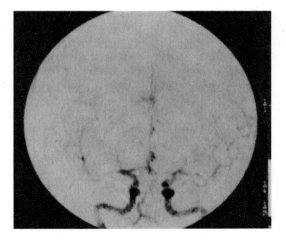

**Figure 23–3**
Digital cerebral angiogram. Vessels appear dark because of computer manipulation. (Courtesy of David Skarbek.)

| **Findings** | **Abnormal Values** | | |
|---|---|---|---|
| | Brain tumor | Arteriosclerosis | Subarachnoid |
| | Fistula | Atherosclerotic | hemorrhage |
| | Arteriovenous | plaque | Stenosis |
| | malformation | Vasospasm, arteritis | Vascular occlusion |
| | Obstruction of the | Cerebral aneurysm | |
| | cerebrospinal fluid | Cerebral edema | |

**Interfering Factors**

- Movement of the head during imaging
- Metal objects in the x-ray field
- Vomiting during the imaging process
- Allergy to iodine

**Nursing Implementation**        **Pretest**

Ask the patient about a history of allergy to iodine, including allergic reactions to seafood such as shellfish or to iodine during previous x-ray studies using contrast medium.

Obtain written consent from the patient or the person legally responsible for the patient's health care decisions.

Instruct the patient regarding the food and fluid restrictions to be implemented before the test. Because some variations occur among institutions, verify the protocol that is to be used by the particular radiology department.

Instruct the patient to discontinue food intake for 6 to 8 hours before the test. The contrast medium can cause nausea. If food is in the stomach, vomiting would result in head movement during the imaging process and blurring of the photographic results.

Most institutions permit the intake of clear fluids during the fasting period (Snopek, 1992). Some limit the amount, and others encourage extra intake of fluids to promote hydration and renal excretion of the contrast medium (Torres, 1993). For the patient who has fluid restrictions, intravenous fluids are started early in the test period so that renal function is optimal.

When this test is to be performed on an outpatient or ambulatory basis, instruct the patient to have a responsible person available for transportation home after the test. The sedative effects of the medications will remain for several hours after the test is completed.

Assist the patient in removing all clothing and putting on a hospital gown. All metal objects and jewelry are removed from the head, hair, neck, and upper torso.

Monitor the baseline vital signs and assess the peripheral pulses. Record the results.

Administer the prescribed pretest sedative and analgesic medications. The purpose of the medications is to decrease central nervous system activity, anxiety, tension, physical activity, and potential agitation. Some of the medications also reduce nausea and the potential for vomiting. The particular combination of drugs varies with the institutional protocol or the choice of the physician. Drugs with a sedative or calming effect include phenobarbital (Luminal), hydroxyzine hydrochloride (Vistaril), promethazine hydrochloride (Phenergan), diphenhydramine (Benadryl), and diazepam (Valium). Choices of analgesics include morphine sulfate, meperidine (Demerol), and fentanyl (Sublimaze) (Snopek, 1992).

### During the Test

Establish an intravenous line for fluid replacement and the electrocardiographic leads for monitoring the heart rate and rhythm. Monitor vital signs at appropriate intervals.

Instruct the patient to keep the head and neck absolutely still during the injection of contrast material and the imaging sequence. Restraints may be used to prevent movement.

Inform the patient that he or she may experience a temporary flushing or burning sensation, a salty taste, headache, or nausea as the contrast medium is injected.

### Posttest

Once the catheter is removed from the artery, use sterile gauze to apply digital pressure to the puncture site for 10 minutes. This should prevent bleeding or hematoma formation. If swelling or redness occurs, apply ice to the area.

Continue to monitor vital signs at frequent intervals until they are stable and in a normal range.

Assess the extremity that is distal to the arterial injection site. Adequate circulation and mobility and intact neurologic function should be present.

Assess the patient's mental status, observing for clarity of thinking, alertness, and intact neurologic function.

Before discharge, instruct the patient to remain on bedrest for the remainder of the day. The extremity used for the arterial injection should be maintained in extension. By the next day, most physical activities may be resumed, but vigorous exercise should be avoided for an additional day or two.

■

*Critical Thinking 23–2*
One hour after cerebral angiography, you note that the patient has one pupil that is sluggish in response to light. What other immediate nursing assessments are indicated?

### Complications

After cerebral angiography, the overall incidence of complication is 0.5% to 3% (Bogousslavsky & Fisher, 1998). Complications include stroke, leg ischemia, excessive bleeding, a reaction to the contrast medium, and possible death. In most instances, the complications occur within 1 to 2 hours after the test.

## Computed Tomography, Cranial, Spinal

**(Tomography)**                    Synonyms: None

The computed tomographic (CT) scan is an effective noninvasive diagnostic procedure to image the structure of the brain and spinal cord. It is used to investigate intracerebral, extracerebral, and spinal lesions. The abnormalities may be congenital, degenerative, inflammatory, vascular, or tumorous in origin. Because the scan produces tomographic axial slices for viewing, the precise location, size, and characteristics of the abnormality can be seen. The procedure is performed with or without the use of contrast material.

Intracranial lesions that are identified by CT are hydrocephalus and aqueduct stenosis, cerebral atrophy, hemorrhage, hematoma, infarction, and edema of the brain. Tumors within the cranium may be (1) intracerebral and often malignant or (2) extracerebral and probably benign. Extracerebral tumors include meningiomas, acoustic neuromas, epidermoid tumors, dermoid tumors, craniopharyngiomas, and pituitary tumors. An extracerebral hematoma can also be identified, and its relationship to a fracture of the skull is visible.

In the spinal column, the CT scan demonstrates the bony and soft tissue abnormalities that compress the cord and nerve roots. It images a bulge in a disc, a degenerative change, the alignment and structure of the vertebrae, spinal infection, and hypertrophy of the ligaments. In addition, the diameter of the spinal cord can be measured. CT is often used to confirm spinal stenosis as a cause of spinal cord disorder.

**Computed Tomographic Angiography.** This invasive procedure uses contrast medium to better visualize the lumens of the intracranial arteries. Because the amount of contrast medium used is less than that used for cerebral angiography, this procedure has a lower complication rate.

**Helical (Spiral) Computed Tomography.** Helical CT angiography uses contrast medium and new CT technology to image the blood vessels of the brain and then reconstruct the data as three-dimensional (3-D) vascular images. Although the procedure is invasive because of the contrast material, less contrast material is used, and the imaging time is more rapid than that of conventional CT. The test can provide very sharp, clear images of cerebral blood vessels and their structural abnormalities, including stenosis, aneurysm, and arteriovascular malformation (Schwartz, 1995).

**Xenon Computed Tomography.** This very new procedure consists of a plain CT scan followed by the administration of xenon and then additional CT scanning for a few minutes. Using a special face mask, the patient breathes a mixture of xenon gas and oxygen. The xenon CT quantifies or measures cerebral blood flow in the brain tissue as part of the initial evaluation in the early period after a stroke. One of the procedure's important capabilities is its ability to define the degree and extent of ischemia of the brain tissue and to distinguish between viable brain tissue and brain tissue that is irreversibly damaged by the stroke. The test value is measured in milliliters of blood flow per 100 g of brain tissue per minute. A value of less than 20 mL/100 g/min indicates ischemia, and a value of less than 10 to 12 mL/100 g/min indicates irreversible ischemia. If the cause of the stroke is a thrombus and the surrounding brain tissue is not irreversibly damaged, the patient may be treated with thrombolytic therapy to restore the circulation (Barker, 1998).

A detailed discussion of CT is presented in Chapter 12.

## Electroencephalography

(Electrophysiology)    Synonyms: Electroencephalogram, EEG

| Normal Values | Normal patterns of electric brain activity are seen. |
| --- | --- |

### Background Information

Electroencephalography (EEG) records the spontaneous brain activity that originates from brain cells on the surface of the brain. The electric activity, called *action potential*, comes from the depolarization along nerve cell membranes. The fluctuations of electric activity from the larger cortical areas of the brain pass through the cranial bones and the scalp. The voltage is detected by the electrodes. Once the impulses are amplified, they can be recorded.

Using the older electroencephalographic methodology, the fluctuations in electric activity are recorded on a moving paper by a series of pens. In several of the newer methodologies, the data are computerized and displayed on a monitor. In the process of *electric brain mapping,* the computer demonstrates trends in particular areas of brain activity. Another alternative electroencephalographic methodology uses the *video electroencephalography monitor.* It combines the recording of the EEG waveforms with videotaping to correlate the behavioral events with electroencephalographic seizure activity. *Ambulatory monitoring,* another variation in methodology, uses a small portable cassette recording device. It is useful for small children who have seizures in school.

During the recording of the EEG, *sensory evoked potentials* can be measured. These are the electric brain responses that occur when a visual, auditory, or somatosensory stimulus is present. One type of visual stimulus is a strobe light, and the response to this stimulus is recorded by an electrode placed over the occipital lobe. The auditory stimulus is a clicking noise, and it may be used to evaluate the integrity of the eighth cranial nerve during surgery to remove an acoustic neuroma. The somatosensory stimulus is an electric shock delivered to the posterior tibial nerve or median nerve. It is used to assess the lower extremities for movement in the paralyzed individual. It may also be used to assess the function of other specific neural pathways. Sensory evoked potentials may also be used to determine cerebral death.

The rhythms of the electroencephalographic recording are identified as delta (the slowest), theta, alpha, and beta (the fastest). The interpretation of the EEG considers the frequency of the predominant rhythm, the amplitude, any abnormal waves or wave groups, and the asymmetry between the right and left hemispheres.

| | |
|---|---|
| **Purpose of the Test** | The major applications of EEG are in the diagnosis of epilepsy and the determination of the type of epilepsy. It can also be used to help diagnose metabolic encephalopathy and to help detect brain injury. |
| **Procedure** | In adults, 21 recording needle electrodes are applied to the scalp in particular groupings, using electric paste to promote conduction. The electrode wires are connected to the electroencephalograph recorder. In neonates, fewer electrodes are used because of the smaller head size (Fig. 23–4). The electroencephalography procedure usually takes 30 to 90 minutes, but the sleep EEG is recorded all night. For the neonate, the test is usually performed in the isolette in the neonatal intensive care unit. |

**Findings**

**Abnormal Values**

| | | |
|---|---|---|
| Epilepsy (grand mal, focal, temporal lobe, myoclonal, petit mal) | Hypoxic, ischemic encephalopathy | Drug withdrawal |
| Intracranial hemorrhage | Cerebral infarct | Toxoplasmosis, rubella, cytomegalovirus, herpes simplex (TORCH) infection |
| Mental retardation | Hypocalcemia | |
| | Hypoglycemia | |
| | Meningitis | |
| | Brain tumor | |

**Interfering Factors**

- Caffeine
- Movements of the hands, body, or tongue

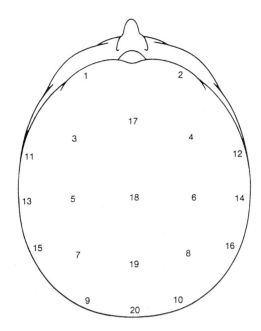

**Figure 23–4**
Placement of electroencephalogram electrodes in the infant.
(Reproduced with permission from Squires, L. A. [1992].
Neonatal seizures. *Critical Care Clinics of North America, 4,* 497.)

- Muscle contractions
- Drug intoxication (heroin, cocaine, marijuana, crack cocaine, lysergic acid diethylamide [LSD])
- Particular medications (narcotics, sedatives, tranquilizers, monoamine oxidase inhibitors, anticonvulsants, antihistamines)

---

**Nursing Implementation**  **Pretest**

Instruct the patient to avoid caffeine before the test, because stimulants alter the electroencephalographic activity. A light meal and fluid intake are encouraged, because a low blood glucose level can also alter the electroencephalographic results.

Instruct the patient to wash his or her hair thoroughly before the test. Hair spray, creams, or oils interfere with the recording of results.

If a sleep-deprived EEG is performed to evaluate sleep disorder or seizures that occur during sleep, advise the patient not to sleep on the night before the test.

At the time of the test, a sedative may be given to promote sleep. If this form of EEG is used, advise the patient to have a responsible person available to drive him or her home after the test is completed.

Because anticonvulsant and other sedative medications alter the electric activity of the brain, these medications may be withheld for 24 to 48 hours before the test begins, as determined by the physician. If the medications cannot be withheld because of the seriousness of the patient's seizure disorder, all medications taken in the 24- to 48-hour pretest period are documented on the requisition slip.

### During the Test

Help the patient to relax in the reclining chair or on the bed.

Inform the patient that a prickly sensation or temporary pain is felt as the electrodes are attached to the scalp. Reassure the patient that the electrodes and wires will not cause a shock or harm the patient.

Instruct the patient not to move the head or body and not to talk during the test. These muscle movements alter the electroencephalographic readings. For the neonate, place the head in a midline alignment.

Reassure the patient that the nurse is nearby with full visibility of the patient during the procedure. If a seizure occurs, the nurse is prepared to provide care during the episode.

### Posttest

Observe the patient for seizure activity.

Remove the electrodes. The electrode paste is cleaned from the hair and scalp with acetone and cotton balls. Acetone is not used in the Isolette because of the limited circulation of air (Squires, 1992).

Anticonvulsant medications that were withheld for the test are not automatically restarted at the same dosage. The previous orders are reviewed by the physician, and a new set of orders are written.

## Electromyography and Nerve Conduction Studies

**(Electrophysiology)**          Synonyms: EMG, NCS, electrodiagnostic studies

| Normal Values | The muscle shows minimal activity at rest. Nerve conduction time is within normal limits. |
|---|---|

## Background Information

Muscle fibers are innervated by a terminal branch of an axon, located near the midpoint of a muscle. With nerve stimulation, depolarization of the nerve, release of acetylcholine by the nerve terminals, and diffusion of the stimulus across the synapse to contract the muscle membrane occur. As the muscle contracts, movement of the body and the performance of work occur.

When a patient complains of muscle weakness, muscle spasms, or paralysis, the cause may be disease of the muscle or nervous system or a problem with neuromuscular transmission at the junction between the nerves and the muscle fibers. Electromyography (EMG) and nerve conduction studies are two diagnostic tests that help identify the physiologic location of the problem.

**Electromyography.**    This procedure records the electric potential of various muscles in a resting state and during voluntary contraction of the muscles. The linear recordings are comparable to electrocardiographic recordings. The normal tracings of muscle potential demonstrate characteristic patterns at rest and during a strong voluntary muscle contraction. The recordings are examined for amplitude, duration, form, and abundance. Characteristic abnormal patterns are seen when the problem is neurologic in origin, such as denervation, or muscular in origin, such as muscle inflammation.

**Nerve Conduction Studies.**    These studies measure motor conduction velocity and sensory conduction. Motor conduction velocity is the timed measurement of conduction along a nerve between two points, as measured by the stimulating and recording electrodes that are applied on the nerve's pathway. Sensory conduction measures the voltage or strength of the nerve stimulus in sensory nerve endings, as measured by recording electrodes applied to a distal area of tissue.

Carpal tunnel syndrome diagnosis provides an illustration of how nerve conduction studies are used. In this disorder, the median nerve is trapped in the bony canal of the wrist. Because of the compression, some loss of nerve conduction occurs, and nerve stimulation of specific muscles in the hand and fingers is diminished. In nerve conduction studies, the nerve stimulus is applied above the area of entrapment and recorded in the distal electrodes of the digits. Because of the nerve entrapment, the time and analysis of the tracings demonstrate a slowing of the impulses and a lower voltage (a decrease in stimulation) in the digits.

The electrodiagnostic tests are somewhat painful, and they provoke some patient anxiety (Kothari, Preston, et al., 1995). The discomfort is sharp, but it is brief and temporary. The pain is caused by the needle insertions and the electric stimuli and is increased with anxiety. Sedation is not recommended because it interferes with voluntary muscle activity.

For infants and children, the process of testing is similar to that for adults, with some modifications because of the smaller body size. The infant or child may have a focal nerve deficit, such as paralysis from a brachial plexus injury that occurred during birth. Other types of problems include generalized hypotonia and weakness that may be congenital or acquired and may involve a systemic or muscular disorder.

When nerve conduction studies must be performed on the infant or small child, the parent may wish to stay and hold the child during the procedure. The presence of a supportive parent can be a comfort to the child. Children older than 5 years are often able to cooperate and participate in the test, thus reducing their anxiety. If the small child cannot cooperate because of a high level of fear or anxiety, sedation with an oral dose of chloral hydrate, 50 to 75 mg/kg, is used for nerve conduction studies.

---

| | |
|---|---|
| **Purpose of the Test** | These tests help distinguish among the causes of weakness and paralysis, differentiating nerve involvement from a muscle disorder. The tests are also used to identify the particular nerve or muscle group that is involved, to localize the site of the abnormality, to evaluate the severity, and to distinguish sensorimotor nerve disorder from pure motor disorder. |

---

| | |
|---|---|
| **Procedure** | Needle electrodes are inserted into muscles and connected to stimulator and recorder devices (Fig. 23–5). As the electric stimulus is initiated, the results appear on an oscilloscope or video screen or are photographed. Linear tracings of the electromyography are made by the electromyographic equipment. |

---

**Findings**

**Abnormal Findings**

Amyotrophic lateral
  sclerosis
Botulism
Muscular dystrophy
Herniated lumbar
  disc
Myasthenia gravis
Guillain-Barré
  syndrome

Poliomyelitis
Carpal tunnel
  syndrome
Inflammatory
  myositis
Brachial plexus injury
Myopathy (endo-
  crine, metabolic,
  toxic, congenital)

Lumbosacral plexus
  injury
Nerve trauma
Glycogen storage
  disease
Hypothyroidism

---

**Interfering Factors**

- Smoking
- Caffeine
- Acute anxiety

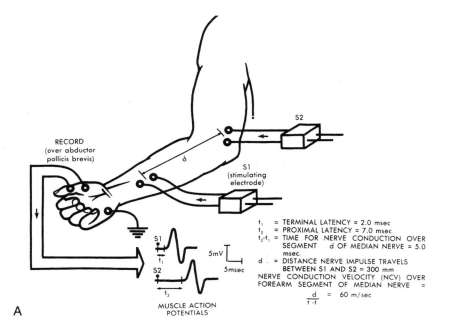

t₁ = TERMINAL LATENCY = 2.0 msec
$t_1$ = TERMINAL LATENCY = 2.0 msec
$t_2$ = PROXIMAL LATENCY = 7.0 msec
$t_2-t_1$ = TIME FOR NERVE CONDUCTION OVER SEGMENT d OF MEDIAN NERVE = 5.0 msec.
d = DISTANCE NERVE IMPULSE TRAVELS BETWEEN S1 AND S2 = 300 mm
NERVE CONDUCTION VELOCITY (NCV) OVER FOREARM SEGMENT OF MEDIAN NERVE =

$$\frac{d}{t-t} = 60 \text{ m/sec}$$

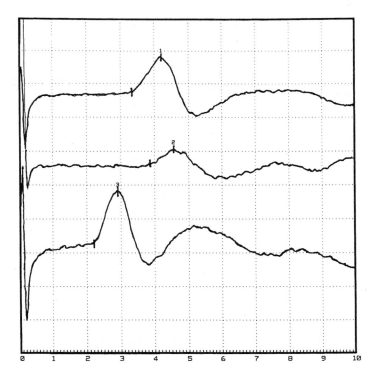

### Figure 23–5

Peripheral nerve conduction studies. *A,* The technique of measurement of motor nerve conduction velocity in the forearm. *B,* The results of sensory nerve conduction velocity. The results are of median nerve *(upper two tracings)* and ulnar nerve *(lower tracing)* conduction in carpal tunnel syndrome. The compression of the median nerve resulted in nerve impairment, with delayed response and low voltage *(second tracing).* (Reproduced with permission from Guberman, A. [1994]. *An introduction to clinical neurology* [pp. 59–60]. Boston: Little, Brown.)

**Nursing Implementation**

### Pretest

Obtain written consent from the patient or the person legally responsible for the patient's health care decisions.

Instruct the patient to refrain from smoking for 24 hours before the test and to avoid caffeine (coffee, tea, cola) for 2 to 3 hours before the test.

Inform the patient that the insertion of the needles can be painful and that the small shocks are also painful. Reassure the patient that these sensations are brief and temporary and can be tolerated.

If possible, encourage the parent of a child patient to comfort the child during the procedure.

### During the Test

Cleanse the skin with antiseptic before inserting the electrodes.

As the electrodes are inserted, again reassure the patient to help reduce anxiety.

For grounding, place a metal plate under the patient's body.

At appropriate intervals during EMG, ask the patient to perform various voluntary muscle contractions.

### Posttest

To avoid additional pain, remove the needle electrodes gently and slowly.

If pain persists at the puncture sites, instruct the patient to apply warm compresses.

## Magnetic Resonance Imaging, Brain, Spinal Cord

**(Magnetic Field Scan)** Synonym: MRI

Magnetic resonance imaging (MRI) is particularly valuable for assessment of the soft tissue of the brain and spinal cord. Although it cannot image the bones of the skull and vertebrae, it provides clear imaging of the organs and tissue contained within these bones. MRI uses magnetic frequencies and radiofrequency waves to assess the movement of concentrations of protons within magnetic fields. The signals emitted from tissues are converted to images. Images from transverse, coronal, and sagittal planes can be obtained to provide additional information. Because no contrast material is used, the procedure is noninvasive.

In the study of the brain, MRI provides images of tumors, cerebral edema, ischemia, multiple sclerosis, and other demyelinating diseases. In the study of the spinal cord, MRI provides images of disc degeneration, spinal cord tumor, epidural fat, and postoperative scar tissue that impinges on the cord or its nerve roots.

**Magnetic Resonance Angiography.** This new methodology provides enhancement of the intravascular and extravascular structures of the brain without the use of an injected contrast material. Once the routine MRI is completed, the computer operations can present the data about the vasculature by suppression of the image of the stationary brain tissue and enhancement of the signal from the blood flow within particular arteries (Fig. 23–6).

A complete discussion of MRI is presented in Chapter 12.

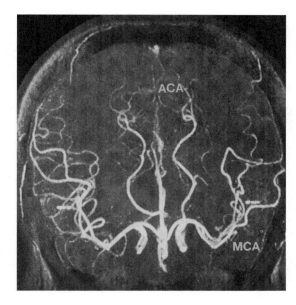

**Figure 23–6**
MR angiogram. An anterior view of the head showing intracerebral vessels, including the anterior cerebral artery (ACA) and the middle cerebral artery (MCA). These images were obtained without injection of any contrast agent. (Reproduced with permission from Mettler, F. A. [1996]. *Essentials of radiology* [p. 9]. Philadelphia: W. B. Saunders.)

## Myelography

**(Radiography)**    Synonyms: Myelogram, low-dose myelography, LDM

| **Normal Values** | No obstruction or structural abnormalities of the spinal canal, discs, cord, or nerve roots are noted. |
|---|---|

## Background Information

As a single procedure, myelography is a radiographic study that uses plain x-ray film with contrast medium to evaluate spinal disorders. More commonly, it is combined with CT (*CT myelography*) in the detection of pathologic conditions of the spine. The combination procedure is particularly useful when the CT examination has not resulted in a clear diagnosis.

Although CT and MRI have replaced myelography in most instances, myelography is still useful in the evaluation of the postoperative spinal surgery patient, the obese patient, and the patient who has a mobile herniated disc that is demonstrated only in a weight-bearing or flexion-extension position.

In myelography, the radiopaque contrast material is instilled in the subarachnoid space using a lumbar puncture needle. The patient is then placed in a prone position with the table tilted to a head-down position. This positioning allows the contrast medium to move up the spinal column. Once the contrast material is in place, the spinal cord, spinal nerve roots, and thecal sac appear radiolucent (Fig. 23–7). X-ray films or a CT scan is used for imaging. The area of the spinal pathology can be anywhere along the spinal column, and the regions are identified as *cervical*, *lumbothoracic*, or *lumbar*.

Several iodinated contrast media are available for use. A water-soluble contrast medium is used because it is better tolerated by the patient; the side effects are nausea, vomiting, and headache.

| | |
|---|---|
| **Purpose of the Test** | Myelography is performed to identify an obstruction or abnormality that impinges on the spinal cord or its nerve roots. |
| **Procedure** | With the patient under local anesthesia, iodinated contrast material, guided by fluoroscopy, is instilled into the lumbar subarachnoid space using a lumbar puncture needle. Once the contrast medium has filled the subarachnoid space or the whole spinal column, the images are taken at the appropriate level. The procedure takes 1 to 2 hours. |

**Findings**

**Abnormal Values**

| | | |
|---|---|---|
| Protrusion of an intervertebral disc | Syringomyelia | Epidural mass or tumor |
| Spinal nerve root injury | Cervical spondylosis | |
| Herniated intervertebral disc | Tumor of the spinal cord | |
| | Lumbar stenosis | |
| | Arachnoiditis | |

**Interfering Factors**

- Allergy to iodine
- Incorrect placement of the needle
- Failure to maintain nothing-by-mouth status

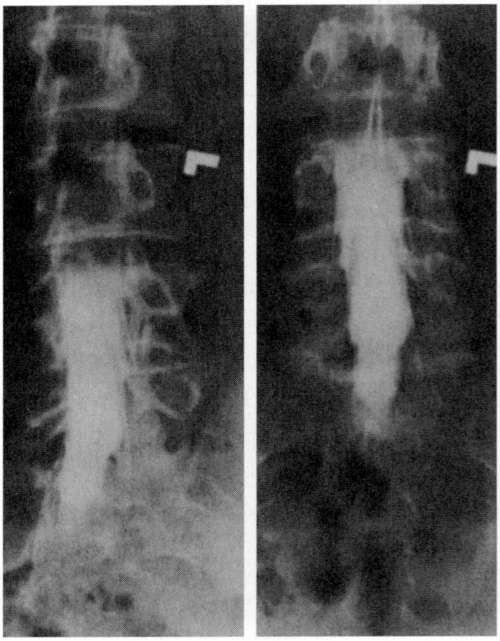

**Figure 23–7**
Lumbar myelogram. Posteroanterior (PA) and oblique views of the spinal column. The contrast material is in the subarachnoid space. (Reproduced with permission from Adler, A. M., & Carlton, R. R. [1994]. *Introduction to radiography and patient care* [Vol. 1, Slide 206]. Philadelphia: W. B. Saunders.)

**Nursing Implementation**    **Pretest**

After the procedure is explained by the physician, obtain a written consent from the patient or the person legally responsible for the patient's health care decisions.

Ask the patient about a history of allergy to iodine or shellfish or of a reaction to contrast material during a previous x-ray study.

Provide a preparatory explanation to the patient, including what the patient will feel during and after the procedure. Concrete information should help to reduce anxiety caused by the unknown (Cason & Sample, 1995). When this procedure is performed in an outpatient setting, instruct the patient to have a responsible adult present to provide transportation home at the end of the procedure.

Instruct the patient about pretest modifications of food and fluid intake. For 8 hours before the test, most institutions require a fast from food and also require that the patient drink extra fluids to maintain hydration status (Torres, 1993). Because some variation exists among institutions regarding the fluid intake and the period for dietary modifications, the protocol of the individual radiology department is followed.

Help the patient to undress completely and put on a hospital gown. Also, assist the patient in moving into the desired positions on the examining table. Most of these patients have problems with back pain and limited mobility because of their spinal injury or disease.

Monitor baseline vital signs and record the results.

If the patient is extremely anxious or has muscle spasms, administer 5 mg of diazepam (Valium) by mouth or intravenously, as prescribed. Most patients do not require pretest medication.

**During the Test**

Position the patient according to the requirements of the radiologist or the anesthesiologist who administers the local anesthesia and performs the lumbar puncture. Alternative positions include (1) seated at the edge of the table with the legs dangling and the back somewhat flexed, (2) in a lateral position with the head and knees flexed toward the chest, and (3) prone, with a small pillow under the abdomen.

If hair is present on the lower back, the skin is shaved before it is cleansed. Assist the physician with the skin preparation, draping, and preparation of the local anesthetic. The skin preparation feels wet and cold to the patient.

Prepare the sterile lumbar puncture tray for the intrathecal administration of contrast medium.

Reassure the patient during the injection of the local anesthetic. It causes stinging pain as it is injected subcutaneously.

Help the patient remain still as the lumbar puncture needle is inserted. Usually, brief pain occurs as the needle penetrates the thecal sac. With a lumbar procedure, the patient feels a tingling sensation during instillation of the contrast material. With a cervical procedure, the instillation is associated with a burning sensation (Cason & Sample, 1995).

After the contrast medium has been instilled, place the patient in a prone position, with a shoulder harness and footrest in place. These are used to help the patient maintain position as the table is tilted.

### Posttest

Place the patient in a slight semi-Fowler position to ease the lumbar pain.

Monitor vital signs at regular, frequent intervals for 1 hour or until the results are stable in a normal range.

Instruct the patient to remain on bedrest at home for 8 to 10 hours. Two pillows are used to elevate the upper torso and head. The pillows prevent the contrast medium from rising up to the head and causing headache.

Encourage the patient to drink extra fluids for the next day or two. The contrast medium eventually diffuses out of the subarachnoid space and is excreted in the urine. Alcohol and caffeine intake are not permitted for 24 hours, however, because they promote rapid diuresis.

Instruct the patient to notify the physician if inability to urinate exists or if onset of fever, drowsiness, stiff neck, paralysis, or seizure occurs.

## Single Photon Emission Computed Tomography Scan, Brain

(Radionuclide Scan)          Synonyms: SPECT brain imaging; SPECT scan, brain

| **Normal Values** | No abnormalities of brain tissue and brain function are noted. |
| --- | --- |

### Background Information

Cerebral single photon emission computed tomography (SPECT) imaging uses a traditional radionuclide that emits gamma rays and a multidetector rotary camera to produce tomographic images of the brain. With the development of new radiopharmaceuticals and better scanning equipment, the SPECT scan produces clear imaging and a shorter imaging time. The results of the SPECT scan are usually compared with the results of the CT or MRI scan to provide additional information about the changes in the patient's brain tissue. Additional discussion of nuclear scans and the SPECT scan is presented in Chapter 10.

In cerebral studies, the radiopharmaceutical technetium 99m is most widely used. Once it is injected into the vascular system, it travels rapidly to the head, crosses the blood-brain barrier, and perfuses into the brain tissue. The tracer undergoes some decomposition so that it cannot recross the blood-brain barrier, and it remains trapped in the brain tissues. The radioactive capability of this tracer has a short half-life of 6 hours.

The imaging is performed about 1 to 2 hours after the radiopharmaceutical is introduced. This interval allows maximal absorption of the radiopharmaceutical into the brain. The normal imaging time is 20 to 30 minutes. From the data received by the SPECT camera, the SPECT computer can produce the images along transaxial, coronal, and sagittal planes, providing visualization of all lobes, tissues, and structures of the brain (Fig. 23–8).

In the investigation of cerebrovascular disease, SPECT can be used for detection of acute ischemia, determination of the cause of stroke, and assessment of a transient ischemic attack. In the study of dementia, this method can help identify the cause of dementia and distinguish among Alzheimer's disease, multi-infarct dementia, and frontal lobe dementia. In epilepsy, this test can help identify the seizure focus in conjunction with other neurologic procedures. In cases of head trauma, SPECT can identify mild head injury that is not visible on the CT scan.

### Purpose of the Test

The SPECT scan is used to investigate cerebrovascular diseases, dementia, epilepsy, and head trauma. It produces images of brain function, based on

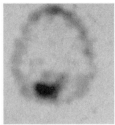

Transverse

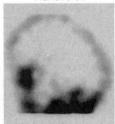

Sagittal

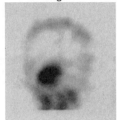

Coronal

**Figure 23–8**
Recurrent brain tumor in the occipital region. The three different views of the SPECT scan demonstrate intense and irregular tracer concentration within the tumor. (Reproduced with permission from Wagner, H. N., Szabo, Z., & Buchanan, J. W. [1995]. *Principles of nuclear medicine* [2nd ed., p. 1138]. Philadelphia: W. B. Saunders.)

physiologic and biochemical processes. It may be used to assess and diagnose a disorder as well as to evaluate the brain's response to treatment.

| Findings | **Abnormal Values** | | |
|---|---|---|---|
| | Stroke | Multi-infarct | Hypertensive enceph- |
| | Human immunodefi- | dementia | alopathy |
| | ciency virus | Transient ischemic | Intracranial trauma |
| | encephalopathy | attack | Alzheimer's disease |
| | Intracranial hemor- | Epilepsy | |
| | rhage | | |

| Interfering Factors | • Movement of the head during imaging |
|---|---|
| | • Failure to remove metal objects from the imaging field |

| Nursing Implementation | **Pretest** |
|---|---|
| | Instruct the patient to avoid caffeine intake (e.g., coffee, tea, cola) for 24 hours before the test. |

After the physician explains the procedure, ensure that written consent is obtained from the patient or the person legally responsible for the patient's health care decisions.

Assist the patient in removing all clothes and putting on a hospital gown. All jewelry and metal objects are removed from the head, hair, and neck.

Place the patient in a recumbent position on the scanning table. Apply a minimal restraint to prevent a fall from a table that has no siderails.

The person who needs a SPECT scan is usually elderly and suffering from dementia or has residual trauma to the brain. The unfamiliar room and the procedure may be confusing or frightening to this type of patient. Instructions may be difficult to follow. If these conditions exist, give simple instructions and close guidance to the patient. Because no radiation hazard to people in the room exists, a member of the family or a familiar person can assist and help calm the patient during the test.

Remind the patient to keep the head still during the injection of the radiopharmaceutical and during the imaging procedure.

Explain that the room will be kept calm for 10 minutes before and after the radiopharmaceutical is administered. During this quiet time, the patient should keep his or her eyes open. Blinking is allowed.

Earplugs are unnecessary.

### Quality Control

> The quiet, stimulus-free environment promotes a resting basal state of brain activity. The patient keeps his or her eyes open during administration of the radionuclide so that the occipital lobes are more clearly visible.

### During the Test

Position the patient's head in body alignment.

Establish the intravenous line for the administration of the radiopharmaceutical.

To maintain a quiet environment, dim the lights in the room, keep noise to a minimum, and prevent traffic in the room.

During the scanning process, the patient will hear the quiet sounds of the scanner, but no pain or discomfort is experienced.

### Posttest

Remove the intravenous line and apply a small bandage to the venipuncture site.

Because the kidneys will remove the radionuclide from the blood and excrete it in the urine, instruct the patient to wash his or her hands after voiding. This prevents radioisotopes from remaining on the skin. By 6 hours after the test, the radioactivity level of the isotope is minimal to none.

## Single Photon Emission Computed Tomography Scan, Spine

**(Radionuclide Scan)**           Synonyms: SPECT scan, spine

Single photon emission computed tomography (SPECT) imaging of bone is one of the more common uses for the SPECT scan. This radionuclide scan is superior to the regular bone scan when used in regions where bones overlap, such as the vertebral body and the neural arch of the spine. It is particularly useful in the investigation of low back pain when the bone abnormality impinges on the nerve roots or the spinal cord.

Abnormalities identified by the SPECT scan include benign or malignant spinal disease, discitis, ankylosing spondylitis, and septic arthritis. It also investigates the cause of low back pain produced by acute stress injury, as in sports injuries.

Additional discussion of the SPECT scan is presented in Chapter 10.

## Ultrasound, Cranial, Neck

**(Ultrasonography)**          Synonyms: None

In infants, the anterior fontanelle serves as a window for the passage of ultrasound waves into the brain (Fig. 23–9). Ultrasound imaging can identify hydrocephalus, hemorrhage, cystic or solid tumors, or infections such as toxoplasmosis, rubella, cytomegalovirus, and herpes simplex (TORCH). This diagnostic procedure is often used in the neonatal intensive care unit when the infant has a suspected intracranial hemorrhage, a low Apgar score, suspected congenital malformations, or an abnormal neurologic examination.

With newer Doppler techniques, ultrasound may be used to evaluate the circulation of the major cerebral arteries. The Doppler probe is placed over the thin layer of temporal bone, over the bony orbits, and posteriorly at the base of the neck. This technique provides visualization of a stenosis of the internal carotid artery and its branches, the vertebral artery, and the basilar artery. It may also identify a vasospasm following a subarachnoid hemorrhage. The vasospasm causes the blood vessel to become narrowed, and the ultrasound can detect the reduced blood flow (Guberman, 1994; Manno, 1997).

Doppler ultrasound is also useful in the assessment of the arteries of the neck. The procedure demonstrates the velocity, turbulence, and direction of blood flow and the patency of the arteries. It is particularly helpful in the

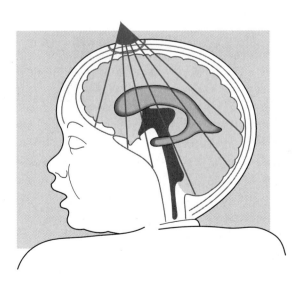

**Figure 23–9**
Pediatric ultrasound. The anterior fontanelle provides the window for imaging the brain of the infant. (Redrawn with permission from Blickman, J. [1992, May]. The inroads of ultrasound, CT, and MR in pediatric imaging. *Applied Radiology, 21,* 39.)

investigation of transient ischemic attacks and in the determination of arterial patency after a carotid thromboendarterectomy or arteriotomy with anastomosis (Foldes, 1993).

A complete discussion of ultrasound is found in Chapter 8 of this text.

## X-Ray, Skull

**(Radiography)**

Synonym: Skull series

Plain x-rays of the skull demonstrate changes in the bony tissue and may demonstrate changes in the brain tissue. A skull fracture can be identified, located, and described. The bone tissue may show erosion or thinning because of chronically increased intracranial pressure or a cerebral tumor. In children, the increased intracranial pressure causes separation of the sutures. Tumors can cause a localized thickening of the bony tissue. Abnormalities of the brain can be visualized when the tissue is calcified, such as in some types of tumor or in the displacement of the pineal gland.

Because the skull x-ray series is helpful but does not provide detailed data, other specialized tests such as the CT scan, MRI scan, or isotope scan are used to obtain better information.

A complete discussion of x-ray studies is presented in Chapter 9.

## X-Ray, Spine

**(Radiography)**

Synonyms: None

The plain x-ray film of the spine can provide helpful data regarding the cause of neurologic disability. Spinal abnormalities include inflammatory lesions such as tuberculosis of the spine, malignant tumor or metastasis, or congenital abnormality of the cervical spine. Fractures and dislocations are also apparent on x-ray film. When bone abnormalities such as these exist, resultant neurologic abnormality may occur as the spinal cord or nerve roots are compressed. In radiologic views of the soft tissues, a protruding disc can be seen, along with narrowing or bony sclerosis of the vertebrae. Intraspinal tumor with erosion of the vertebral body is also evident.

As with the x-ray series of the skull, the x-ray film of the spine does not provide sufficient detail about the neurologic problem. Follow-up with myelography, CT, or MRI provides better visualization and accurate diagnosis of a spinal pathologic condition.

A complete discussion of radiology is presented in Chapter 9.

## References

Adams, R. D., Victor, M., & Ropper, A. H. (1998). *Principles of neurology* (6th ed.). New York: McGraw-Hill.

Barker, E. (1998). The xenon CT: A new neuro tool. *RN, 61*(2), 22–26.

Bentz, J. S. (1995). Neurology I. Laboratory investigation of multiple sclerosis. *Laboratory Medicine, 26*(6), 393–399.

Blickman, J. G. (1992). The inroads of ultrasound, CT, and MRI in pediatric imaging. *Applied Radiology, 21*, 38–47.

Bogousslavsky, J., & Fisher, M. (1998). *Textbook of neurology.* Boston: Butterworth-Heinemann.

Bonebreak, K. J. (1996). A sound way to induce relaxation and natural sleep—a safe alternative to sedation. *American Journal of EEG Technology, 36*(4), 264–268.

Brady, S., Thornhill, A., & Colapinto, E. (1997). Stereotactic biopsy procedures for brain tumor diagnosis. *AORN Journal, 65*(5), 890, 892, 894–895, 898, 900.

Brunzel, N. A. (1994). *Fundamentals of urine and body fluid analysis.* Philadelphia: W. B. Saunders.

Burtis, C. A., & Ashwood, E. R. (1999). *Tietz textbook of clinical chemistry* (3rd ed.). Philadelphia: W. B. Saunders.

Calder, H. B., & White, D. E. (1996). Facial nerve EMG monitoring. *American Journal of Electrodiagnostic Technology, 36*(1), 28–46.

Cason, C. L., & Sample, J. G. (1995). Preparing information for myelogram. *Journal of Neuroscience Nursing, 27*(3), 182–187.

Chestnut, R. M. (1994). Computed tomography of the brain: A guide to understanding and interpreting normal and abnormal images in the critically ill patient. *Critical Care Nursing Quarterly, 7*, 33–50.

Foldes, M. (1993). The role of duplex and color Doppler imaging in the operating room. *Journal of Vascular Nursing, 11*, 108–110.

Guberman, A. (1994). *An introduction to clinical neurology.* Boston: Little, Brown.

Hinkle, J. L. (1997). New developments in managing transient ischemic attack and acute stroke. *AACN Clinical Issues: Advanced Practice in Acute and Critical Care, 8*(2), 205–213.

Hudak, C. M., & Gallo, B. M. (1997). Quick review of neurodiagnostic testing. *American Journal of Nursing, 97*(7), 16CC–16DD, 16FF.

Kothari, M. J., Preston, D. C., Plotkin, G. M., Venkatesh, S., Shefner, J. M., & Logigian, E. L. (1995). Electromyography: Do the diagnostic ends justify the means? *Archives of Physical Medicine and Rehabilitation, 76*(10), 947–949.

Kothari, M. J., Rutkove, S. B., Logigian, E. L., & Shefner, J. M. (1995). Coexistent entrapment neuropathies in patients with amyotrophic lateral sclerosis. *Archives of Physical Medicine and Rehabilitation, 77*(11), 1186–1188.

Manno, E. M. (1997). Transcranial Doppler ultrasonography in the neurocritical care unit. *Critical Care Clinics, 13*(1), 79–104.

Newberry, A. B., & Alavi, A. (1996). Neuroimaging in patients with traumatic brain injury. *Journal of Head Trauma Rehabilitation, 11*(6), 65–79.

Rupright, J., Woods, E. A., & Singh, A. (1996). Hypoxic brain injury: Evaluation by single photon emission computed tomography. *Archives of Physical Medicine and Rehabilitation, 77*(11), 1205–1208.

Schwartz, R. B. (1995). Helical (spiral) CT in neuroradiologic diagnosis. *Radiologic Clinics of North America, 33*(5), 981–995.

Snopek, A. M. (1992). *Fundamentals of special radiographic procedures* (3rd ed.). Philadelphia: W. B. Saunders.

Stewart-Amidei, C. (1996). Spiral CT scanning. *Journal of Neuroscience Nursing, 28*(5), 339.

Squires, L. A. (1992). Neonatal seizures. *Critical Care Nursing Clinics of North America, 4*, 495–506.

Thornbury, J. R., Fryback, D. G., Turski, P. A., Javid, M. J., McDonald, J. V., Beinlich, B. R., Gentry, L. R., Sackett, J. F., Dasbach, E. J., & Martin, P. A. (1993). Disk-caused nerve compression in patients with acute low back pain: Diagnosis with MR, CT myelography and plain CT. *Radiology, 186*(3), 731–738.

Tietz, N. W. (1995). *Clinical guide to laboratory tests* (3rd ed.). Philadelphia: W. B. Saunders.

Torres, L. S. (1993). *Basic medical techniques and patient care for radiologic technologists.* Philadelphia: J. B. Lippincott.

Wang, H. (1995). Radiologic assessment of the spine. *Physical Medicine and Rehabilitation, 9*(3), 605–617.

# CHAPTER 24

# Musculoskeletal Function

The musculoskeletal system consists of bones, joints, cartilage, ligaments, tendons, muscle, fascia, and bursae. An integrated system, the skeleton, muscle, and connective tissue function to provide support, protection, movement, and blood formation for the body. The musculoskeletal system is subject to many disorders caused by trauma, malignancy, inflammation, metabolic change, degeneration, or vascular deficiency.

In this chapter, the section on laboratory tests examines testing of blood and synovial fluid. In many cases, no one test can diagnose an autoimmune disorder or cause of inflammation. The diagnosis is confirmed or excluded by a combination of laboratory tests, diagnostic procedures, and clinical findings. The laboratory tests are also used to evaluate the severity of disease and to monitor the effects of treatment.

Most of the diagnostic procedures discussed in this chapter allow visualization of the bones or joints. Other procedures are used to obtain samples of tissue or fluid. These specimens are stained or cultured and analyzed microscopically. The diagnostic procedures provide specific data regarding the cause or extent of pathologic change in the bone or joint.

## Laboratory Tests

## Anti-DNA

**(Serum)**

Synonyms: DNA antibody, antibody to double-stranded DNA (anti-ds-DNA), antibody to single-stranded DNA (anti-ss-DNA), antibody to native DNA (n-DNA)

### Normal Values

Enzyme immunoassay method: Negative; <70 IU/mL
Indirect immunofluorescent method: <1:10

## Background Information

In autoimmune disease, antibodies attach to and destroy nuclear or cytoplasmic antigens of one's own body tissue. The autoimmune response causes inflammation, fibrosis, and destruction of a single target organ, or the process becomes disseminated and affects many different organs or tissues of the body.

The anti-DNA antibody test is one of the specific antinuclear antibody (ANA) tests. Antibodies to single-stranded or double-stranded DNA are found in the serum of 60% to 70% of patients with active systemic lupus erythematosus (Bryant, 1992). It is present to a much lesser degree in patients with other collagen vascular or autoimmune diseases.

The different laboratory methods use binding assay to detect the antibodies in the serum. Although the normal values are expressed differently according to the method of analysis, high levels of antibodies are abnormal and confirm the diagnosis of systemic lupus erythematosus. By enzyme-linked immunosorbent assay, a value of 70 to 200 IU/mL is considered to be a borderline result, and a value greater than 800 IU/mL is specific for systemic lupus erythematosus (Tietz, 1995). By the indirect immunofluorescent technique, the antibody is detected in a titer with a dilution greater than 1:10.

| | |
|---|---|
| **Purpose of the Test** | The anti-DNA test confirms the diagnosis of systemic lupus erythematosus. It is also used to monitor the response to treatment. |

| | |
|---|---|
| **Procedure** | A red-topped tube is used to collect 10 mL of venous blood. |

**Findings**

**Elevated Values**

| | | |
|---|---|---|
| Active systemic lupus erythematosus | Other collagen vascular or rheumatic disorders | Infectious mononucleosis |
| Discoid lupus erythematosus | Chronic active hepatitis (lupoid hepatitis) | Biliary cirrhosis |
| Rheumatoid arthritis | | |

**Interfering Factors**

- Administration of radioactive isotopes in the preceding 7 days
- Warming of the specimen

**Nursing Implementation**

The nursing implementation includes care of the venipuncture site.

**Pretest**

Schedule this test for before any radioactive isotope test.

**Posttest**

Arrange for prompt transport of the specimen to the laboratory, because the specimen will require chilling.

## Antinuclear Antibody

(Serum)    Synonyms: ANA, fluorescent antinuclear antibody, FANA, ANF

| | |
|---|---|
| **Normal Values** | Negative at a 1:20 dilution |

## Background Information

Autoimmune diseases are disorders that produce tissue injury because of an immunologic reaction against one's own tissue antigens. When the antibodies attack one or more antigens in the cell nuclei, the antibodies are called *antinuclear antibodies,* or ANA. Of the many different autoimmune disorders, some affect cell nuclei of a single organ and others cause systemic disease, affecting the cell nuclei of many tissues.

In disorders that are organ specific, the autoimmune response is directed at the antigen of DNA, at other nuclear antigens, and at the mitochondria within the nuclei. Organ-specific autoimmune diseases can affect the blood; endocrine, neuro-logic, or intestinal systems; kidneys; liver; muscle; eyes; skin; or other target organs.

In systemic autoimmune diseases, the pathophysiologic process deposits immune complexes in the capillaries of multiple organs. These complexes contain tissue components and complement. The presence of complement results in inflammatory reactions and tissue destruction.

The laboratory technique of indirect immunofluorescence visually demonstrates the presence of ANA in the serum and provides quantitative data regarding the concentration of antibody in the serum. If ANA is present in the serum, it will bind to the antigen, forming antigen-antibody com-

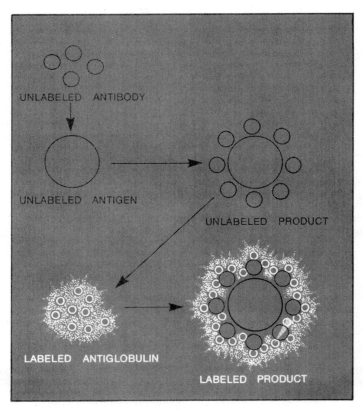

**Figure 24–1**

Indirect fluorescent antibody procedure. (Reproduced with permission from Bryant, N. J. [1992]. *Laboratory immunology and serology* [3rd ed., p. 101]. Philadelphia: W. B. Saunders.)

plexes. Fluorescein-labeled antiglobulin is added to give a fluorescent stain to the newly formed complexes (Fig. 24–1). The patterns of fluorescence of the nuclei (speckled, outline, homogenous, or nucleolar) are demonstrated under fluorescent microscopy. Additionally, the amount of antibody is measured by the presence of a high serum titer.

Positive ANA results identify the presence of the antitissue antibodies of various systemic rheumatic diseases, but the test cannot identify a specific disease. As a screening tool, however, ANA is particularly relevant in the detection of systemic lupus erythematosus because of a greater than 95% accuracy rate in detection of this particular antibody (Tietz, 1995).

**Antinuclear Antibody Subtypes.**    For more specific information, a *precipitin panel* may be ordered to test for some specific subtypes of ANA. These subtypes include anti-ds-DNA, anti-ss-DNA, anti-Ro, anti-La, anti-RNP, and anti-Smith autoantibodies. When present, the subtype is highly specific for a particular rheumatic disease.

The ANA immunofluorescence test can produce false-positive results because of medications, including procainamide (Pronestyl) and hydralazine (Apresoline). It can produce false-positive results in normal individuals, particularly normal elderly individuals (Jacobs et al., 1996; Slater, Davis, & Shmerling, 1996).

| | |
|---|---|
| **Purpose of the Test** | The ANA test is used as a screen to detect autoimmune systemic rheumatic diseases or systemic lupus erythematosus, or both. It is also used to monitor the effectiveness of medication in the treatment of systemic lupus erythematosus. |

| | |
|---|---|
| **Procedure** | A red-topped tube is used to collect 7 to 10 mL of venous blood. |

**Quality Control**

Venipuncture technique must be smooth, with a blood flow that fills the vacuum tube rapidly. If the blood has excessive turbulence because of flawed venipuncture technique, the hemolysis of the erythrocytes will alter the test results.

**Findings**

**Elevated Values**

SYSTEMIC AUTOIMMUNE DISEASES

| | | |
|---|---|---|
| Systemic lupus erythematosus | Necrotizing angiitis | Mixed connective tissue disease |
| Rheumatoid arthritis | Polymyositis | Sjögren's syndrome |
| Ankylosing spondylitis | Dermatomyositis | |
| | Progressive systemic sclerosis | |

AUTOIMMUNE DISEASES OF BLOOD AND TARGET ORGANS

| | | |
|---|---|---|
| Hashimoto's thyroiditis | Leukemia | Gluten-sensitive enteropathy |
| Myxedema | Chronic renal failure | Pemphigus vulgaris |
| Thyrotoxicosis | Multiple sclerosis | |
| Hepatic or biliary cirrhosis | Pernicious anemia | |
| | Regional ileitis | |
| | Ulcerative colitis | |

**Interfering Factors**

- Hemolysis of the blood specimen

**Nursing Implementation**     Nursing implementation includes care of the venipuncture site.

### Pretest

List any medications taken by the patient.

### Posttest

Arrange for prompt transport of the specimen to the laboratory. The cells must be extracted from the serum promptly to prevent contamination of the specimen because of hemolysis.

## C-Reactive Protein

**(Serum)**                    Synonym: CRP

| **Normal Values** | <1 mg/dL *or* SI <10 mg/L |
|---|---|

### Background Information

C-reactive protein is a globulin, a serum protein that is synthesized by the liver. Normally, it is not present in the blood, except when tissue necrosis, trauma, inflammation, or infection exists. Its synthesis and rise in serum values are triggered by the presence of antigens, immune complexes, bacteria, and fungi. Once it enters the blood, this protein attaches to the surface of many bacteria, fungi, or other microorganisms and initiates the pathway of complement as part of the immunologic response. It is believed that the function of C-reactive protein is to act as an early defense mechanism against infection or to detoxify and remove products of tissue degradation (Tietz, 1995).

The serum level of C-reactive protein rises rapidly in response to bacterial infection and acute inflammation. The progressive rise in value reflects increasing infection, inflammation, or tissue damage. Equally, the progressive fall in the serum value indicates healing or the effectiveness of antibiotic or anti-inflammatory medication. In a normal postoperative response, the C-reactive protein value demonstrates a sharp rise by the third postoperative day. If no bacterial sepsis is present, the value falls by the seventh day.

Serial testing for C-reactive protein may be used to monitor infection. A rising or persistently high C-reactive protein level may indicate antibiotic treatment failure or the onset of a postoperative infection (Smith, Lipworth, Cree, Spiers, & Winter, 1995). Because the protein level does not rise in the presence of viral infection, the test may be used to differentiate between viral and bacterial sources of infection.

**Purpose of the Test**     C-reactive protein is used as a nonspecific indicator of infection or inflammation and also is used to monitor the response to antibiotic or anti-inflammatory medication. It is commonly used to help with the diagnosis of rheumatoid arthritis and rheumatic fever, particularly when the erythrocyte sedimentation rate (ESR) and other test results are inconclusive.

**Procedure**     A red-topped tube is used to collect 10 mL of venous blood.

**Quality Control**

Venipuncture technique must be smooth, with a blood flow that fills the vacuum tube readily. If the blood has excessive turbulence because of flawed venipuncture technique, the hemolysis of the erythrocytes will alter the test results.

| Findings | **Elevated Values** | | |
|---|---|---|---|
| | Rheumatoid arthritis | Bacterial sepsis | Crohn's disease |
| | Rheumatic fever | Tuberculosis | Myocardial infarction |
| | Systemic lupus erythematosus | Pneumococcal pneumonia | |

**Interfering Factors**

- Oral contraceptives
- Intrauterine device
- Hemolysis

**Nursing Implementation**

Nursing intervention includes care of the venipuncture site.

**Pretest**

Instruct the patient to fast from food for 4 to 8 hours before the test. Fluids are permitted. Fasting is necessary because it is desirable to have the level of serum lipids as low as possible.

**Posttest**

No specific intervention is necessary.

## Erythrocyte Sedimentation Rate

**(Blood)**                    Synonyms: ESR, sed rate

**Normal Values**

**Adult <50 Years**
    Male: 0–15 mm/hr
    Female: 0–20 mm/hr
**Adult >50 Years**
    Male: 0–20 mm/hr
    Female: 0–30 mm/hr
**Child:** 0–10 mm/hr

## Background Information

The erythrocyte sedimentation rate (ESR) test is a nonspecific measurement of infection or inflammation in the body. The rate particularly rises when elevated levels of fibrinogen or globulins, or both, are present in the blood.

When venous blood is placed in a vertical

tube, the erythrocytes act like sediment; over time, they fall to the bottom of the tube. In normal conditions, as the erythrocytes settle, they exhibit a characteristic *rouleau formation,* meaning that they form a stack.

**Elevated Values.** In conditions that produce greater amounts of fibrinogen or globulins, the rouleau formation is greater, the sedimentation rate is faster, and the ESR is elevated. In rheumatic disorders such as rheumatoid arthritis and systemic lupus erythematosus, the severity or rise in the ESR is usually reflective of the severity in the inflammatory condition (Shmerling, 1996). Anemia also increases the ESR, because fewer erythrocytes are present in the plasma.

**Decreased Values.** Microcytes have a slower sedimentation rate than do macrocytes. Additionally, erythrocytes with irregularities or abnormal shape exhibit less rouleau formation. When a low plasma fibrinogen level exists, the ESR value is proportionately lower. These conditions demonstrate less erythrocyte sedimentation.

---

**Purpose of the Test**

The erythrocyte sedimentation test is useful in identifying and monitoring disease activity in infectious, inflammatory, and neoplastic conditions. It is especially useful in rheumatic and collagen diseases.

---

**Procedure**

A lavender-topped tube is used to collect 7 mL of venous blood.

**Quality Control**

Venipuncture technique must be smooth, with a blood flow that fills the vacuum tube readily. If the blood has excessive turbulence because of flawed technique, the hemolysis of erythrocytes will alter the test results.

---

**Findings**

**Elevated Values**

Rheumatoid arthritis
Multiple myeloma
Rheumatic fever
Waldenström's
    macroglobulinemia
Inflammation

Anemia
Temporal arteritis
Pregnancy
Polymyalgia rheu-
    matica

**Decreased Values**

Sickle cell anemia
Polycythemia

Spherocytosis
Hypofibrinogenemia

---

**Nursing Implementation**

**Pretest**

Because many medications, including salicylate, can alter laboratory values, list all medications taken by the patient on the requisition slip. In some cases, the medication may be withheld until after the test.

**Posttest**

Ensure that the specimen is sent promptly to the laboratory. The specimen must be analyzed within 4 hours of collection.

## Human Leukocyte Antigen B-27

**(Blood)**　　　　　　　Synonym: HLA B-27

The human leukocyte antigens (HLA) are gene products from specific loci on the short arm of the sixth chromosome. Their loci are labeled A, B, C, and D. These antigens appear on all nucleated cells and are the major antigens of white blood cells and platelets. It is believed that the HLA antigens play a major role in the genetic regulation of the immune response (Henry, 1996). HLA B-27 is one of many different antigens in the HLA group.

HLA B-27, an inherited antigen, has a statistically high correlation with ankylosing spondylitis and Reiter's syndrome. Ninety-five percent of patients with ankylosing spondylitis and 80% of those with Reiter's syndrome have the inherited antigen HLA B-27, confirming the genetic linkage to this disorder (Shmerling, 1996).

The significance of this genetic marker is not well understood. Although HLA B-27 is not the cause of the disease, it is a marker of disease susceptibility. Infection or environmental stimuli may alter HLA B-27 and initiate a complex autoimmune response. Ultimately, injury or destruction of the tissue of one's own cells, such as synovial or cartilage tissue, occurs.

HLA B-27 may be used clinically to assess the disease state of ankylosing spondylitis. A heparinized, green-topped tube is used to collect 10 mL of venous blood.

A complete discussion of the HLA antigens is presented in Chapter 17.

## Lupus Erythematosus Test

**(Serum)**　　　　　　　Synonyms: LE prep, LE cell test, lupus test, lupus erythematosus cell test

| **Normal Values** | Negative; no LE cells are present. |
| --- | --- |

## Background Information

In autoimmune disease, the serum contains the antibodies that are directed against cell nuclei of one's own body tissues. In systemic lupus erythematosus (LE), the antinuclear antibody is usually immunoglobulin G (IgG) and is called the *LE factor.* The antibody reacts by attaching to the nuclei of leukocytes and infiltrating them. The altered cell is called an *LE body.* Other neutrophils and phagocytes surround the LE body and engulf it by phagocytosis. The final cell, the *LE cell,* is a polymorphonuclear leukocyte with a lysed nucleus (Bryant, 1992). In systemic lupus erythematosus, the LE cells are found in the bone marrow and peripheral blood.

In the LE test, the laboratory sample blood cells are ruptured by using glass beads to release nuclear material. The patient's serum is then mixed and incubated with this nuclear material. If the LE factor is present, the antibody interacts with the sample nuclear material, and the altered nuclei undergo phagocytosis. The specimen is stained and prepared for microscopy. The presence of lavender-stained LE cells is considered a positive result.

The LE test is an indirect measure used to detect one of the antinuclear antibodies. The value of the test is limited, because it is less sensitive than the fluorescent ANA test. A positive LE test result is useful in the diagnosis of lupus erythematosus, but many patients who are acutely ill with this disease have negative test results. Additionally, numerous medications, including phenytoin (Dilantin), produce a false-positive result. The LE test is rarely used today because of the time-consuming methodology and the insensitivity of the test.

| | |
|---|---|
| **Purpose** | The LE test is used to help diagnose lupus erythematosus and to monitor the response to treatment. |

| | |
|---|---|
| **Procedure** | A green-topped tube is used to collect 10 mL of venous blood. |

**Findings**

**Positive Values**

Systemic lupus
  erythematosus
Rheumatoid arthritis
Chronic active
  hepatitis (lupoid
  hepatitis)

Scleroderma
Drug hypersensitivity
Drug-induced lupus
  syndrome

**Interfering Factors**

- Severe leukopenia, neutropenia
- Heparin
- Inadequate volume of blood (<6 mL)

**Nursing Implementation**

**Pretest**

If heparin has been administered, schedule the test for 2 days after the heparin is discontinued. Heparin can cause a false-negative result.
On the laboratory requisition slip, list the medications taken by the patient.

**Posttest**

Arrange for transport of the specimen to the laboratory within 30 minutes.

## Myoglobin, Urine

(Urine)

Synonyms: None

| | |
|---|---|
| **Normal Values** | Qualitative method: Negative<br>Quantitative method: <0.4 mg/dL *or* SI <4 mg/L |

## Background Information

*Rhabdomyolysis* is the breakdown of striated muscle tissue with a release of myoglobin in the urine. With severe injury or ischemia, skeletal or cardiac muscle tissue releases myoglobin into the blood. The kidneys filter the blood rapidly, and the myoglobin is excreted in the urine.

*Myoglobinuria* (myoglobin in the urine) in large quantities causes the urine to become a shade of red, to dark red, to a darker brown color similar in appearance to a cola beverage. It is difficult to distinguish by appearance between hemoglobin and myoglobin in the urine because the color change is similar. In addition, myoglobin will cause a false-positive value for hemoglobin or for occult blood when tested by dipstick.

In laboratory testing, qualitative methods identify an abnormally elevated value as *positive* or *present*. Quantitative methods measure the amount of myoglobin that is present. In normal individuals, little or no myoglobin should be present.

Myoglobinuria has many possible causes. The myoglobin is released after skeletal or cardiac muscle is damaged. In skeletal muscle damage, the underlying cause may be muscle trauma, such as after a "crush injury," severe exercise, or seizure; or immobility, such as from muscle compression during a coma or prolonged unconsciousness. It may also result from metabolic causes, such as electrolyte imbalance, or from toxic exposure, such as carbon monoxide inhalation, poisoning, or alcohol or cocaine ingestion.

Myoglobin is nephrotoxic. Large quantities of this protein can occlude the renal tubules and result in acute tubular necrosis and acute renal failure (Burtis & Ashwood, 1999; Henry, 1996). For information on serum myoglobin and its relation to cardiac disorder, see Chapter 15.

---

**Purpose of the Test**

This test is used to identify the presence of myoglobinuria and to investigate for the cause of the problem.

---

**Procedure**

Either a random sample of urine is collected in a plastic container or a 24-hour urine specimen is collected.

---

**Findings**

**Elevated Values**

| | | |
|---|---|---|
| Severe muscle trauma | Severe electrical shock | Carbon monoxide poisoning |
| Arterial insufficiency to a large muscle mass | Thermal injury | Muscular dystrophy |
| Severe exercise | Prolonged immobility | Dermatomyositis |
| Surgical muscle trauma | Drug toxicity (alcohol, barbiturates, amphetamines) | Electrolyte imbalance (potassium, magnesium, phosphate) |
| Myocardial infarction | | |

---

**Interfering Factors**

- Ascorbic acid
- Renal failure

---

**Nursing Implementation**

**Pretest**

If the patient is conscious, request a urine specimen, collected in a plastic container.

If the patient is unresponsive or cannot assist, obtain the specimen from the port in the urinary catheter.

For a 24-hour urine collection, plan to collect all urine for a 24-hour period (see Chapter 2 for procedure guidelines).

**Posttest**

Send the speciment to the laboratory without delay. If the result is very elevated, treatment, including rehydration and restoration of electrolyte balance, must be done quickly to protect and preserve renal function.

## Rheumatoid Factor

(Serum, Synovial Fluid)     Synonyms: RF, RA factor

| Normal Values | Negative |
|---|---|

### Background Information

Rheumatoid factor is a group of immunoglobulins that are directed against the Fc fragment of IgG molecules. Stated simply, rheumatoid factors are anti-antibodies.

At a titer level of 80 IU/mL or higher, rheumatoid factor is present or positive in the serum of the majority of patients with rheumatoid arthritis and some other rheumatic conditions. Although a high correlation exists between the presence of rheumatoid factor and rheumatoid arthritis, the exact nature of the relationship is unknown.

Rheumatoid factor can be detected by the latex fixation method or the sheep cell agglutination method. In the latex fixation method, latex beads are coated with human IgG. In the sheep cell agglutination test, sheep erythrocytes are coated with rabbit IgG. Either of these two antigens is mixed with diluted serum from the patient. If the serum has antibody against IgG, a visible agglutination (clumping) indicates a positive result. Synovial fluid can also be analyzed for rheumatoid factor, using the patient's joint fluid instead of serum. The test results are comparable.

The titer is the highest dilution in which agglutination or a positive result exists. In rheumatoid arthritis, the highest titers occur in patients who have severe active disease. Additionally, Sjögren's syndrome demonstrates high titers of rheumatoid factor. Positive results at low titers (titers of 80 IU/mL or lower) occur in normal elderly individuals, in those with infectious mononucleosis, or in those with acute inflammation from another cause.

| Purpose of the Test | The test for rheumatoid factor is used in the diagnosis and prognosis of rheumatoid arthritis. |
|---|---|

| Procedure | A red-topped tube is used to collect 10 mL of venous blood. |
|---|---|

### Findings

**Positive Values**

Rheumatoid arthritis
Sjögren's syndrome
Systemic lupus
  erythematosus
Dermatomyositis
Scleroderma

Polymyositis
Waldenström's
  disease
Sarcoidosis
Infectious mono-
  nucleosis

Subacute bacterial
  endocarditis
Tuberculosis
Chronic lung disease
Chronic liver disease

| Interfering Factors | • Severe lipemia<br>• Circulating immune complexes |
|---|---|

| Nursing Implementation | Nursing care includes care of the venipuncture site. No other special nursing measures are required. |
|---|---|

## Uric Acid

**(Serum)**                    Synonym: Urate

**Normal Values**

**Adult <60 Years**
Male: 4.4–7.6 mg/dL *or* SI 262–452 µmol/L
Female: 2.3–6.6 mg/dL *or* SI 137–393 µmol/L
**Adult 60–90 Years**
Male: 4.2–8 mg/dL *or* SI 250–476 µmol/L
Female: 2.2–7.7 mg/dL *or* SI 208–434 µmol/L
**Child <12 years:** 2.0–5.5 mg/dL *or* SI 119–327 µmol/L

### Background Information

Uric acid is the end product of protein metabolism and is excreted from the body by the kidneys and bowels. The production of uric acid comes from a combination of dietary intake of protein and purine foods, purine biosynthesis, and catabolism of body tissues. The normal excretion of uric acid by the kidneys should eliminate two thirds of the uric acid from the blood daily. The remaining one third is in the bile and intestinal secretions. The intestinal bacteria act on the secretions by uricolysis, and the wastes are excreted in feces. The level of uric acid in the blood is maintained by a balance between the amount that is produced and the amount that is excreted (Fig. 24–2).

Under normal conditions, a temporary rise in the serum uric acid level can occur after ingestion of foods that are rich in purine (organ meats, legumes, meat, and some fish), after strenuous exercise or heavy alcohol ingestion, or during periods of stress. This type of rise is temporary, and the blood level returns to normal within a day.

**Elevated Values.** *Hyperuricemia,* an elevated level of uric acid in the blood, results from excessive production of uric acid or impaired excretion of uric acid, or a combination of the two causes. The conditions of abnormal overproduction include abnormal metabolism of purines and amino acids, excessive catabolism of body tissues, destruction of nucleoproteins, some cancers before and after chemotherapy or radiation, some endocrine and hemolytic disorders, and conditions that cause acidosis or lactic acidosis. Impaired excretion or urate retention is usually a result of renal disease that affects tubular secretion and reabsorption. It may also be caused by reduced renal blood flow and decreased renal filtration of the blood.

Gout is a genetic disorder of purine metabolism that usually produces a high level of uric acid in the blood and monosodium urate crystal deposits throughout the body. The deposits are located in the joints, cartilage, bones, bursae, and subcutaneous tissue. Some patients, however, develop gout with lower elevations of serum uric acid, and some patients have high levels of serum uric acid and do not acquire this inflammatory disease. The urate crystals can also accumulate in the renal pelvis and cause uric acid kidney stones to form.

**Decreased Values.** *Hypouricemia,* the abnormally low level of uric acid in the blood, usually results from defects in renal tubular absorption. The disorder can be congenital or acquired, but an increased urinary loss of urate, and therefore a low level of uric acid in the blood, occurs.

**Purpose of the Test**    The elevated level of uric acid is used to confirm the diagnosis of gout and helps detect renal impairment that causes prerenal azotemia and renal failure.

**Procedure**    A red-topped tube is used to collect 10 mL of venous blood.

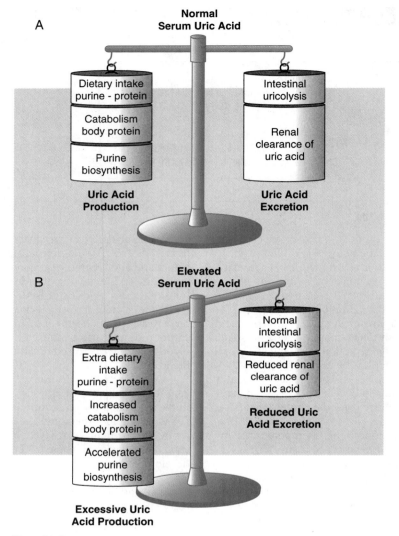

**Figure 24–2**
Uric acid production and excretion. *A,* Normal physiology. *B,* Pathophysiology of hyperuricemia.

**Findings**

**Elevated Values**

| | | |
|---|---|---|
| Gout | Leukemia | Lead poisoning |
| Diabetic ketoacidosis | Glycogen storage | Polycythemia vera |
| Renal failure |   disease | Acute alcohol |
| Shock | Lymphoma |   ingestion |
| Polycystic kidney | Lesch-Nyhan syndrome | Psoriasis |
|   disease | Toxemia of pregnancy | Pernicious anemia |
| Down syndrome | Hemolytic anemia | Tumor lysis syndrome |

**Decreased Values**

| | | |
|---|---|---|
| Fanconi's syndrome | Multiple myeloma | Xanthinuria |
| Wilson's disease | Bronchogenic | |
| Hodgkin's disease | carcinoma | |

---

**Interfering Factors**

- Starvation
- High purine diet
- Stress
- Caffeine or vitamin C ingestion

---

**Nursing Implementation**

Nursing intervention includes care of the venipuncture site.

### Pretest

When the laboratory protocol specifies a fasting specimen, instruct the patient
to discontinue all food and fluids for 8 hours.
On the requisition slip, list all medications taken by the patient. Many drugs
cause either a false-positive or a false-negative result.

### Posttest

No specific nursing intervention is required.

---

**Critical Value**

> **>12 mg/dL (SI >714 µmol/L)**
>
> Severe hyperuricemia is dangerous, because the urate crystals can accumulate in the
> renal tubules and ureters, resulting in obstruction and renal failure. This crisis can
> occur after administration of cytotoxic drugs, after a malignancy is irradiated, as
> a result of acute alcohol ingestion, or with adult respiratory distress syndrome. The
> physician must be notified of this critical elevation that is a marker of cell injury crisis.
> The interventions will depend on the cause of the cell destruction.

---

## Diagnostic Procedures

## Arthrocentesis and Synovial Fluid Analysis

**(Synovial Fluid)**            Synonym: Joint fluid analysis

**Normal Values**

> **Synovial Fluid Analysis**
> Appearance: Crystal clear, transparent, pale yellow
> Viscosity: High
> Volume: <3.5 mL
> Red blood cells: Absent
> White blood cells: 0–200/mm³ *or* SI 0–200 × 10⁶/L
> Nucleated cell count: <200/µL *or* SI <200 × 10⁶/L
> Granulocytes: <25% of nucleated cells
> Protein: 3 g/dL *or* SI 30 g/L
> Uric acid: <8 mg/dL *or* SI 476 µmol/L
> Glucose (fasting): 70–110 mg/dL *or* SI 3.9–6.1 mmol/L
> Blood–synovial fluid glucose difference: <10 mg/dL *or* SI <0.56 mmol/L
> Fibrin clot: Negative or absent
> Mucin clot: Positive or abundant
> Mucin string test: Formation of a long string
> Culture: No growth

## Background Information

*Arthrocentesis,* needle aspiration of the joint, is used to obtain a sample of synovial fluid. Normally, the joint contains little fluid volume. In inflammation, infection, trauma, or irritation of the joint, cartilage, or synovial membrane, the fluid fills or distends the joint capsule. Analysis of the aspirated fluid provides data regarding the cause of the swelling and the increased fluid production.

Few to no red blood cells should be present in the fluid. If the specimen is grossly bloody, it indicates hemorrhage into the joint such as from fracture, hemophilia, trauma, or a traumatic tap.

An abnormal leukocyte count can be mildly to dramatically elevated. Virtually all the diseases listed in the Findings section demonstrate a high white blood cell count in the synovial fluid.

Protein increases in the synovial fluid because of inflammation. When the patient has gout, the uric acid level is elevated. The glucose level should be equivalent to or less than a 10-mg difference between the blood value and the synovial fluid value. A decrease in the synovial fluid glucose level is indicative of inflammatory arthritis. For the glucose analysis, the patient is usually in a fasting state before the test is performed. This provides a stable baseline value for both the blood and the synovial fluid.

A fibrin clot should not be present, because normal synovial fluid has no fibrinogen. When clotting occurs, it is a sign of inflammation. A mucin clot and a favorable string test are indications of normal viscosity. Inflammation and excessive synovial fluid lessen the viscosity. When the fluid is poured, only a short string can form.

Culture of the fluid may identify the pathogen that caused the infection. Microscopic examination of the fluid is also performed to identify cells, sediment, or crystals in the fluid.

## Purpose of the Test

Synovial fluid analysis helps in the diagnosis of rheumatic diseases, infection, or other diseases that cause swelling of the joint, increased production of fluid, or damage to the joint space.

## Procedure

**Joint.**  Under sterile conditions, an aspiration needle is inserted into the joint space, and fluid is withdrawn. The fluid specimen is placed into one green-topped tube with heparin and two red-topped tubes.

**Blood.**   A red-topped tube is used to obtain 10 mL of venous blood for a serum chemistry profile. If additional tests are to be performed, a second red-topped tube is filled. The blood is drawn at the same time as the joint aspiration is performed.

**Culture.**   If gonococcus is suspected, some synovial fluid is inoculated onto a plate that contains Thayer-Martin culture medium. This is carried out immediately after the arthrocentesis is completed. Other cultures are started in the laboratory.

| Findings | **Abnormal Values** | | |
|---|---|---|---|
| | Rheumatoid arthritis | Traumatic arthritis | Hemophilic arthritis |
| | Rheumatic fever | Lyme disease | Pseudogout |
| | Infectious arthritis | Osteoarthritis | Systemic lupus |
| | Tuberculosis | Gout | erythematosus |

**Interfering Factors**

- Failure to maintain nothing-by-mouth status

**Nursing Implementation**

### Pretest

Inform the patient about the procedure and obtain written consent from the patient or the person legally designated to make health care decisions for the patient.

Instruct the patient to fast for 6 to 8 hours before the test.

Inform the patient that the procedure is performed with local anesthesia. Mild discomfort may be felt as the anesthetic is injected and as the joint capsule is penetrated.

### During the Test

Assist with positioning of the extremity. The skin is cleansed with antiseptic, and the area is covered with a sterile drape.

Assist with the preparation of the local anesthetic and the collection of all specimens.

### Posttest

After the needle is withdrawn, apply a pressure dressing to the aspiration site to prevent hematoma.

An elastic binding may be applied to the joint for 8 to 24 hours to increase the stability of the joint. Instruct the patient to apply a cold pack to the joint for 24 to 36 hours to decrease the swelling. The extremity may be elevated on pillows.

Teach the patient to avoid excessive use of the joint for 2 to 3 days. This will help prevent stiffness, pain, and swelling.

Arrange for immediate transport of the specimens to the laboratory.

**Complications**

Infection is a possible complication of arthrocentesis or any other procedure that opens the joint capsule. The infection can be introduced from environmental contamination or from aggravation of infection already present in the joint

**Table 24–1 Complications of Arthrocentesis, Arthroscopy, and Synovial Biopsy**

| Complication | Nursing Assessment |
|---|---|
| Infection of the joint | Fever |
| | Joint swelling |
| | Pain |
| | Purulent, malodorous drainage |

tissues. The drainage is purulent, and the dressing is contaminated by the secretions. The nursing assessment for complications of arthrocentesis is presented in Table 24–1.

## Arthrography

**(Radiology)**  Synonyms: None

---

**Normal Values**  Normal joint capsule and ligament structure; no abnormalities noted

---

### Background Information

The articulating bones, cartilage, and ligaments form the joint and its capsule. The inner surface of the joint capsule is lined by cartilage and synovia. The small amount of synovial fluid provides lubrication for easy joint motion.

The knee and shoulder joints are heavily bound by ligaments and tendons. They are subject to injury or trauma when they are forced beyond the normal range. Injury to the muscles, ligaments, tendons, bursae, synovial tissue, cartilage, or bone alters the structure of the joint capsule and limits the function of the joint.

---

### Purpose of the Test

Arthrography is performed to evaluate suspected adhesion, cartilage tear, or other abnormality of the joint capsule.

---

### Procedure

Using sterile technique and local anesthesia, a needle is inserted into the joint space to remove the synovial fluid and to inject air and iodinated contrast material. Fluoroscopy is used to guide the placement of the needle, and x-ray films are taken to document the interior structure of the joint capsule. The time needed for this test is 1 to 2 hours.

---

### Findings

**Abnormal Values**

| | | |
|---|---|---|
| Damage or deterioration of the cartilage | Torn collateral or cruciate ligaments of the knee | Tear or laceration of the medial meniscus of the knee |
| Disruption of the joint capsule | | |

| | | |
|---|---|---|
| Rotator cuff tear of the shoulder | Tenosynovitis | Chondromalacia patellae |
| Synovial abnormality | Osteochondritis dissecans | |
| Adhesions of the joint capsule | Osteochondral fracture | |

| | |
|---|---|
| **Interfering Factors** | • Incomplete removal of synovial fluid<br>• Incorrect placement of the contrast medium<br>• Allergy to iodine |

**Nursing Implementation**

### Pretest

Ask the patient about any history of allergy to iodine or shellfish or of a reaction to a previous x-ray test that used dye.

Once the physician has explained the test and the procedure, obtain written consent from the patient or the person legally designated to make the patient's health care decisions.

Inform the patient that the procedure is performed with local anesthesia. Mild pain is felt as the anesthetic is injected, and a tingling or a sensation of pressure is experienced when the contrast medium is injected. Once the needle is removed, the patient will be asked to move the joint to various positions. This distributes the contrast material until all structures are visible on the x-ray film.

### During the Test

Place the synovial fluid in a sterile specimen container and send it to the laboratory for analysis.

### Posttest

Monitor the patient's vital signs to ensure that the blood pressure and pulse readings are within normal limits.

Ensure that the pressure dressing or elastic bandage is intact and dry.

Instruct the patient to rest the joint for 12 hours and apply ice packs to the joint to reduce the swelling. The inflammation usually subsides in 1 to 2 days.

Mild pain medication is be taken to relieve any discomfort.

Generally, the pain is present for 2 to 3 days after the test is completed.

Advise the patient that a crackling sensation (crepitus) in the joint is expected for 1 to 2 days until the air contrast is fully absorbed. The iodinated contrast material is a water-soluble medium and is quickly absorbed from the joint by normal body processes.

## Arthroscopy

**(Endoscopy)**      Synonyms: None

| | |
|---|---|
| **Normal Values** | No tissue or structural abnormalities of the joint space are noted. |

## Background Information

The arthroscope—a thin, flexible fiberoptic endoscope—provides direct visualization of the joint structures and tissues in the joint space (Fig. 24–3). The instrument has light, fiberoptics, and lenses to allow inspection of the interior of the joint and any abnormalities that are present. The arthroscope is attached to a video camera so that the images can be shown on a monitor and videotaped for further study. The arthroscope contains a small camera that can photograph areas of interest. The special accessory instruments can be used to obtain biopsy specimens or to aspirate synovial fluid.

The joint and its interior ligaments, structures, synovial lining, and bony surfaces can develop

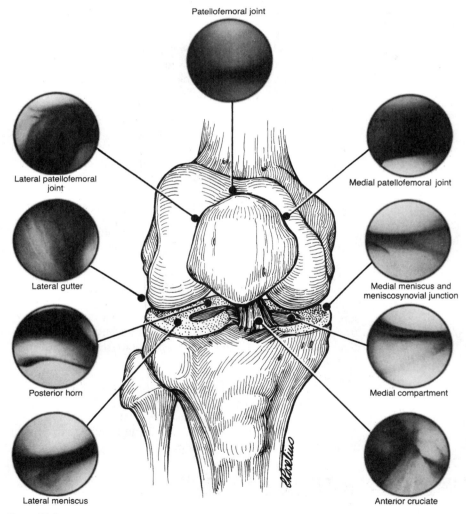

**Figure 24–3**
Arthroscopy. Anterior view of the knee showing each section as it appears with arthroscopy. (Reproduced with permission from Scott, W. N. [1990]. *Arthroscopy of the knee: Diagnosis and treatment* [p. 63]. Philadelphia: W. B. Saunders.)

infection, inflammation, tumor growth, or injury from trauma. When the pathologic change in the joint is not fully explained by more simple laboratory tests and diagnostic procedures, arthroscopy may be needed to confirm the diagnosis and evaluate the extent of the problem. The knee is the most common joint to be examined by arthroscopy, but the shoulder and other joints also can be examined by this method.

Diagnostic arthroscopy is performed as a same-day surgical procedure. Either local or general anesthesia may be used. Arthroscopy is an invasive procedure because surgical openings are made into the joint capsule to allow the insertion of the endoscope. Following the diagnostic phase, arthroscopic surgical repair of the torn or damaged tissue may be performed.

| | |
|---|---|
| **Purpose of the Test** | Arthroscopy provides direct visualization of the interior of the joint and tissue surfaces. It is used to detect torn tendon or ligament, injured meniscus, abnormal synovial tissue, pannus formation, and damaged cartilage. |
| **Procedure** | Two surgical incisions are made in the skin. A trocar is inserted into the joint capsule through one incision, followed by insertion of the arthroscope. A probe or the accessory instruments are inserted through the other incision. The joint capsule is filled and distended with saline or Ringer's lactate solution to promote visualization. Additional incisions may be needed to visualize all aspects of the joint. Tissue and fluid samples may be collected for laboratory analysis. Once the fluid is drained and the instruments removed, sutures or tape strips are used to close the incisions (Long, 1996). The total time needed for the procedure is 2 to 3 hours. |

**Findings**

**Abnormal Values**

| | | |
|---|---|---|
| Torn anterior cruciate or tibial collateral ligaments of the knee | Synovitis | Gout or pseudogout |
| | Loose bodies | Ganglion or Baker's cyst |
| Torn medial or lateral meniscus of the knee | Subluxation, fracture, or dislocation of the bone | Torn rotator cuff of the shoulder |
| Degenerative articular cartilage | Chondromalacia | |
| | Osteochondritis dissecans | |
| | Arthritis | |

| | |
|---|---|
| **Interfering Factors** | • Failure to maintain nothing-by-mouth status |

**Nursing Implementation**     **Pretest**

In preoperative teaching, the patient learns about the procedure, the anesthetic, the tests that will be done, the incisions, and the postoperative inflammation. Mild postoperative pain will occur, but it will be controlled with analgesics (Long, 1996). Once the procedure has been explained by the physician, obtain written consent from the patient or the person legally designated to make health care decisions for the patient.

■
*Critical Thinking 24–1*
The patient will undergo arthroscopy of the knee. In your
discussion of posttest activity
restrictions, he states that
his bedroom and bathroom are on
the second floor of his home.
What modifications can you
suggest?

Instruct the patient to discontinue all food and fluids for 8 hours before the
procedure.
Instruct the patient to have a responsible person available to provide transportation after the procedure.
Monitor baseline vital signs and record the results.

### During the Test

Position the patient, including possible placement of a stabilizing support
mechanism. The extremity is prepped and draped.
The arthroscopy equipment is set up and operational, including the irrigation
system and suction unit.
On completion of the procedure, bulky sterile dressings are applied and
covered with an elastic bandage. An immobilizer may also be applied (Moye
& Carpenter, 1994).

### Posttest

If general anesthesia was administered, monitor vital signs immediately and
thereafter every 15 minutes for the first 2 hours, then every 30 minutes
for 1 hour, and then every hour for 2 hours or until discharge from the post-
anesthesia unit.
If intravenous sedation and local anesthesia were administered, monitor initial
vital signs and repeat monitoring at regular intervals thereafter.
Assess for neurovascular function in the distal extremity every 15 minutes, and
compare the results with assessment of the unaffected side. The distal pulse
should be strong, and the skin should be cool to warm with satisfactory
color. Movement and sensation should be present in the fingers or toes.
Assess for pain and provide the prescribed medication for relief of pain, as
needed.
Check the elastic compression dressing for any signs of excessive bleeding, con-
striction, or excessive swelling of the joint or distal extremity.
For discharge instructions, remind the patient to keep the extremity elevated
for 24 to 48 hours to reduce the swelling. Ice should be applied for 24
hours.
With arthroscopy of the knee, remind the patient that walking is permitted, but
that no exercise or excessive use of the joint should occur for 24 hours. The
patient may be instructed to use crutches to keep all weight off the knee or to
walk only with a partial weight-bearing gait.
With arthroscopy of the shoulder, the arm is placed in a sling. Activity requirements or restrictions depend on the type of injury and any surgical repair
that may have been done following the diagnostic phase of the test.
Range-of-motion exercises are usually started on the second to third postoperative day, and physical therapy may be instituted to strengthen the muscles.
Provide the prescriptions for medications to be taken at home. Pain is usually
minimal and can be relieved by nonsteroidal, anti-inflammatory medications and nonnarcotic analgesics.

---

**Complications**

The complications of diagnostic arthroscopy are rare, but infection can occur.
Instruct the patient to report any sign of infection to the physician. The complications of arthroscopy are found in Table 24–1.

## Bone Biopsy

**(Tissue Biopsy)**          Synonym: Bone needle aspiration cytology

| Normal Values | Bone tissue is normal, with no tumor cells present. |
|---|---|

### Background Information

Benign bone tumors are characterized by their uniform density and well-defined margins.
The most common benign tumor is the giant cell tumor, often located in the end of a long bone near a joint.

Malignant primary bone tumors are characterized by borders that extend outward into surrounding fat or muscle tissue or inward into the marrow and medullary cavity, or both (Fig. 24–4). The most common primary bone malignancy is osteogenic sarcoma, which is often located in the region of the knee.

Malignant bone tumors may also be metastatic tumors, with the primary site located elsewhere in the body (Table 24–2). Most bone metastases are in multiple sites, usually located in the vertebrae, ribs, sternum, or pelvis.

When bone tumor is suspected, a bone scan or computed tomographic (CT) scan is performed first. These preliminary tests are used to verify the presence of the tumor and identify the site for bone biopsy. These preliminary tests are also used to identify additional metastatic sites and to help assess the extent of growth or invasion of the tumor. Unlike biopsy, the preliminary tests cannot distinguish benign from malignant disease.

### Purpose of the Test

Bone biopsy is performed to examine a specimen of bone tissue for its cell type and to distinguish benign from malignant bone tumor.

### Procedure

With local anesthesia, a small incision is made in the skin, and a bone biopsy needle is drilled or pushed into the bone. Once it is in place, the biopsy needle is rotated 180 degrees to obtain a core sample of the tissue. The specimen is placed on a slide with fixative or in a specimen jar with 95% alcohol as a fixative, or both procedures are carried out. The time needed for this procedure is 30 minutes or more.

### Findings

**Abnormal Values**

MALIGNANT

Osteogenic sarcoma          Angiosarcoma
Ewing's sarcoma          Multiple myeloma
Reticulum cell          Metastatic
  sarcoma          tumor

BENIGN

Giant cell tumor          Osteoid osteoma
Osteoma          Chondroma

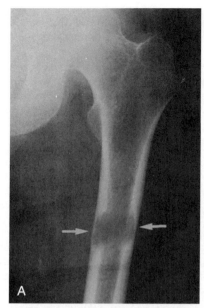

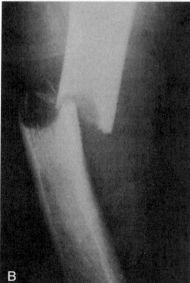

**Figure 24–4**

X-ray of bone metastasis. *A,* View of the femur in a patient with known lung cancer shows a destructive lesion expanding from the marrow space and thinning the bone cortex *(arrows).* The lesion has no defined, clear margin to distinguish it from normal bone. It is important to find lesions such as this in weight-bearing bones so that treatment can be undertaken to prevent pathologic fracture. *B,* View of the femur of the same patient who returned 2 weeks later with a pathologic fracture. (Reproduced with permission from Mettler, F. M. [1996]. *Essentials of radiology* [p. 342]. Philadelphia: W. B. Saunders.)

**Table 24–2    Primary Sites of Metastatic Bone Tumors**

| | |
|---|---|
| Breast | Lung |
| Prostate | Lymphoma |
| Thyroid | Kidney |
| Neuroblastoma | |

| Interfering Factors | • Failure to obtain an adequate sample of tissue<br>• Failure to send the specimen to the laboratory immediately |
|---|---|

**Nursing Implementation**

### Pretest

After the procedure has been explained to the patient by the physician, obtain written consent from the patient or the person legally designated to make the patient's health care decisions.

Instruct the patient to remove all clothing and put on a hospital gown.

Monitor baseline vital signs and record the results.

Shave the skin at the biopsy location and cleanse it with antiseptic.

Use a calm, reassuring approach with the patient. The procedure and possible results can cause anxiety.

### During the Test

Provide support to the patient as the skin and subcutaneous tissue are anesthetized and as the biopsy needle is inserted. Despite the local anesthetic, momentary pain is experienced as the needle penetrates the periosteum and enters the bone.

Label all specimen containers and slides with the patient's name and the tissue source.

Complete the requisition form for a tissue cytologic study.

The requisition slip states the patient's name and age, any history of carcinoma or infection, and the site of biopsy.

Send the slides or specimen, or both, to the laboratory without delay.

### Quality Control

The final preparation of the slides must be performed within 6 hours after specimen collection to prevent deterioration of the tissue.

### Posttest

The patient is instructed to rest quietly with an ice pack over the dressing for about 2 hours.

Assess vital signs and monitor them at regular intervals until they are stable.

Ensure that the pressure dressing remains clean, dry, and intact.

In preparation for discharge from the ambulatory setting, instruct the patient to resume routine activity but to avoid strenuous physical activity for a few days. The pressure dressing may be changed to a small adhesive bandage on the day after the procedure, and a shower is permitted. Mild discomfort is common, and the patient can take an analgesic medication as needed (Kim, 1994).

**Complications**

Infection of bone is a possible complication. Instruct the patient to notify the physician if untoward symptoms occur. The complications of bone biopsy are presented in Table 24–3.

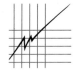

### Table 24–3 Complications of Bone Biopsy

| Complication | Nursing Assessment |
|---|---|
| Infection of bone | Fever |
| | Bone pain |
| | Headache |
| | Pain on movement |
| | Redness |
| | Drainage |
| | Purulence or abscess |
| | Elevated leukocyte count |

## Bone Scan

**(Radionuclide Scan)**     Synonyms: None

**Normal Values**     Symmetry of uptake of the radionuclide, with no bone abnormalities noted

### Background Information

Radionuclide bone studies produce sensitive, high-resolution images of the skeleton and joints. Because of the effectiveness of bone-seeking radio-pharmaceuticals, the bone scan is sensitive to changes in bone. It can detect early stages of bone disease before other radiologic procedures can.

Bone tissue is metabolically active, with a large number of nutrients exchanged in the blood vessels that supply the bones. A continual renewal of bone tissue is maintained by a balance between *osteogenesis,* the manufacture of new bone, and bone reabsorption. This renewal process is called *bone turnover.*

The bone scan procedure uses the physiology of bone turnover to ensure uptake of the radiopharmaceutical into the bone. Technetium 99m is a radioisotope that can be combined with an analogue of calcium, hydroxyl group, or phosphate to become a bone-seeking radioisotope. Once this radioactive substance is in the blood, it will be taken up by the bones and detected by the scintillation camera or scanner. To achieve adequate uptake by the bones, (1) adequate blood supply and (2) metabolic activity (bone turnover) are necessary.

**Bone Imaging.** The normal scan demonstrates symmetrical activity throughout the skeleton. In children, greater uptake occurs in the growth regions of the epiphyses, cranial sutures, and joints of the pelvic bones.

The abnormal scan presents "hot" spots or "cold" spots and an asymmetrical uptake of the radiopharmaceutical. A *hot spot* is an area of increased uptake of the radiopharmaceutical that indicates increased osteogenic activity (Fig. 24–5). The cause may be a primary or metastatic malignancy, Paget's disease, infection, healing activity in the repair of a fracture, or other conditions that accelerate osteogenesis. A *cold spot* indicates decreased uptake because of an absence of osteogenic activity. Causes of decreased or absent activity include a lack of blood supply to the area of bone or destruction of bone tissue by tumor, an inflammatory mass, or irradiation.

**Joint Imaging.** Because joints can be imaged, the bone scan can evaluate inflammatory joint disease. The radionuclide collects in tissues with increased blood flow, such as in the increased vascularity of synovitis or degenerative arthritis. Often, early joint inflammation is detected by radionuclide scan before it can be seen on x-ray film.

Additional discussion of nuclear scans is presented in Chapter 10.

**Purpose of the Test**

The bone scan is used to detect the presence and extent of metastatic disease of the bones. In addition, it is used to monitor degenerative bone diseases, detect osteomyelitis, determine bone viability, identify bone biopsy sites, and evaluate difficult fractures or fractures in battered children.

**Procedure**

An intravenous injection of a technetium radiopharmaceutical is followed by scanning with a gamma camera 1 to 4 hours later. The time variable depends on the type of radiopharmaceutical that is used. Scans are taken of anterior and posterior views. The images are seen on the monitor and are photographed for further study. The scanning process takes 1 hour to complete.

**Quality Control**

When administering the radiopharmaceutical, the needle must be placed correctly in the vein lumen. If leakage into the surrounding tissue occurs, the scanner detects the pooled isotopes. The localization may be interpreted as a false-positive finding.

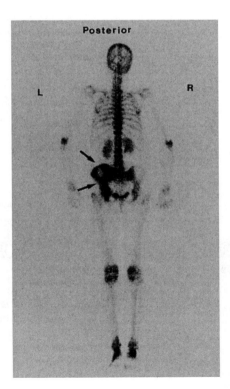

**Figure 24–5**

Bone scan of Paget's disease. This posterior view shows a darkened area (*arrows*) on the left side of the patient's iliac crest and pelvis. The increased uptake of radionuclide in the affected area is due to the markedly increased bone activity and increased blood flow that occur in Paget's disease. (Reproduced with permission from Mettler, F. M. [1996]. *Essentials of radiology* [p. 332]. Philadelphia: W. B. Saunders.)

| Findings | Abnormal Values | | |
|---|---|---|---|
| | Primary malignant bone tumor | Paget's disease | Soft tissue activity |
| | Osteomyelitis | Fractures | Aseptic necrosis |
| | Metastatic tumors | Arthritis | Post radiation therapy |
| | | Loose prostheses | |

| Interfering Factors |  |
|---|---|
| | • Metallic objects |
| | • Full or enlarged bladder |
| | • Pregnancy |

**Nursing Implementation**

### Pretest

Explain the procedure to the patient and obtain written consent from the patient or the person legally designated to make health care decisions for the patient. Ensure that the patient is not pregnant, because the radioactivity presents a potential danger to the fetus.

The radiopharmaceutical is a radioactive substance, but it is of low dosage and has a short half-life. The phosphate radiopharmaceutical is excreted rapidly from the body by the kidneys and bladder so that radiation exposure is minimal.

Instruct the patient to remove all clothing and jewelry and put on a hospital gown. The bladder must be emptied before the start of the procedure, because retained urine will contain the radiopharmaceutical and prevent a clear view of the pelvis.

### During the Test

The radiopharmaceutical is injected intravenously, usually in an arm vein.

Help the patient drink several glasses of water after the injection, before the scanning process begins. These extra fluids will help the patient void at the end of the procedure.

### Posttest

If the venipuncture site is sore or swollen, instruct the patient to apply moist compresses every 2 to 4 hours.

## Computed Tomography, Bones and Joints

**(Tomography)**

Synonym: CT scan

In orthopedics, the computed tomographic (CT) scan is particularly useful because the bone tissue is dense and absorbs many of the x-ray photons. Thus, the image of the bones appears white or bright on the film. The scan gives accurate definition of the structure of the bones and demonstrates subtle pathologic changes such as the small linear fracture, stenosis of a bony canal, or erosion of the bone.

Traditional CT may also be used to assess the spinal column, confirming the presence of bony or soft tissue changes that affect the vertebrae or spinal canal. CT detects congenital malformation, bony overgrowth, bone spurs, lumbar stenosis, cervical spondylosis, degenerative changes, a bulging disc, and ligament hypertrophy.

For other orthopedic problems, CT provides excellent images of bone and joint changes such as complex or subtle fracture, bone erosion, subluxation, dislocation, calcification, neoplasm, and scoliosis, including precise measure of the spinal curvature.

**Helical Computed Tomography.**    The helical CT scan has the ability to reconstruct a two- or three-dimensional image. This procedure is particularly useful in cases of cervical spine trauma with a suspected fracture, subluxation, or dislocation that could result in compression of the spinal cord (Kathol, 1997). It is also very useful in cases of massive or multiple fractures such as trauma to the pelvis involving the pelvic and hip bones. Helical CT also is used to identify abnormality in the bone due to neoplasm, infection, degenerative disease of the spine, and postsurgical difficulty with a spinal repair of the lumbar spine (Wang, 1995).

**Quantitative Computed Tomography.**    Another CT application is quantitative CT (QCT), which is used to measure or quantify the density of specific bone tissue. This specialized analysis uses the CT scan and mathematical calculations to assess bone mineral content, particularly of the vertebrae in the lower back (T4–L3). The quantitative analysis may be used to assess for osteoporosis or to evaluate the results of medical therapy and its effect of a decrease or increase in the density of the bones. Because this procedure is costly and difficult to schedule, an alternative method to measure bone density, such as dual-energy x-ray absorptiometry (DEXA), may be selected.

A complete discussion of CT is presented in Chapter 12.

## Dual-Energy X-Ray Absorptiometry

**(Radiology)**                    Synonyms: DEXA, DXA, bone densitometry

| **Normal Values** | Within 1.0 standard deviation (SD) of the average value |
| --- | --- |

## Background Information

Osteoporosis is a metabolic bone disease that causes the bones to become more porous or less dense. Because the bones become "thin" or brittle, they are at risk for fracture. Osteoporosis has the greatest incidence in postmenopausal women older than 65 years. When osteoporosis occurs, it affects all bones, but the bones that are most likely to fracture are the femoral neck (hip), vertebrae (spine), distal radius (wrist), and proximal humerus (upper arm–shoulder).

Dual-energy x-ray absorptiometry (DEXA) is a new, valid, and valuable procedure that can detect a decrease in bone mineral density at a very early stage, before osteoporosis or fractures occur. If the procedure is done only once, the measurement of the patient's bone mineral density (BMD) is compared with the values of the general population. If the patient has follow-up procedures performed over the years, it may be possible to compare the results with previous findings and determine whether additional loss or improvement has occurred in response to therapy.

**Understanding the Test Results.**    The patient's bone mineral density measurement is usually compared with the average test value of young normal individuals (T score). It can also be compared with the average test value of individuals who are the same sex and age (Z score) (Lindsay, 1998). The standard deviation (SD) is a statistical measurement that represents how much the patient's value is above (+) or below (−) the average, or mean, value.

**Decreased Values.** A test result that is between 1.0 and 2.5 SD below the mean (written as −1.0 SD to −2.5 SD) indicates a low bone mass, or osteopenia. A test result that is more than 2.5 SD below the average value (>−2.5 SD) indicates osteoporosis. If the level is this low and a fracture has already occurred, the osteoporosis is severe. With osteopenia, the patient may opt to begin preventive therapy. Once the test level reaches a value of −2.5 SD or more, therapy to prevent osteoporosis should be started (Raisz, 1995).

The most common cause of a loss of bone mineral density is the postmenopausal lack of estrogen. Osteoporosis has a silent onset. Except for some complaints of low back pain, the patient does not notice any difficulty until a fracture occurs. A simple x-ray cannot detect osteoporosis until 40% of the bone mass has been lost. For these reasons, the DEXA procedure is recommended for all women a few years after menopause or, at the latest, by age 60 to 65 years. A follow-up DEXA test may be recommended in 2 to 3 years. For the woman with multiple risk factors for osteoporosis, the procedure should be done at the time of menopause (Lindsay, 1998).

Steroid therapy and some diseases also cause bone loss, resulting in osteopenia or osteoporosis. Patients with these problems should also have a DEXA procedure. If bone loss has occurred, the patient's test value will be lower than normal.

---

**Purpose of the Test**

Dual-energy x-ray absorptiometry is used to measure bone mineral density and compare it with measurement standards of the population. The purpose is to identify osteopenia and osteoporosis at an early stage.

---

**Procedure**

Dual x-ray beams above and below the patient scan designated areas of bone. The usual areas are the vertebrae of the lumbar spine, the femoral neck (hip), and the forearm (wrist). From the data, computer calculations measure the bone density and quantify the results, compared with standardized normal values.

---

**Findings**

**Decreased Values**

| | | |
|---|---|---|
| Osteoporosis | Multiple myeloma | Chronic immobility |
| Steroid therapy | Hyperparathyroidism | |
| Osteopenia | Chronic gastrointesti- | |
| Cushing's syndrome | nal malabsorption | |
| Osteomalacia | Hyperthyroidism | |

---

**Interfering Factors**

- Calcified aortic aneurysm
- Previous bone fracture
- Metal prosthetic device
- Metallic items on the clothing or the body in the imaging area

---

**Nursing Implementation**   **Pretest**

Instruct the patient to remove any jewelry or clothing that contains metal (buttons, belt, zipper) in the area to be imaged. It is not necessary to disrobe completely.

Explain that no noise, pain, or discomfort is associated with the procedure. Although the procedure uses radiation, the exposure and dose are minimal.

### During the Test

The patient is positioned on an imaging table. For measurement of the bone density of the vertebrae, the patient is in the supine position, with the lower legs elevated on a boxlike cushion. This aligns the pelvis and spine in a flat position on the table. For measurement of the bone density of the femoral neck, the patient is supine, with the nondominant leg braced in a position of internal rotation. The patient is seated for bone mass measurement of the arm and wrist.

### Posttest

No special measures are needed.

■
*Critical Thinking 24–2*
You are assigned to present a class to older women on the topic of osteoporosis. What health promotion measures should you include?

## Magnetic Resonance Imaging

**(Tomography)**                           Synonym: MRI

Magnetic resonance imaging (MRI) using a whole body scanner has limited use in orthopedics, because the bone tissue produces a weak signal and therefore a poor image. MRI is very useful, however, in the evaluation of soft tissue within the bones or joints, such as a torn rotator cuff in the shoulder and the meniscus and ligaments of the knee. It can demonstrate a tumor or other abnormalities of the anterior or posterior cruciate ligaments. MRI can also be used to diagnose spinal stenosis and to evaluate the soft tissues of the spine (Kathol, 1997). MRI demonstrates degenerative disc changes, epidural fat, and postoperative scar tissue and ligament injury that affect spinal or neural function.

In more recent technology, the *extremity MRI* uses smaller equipment that is dedicated to imaging the distal upper and lower extremities. With this equipment, the MR images can demonstrate small fractures of the wrist or ankle that are not always seen with x-ray or CT. In addition to traumatic injury to the joints, this technology can image the bone marrow, inflammation of joints, bone erosion, and osteomyelitis in the bones of the distal extremities (Peterfry, Roberts, & Genant, 1997).

A complete discussion of MRI is presented in Chapter 12.

## Roentgenography, Bones and Joints

**(Radiology)**                           Synonym: X-ray

X-ray films of bones and joints can identify fractures and monitor the degree of healing. This radiology procedure also demonstrates pathologic changes in bone such as abnormal structure, decreased bone density, tumor, arthritic change, and avascular necrosis (Fig. 24–6). Changes in the joints include narrowing of the joint spaces, bony overgrowth, loose bodies, erosion of the joint margins, subluxation, and dislocation. A complete discussion of roentgenography is presented in Chapter 9.

## Synovial Membrane Biopsy

**(Tissue Biopsy)**                           Synonyms: None

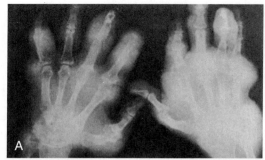

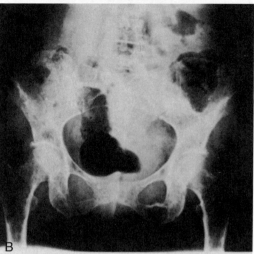

**Figure 24–6**
Radiographic visualization of osteolytic changes in bones. *A,*
Osteolytic changes have resulted from bone destruction owing to
the disease process known as gout. Note the soft tissue swelling
and bone destruction in the joints of both hands. *B,* Multiple
myeloma produces osteolytic changes as the result of metastases.
Radiolucent areas can be seen throughout the pelvis. (Reproduced with permission from Thompson, M. A., Hattaway,
M. P., Hall, J. D., & Dowd, S. B. [1994]. *Principles of imaging
science and protection* [Vol. 2, Slide 293]. Philadelphia:
W. B. Saunders.)

| Normal Values | Normal cells of the synovial membrane |
|---|---|

## Background Information

The synovial membrane forms the inner lining of
the joint capsule and secretes small amounts of
synovial fluid within the joint cavity. The fluid
is a thickened liquid that lubricates the joint surfaces and provides nourishment to the joint
cartilage. The volume of synovial fluid is minimal,
because the surrounding tissue absorbs the
excess fluid and electrolytes on a continual basis.

The synovia is subject to inflammation, granulation, or degeneration from a variety of causes,
including infection, trauma, and inflammatory
or arthritic changes to the joint itself. When
the synovia is infected or inflamed, excess produc-

tion of fluid occurs. The edema and congestion in
the joint tissues prevent the absorption of the fluid,
and the joint capsule becomes swollen and
painful. Following the inflammatory stage, granulation and fibrosis develop as the synovial tissue
heals. Eventually, the synovial tissue can be
destroyed by an ongoing pathologic process.

The synovial membrane biopsy procedure can
be performed on the affected knee, elbow, wrist,
ankle, or shoulder joint. From the tissue specimen,
histologic examination looks for evidence of inflammation. Synovial fluid is collected during the
procedure and is sent for culture.

| | |
|---|---|
| **Purpose of the Test** | Synovial membrane biopsy procedure is used to help differentiate among the various types of arthritis, collagen diseases, infections, and other disorders that cause inflammation of the joint and its synovial lining. |
| **Procedure** | Using sterile technique and local anesthesia, a trocar is pushed into the joint capsule. A special synovial biopsy needle is inserted through the trocar, and a small sample of synovial tissue is aspirated into a syringe. The tissue is sent to the laboratory for analysis. The procedure requires 30 minutes to complete. |

**Findings**

**Abnormal Values**

| | | |
|---|---|---|
| Coccidioidomycosis | Rheumatoid arthritis | Tumor |
| Gout | Reiter's disease | Systemic lupus |
| Lyme disease | Synovitis | erythematosus |
| Pseudogout | Sarcoidosis | |

**Interfering Factors**

• None

**Nursing Implementation**

**Pretest**

After the physician explains the procedure to the patient, obtain written consent from the patient or the person legally designated to make the patient's health care decisions.

Inform the patient that the local anesthetic is injected and that the procedure is not started until the tissue is numb. Brief pain is felt, however, as the trocar is inserted into the joint capsule.

Assess baseline vital signs and record the results.

**During the Test**

Assist with the positioning of the patient's extremity, cleansing of the skin, application of the drape, and instillation of the anesthetic.

Place the biopsy tissue in a sterile container with preservative. Label the container with the patient's name, the date, and the source of the tissue.

**Posttest**

Monitor the patient's vital signs at regular intervals until they are stable.

Check the compression dressing. The elastic bandage should be intact without constricting the circulation in the extremity. No evidence of swelling or bleeding should be present. The neurovascular assessment should be normal, including the presence of a distal pulse.

Send the specimen and requisition slip to the laboratory.

Instruct the patient to rest the joint for 24 hours to prevent hemorrhage or effusion.

Advise the patient to notify the physician about excessive swelling, pain in the joint, or bleeding, because hemorrhage or effusion can occur. Infection in the joint can also occur, and the patient must report any problems of fever, malodorous drainage, or purulent drainage. The complications of synovial biopsy are presented in Table 24–1.

## Ultrasound, Quantitative

**(Ultrasound)**                    Synonym: QUS

One newer technology to identify osteoporosis is quantitative ultrasound (QUS). The equipment is cost-effective compared with that of quantitative CT (QCT) or dual-energy x-ray absorptiometry (DEXA) methodologies. The ultrasound equipment is less expensive to purchase, and the test is less costly to the patient. Additionally, this type of ultrasound is portable and can be used in various locations that are accessible to the patient (Raisz, 1995; Torgerson, 1998).

Because the results of this test are less precise than those of DEXA or CT, the ultrasound method is best used as a screening device to detect osteoporosis. The ultrasound device accurately estimates the bone mineral density in the calcaneus (heel) or patella (kneecap). This method is not precise enough to measure bone loss over time or bone changes after treatment for osteoporosis. Research findings of the future will focus on using this technology to estimate the risk of bone fracture (Torgerson, 1998).

## References

Anderson, L. G. (1998). Aspirating and injecting the acutely painful joint. *Emergency Medicine, 30*(1), 16–18, 23, 28, 30, 35–36, 38.

Blumsholm, A., Hannon, R. A., & Eastell, R. (1995). Biochemical assessment of skeletal activity. *Physical Medicine and Rehabilitation Clinics of North America, 6*(3), 483–505.

Bryant, N. J. (1992). *Laboratory immunology and serology* (3rd ed.). Philadelphia: W. B. Saunders.

Burtis, C. A., & Ashwood, E. R. (Eds.). (1999). *Tietz textbook of clinical chemistry* (3rd ed.). Philadelphia: W.B. Saunders.

Cautilli, R. (1997). Introduction to the basics of arthroscopy of the knee. *Clinics in Sports Medicine, 16*(1), 1–16.

Christiansen, C. (1998). Practical application of risk assessment. *Osteoporosis International, 8*(Suppl. 1), S43–S46.

DeNuccio, M. A. (1994). Recognizing gout and pseudogout in hospitalized patients. *Journal of Musculoskeletal Medicine, 11*(10), 38–40, 42–44.

Gutierrez, M. J., & Edwards, N. L. (1996). Arthrocentesis and joint injection: Procedures and pitfalls. *Journal of Musculoskeletal Medicine, 13*(10), 41–48.

Henry, J. B. (Ed.). (1996). *Clinical diagnosis and management by laboratory methods* (19th ed.). Philadelphia: W. B. Saunders.

Jacobs, D. S., Dermott, W. R., Grady, H. J., Horvat, R. T., Huestis, D. W., & Kasten, B. L. (Eds.). (1996). *Laboratory test handbook* (4th ed.). Baltimore: Williams & Wilkins.

Jahng, J. S., & Lee, W. I. (1996). Measurement of bone mineral density in osteoporotic fractures in the spine, using dual energy x-ray absorptiometry. *Orthopedics, 19*(11), 951–954.

Kao, S. C. S., & Smith, W. L. (1997). Skeletal injuries in the pediatric patient. *The Radiologic Clinics of North America, 35*(3), 727–746.

Kathol, M. H. (1997). Cervical spine trauma. What is new? *The Radiologic Clinics of North America, 35*(3), 507–532.

Katz, R. T., & McCulla, M. M. (1995). Impedance plethysmography as a screening procedure for asymptomatic deep venous thrombosis in a rehabilitation hospital. *Archives of Physical Medicine and Rehabilitation, 76*(9), 833–839.

Kim, T. S. (1994). Primary hyperthyroidism. *Orthopaedic Nursing, 13*(3), 17–28.

Koepke, J. A. (1997). Is ESR useful? *Medical Laboratory Observer, 29*(1), 14.

Lehmann, C. A. (1998). *Saunders manual of clinical laboratory sciences.* Philadelphia: W. B. Saunders.

Lindsay, R. (1998). Risk assessment using bone mineral density determination. *Osteoporosis International, 8*(1), 28, 31.

Long, J. S. (1996). Shoulder arthroscopy. *Orthopaedic Nursing, 15*(2), 21–31.

Mettler, F. M. (1996). *Essentials of radiology.* Philadelphia: W. B. Saunders.

Moye, C. E., & Carpenter, R. J. (1994). Diagnostic modalities for orthopaedic disorders. In Maher, A. B., Salmond, S. W., & Pellino, T. A. *Orthopaedic nursing.* Philadelphia: W. B. Saunders.

Nakamura, R. M. (1995). R F latex test. *Medical Laboratory Observer, 27*(2), 11–12.

Nakamura, R. M. (1996). Mucin clot test. *Medical Laboratory Observer, 28*(1), 15.

Norris, M. K. G. (1994). Measuring antinuclear antibodies. *Nursing94, 24*(4), 27.

Peterfry, C. G., Roberts, T., & Genant, H. K. (1997). Dedicated extremity MR imaging: An emerging technology. *Radiologic Clinics of North America, 35*(1), 1–20.

Pretorius, E. S., & Fishman, E. K. (1995). Helical (spiral) CT of the musculosskeletal system. *Radiologic Clinics of North America, 33*(5), 949–979.

Raisz, L. G. (1995). Osteoporosis: 13 questions physicians often ask. *Consultant, 35*(7), 1039–1046.

Schaffer, T. C. (1993). Joint and soft tissue arthrocentesis. *Primary Care: Clinics in Office Practice, 20*(4), 757–70.

Shmerling, R. H. (1996). Rheumatic disease: Choosing the most useful diagnostic tests. *Geriatrics, 5*(11), 22–24, 26, 29–30.

Slater, C. A., Davis, R. B., & Shmerling, R. H. (1996). Antinuclear antibody testing. *Archives of Internal Medicine, 156*(7), 1421–1425.

Smith, R. P., Lipworth, B. J., Cree, I. A., Spiers, E. M., & Winter, J. H. (1995). C-reactive protein: A clinical marker in community-acquired pneumonia. *Chest: The Cardiopulmonary Journal, 108*(5), 1288–1291.

Soni, N., Sheldon, J., & Yentis, S. (1997). C-reactive protein. *Care of the Critically Ill, 13*(1), 14–18.

Tietz, N. W. (1995) *Clinical guide to laboratory tests* (3rd ed.). Philadelphia: W. B. Saunders.

Torgerson, D. J. (1998). Is there a future for non-menopausal screening strategies for osteoporosis prevention? *Osteoporosis International, 8*(Suppl. 1), S57–S61.

Wang, H. (1995). Radiologic assessment of the spine. *Physical Medicine and Rehabilitation, 9*(3), 605–617.

Williams, R. C. (1996). Rheumatoid arthritis: Using laboratory tests in diagnosis and follow-up. *Journal of Musculoskeletal Medicine, 13*(1), 14–16, 19–20, 23.

# Sensory Function

This chapter contains the diagnostic procedures that assess the sensory organs of the eyes, ears, and skin (Table 25–1). Because of the distinctly different nature of these diagnostic procedures, they are organized in sections for each organ system.

The diagnostic procedures are used to identify and locate abnormality as well as to assess the extent of change or impairment. Abnormality is caused by a change in the structure or the function of the organ system, or both. Many of these tests can supply data early in the course of the disorder, which provides accurate information and guidance for prompt treatment. In some conditions, the treatment results in cure or correction to overcome the problem. In other conditions, early diagnosis and treatment can minimize the deficit or loss of sensory function.

## Diagnostic Procedures: Eye Testing

## Computed Tomography, Eye, Orbits

**(Tomography)**                Synonym: CT scan

The computed tomographic (CT) scan with contrast medium is the primary imaging procedure used to examine the eye orbits and their contents. It provides visual information about the eyes and the bones and soft tissues surrounding the eyes (Fig. 25–1). The use of tomographic slices and different visual planes allows the assessment of the parts in a complex anatomic area. The procedure has an additional advantage because it can be performed rapidly. This is beneficial when a small child or an uncooperative patient requires an examination but cannot remain still for a long period of imaging.

In imaging the bones of the orbits, the CT scan identifies abnormalities caused by abscess, calcification, fracture, trauma, and metastatic lesion (Fig. 25–2). In the assessment of the orbital contents, the CT scan can image the globe, lens, ocular muscles, and optic nerve. Abnormalities that are clearly defined include retinoblastoma, meningioma, granuloma, penetrating foreign

**Table 25–1    Laboratory Tests According to Organ Involvement**

| Organ | Test |
| --- | --- |
| Eye | Computed tomography, eye, orbits |
| |    Helical (spiral) computed tomography |
| | Fluorescein angiography |
| | Magnetic resonance imaging, eye |
| | Orbital radiography |
| | Ultrasonography, eye |
| | Visual acuity testing |
| |    Distance vision |
| |    Near vision |
| |    Astigmatism |
| | Visual field testing |
| |    Amsler's grid |
| |    Tangent screen test |
| Ear | Audiometry |
| |    Pure tone audiometry |
| |    Speech audiometry |
| | Computed tomography, labyrinth system |
| | Electronystagmography |
| Skin | Biopsy, skin |
| | Patch test, skin |

bodies, orbital hematoma, some vascular lesions, and the muscle changes associated with the exophthalmos of Graves' disease.

**Helical (Spiral) Computed Tomography.**    With this newest refinement of the technology, the CT images can be obtained more rapidly than with conventional CT. The shorter imaging time, reduced radiation, and reduced dosage of the contrast medium are particularly helpful in the imaging of children (Cantore & Goldberg, 1996).

A complete discussion of CT is presented in Chapter 12.

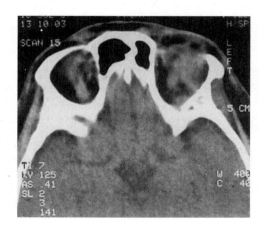

**Figure 25–1**

Orbital metastasis. Transverse computed tomographic (CT) section showing a tumor mass in the left orbit. The enlarged size and irregular shape of the left orbit are the result of metastasis from ovarian cancer. (Reproduced with permission from Bomanji, J., Glaholm, J., Hungerford, J. L., Mather, S. J., Granowska, M., Britton, K. E., & Whitelock, R. [1990]. Radioimmunoscintigraphy of orbital metastases from ovarian carcinoma. *Clinics in Nuclear Medicine, 15,* 825–827.)

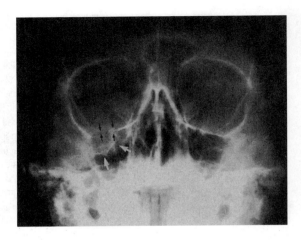

**Figure 25–2**
Inferior blowout fracture of the orbit. An x-ray anteroposterior (AP) view of the face shows air in the right orbit and discontinuity of the floor of the right orbit (*black arrows*), as well as a soft tissue mass hanging down from the orbit into the maxillary sinus (*white arrows*) and blood in the dependent part of the sinus. (Reproduced with permission from Mettler, F. A. [1996]. *Essentials of radiology* [p. 38]. Philadelphia: W. B. Saunders.)

## Fluorescein Angiography

**(Photography with Contrast)**   Synonyms: Intravenous fluorescent angiography, IVFA

| Normal Values | Retinal blood vessels are intact, with normal circulation and no evidence of leakage. |
| --- | --- |

### Background Information

The normal circulation of the retina consists of the central retinal artery and the central retinal vein, their four main branches, arterioles, venules, and capillaries. Behind the retina is the vascular choroid layer that allows the retinal exchange of oxygen, nutrients, and metabolic waste products. When local or systemic disease alters the retinal circulation, the changes can be seen in the retina and the blood vessels. Fluorescein angiography photographs the changes to document the location and extent of the circulatory abnormality.

The dye used in the examination illuminates the blood vessels by its fluorescence. When rupture or leakage of the blood vessel exists, the dye leaks into the vitreous humor, producing a hyperfluorescent area. Retinal arterial stenosis or occlusion demonstrates an area of hypofluorescence or prolonged venous drainage. Abnormal vascular patterns are characteristic of other retinal and circulatory problems, and the findings are used to diagnose the retinal condition.

**Purpose of the Test**   This test is used to highlight the retinal circulation as part of the evaluation of retinopathy. The retinopathy is the result of a systemic, intraocular, or retinal pathologic change.

**Procedure**   After pupillary dilation, the fluorescent dye is injected intravenously. A rapid series of 20 to 30 photographs is taken at 1- to 2-second intervals to document the retinal circulation. After a rest period, a second series of photographs may be obtained to document the retinal findings.

| Findings | **Abnormal Values** | | |
|---|---|---|---|
| | Microaneurysm | Capillary heman- | Ruptured blood |
| | Arteriovenous shunt | gioma | vessel |
| | Occlusion (arterial, | Hypertensive reti- | Papilledema |
| | venous) | nopathy | |
| | Neovascularization | Tumor | |
| | Tortuosity of blood | Edema (retinal, | |
| | vessels | macular) | |

**Interfering Factors**

- Allergy to the iodinated contrast medium
- Cataracts
- Insufficient dilation of the pupils
- Movement of the head, eyes, or eyelids

**Nursing Implementation**

### Pretest

Obtain written consent from the patient or the person who is legally responsible for the patient's health care decisions.

Inquire about past history of allergy to iodine or seafood or of a previous reaction to contrast material during a radiographic examination.

If the patient has glaucoma, instruct him or her to omit eye drop medication on the morning of the test. Glaucoma medication constricts the pupils, so the pupillary dilation needed for the test would be difficult to accomplish.

Assess the patient's baseline vital signs and record the results.

### During the Test

Dilate the pupils with mydriatic eye drops.

Insert the intravenous line into a vein of the antecubital fossa. A scalp vein needle commonly is used.

Instruct the patient to sit in a chair with the chin and forehead resting against supports. The camera is positioned in front of the eye and is focused on the retina.

Instruct the patient to keep the head immobile and to stare straight ahead. Normal breathing and blinking are carried out during the photography phase.

Inform the patient that nausea, hot flashes, or a sensation of warmth may be experienced as the fluorescein dye is injected. Vomiting can occur.

After the photographs are taken, remove the intravenous needle and instruct the patient to rest for 20 to 60 minutes. If a second series of photographs is taken after the rest interval, no additional dye is needed. The dye has recirculated so that the retina is clearly visible.

### Posttest

Inform the patient that the skin and sclera may appear yellow because of the dye circulation, but that the yellow color disappears in 4 to 6 hours. The urine will be fluorescent yellow-orange for about 24 hours as the dye is excreted from the body.

■
*Critical Thinking 25–1*
At the urban diagnostic eye center, the patient has just completed a fluorescein angiography examination. She tells you that she and her friend are going shopping. What precautionary advice can you provide?

Instruct the patient to drink extra fluids to help with the renal clearance of the dye.

Because the pupils remain dilated for a few hours, instruct the patient to wear sunglasses to protect the eyes from the glare of sunlight. Instruct the patient to avoid driving a car until the vision is clear.

## Magnetic Resonance Imaging, Eye

**(Tomography)**           Synonym: MRI

Although magnetic resonance imaging (MRI) cannot image the bones or calcification of the orbits, it provides exceptional visualization of the soft tissue structures of the eye. It is often used as a supplement to the CT scan, particularly in the evaluation of a soft tissue tumor, the extraocular muscles, or the optic nerve. MRI can distinguish among solid tumor, subretinal fluid, and effusion. It is also useful in determining the cause of visual disturbance when the origin of the problem is brain infarct, brain tumor, inflammation of the brain, or demyelinating disease.

A complete discussion of MRI is presented in Chapter 12.

## Orbital Radiography

**(Radiography)**           Synonym: X-ray of orbits

Plain radiography of the bony orbits may be used to investigate possible orbital fracture. When resulting from facial trauma, the fracture may be linear or with displacement of bone fragments. Severe facial fracture may result in a widening of the protective bones that surround the eyes, which can be seen on x-ray film. Increased bone density is indicative of metastatic cancer, Paget's disease, or meningioma. Because of the superior ability of the computed tomography (CT) scan to provide images from many tomographic planes, it is the preferred modality to investigate problems of the bony orbits.

A complete discussion of radiography is found in Chapter 9.

## Ultrasonography, Eye

**(Ultrasound)**           Synonyms: None

Ultrasonography of the eye and orbit provides an accurate assessment of retinal detachment and can detect fluid leakage or hemorrhage within the eye or behind the retina. It can also identify the presence of an intraocular tumor. Ultrasound may be used to assess and measure extraocular muscles or other eye structures that are altered because of inflammation, infection, or edema. It is also used to locate a nonmetal foreign body in the eye (Fleischer & Kepple, 1995).

A complete discussion of ultrasound is presented in Chapter 8.

## Visual Acuity Testing

**(Vision Test)**           Synonym: VA

**Normal Values**

Distance vision: 20/20 vision or better in each eye
Near vision: 14/14 vision or better in each eye
Astigmatism: All lines seen as clear and of equal blackness

## Background Information

*Central vision* is a function of the fovea in the center of the macula. This retinal tissue provides the sharp image of both distant and near objects, aided by the functions of the cornea and lens.

**Distance Vision.**   This type of vision is assessed by the use of Snellen's chart (Fig. 25–3). Each eye is tested separately, without and then with the use of corrective lenses. By tradition, the right eye is tested first.

The test results are written in fraction form (e.g., 20/20 vision). The first number, or the numerator, represents the distance between the patient and Snellen's chart. The second number, or the denominator, represents the lowest line on Snellen's chart that is read correctly by the patient. When the patient stands at a distance of 20 ft from the chart and reads line 20 correctly with one eye, the result is recorded as 20/20 for that eye. The interpretation is that the patient sees at 20 ft what other individuals see at 20 ft. If the patient has a result of 20/80 in one eye, it means that the patient sees at 20 ft what other individuals see at 80 ft.

The legal definition of blindness is 20/200 or

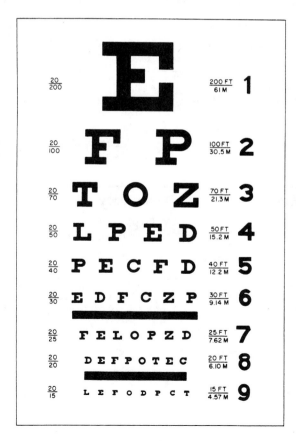

**Figure 25–3**
Snellen's chart. This chart is used to assess distance vision.

worse with corrective lenses. If the patient cannot see the large letter E (line 200) on Snellen's chart at a distance of 20 ft, the patient is retested at a distance nearer the chart. Thus, when the patient can see the letter E at a distance of 10 ft, the result is 10/200.

For the patient who cannot see the letter E at any distance, additional assessment is performed. The patient may be able to count fingers (CF) that are 1 ft in front of his or her face. The recording of the vision is 1/CF. If this test is unsuccessful, the patient may be able to see hand movement (HM) at a 1-ft distance. The result is written as 1/HM. If this test is unsuccessful, light perception (LP) is tested. While a bright light shines in the patient's eye, he or she is asked to state if the light is off or on. The affirmative response is recorded as 1/LP, meaning that light perception exists at a 1-ft distance. The negative response is recorded as no light perception (NLP).

**Near Vision.** This is tested to determine the patient's ability to focus on small details that are in close range. At rest, the normal eye is adapted for distance vision. If a need exists to focus on fine details, the eye must accommodate or change. This is carried out by contraction of the ciliary muscles and a change in the shape and thickness of the lens. Patients older than 40 years may have a loss of elasticity of the lens, resulting in difficulty with accommodation, or *presbyopia*. Near vision testing assesses the power of accommodation and is performed by requiring the patient to read small print or focus on small objects.

**Astigmatism.** This is the blurring of vision caused by the irregular curvature of the cornea or lens. Because of the irregularity, part of the view is clear and part is blurred. The astigmatism test chart is used to measure the clarity of vision in different axis areas of the cornea and lens. When astigmatism is present, the patient sees some of the axis lines on the chart as blurred or distinctly darker than other lines.

---

**Purpose of the Test**     Visual acuity testing is performed to assess the sharpness of central vision.

---

**Procedure**     **Distance Vision.** Testing each eye separately, the patient is asked to read the lines of Snellen's chart from a distance of 20 ft.
**Near Vision.** From a distance of 14 in, the patient is asked to read small print or to identify the location of the opening in each letter C in a series.
**Astigmatism.** The patient looks at the test chart and identifies any lines that are blurred or darker in tone.

---

**Findings**     **Abnormal Values**

| | | |
|---|---|---|
| Hyperopia | Corneal opacity | Retinal detachment |
| Macular degeneration | Presbyopia | Optic nerve |
| Myopia | Advanced cataracts | impairment |

---

**Interfering Factors**     • Failure to bring corrective lenses to the test
• Use of improperly prescribed or outdated lenses

---

**Nursing Implementation**     **Pretest**

**Snellen's Chart**

Place the patient 20 ft from the chart. The patient may stand or sit for the test. Plan to test the vision first without corrective lenses and then with the corrective lenses used for distance vision.

### During the Test

#### Snellen's Chart

Have the patient occlude the left eye, and begin testing the right eye.

Ask the patient to read the letters for each line, starting at the top line or starting at a lower line where the patient can see the letters clearly.

If the chart uses the letter E, ask the patient to position the fingers in the same direction as the E on a particular line of the chart. If the chart has numbers or objects, the patient identifies them.

Ask the patient to continue reading the progressively smaller lines until errors are made on more than half the letters or until the line marked 20 is completed.

If the patient with corrective lenses cannot see the line marked 400 (the large E) from 20 ft away, walk the patient toward the chart until the letter can be identified. Record the distance from the chart. If necessary, assess the ability of the patient to count fingers, see hand movement, or perceive light, usually from a distance of 1 ft.

Repeat the test for the other eye.

#### Near Vision

Test each eye separately.

Request that the patient use the corrective lenses to read a sample of tiny print from a distance of 14 in. As an alternative, ask the patient to use a finger to point in the same direction as the opening of the letter C.

#### Astigmatism

Test each eye separately, first without and then with corrective lenses.

Instruct the patient to look at the center of the figure with the radial black lines.

Ask the patient to identify any blurred lines or any lines that look darker than the others.

#### Posttest

Record the results for each eye, without and then with the corrective lenses.

## Visual Field Testing

**(Vision Test)**    Synonyms: None

**Normal Values**

Amsler's grid: The black dot, the four sides of the grid, and all squares within the grid are seen.

Tangent screen test: The test object remains visible in all areas of central vision.

## Background Information

The visual field is the total extent of vision out to the periphery. The two areas that combine to make the total are the central and the peripheral areas of the visual field. The central portion contains the fovea centralis retinae, the retinal area of visual acuity. It provides sharp focus in an area of 25 degrees surrounding a fixation point. The peripheral visual field is the larger area that has vision but little acuity or focus. The peripheral field extends out to 60 degrees on the nasal side and to 85 degrees on the temporal side of each retina.

**Amsler's Grid.**   This is a screening test that assesses the central portion of the total visual field (Fig. 25–4A). When deterioration or damage to the central visual field, the fovea centralis retinae, or the macula exists, the patient may be unable to see the central black dot or may not see all four sides of the grid (Fig. 25–4B). Some of the grid may be seen as blurred or distorted instead of as horizontal and vertical black lines that form squares.

**Tangent Screen Test.**   This measures the central portion of the visual field by mapping the boundaries of the central vision of each eye (Fig. 25–5). After mapping the perimeter, the optic disc area is located, and its boundary is mapped. Because the optic disc has no photoreceptors, it acts like a small blind spot in the central visual field. Once the mapping of the outer and inner boundaries is completed, each eye is tested to verify that visual acuity exists in all areas within the boundaries. This method can provide some data, but in patients who have a deficit in central visual acuity, more precise automated or computerized equipment is used to measure the abnormality.

| | |
|---|---|
| **Purpose of the Test** | These tests detect a loss of acuity in part of the central visual field and estimate the location and extent of the retinal change. |
| **Procedure** | Amsler's grid is placed 13 to 14 in from the patient, and the vision of each eye is tested separately. The patient is asked to describe what is seen.<br><br>    The tangent screen hangs on a wall, 40 in from the patient, and the vision of each eye is tested separately. The patient states when he or she sees the test object, which is a disc with a black side and a white side. The black side is used when the tangent screen has a white background, and the white side is used when the screen has a black background. The results are mapped to define the perimeters of the central visual field and any areas of deficit within the normal field. |

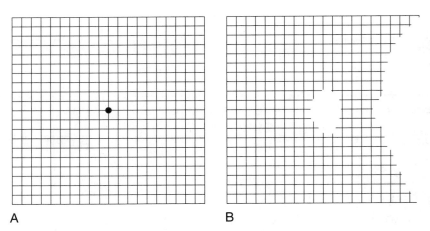

A

B

**Figure 25–4**

A, Amsler's grid. B, Loss of visibility of some lines or of the dot indicates retinal abnormality, particularly in the area of the macula.

NAME _____ DATE _____

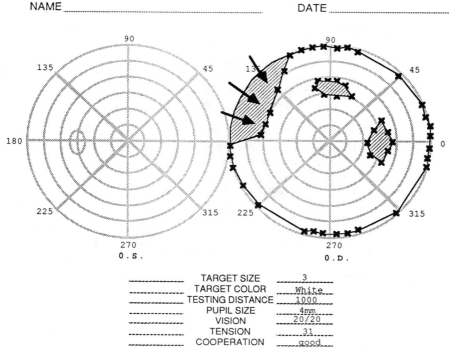

| | | |
|---|---|---|
| _____ | TARGET SIZE | 3 |
| _____ | TARGET COLOR | White |
| _____ | TESTING DISTANCE | 1000 |
| _____ | PUPIL SIZE | 4mm |
| _____ | VISION | 20/20 |
| _____ | TENSION | 31 |
| _____ | COOPERATION | good |

**Figure 25–5**

Tangent screen recording form. The test provides a mapping of the visual field of each eye. For the left eye (OS), a record has not yet been made on the form. For the right eye (OD), the chart is filled in and shows a superior nasal step, an arcuate scotoma, and vertical enlargement of the blind spot such as might be found in glaucoma. (Reproduced with permission from Carlson, N. B., Kurtz, D., Heath, D. A., & Hines, C. [1996]. *Clinical procedures for ocular examination* [2nd ed., p. 315]. Stamford, CT: Appleton & Lange.)

---

**Findings**  **Abnormal Values**

Macular degeneration  Cerebral aneurysm  Retinal detachment
Hemianopsia  Cerebral vascular  Retinitis pigmentosa
Pituitary tumor  accident
Meningioma  Glaucoma

---

**Interfering Factors**
- Severe loss of vision or blindness
- Failure to focus on the central dot or object on the screen

---

**Nursing Implementation**  **Pretest**

Instruct the patient to wear corrective lenses for each of these tests.
Provide an occluder or a folded tissue to cover one eye as the other eye is tested.

### During the Test

#### Amsler's Grid

Place the patient about 13 in from Amsler's grid.

Request that the patient keep his or her eye focused on the black dot.

Ask the patient the following questions: Is the black dot visible? Are the four sides of the grid visible? Are all lines and squares visible?

Repeat the test on the other eye.

#### Tangent Screen

Ask the patient to sit down for the examination. The chair is placed 40 in from the wall where the screen is hung.

Stand at the side of the screen and ensure that the patient's eye remains centered and does not search for the test object.

Ask the patient to fix his or her eye on the center of the screen and state when the test object first comes into view on the screen.

Use a handheld wand with the test object on the tip to do the mapping. Along each tangent line, bring the object into view, from the periphery toward the center.

Place a pin on each tangent line where the patient states the test object is first seen. These pins mark the outer boundary of the central visual field.

Identify and map the boundaries of the optic disc. In a small area on the nasal side of each visual field, the patient sees the disc along several tangent lines; first it disappears, and then it reappears. Mark the places of disappearance and reappearance until the circular area is completed. This is the area of the optic disc.

Now that the boundaries are completed, use the test object to confirm visual acuity throughout the visual field.

In each sector defined by the tangent lines, place the black test object on the black field. Turn the test object so that the white side shows. Ask the patient to state when the object appears. Repeat this maneuver in each sector (Carlson, Kurtz, Heath, & Hines, 1996).

If an area is not identified, repeat the maneuver with a test object of a different color or one of a larger size.

Record the results on the special test sheet and then repeat the test on the other eye.

### Posttest

Patient variables of inattention, difficulty in following instructions, lens opacities, or other vision difficulties can interfere with the accuracy of results.

If problems cannot be overcome, that information should be recorded in the patient's chart (Hupp, 1993).

---

## Diagnostic Procedures: Ear Testing

## Audiometry
**(Hearing Test)** — Synonyms: Hearing test, audiometric test, audiogram

**Normal Values**

> **Pure tone average:** 0–20 dB
> **Speech reception threshold:** Ability to repeat 50% of the words correctly, in a range of 0–20 dB
> **Word discrimination threshold test:** >90% of the words repeated correctly

## Background Information

Hearing occurs by bone, air, and nerve conduction of sound waves. *Conductive hearing loss* occurs when interference with air conduction is caused by problems in the external or middle ear. *Sensorineural hearing loss* occurs because of interference with nerve transmission caused by problems of the inner ear, cochlea, or acoustic nerve, or a combination of these. A *mixed hearing loss* involves some impairment of both bone and air conduction.

*Audiometry* is a test that measures the degree of hearing or hearing loss in response to pure tones and speech. The audiometer is the diagnostic instrument that produces sounds in different intensities (degrees of loudness) and different frequencies (degrees of pitch). Intensity is measured in decibels (dB), and frequency is measured in hertz (Hz) or cycles per second.

**Pure Tone Audiometry.** In this method of testing, the audiometer emits a series of tones at different frequencies. For the assessment of air conduction, the patient wears headphones and indicates when the different tones are heard. For the assessment of bone conduction, a vibrator is placed at the mastoid bone and emits the different tones. The tones that are heard identify the patient's hearing thresholds. A *hearing threshold* is the lowest decibel level at distinct frequencies when at least 50% of the tones are heard.

As the patient indicates that a sound is heard, the examiner plots the response on an audiogram (Fig. 25–6). The normal range of hearing is 0 to 20 dB at all tested frequencies. The patient with a hearing loss requires a higher decibel level to obtain a threshold response. Impaired hearing is measured in terms of decibel loss, such as a 40-dB loss. Some patients have a decibel loss only at particular frequencies, usually the higher-level frequencies. Each ear is tested separately, starting with the better ear.

In sensorineural hearing loss, both air and bone conduction thresholds demonstrate higher decibel ratings (or a greater decibel loss). In conductive hearing loss, the air conduction threshold has a higher decibel rating (or a greater decibel loss), but bone conduction is normal. In a mixed hearing loss, both air and bone conduction have higher decibel ratings, but air conduction is worse than bone conduction.

**Speech Audiometry.** Hearing for speech measures the *speech reception threshold* and the *word discrimination threshold*. The speech reception threshold test is a spoken word test that measures sound intensity. It helps detect conduction hearing loss. The word discrimination threshold test measures the client's ability to understand spoken words (Martin, 1997). It helps detect sensorineural hearing loss.

The speech reception threshold measurement uses *spondiac* words. These are easily understood words of two syllables, such as *airplane, hardware, woodchuck,* and *birthday*. The speech reception threshold identifies the decibel level at which the patient can repeat 50% of the words accurately. The decibel level of the speech reception threshold is usually similar to the results of tone testing for air conduction hearing.

The word discrimination threshold test uses familiar, one-syllable words that are balanced phonetically, such as *day, stove,* and *run*. The patient hears the words at an intensity of about 30 dB above the speech reception threshold and repeats the words. The normal score is greater than 90% accuracy, but individuals with normal hearing often have 95% to 100% accuracy.

The patient with sensorineural hearing loss has a below-normal score on the word discrimination threshold test no matter what decibel level is

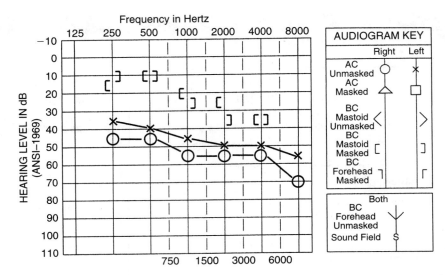

**Figure 25-6**

Audiogram. Audiometry provides precise measurement of hearing of pure tones and speech for each ear. (From Martin, F. N., *Introduction to audiology: A review manual 4/e.* Copyright © 1997 by Allyn & Bacon. Reprinted by permission.)

used. This patient might describe the hearing loss as "hearing the sounds but having difficulty understanding the words." In contrast, the patient with conductive hearing loss will have a good response on this test at the higher decibel levels. This patient might describe the hearing loss as "hearing the words as long as they are loud enough."

| **Purpose of the Test** | Audiometry tests determine the type and extent of hearing loss. |
| --- | --- |

**Procedure**

**Pure Tone Audiometry.** Sounds of differing intensity and frequency are emitted through earphones and a vibrator that is placed on the mastoid bone. When the sounds are heard, the patient's responses are charted on an audiogram.

**Speech Audiometry.** Words are spoken through earphones at different decibel levels. As the patient repeats the words, the accuracy is recorded and the overall measurement is calculated in percentage of accurate answers.

**Findings**

**Abnormal Values**

Otitis media
Cerebral infarction
Otosclerosis
Kernicterus
Ruptured tympanum

Multiple sclerosis
Acoustic neuroma
Mastoiditis
Meniere's disease
Labyrinthitis

Infection, inflammation
Ototoxicity
Hypothyroidism

**Interfering Factors**

• Impacted cerumen in the external auditory canal
• Background noise

- Inattention or mental confusion
- Extraneous cues from the examiner
- Recent ear or upper respiratory tract infection

## Nursing Implementation

### Pretest

Examine the external auditory canal and remove any impacted cerumen.
Provide an overview of the examination, including what to expect and how to respond. This promotes the patient's cooperation and responsiveness.
Instruct the patient to remove hearing aid, hat, and eyeglasses and then to sit in the soundproof booth or room.

### During the Test

Place the headphones on the patient and adjust them to fit properly.
Before each test, repeat the specific instructions so that the patient knows how to respond.

### Posttest

No specific nursing interventions are needed.

## Computed Tomography, Labyrinth System

**(Tomography)**        Synonym: CT scan

The computed tomographic (CT) scan is used to evaluate the labyrinth system as part of the investigation of dizziness. It provides visualization of congenital abnormality, tumor, abscess, bony changes, temporal bone fracture, and inflammatory disease.
A complete discussion of CT is presented in Chapter 12.

## Electronystagmography

**(Electric Monitoring)**        Synonym: ENG

## Normal Values

Electronystagmography: Normal waveform patterns; no nystagmus present
Caloric test: Normal waveform pattern
Cold stimulation: Nystagmus present in eye opposite the stimulated ear
Warm stimulation: Nystagmus present in eye on same side as stimulated ear

## Background Information

Electronystagmography is used to help determine the cause of dizziness, vertigo, tinnitus, and unexplained hearing loss. Some sources of these symptoms are abnormalities in the labyrinth system, the eighth cranial (acoustic) nerve, the cerebellum, or the brain stem.

The interaction between the vestibular system and oculomotor function is regulated by the vestibulo-ocular reflex. The regulation allows the eyes to maintain visual fixation while the head turns. In normal function, lateral nystagmus occurs only when the head is turned to an extreme lateral position or when the eyes move into an extreme lateral position. The eyes then return rapidly to a normal position with no further nystagmus. Abnormal nystagmus occurs at rest (spontaneously), or it persists after head turning or other evoked stimulus.

With this test, the measurement of eye movements is based on the recording of changing electric potentials. The cornea of the eye has a positive electric charge, and the retina has a negative electric charge. The electrodes detect the changing position of the eyes, and the results are recorded as linear patterns on graph paper. One benefit of the test is that it records the nystagmus even when the patient's eyes are closed ("An Adjunctive Test for Acute Dizziness," 1994).

An electrode is placed near the outer canthus of each eye to detect lateral nystagmus. Additional electrodes are placed above and below one eye to detect vertical nystagmus. One electrode is placed above the bridge of the nose to minimize noise interference (Fig. 25–7).

---

**Purpose of the Test**

These tests are used to verify the problem of dizziness and vertigo and to help identify the location of the abnormality.

---

**Procedure**

A number of different test maneuvers are performed during the examination. Most are carried out with the patient in a seated position and involve having the patient move the eyes, fix on or follow a light with the eyes, move the head, or move the body. The test battery includes the spontaneous nystagmus test, gaze nystagmus test, position tests, pendulum tracking test, optokinetic test, and *caloric test*.

In the caloric test, the patient lies supine with the head elevated 30 degrees. Cool water (30°C) and then warm water (44°C) are instilled in

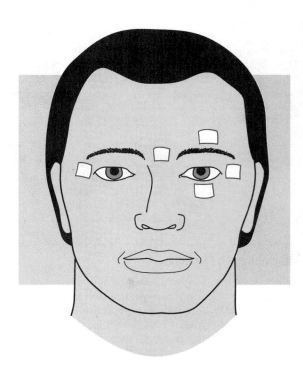

**Figure 25–7**

Placement of the electrodes for electronystagmography. The needle electrodes are inserted under the skin and are held in place with squares of adhesive tape. During the testing process, these electrodes transmit data that identify horizontal or vertical nystagmus.

each ear. The nystagmus response to the stimulus of temperature differences between the water and the patient's ear canal is recorded (Luxon, 1995).

**Findings**

**Abnormal Values**

| | | |
|---|---|---|
| Meniere's disease | Cerebral infarction | Ototoxicity |
| Congenital malfor- mation | Infection, inflam- mation | Otosclerosis |
| Lesion or tumor of the cerebellopon- tine angle | Ischemic neuritis | Temporal lobe epilepsy |
| | Head injury | Acoustic nerve tumor |
| | Posterior fossa mass or deformity | Hypothyroidism |
| Multiple sclerosis | | Labyrinthitis |

**Interfering Factors**

- Perforated tympanum
- Cardiac pacemaker
- Intake of caffeine or alcohol
- Poor eyesight
- Inability to comply with test instructions
- Back or neck disorder

**Nursing Implementation**

**Pretest**

Ask if the patient has a pacemaker, neck or back disorder, ruptured eardrum, or other problem that would interfere with the procedure.

Obtain written consent from the patient or the person legally responsible for the patient's health care decisions.

Instruct the patient to avoid a heavy meal and the intake of alcohol and caffeine on the day of the test. The alcohol and caffeine alter the nerve potentials, and the heavy meal is avoided because the test can cause nausea and vomiting.

Many medications subdue the neurologic responses and are often omitted for 24 to 48 hours before the test. These include antivertigo and anti-inflammatory drugs, aspirin, depressants, tranquilizers, sedatives, and stimulants. If the patient has been instructed by the physician to continue with these medications, record them on the requisition slip.

If a caloric test is planned, use the otoscope to examine the external auditory canal for a perforation of the tympanum and the presence of cerumen. An opening in the tympanum is a contraindication for this test. If an impaction exists, the cerumen must be removed.

Explain that dizziness and nausea can occur during the tests but that they subside after the tests are completed.

Provide reassurance that the examiner or nurse will remain nearby to prevent a fall. Position the patient comfortably in a chair.

**During the Test**

Before the placement of the electrodes, cleanse the skin with alcohol to reduce the electric impedance caused by skin oil.

To improve conduction, apply the electrode paste to the five sites. Insert the skin electrodes. Inform the patient that the electrodes on the face will feel uncomfortable.

As each test preparation is ready, provide specific instructions to the patient. These instructions include looking at the light, following the light with the eyes, opening or closing the eyes, and changing the head or body position. Assess the patient for nausea, dizziness, weakness, or vomiting throughout the test period.

### Posttest

Remove the electrodes and paste from the skin.
Assist the patient to a chair or couch to rest until the symptoms subside.

---

## Diagnostic Procedures: Skin Testing

## Biopsy, Skin

(Tissue Biopsy)                 Synonym: Gross and microscopic pathology, skin

| Normal Values | Benign; no malignant cells are present. No infectious organisms are present. |
|---|---|

### Background Information

When a skin lesion is present and the clinical diagnosis is uncertain or must be verified, a skin biopsy is carried out to determine the cellular composition of the lesion or the presence of infection. Skin biopsy can be performed by three different types of technique, all of which cause minimal amounts of discomfort, scarring, and bleeding (Jacobs, et al., 1996). The methods are *shave biopsy, punch biopsy,* and *elliptical excision* (Fig. 25–8).

**Shave Biopsy.** This procedure is used when a small, raised growth or lesion is present. The scalpel is placed parallel to the surface of the growth, and a shallow cut is used to remove some of the superficial tissue layers.

**Punch Biopsy.** This technique is used when the lesion extends into the middle to lower portion of the dermis. A circular cutting tool is rotated with downward pressure to cut and remove a core sample of the tissue. The small hole may be closed with a suture or allowed to heal by granulation.

**Elliptical Excision Biopsy.** This method is used when the lesion or growth is greater than 4.5 mm in diameter or is thought to extend deeper than the mid-dermis. A scalpel is used to excise the tissue to a depth that includes some subcutaneous fat. The tissue defect is closed with sutures.

| Purpose of the Test | Skin biopsy is performed to differentiate a benign from a malignant growth. It is sometimes used to diagnose particular bacterial or fungal infections. |
|---|---|

| Procedure | After local anesthesia is administered, a small sample of skin tissue is removed surgically for histologic and microbiologic examination. |
|---|---|

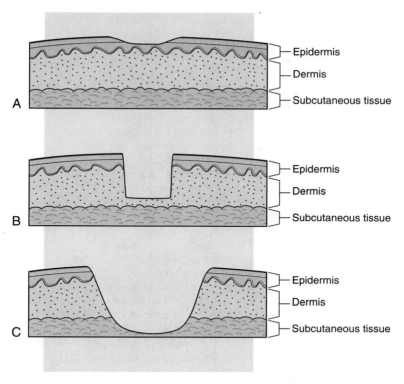

**Figure 25–8**
Skin biopsy. The depth of tissue removal for (A) shave biopsy, (B) punch biopsy, and (C) elliptical excision biopsy.

| Findings | Abnormal Values | | |
|---|---|---|---|
| | Malignant melanoma | Squamous cell | Bacterial infection |
| | Seborrheic dermatitis | carcinoma | Dermatofibroma |
| | Basal cell carcinoma | Cyst | Fungal infection |
| | Keloid | Neurofibroma | Mole |

| Interfering Factors | • Failure to identify the specimen<br>• Inaccurate identification of the specimen |
|---|---|

**Nursing Implementation**

**Pretest**

Obtain written consent from the patient or the person legally responsible for the patient's health care decisions.

Instruct the patient to remove the necessary clothing to expose the biopsy site. A hospital gown may be worn as needed.

Assess the patient's vital signs and record the results.

Depending on the site of the lesion, instruct the patient to sit or lie on the examining table.

### During the Test

Cleanse the skin site with a surgical antiseptic.

Assist with the application of the surgical drape and the preparation of the local anesthetic (lidocaine 1%).

Once the tissue sample has been removed, place it in a sterile, covered container with formalin or other tissue preservative.

If a tissue sample is needed for culture, place a small amount of tissue in a sterile container *without preservative.*

Close and label each container accurately, including the patient's name, the date, and the tissue source. Place the same information on the requisition slip.

After the bleeding ceases, place a small sterile dressing over the biopsy site.

### Posttest

■

*Critical Thinking 25–2*
Prepare a teaching plan that will help a female patient and her family prevent skin cancer (non-melanoma) from exposure to sunlight.

Monitor the patient's vital signs and record the results.

Assess the dressing for signs of bleeding. It should be clean, dry, and intact.

Ensure that the specimens are transported to the laboratory promptly. Microbiologic specimens must be sent immediately, because they can dry out. The specimens in preservative are sent on a routine basis.

Instruct the patient to keep the dressing clean and dry.

If sutures are in place, instruct the patient to return to the physician for their removal. Facial sutures are removed in 3 to 5 days. For other sites, the time of removal is 7 to 14 days.

## Patch Test, Skin

**(Skin Sensitivity Test)**        Synonyms: None

**Normal Values**        Negative; no abnormal skin reactions are noted.

### Background Information

Allergic contact dermatitis is an eczematous skin change that occurs as an inflammatory response to contact with a particular antigen. The person is sensitized to the antigen over time, without the immediate development of a skin reaction. Eventually, reexposure to the antigen induces a vigorous cell-mediated immune (allergic) response at the site of contact with the antigen (Lynch, 1994).

Because one part of the treatment of the skin eruption is to remove the patient from further contact with the antigen, the antigen must be identified.

In some cases, a patch test is used to identify one or more suspected antigens by evoking a skin reaction.

The patch test may be carried out by placing the suspected allergen, such as a small piece of clothing, a bit of a cosmetic substance, or a diluted solution of chemical components, on the skin. Industrial substances or laboratory chemicals are never used in testing, because they can produce an irritant dermatitis or a chemical burn. The most common allergens or sources of contact dermatitis are listed in the Findings section.

**Abnormal Values.** In reading the results of the testing, the reactions are graded according to severity. An *undecided*, *doubtful*, or *weak* result is an erythematous (red), macular (flat), or papular (raised) lesion. A *strongly positive* reaction is an erythematous, edematous, papular, or vesicular (fluid-filled) area of skin where a particular allergen was placed. An *extreme* reaction is one that has a raised, red, edematous area with large vesicles, bullae (fluid-filled blisters), or possible ulceration (Arndt, 1995).

---

**Purpose of the Test**

This test is used to identify the particular allergen that causes contact dermatitis. It is also used to differentiate contact dermatitis from other causes of eczematous disease.

---

**Procedure**

Samples of selected allergens used by the patient or of a number of standard allergens are taped to the patient's skin for 48 hours of contact (Fig. 25–9). The readings of the results are performed after 48 hours and again after 72 hours to 7 days, as prescribed.

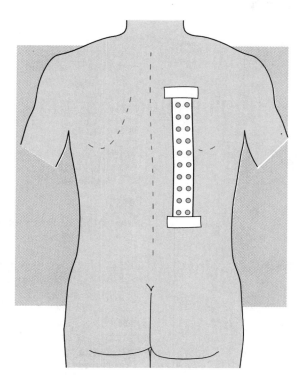

**Figure 25–9**

Patch test. Various allergens are applied to the skin of the patient's back. Those allergens that cause an allergic skin response are identified as the sources of contact dermatitis.

| Findings | **Abnormal Values** |
|---|---|

SOURCES OF CONTACT DERMATITIS

Nickel (snaps, belt buckles, rings, watchbands, bracelets, earrings)

Formaldehyde (permanent-press clothing, skin and nail products)

Chromates (cement, cutting oil)

Topical medication with neomycin, benzocaine, or ethylenediamine (plastics, topical creams)

Epoxy resins (adhesives, glues)

Hair dyes

Lanolin

Chemicals in sunscreen creams

Permanent-wave solutions

Fragrances in perfumes and soaps

| **Interfering Factors** | • Concurrent dermatitis from another source |
|---|---|
| | • Exposure of the patch site to water or excessive perspiration |
| | • Inaccurate interpretation of the results |
| | • Inaccurate timing for reading of the results |

## Nursing Implementation

### Pretest

Schedule this test for after acute dermatitis has subsided and after treatment with corticosteroids has ceased.

If the products the patient uses are to be tested, instruct the patient to bring them in beforehand. The patch test must be prepared, and a detailed list of the ingredients must be written.

Obtain written consent from the patient or the person legally designated to make the patient's health care decisions.

### During the Test

Tape the allergen patch to the patient's upper back between the scapula and the spinal column.

Make a diagram on paper to identify the location of each allergen.

### Posttest

Instruct the patient to refrain from showers and physical exercise during the following 48 hours. Water and perspiration will loosen the tape of the patch.

Inform the patient that if itching, irritation, or pain occurs under one of the discs of allergen, it should be removed immediately (Arndt, 1995).

Instruct the patient to return in 48 hours for the first evaluation of the results. The patch is removed at that time. After a 30-minute to 1-hour wait, the skin is assessed for any reaction in the area of the allergens (Guin, Lowery, Veazey, & Kincannon, 1997).

Instruct the patient to return for the second appointment to reevaluate the skin. Sometimes, a delayed reaction occurs. This second reading is done at 96 hours (4 days) after the patch is applied.

Advise the patient that exercise and showers are permitted while waiting for the second evaluation, but that soap must not be used, and that the patient must not scrub, scratch, or rub the skin in the test area.

## References

An adjunctive test for acute dizziness . . . electronystagmography. (1994). *Emergency Medicine, 26*(3), 26–28.

Arndt, K. A. (1995). *Manual of dermatologic therapeutics* (5th ed.). Boston: Little, Brown.

Cantore, W. A., & Goldberg, S. H. (1996). Orbital imaging techniques. *Current Opinion in Ophthalmology, 7*(5), 48–53.

Carlson, N. B., Kurtz, D., Heath, D. A., & Hines, C. (1996). *Clinical procedures for ocular examination* (2nd ed.). Stamford, CT: Appleton & Lange.

Cranford, J. L., Thompson, N., Hoyer, E., & Faires, W. (1997). Brief tone discrimination by children with histories of early otitis media. *Journal of the American Academy of Audiology, 8*(2), 137–141.

Fleischer, A. C., & Kepple, D. M. (1995). *Diagnostic sonography* (2nd ed.). Philadelphia: W. B. Saunders.

Gravel, J. S., & Ellis, M. A. (1995). The auditory consequences of otitis media with effusion: The audiogram and beyond. *Seminars in Hearing, 16*(1), 44–59, 113–114.

Guin, J. D., Lowery, B. J., Veazey, M. C., & Kincannon, J. M. (1997). Patch testing for contact dermatitis. *Dermatology Nursing, 9*(3), 178–181, 185, 188.

Hupp, S. L. (1993). Visual fields in neuro-ophthalmology. *Journal of Ophthalmology, 112*(6), 259–265.

Jacobs, D. S., Dermott, W. R., Grady, H. J., Horvat, P. T., Huestis, D. W., & Kasten, B. L. (1996). *Laboratory test handbook* (4th ed.). Baltimore: Williams & Wilkins.

Keith, R. W. (1996). Understanding central auditory processing disorders: Diagnosis and remediation. *Hearing Journal, 49*(11), 19–20, 22, 24.

Luxon, L. (1995). Comparison of assessment of caloric nystagmus by observation, of duration and by electronystagmographic measurements of slow phase velocity. *British Journal of Audiology, 29*(2), 107–116.

Lynch, P. (1994). *Dermatology* (3rd ed.). Baltimore: Williams & Wilkins.

Martin, F. N. (1997). *Introduction to audiology* (4th ed.). Boston: Allyn & Bacon.

Schushard, R. A. (1993). Validity and interpretation of Amsler grid reports. *Archives of Ophthalmology, 111,* 776–780.

Sherertz, E. F., & Byers, S. V. (1997). Common patch test allergens: General guidelines for avoidance. *Dermatology Nursing, 9*(2), 122–126.

Sigler, B. A., & Schuring, L. T. (1993). *Ear, nose and throat disorders.* St. Louis: C. V. Mosby.

Silverstein, H., Wolfson, R. J., & Rosenberg, S. (1992). Diagnosis and management of hearing loss. *Clinical Symposia, 44,* 2–32.

Swartz, S. M., & Sherertz, E. F. (1993). The technique of patch testing: The role of the office staff. *Dermatology Nursing, 5,* 133–137, 144.

# Critical Thinking Discussions

## Chapter 1: The Nursing Role

### Critical Thinking 1–1

One risk of improper identification of the patient is that the wrong patient may have a test that is not needed or intended. If another patient was supposed to have the test, he or she would not receive it, and treatment would be delayed because of the lack of test results. If incorrect patient identification of the specimen and the report occurs, incorrect data could be used to diagnose and treat the patient.

When incorrect identification of the specimen or a difference between the identification on the specimen and on the requisition slip exists, the specimen is declared invalid. The specimen collection must be repeated. This is not so serious when it is a urine test, but it is very serious when a biopsy or other invasive procedure is involved. To prevent errors, careful identification procedures must be followed and rechecked several times.

### Critical Thinking 1–2

First, look for patterns of error. Are all or some of the specimens rejected for the same reason, such as insufficient quantity of the specimen, mislabeling of the requisition slips, or delay in delivery of the specimen to the laboratory? The nurse can consult with laboratory personnel for additional input and suggestions.

Particular individuals may be making errors, or several individuals may perform a procedure incorrectly. Individuals can be counseled, retaught, and more closely supervised until the corrections are well established. When several people make the same mistake, the correct procedure should be reviewed with them, perhaps in a group.

If the series of rejections has no pattern or identified individual, a staff meeting can be called to discuss the problem with everyone. Heightened awareness can help with attention to detail. In addition, group discussion can identify solutions, such as a need for employee training, continuing education, or recertification.

## Chapter 2: Specimen Collection Procedures

### Critical Thinking 2–1

If a complication such as arterial spasm or thrombus occurs, a strong artery with good circulation and good collateral circulation will still be able to provide blood flow to distal tissue in the hand and fingers.

### Critical Thinking 2–2

Fainting, or syncope, can occur when the patient sees blood or thinks about blood. It is not possible to predict who will faint, so safety practices are used for all patients to protect them from injury.

Before the venipuncture is started, have the patient sit in a sturdy chair or in bed. If the patient describes previous faints during venipuncture or indicates apprehension, have the patient lie down for the procedure. Never draw blood while the patient is standing or seated on a high stool.

Remain aware of the patient during the procedure. The patient may provide a warning, such as a complaint of dizziness or of feeling faint. If so, remove the needle from the vein. Have the patient lower his or her head between the knees until the sensation passes. If the patient actually faints, smelling salts can help restore consciousness.

Do not permit the revived patient to get up quickly and walk without support. The dizziness can return, and the patient can be injured in a fall.

### Critical Thinking 2–3

If a specimen was lost during the night, the 24-hour collection is incomplete and therefore invalid. Provide reassurance to the mother that she was correct to tell you of the problem. Explain that a new 24-hour collection must be done. How can another nighttime problem be avoided? Perhaps the mother could wake the child every few hours to urinate in the container. If the child permits it, a pediatric urine collection bag could be applied for one night.

## Chapter 3: Urinalysis Screen
### Critical Thinking 3–1
The nurse should assess to determine the underlying cause of the patient's response. He may have a lack of knowledge and fail to comprehend why the abnormal test result must be investigated further. He may use denial because he fears that the positive result is ominous.

To understand the reason for the patient's objection, the nurse can explore and clarify the issue with the patient. In this early stage of testing, however, the primary nursing goal is to help the patient follow through with the additional tests. The nurse provides reassurance and hope by using a calm, supportive approach to help the patient reach this goal. Hematuria has many possible causes. With follow-up testing and an accurate diagnosis, effective treatment can be initiated.

### Critical Thinking 3–2
In acute glomerulonephritis, urinary abnormalities include hematuria, with the presence of red blood cells and red blood cell casts. The urine's color and clarity change, and it appears smoky or brownish. White blood cells and white blood cell casts may be present. Usually, protein is excreted in the urine, and the amount varies directly with the severity of the glomerular disease.

The nurse monitors the urinalysis results for improvement. The color should lighten and begin to clear. Fewer cells and casts should be present. As the patient recovers, a gradual decrease of protein in the urine should occur. A sustained, high level of proteinuria is a sign of the onset of nephrotic syndrome.

## Chapter 4: Hematology Screen
### Critical Thinking 4–1
In support of a nursing diagnosis of fluid volume deficit, the complete blood count results that would be elevated are the red blood cell count, the hemoglobin value, and the hematocrit value. In dehydration, the blood becomes more concentrated because less plasma fluid exists for the same number of red blood cells. With a greater concentration of red blood cells, the hemoglobin and hematocrit values demonstrate a proportionate elevation.

### Critical Thinking 4–2
Two areas of assessment are a physical assessment of the child and a nutritional assessment done by interviewing the mother. The child may demonstrate pallor and a lack of energy. The weight and height may be less than normal. The nutritional interview should identify the child's intake of foods and the amounts taken in a 24-hour period. Does the child take vitamins with iron supplement? One common source of nutritional deficiency in toddlers is continued milk or formula feeding and the lack of solid food, particularly foods that contain iron. The child may exhibit pica, the eating of strange substances such as clay or laundry starch. This behavior is symptomatic of iron deficiency anemia.

### Critical Thinking 4–3
With a low platelet level, the patient is at risk to bleed, with difficulty forming a clot to stop the bleeding. Nursing actions include teaching the patient how to protect from bruises, falls, and cuts and to avoid aspirin or aspirin-containing medications. The nurse should institute assessment measures to monitor for signs of bleeding in the skin, urine, intestines, and gingiva. Care should be taken to perform blood pressure testing smoothly and quickly, avoiding inflation of the cuff to very high levels.

### Critical Thinking 4–4
With a dangerous decrease in white blood cells, the nurse acts to protect this immunosuppressed patient from infection. Provide an explanation of the plan to the patient so that he or she can participate and assist with the protection. Measures include extra vigilance in hand-washing by all health care personnel before they work with the patient. Institute protective isolation procedures according to the institution's policy, and teach the patient, the family, and other visitors what to do. Maintain the patient's skin integrity. Teach the patient to use a mouthwash or sponge sticks to protect the oral cavity from abrasion. Administer antibiotics as prescribed, and monitor the patient for early or subtle signs of infection. Continue to monitor the white blood cell reports for indications of changes in the white blood cell values (Borton, 1996).

## Chapter 5: Serum Electrolytes
### Critical Thinking 5–1
The patient demonstrates hypercapnia, a serious elevation of the total carbon dioxide level. Given his medical diagnosis, the carbon dioxide retention is likely a result of impaired function of the lungs or inadequate respiratory exchange.

The nursing goal is to improve the quality of breathing. This will help promote better gas exchange in the lungs and increase the exhalation of retained carbon dioxide.

To promote better expansion of the lungs, interventions include changes of body position to semi-Fowler's position or higher, turning from side to side every 2 hours, and ambulating or sitting in a chair at intervals.

The patient should be taught and reminded to perform breathing exercises that promote prolonged exhalation, such as pursed lip breathing and diaphragmatic breathing, to help empty the alveoli of the retained carbon dioxide.

To remove mucus from the air passages and to increase the diameter of the airways, interventions include prompt administration of medications such as nebulized bronchodilators and use of positive-pressure air flow or positive end-expiratory pressure devices as prescribed. Coughing and deep breathing activity should be supervised every 2 hours, and the upper airway should be suctioned as needed. Postural drainage or chest physiotherapy may be prescribed.

## Critical Thinking 5–2

Why is the patient's calcium level low? Ask about her eating habits and cooking practices and specifically about her intake of milk and milk products. Her answers provide direction for modifications.

Provide motivation to increase her calcium intake. Include the information about her current low level of calcium and the associated health risks that can occur in older age.

Do cultural influences guide her food choices? Can these be incorporated into the teaching plan?

Encourage the intake of foods that are rich in calcium. If some foods are a problem, suggest alternatives. Encourage cooking with milk or milk products.

If it seems unlikely that the patient will modify her diet, calcium tablets can be suggested as an alternative source of replacement.

## Critical Thinking 5–3

The teaching plan should include the following:

1. Explanation of how fluid losses affect the potassium level and suggestions for prevention of the losses.
2. Encouragement to eat high-potassium foods for dietary replacement. A list of these foods should be provided.
3. Guidance to take all medications regularly as prescribed. The medications and schedule are reviewed so that the patient has full understanding.

## Chapter 6: Coagulation Screen

### Critical Thinking 6–1

The patient is excessively anticoagulated and at risk for a bleeding episode. Ask if the patient is having any dizziness or weakness. Look at the skin for bruising or seepage of blood in any area where the skin is broken. Look for oozing of blood from the mouth or nose or any other area of mucous membrane. Take vital signs. Lastly, check the intravenous infusion for accuracy in the dose of heparin that was added, and check that the infusion is dripping at an accurate rate. The physician must be notified of the test result immediately.

### Critical Thinking 6–2

Introduce the topic and explain why aspirin must be avoided while taking anticoagulants. Understanding the risk can help the patient to be careful of this harmful drug interaction.

Explain how aspirin is added to many nonprescription medications, particularly those to treat fever, colds, flu, inflammation, headache, aches and pains, and "upset stomach." The aspirin may be identified as aspirin, ASA, or acetylsalicylic acid. The patient must read the label to identify whether aspirin is in the preparation. If in doubt, the patient can ask the pharmacist for assistance.

Bring two to three examples of over-the-counter pill containers that contain aspirin. Let the patient practice looking for the information. Go to a supermarket or pharmacy yourself to make a list of common brand-name preparations that have aspirin. Give the list to the patient for easy referral.

## Chapter 7: Microbiologic Tests

### Critical Thinking 7–1

Analytical thinking requires weighing the risks and benefits of each technology and considering the costs and the feasibility of the alternatives.

The risk involved with using serology tests is that a newly infected person will not demonstrate human immunodeficiency virus (HIV) antigen or antibody for several weeks. If blood is donated before seroconversion occurs, the infection would not be detected. If it is in the blood, HIV would be transmitted to the recipient of the blood transfusion.

The benefit of using the current system of testing for HIV-1 and HIV-2 antigen and antibodies is that only 1 in 500,000 transfusions transmits HIV via a unit of infected blood (Speicher, 1998). The current testing methods are also rapid, inexpensive, and available.

Testing the blood for HIV genetic material provides for earlier detection of the virus, before antibodies have formed. Unfortunately, the tests are prohibitively expensive. In addition, the application of this technology for a very large volume of tests is probably not possible. With current techniques, the completion of one of these tests takes days, and relatively few laboratories are equipped to do the work.

In the state of current laboratory technology, the present methods of antigen and antibody testing provide clear benefits with little risk at a relatively low cost.

### Critical Thinking 7–2

The task requires organization, communication, teaching, and follow-up plans.

To organize, how can the nurse keep track of the steps in the process, such as orientation and distribution of containers, specimens, and results? What materials or supplies must be ordered?

Communication with the parents is essential. Contact with the parents could be by letter, by telephone, or in person. Depending on circumstances, such as culture and availability of the parents, would a certain method of communication work better than another? How would the nurse deal with possible variables, such as distance from the clinic, language, literacy, or awareness of clinic services?

What content is needed in the teaching plan? What particular teaching methods might be helpful? What are the considerations in establishing a schedule for classes or individual conferencing?

In follow-up, has 100% participation been achieved? What can be done to help the remaining parents complete their part? When the results are available, how will the nurse and physician communicate with the parents? What additional health care measures may be needed?

## Critical Thinking 7–3

Assess the stool for its characteristics (color, consistency, odor, etc.), and determine the frequency of bowel movements. If the patient is also vomiting, that information is recorded.

Because the patient is probably losing fluids and electrolytes, assess for signs of dehydration and electrolyte imbalance. Record fluid intake and output data.

Some sources of diarrhea are profoundly infectious and enterotoxic to the patient. Monitor vital signs, including temperature, pulse, respirations, and blood pressure. Septic shock can result in a rapid onset of hypotension and tachycardia. Fever may or may not be present.

In the nursing history, the patient may describe a possible source of the infection, such as drinking water from an unpurified source or eating a suspicious food. Common foods that can be contaminated by bacteria include undercooked beef, apple cider, shellfish, seafood, egg or tuna salad, chicken, spoiled canned food, lettuce, salads, fruits, and pastries (Mahon & Manuselis, 1995).

## Critical Thinking 7–4

The maximum number of blood cultures is four. The request by different physicians indicates that a lack of communication and coordination may exist among them. Each physician can be reminded to check the physicians' order sheet to see what has been ordered and already completed. The physician responsible for the patient's care should be informed of the multiple requests, so that future medical requests are coordinated. Performance of four blood cultures in 1 day is acceptable, but usually a plan for timing of the blood draws is determined. If duplicate requests are carried out, the patient could lose a larger volume of blood, and cultures might not identify the organism.

## Critical Thinking 7–5

This is a case of suspected child sexual abuse. The infection is transmitted by an infected male to the child during oral sex. The nurse should consult with the physician and immediate supervisor about the findings. The case must be reported to the particular state or local agency that investigates allegations of child abuse. Any of the professional health care workers involved with the case can file the report. If this has not been done, the nurse has a professional and, in some states, legal obligation to report the suspicious finding. The child welfare agency or the police follow up with an investigation.

## Chapter 8: Ultrasonography

### Critical Thinking 8–1

Reassure the pregnant woman that ultrasound presents no danger to her or to the fetus. Radiation is not used. Ultrasound is based on sound impulses that cause no risk or harm.

A comforting adult is always welcome to stay with the patient during the ultrasound procedure. Her presence can help keep the patient calm and oriented. Provide a chair so that the daughter can sit near the patient, hold her hand, and provide reassurance.

### Critical Thinking 8–2

The goal is to complete the procedure without increasing the child's fear. The child of this age will respond positively to verbal reassurance and simple explanations. When providing an explanation of the procedure, appeal to the child's imagination by calling the transducer a "magic wand" that will make a picture on the "TV screen." Show the child the transducer. Allow the child to touch it or to hold it. Explain the procedure simply, including that jelly is applied and how the transducer moves over the skin. Make it clear that the procedure does not hurt. Invite the child to watch the TV screen for the picture.

The parent may stay in the room. The child can hold a favorite toy or blanket. The room should be dark for the procedure, but if this distresses the child, keep the light on.

Provide constant reassurance, and praise the child for being a good helper.

## Chapter 9: Radiography

### Critical Thinking 9–1

The goals are to help the patient feel comfortable and to promote her cooperation.

Many elderly patients are thin and are uncomfortable on the hard radiology table. A radiolucent pad can be placed on the table before the patient lies down. This creates a softer surface, which is particularly desirable during a lengthy procedure (Adler & Carlton, 1994).

Frequently, an elderly patient feels the cold, particularly when she is in a hospital gown in an air-conditioned area. Offer a blanket to help warm her while she waits. In addition, re-cover her with the blanket during any waiting time between filming episodes. If the patient is physically comfortable, she is more likely to cooperate and to remain still when the radiographs are taken.

Many patients do not like to have tests done. They may be apprehensive about the unknown and fear the outcome of the test. It is sometimes easier for the patient to complain about little things to gain some control in the situation. Kindness and meeting basic comfort needs are ways to provide support for the patient (Torres, 1993).

## Critical Thinking 9–2

What are the risks for a fall and possible hip fracture? The elderly person may fall in the dark, fall after tripping over an obstacle in the room, or fall after becoming dizzy or disoriented, particularly at night. You should begin the plan by assessing the patient for risk of a fall.

Part of your teaching could include use of a night-light in the bedroom, removal of small objects from the floor, and ensuring that rugs are flat. Is the patient's vision impaired? When did she last have an eye examination? Poor vision contributes to the risk of a fall. If the patient is dizzy on arising from bed, encourage sitting up for a minute before standing and walking. Ask about the use of long-acting sedatives and, if excessive, discourage their use (Cummings, 1998).

What are other measures that help strengthen the bones? If the patient smokes, teach her that smoking is a risk factor that makes osteoporosis worse. After assessing her strength and mobility, encourage her to exercise according to her ability. Walking is recommended.

What is the patient's daily intake of calcium in foods or in tablet form? Based on your nutritional assessment, emphasize the importance of calcium intake and review dietary choices. She also may need a referral to her physician or nurse practitioner for a bone density scan and additional pharmacologic treatment.

## Chapter 10: Nuclear Imaging

### Critical Thinking 10–1

In assessment, the whole patient is considered, including the physical, psychologic, social, and financial aspects of the situation. All these dimensions can be sources of either stress or strength in coping behaviors.

Physically, how is the patient's health since the fracture occurred? Has he been active even though he must use crutches? What physical problems are due to the impaired mobility? How has he managed to cope?

Emotionally, how does he feel about the nonhealing fracture and the need for a different treatment approach? Does he seem hopeful or accepting of the need for additional treatment? Does he exhibit other emotions such as anger, frustration, or sadness? What interview techniques can help him explain his feelings?

How will the continued immobility and pending surgery affect his schooling? What help does he require to continue with his studies? Does he have friends or significant others who can be of assistance? What services can the college provide to help him while he is disabled?

Has he discussed his problem with his parents? Are they available and able to provide support and assistance? Does he have financial concerns related to medical costs or loss of income? If so, how can these concerns be addressed?

Once the assessment is complete, specific goals can be established to help him cope with the additional problems.

## Chapter 11: Angiography

### Critical Thinking 11–1

The patient who is at greater risk for an allergic reaction has had a previous reaction during a radiologic study that used an iodine-based contrast medium. In addition, the patient with a history of allergy to iodine in foods or medication (such as shellfish, cough medication, and kelp) is also more vulnerable. What happened, or what did the patient feel, when the allergic reaction occurred? Did the patient experience hives, itching, mild bronchospasm, low blood pressure, or more severe respiratory and cardiac problems?

Other people who are more vulnerable have a history of severe allergic reactions to foods and medications or have asthma or an unstable cardiac condition, such as a recent heart attack.

The nurse should document the pertinent history in the chart and inform the radiologist of the information.

## Chapter 12: Tomography

### Critical Thinking 12–1

Start by establishing rapport quickly. In all communications and interactions, use an approach of gentle kindness with a calm, reassuring manner. With the establishment of trust, the patient will be more able to listen and follow instructions.

An adolescent will respond to logical explanations. If he has questions about the scan, answer them. Provide a brief explanation about the procedure, what the patient will experience, and the pretest instructions. At this age, emotional control and maturity may not be well developed. The patient may cry, appear withdrawn, remain confused, or express his feelings in other ways. Accept the behavior and help him complete the computed tomographic (CT) scan as quickly as possible.

### Critical Thinking 12–2

The nurse can reassure the young man that magnetic resonance imaging (MRI) has excellent ability to image the knee joint, the ligaments, and the meniscus. The pictures are very clear and accurate. The images will help the physician diagnose the extent of the injury and determine the course of treatment that will be needed.

Regarding the patient's anxiety about his future athletic ability, the nurse cannot comment on the potential impact of the injury or predict the future. At this time, effective nursing interventions include listening, providing emotional support, and expressing hope for the future. The nurse can encourage the patient to address the problems one at a time. The physician's physical examination and the diagnostic testing are priorities in this process.

## Chapter 13: Genetic Testing

### Critical Thinking 13–1
Explain to your neighbor that the physician has recommended an amniocentesis because of her age. Help your neighbor explore her options. She does have the right to refuse the procedure. Suggest that she consider the amniocentesis as a way to identify that there may not be a problem with Down syndrome. Remind her that if the infant has Down syndrome, the amniocentesis will give her and her family time to adjust to the diagnosis and plan for the infant's care.

## Chapter 14: Pulmonary Function

### Critical Thinking 14–1
The patient needs to know that the serum angiotensin-converting enzyme (SACE) test results indicate that the hypertension is because of the conversion of angiotensin I to angiotensin II. Angiotensin II is a potent vasoconstrictor. By taking an angiotensin-converting enzyme (ACE) inhibitor, the enzyme that is necessary for the conversion is blocked. With a decrease in angiotensin II, the patient will have a decrease in blood pressure.

### Critical Thinking 14–2

$$(140 + 5) - (30 + 100) = 15$$

An increase in the anion gap is present if a newer automated laboratory system is being used. You should assess for indications of shock and hyperglycemia. You should also evaluate laboratory results of other electrolytes.

### Critical Thinking 14–3
Anaerobic metabolism, which occurs in shock states, will cause an increase in lactic acid. The lactic acid will be buffered, so a gap is expected. A normal anion gap in a patient in severe shock may be the result of hypoalbuminemia. Check the patient's albumin level and report the finding to the physician. Low albumin levels will influence the physician's choice of fluid replacement, because low albumin levels will decrease the oncotic pressure in the extracellular fluid compartment.

### Critical Thinking 14–4
Two arteries normally are responsible for perfusion to the hands. If the patient for some reason has only one functional artery, the remaining artery must be protected. If an arterial puncture is done, this vessel is at risk. A hematoma could form, occluding the artery. With no blood perfusing to the hand, loss of function and even necrosis may occur.

### Critical Thinking 14–5
The respiratory drive of patients with chronic obstructive pulmonary disease (COPD) is stimulated by low $P_{O_2}$ levels, not by high $CO_2$ levels, which are the normal stimulant for respiration. If a patient with COPD is given high levels of oxygen, the arterial oxygen level will rise, and the stimulation to breathe will cease. This is called oxygen-induced hypoventilation. The old term for this problem was $CO_2$ narcosis, because as the patient hypoventilates, $CO_2$ accumulates in the blood. This can be a lethal event. To prevent oxygen-induced hypoventilation, encourage the COPD patient to wear a Medi-Alert bracelet or medal. This will inform emergency personnel to administer only low-dose oxygen if the patient becomes hypoxic. Before giving oxygen, the nurse should always assess for COPD. This includes questioning the patient or family, if possible, and observing for barrel chest, clubbing of the fingers, and nicotine stains on the fingers and mouth.

### Critical Thinking 14–6
Lactate will increase whenever cells do not receive adequate oxygen. A tourniquet causes distal hypoperfusion and, thus, localized tissue hypoxia. The blood drawn would not reflect the body's lactic acid level.

### Critical Thinking 14–7
A drop in the $S_{VO_2}$ level to less than 40% indicates that the activity (turning) has increased the patient's oxygen consumption without a corresponding increase in cardiac output to meet the body's oxygen need. You need to limit activity (decrease oxygen consumption) and assess delivery (blood pressure, cardiac output, pulse) and supply (factors that interfere with adequate arterial oxygenation). In addition, you should observe and document the recovery time to plan future care activities.

### Critical Thinking 14–8
You can help reduce anxiety in patients undergoing bronchoscopy by eliminating the unknown, instructing the patient on the purpose and procedures, and describing the sensations the patient will feel and experience. You should reassure the patient of your support and of the doctor's presence. You may explore complementary modalities with the patient. Music has been shown to improve patient perceived comfort level during outpatient

bronchoscopy (Dubois, Bartter, & Pratter, 1995). Before the procedure, allow the patient to select the music to be played. Other potential modalities include relaxation techniques and imaging.

## Critical Thinking 14–9

A tracheal shift is the cardinal sign of a tension pneumothorax. As inspired air enters the pleural space and is trapped there, the mediastinum is pushed to the unaffected side. This is observed in patients by a shift of the trachea from midline to the unaffected side. The physician must be notified *immediately,* and a stat chest x-ray will be ordered. Any delay may endanger the patient, because cardiac output will decrease as the preload decreases from increasing intrathoracic pressure.

## Critical Thinking 14–10

When the capnographic waveform disappears, it means that accidental extubation, obstruction, or cessation of breathing has occurred. Immediately initiate the ABCs of resuscitation: Airway, Breathing, and Circulation. Remember to call for assistance.

## Critical Thinking 14–11

With hemodynamic monitoring, a catheter is inserted into the pulmonary arterial system. A pulmonary vascular resistance index (PVRI) can be measured. A PVRI of more than 425 dynes/s/cm$^{-5}$ indicates pulmonary hypertension.

## Critical Thinking 14–12

Pulmonary function studies require full cooperation and *maximum* effort by the patient. To prevent fatigue from interfering with maximum effort, the morning after a restful night's sleep is the best time to schedule the studies for most patients.

## Critical Thinking 14–13

An $Spo_2$ value alone is inadequate for assessing patient oxygen needs. $Spo_2$ measures the amount of oxygen carried by the hemoglobin (Hgb). The nurse should evaluate the $Spo_2$ in relation to the person's Hgb level. This can be done by evaluating the patient's oxygen-carrying capacity. The formula for this is $1.34 \times$ Hgb $\times Spo_2$. 1.34 mL is the amount of oxygen each gram of Hgb is able to carry. If two patients have an $Spo_2$ of 95%, but their Hgb levels are 15 and 11, their oxygen-carrying capacities would be

$$1.34 \times 15 \times 0.95 = 19.09$$
$$1.34 \times 11 \times 0.95 = 14$$

The normal oxygen-carrying capacity is 19 to 20 mL/dL, so one patient has a normal carrying capacity, and the other does not have the necessary oxygen.

## Critical Thinking 14–14

Mechanical ventilation may influence the course of recovery following a thoracoscopy. The ventilator may increase the time needed for pleural healing and may prolong the time of air leaks (Davidson & Colt, 1997). A chest tube is used after a thoracoscopy to restore intrapulmonic pressure. Once the chest tube is clamped, the patient on a ventilator is at risk for a tension pneumothorax. For patients on volume-controlled ventilators, in addition to clinical signs, the nurse should observe for (1) exhaled tidal volume less than the inspiratory tidal volume and (2) increases in airway pressures.

# Chapter 15: Cardiac Function

## Critical Thinking 15–1

Cardiac enzyme protocols require that enzymes and isoenzymes be determined at certain frequencies and times. Because the initial specimen is taken on admission and the protocol calls for two more specimens to be drawn at 8 and 16 hours after the initial specimen is drawn, the times for these collections vary with each patient. This usually leads to the blood not being drawn as required or being drawn at the wrong times. Each nursing unit needs to develop a system for collecting these specimens. It may be as simple as taping a reminder on the wall over the patient's bed, placing notes on the medication sheet, or programming the times into a computer. Look at the environment of the unit. Where can exceptions to routine specimen collection be seen by the person responsible for drawing blood?

## Critical Thinking 15–2

Most myocardial infarctions are due to athelerosclerosis. This process occurs long before the cardiac event. It is also known that control of low-density lipoprotein (LDL) by diet, exercise, or medications will reduce the risk of heart attacks. When a specific person should have the serum lipid level determined depends on family history, secondary diagnosis (such as diabetes mellitus), and sex. A strong family history and being male indicates that the test should be done in early adulthood. Some recommend that children with a strong family history of lipidemia be tested. Women, because of their estrogen, usually do not have difficulties controlling lipid levels until menopause. Estrogen replacement therapy continues this protection. Again, family history, the age at menopause, and secondary diagnosis will influence the decision as to when lipid evaluation should be done.

## Critical Thinking 15–3

The cardiac catheterization laboratory is a high-technology area. Patients are brought into this unfamiliar environment in a vulnerable position (on a stretcher, wearing just a hospital gown). Patients are aware that the results of this test will determine whether they will need surgery or invasive procedures or can lead a "normal life."

As the patient enters the laboratory, you should greet the patient by name, touch the person's hand, identify yourself, and reassure the patient that you will be there throughout the procedure. Small things will add to the patient's comfort. Ask the patient if he or she needs help getting on the x-ray table. Show concern that the patient is comfortable. Offer a blanket. Listen to verbal statements and observe for nonverbal clues as to how much the patient wants to know about the procedure and equipment. Inform the patient of expected sensations (noises, pressure). The patient has placed his or her life in your hands. Competency will reassure the patient that trust in you is warranted.

## Critical Thinking 15–4

An ejection fraction less than 20% indicates inadequate cardiac functioning. This patient is a "cardiac cripple." Such patients can be maintained at home with certain accommodations, such as eliminating stair climbing and positioning the bed close to the bathroom.

In the hospital, you need to adapt patient care to prevent exhaustion and hypoxia. You must plan care to allow periods of rest; for example, the bath is given in the middle of the morning to allow the patient to rest from breakfast and then to rest before lunch. The patient may need to be fed if fatigue occurs during meals. Encourage family and friends to space their visits and limit time with the patient. Coordinate tests and procedures ordered for the patient to allow rest periods.

## Chapter 16: Peripheral Vascular Function

### Critical Thinking 16–1

The first step is to validate that the patient is anxious. Ask her how she is feeling and listen attentively to the response. Observe her facial expressions and physical movements.

If anxiety is a problem, try to discover the cause. Is it simple concern about the Doppler test? Other common sources of anxiety for a preoperative patient include fear of the surgery, the anesthesia, or the outcome of the surgery or other fears that are individual to the patient.

Based on the patient's statements, you can proceed with the appropriate intervention. The patient may need additional explanation by the surgeon or anesthesiologist. You may be able to help with clarification, information, support, reassurance, or listening, depending on the need.

If the anxiety is focused only on the Doppler testing, explain the procedure first, including the purpose and what the patient will feel. Because the procedure is non-invasive and painless, it should present no problems.

## Critical Thinking 16–2

The two areas of focus are observation for signs of complication and validation that the patient is following posttest instructions.

Teach the aide to look at the infusion site in the groin or dorsal aspect of the foot to ensure that no swelling or bruising has occurred. The vital signs should be stable. The patient should rest in bed for a few hours,

drink fluids, and urinate. If the patient demonstrates a problem in these areas, instruct the aide to report them to you. You should then perform a repeat assessment, further evaluate the status of the patient, and intervene as needed.

## Chapter 17: Hematologic Function

### Critical Thinking 17–1

One way the nurse can evaluate the response to vitamin $B_{12}$ therapy is to monitor the posttreatment laboratory results and compare them with pretreatment values.

The laboratory results that were decreased during illness and now show a rise or correction into a normal range are the platelet count, the leukocyte count, the hematocrit level, and the reticulocyte count. The results that were elevated during illness and now show a decline into the normal range are two of the red cell indices: red cell distribution width (RDW) and mean corpuscular volume (MCV).

With effective treatment, all these laboratory results improve within 6 to 20 days (Rodak, 1995).

### Critical Thinking 17–2

In a follow-up to a positive sickle cell test result, education and genetic counseling should be offered. For the individuals who are heterozygous HgbS (have the sickle cell trait), the content should include the following:

1. A clear distinction between sickle cell trait and sickle cell disease
2. Reassurance about the normal health status of those with the sickle cell trait
3. Information about the risks or odds of having a future child with sickle cell disease, based on the genetic analyses of the couple
4. An offer to test other members of the family if they desire to be tested

The education and counseling should be done with sensitivity and awareness that the person being counseled is likely to feel anxious. The communication approach should be open so that the person can ask questions. Repeat explanation and clarification may be needed. Scheduling an additional counseling session may be necessary.

### Critical Thinking 17–3

Any error in the identification process could result in transfusion of the wrong blood to the patient. Two errors can occur in this situation. The first error is that the transfusion identification wristband is on the bed and is not attached to the patient's body. The second problem is that the identification band has the wrong information.

Based on either of these problems of identification, the blood transfusion unit must not be administered. The blood is returned to the blood bank. A new identification process, a new blood sample, and a new type and crossmatch procedure must be done.

You must notify the blood bank of the errors so that this department can determine how the errors occurred. You should ask the patient how the identification band was placed on the bed. A discussion and review of correct procedure should be held with the nurse assigned to the patient. An alert, knowledgeable nurse would have recognized and reported this problem immediately.

### Chapter 18: Gastrointestinal Function

### Critical Thinking 18–1

A child of this age is easily frightened by strange procedures and intrusive medical devices such as the venipuncture. To obtain the child's cooperation, various alternatives can be tried. The alternatives are based on the child's developmental and cognitive level. The establishment of trust and the maintenance of a nonthreatening approach are essential.

The parent can help the child feel protected and less anxious. Allow the child to sit in the parent's lap. The parent may be the best person to encourage the child to drink the D-xylose liquid.

Look for ways to distract the child, such as offering a favorite book or providing crayons and paper to play with as soon as the glass of "sweet water" is finished. Maintain a calm and reassuring attitude to help the child complete the test. In simple words, let the child know what she needs to do to help. Praise the child for cooperative behavior.

If the child protests about the "needle," allow the child to explain the problem. Let the child know that it is all right to be afraid or to cry. Set limits on the child's fear by providing brief information or explanations about what will happen.

### Critical Thinking 18–2

When the nasogastric tube does not drain gastric fluid, you can use a "trouble shooting" approach to solve the problem. Each part of the equipment is checked methodically, from inspecting the cord in the electrical outlet to ensuring that each connection from the collection bottle to the tubing is secure and that the tubing is not kinked. Next, the nasogastric tube is aspirated manually. If it will not aspirate, the tube can be irrigated with a small amount of normal saline. This should solve the problem when previous measures were ineffective. In the gastric stimulation test, the nasogastric tube must be patent and functional. If the nasogastric tube remains inoperative, notify the physician. The test cannot be started until the problem is corrected or the tube is replaced.

### Critical Thinking 18–3

A thorough bowel cleansing is essential to provide clear x-ray images, but this patient seems to be unable to complete the regimen as prescribed.

One approach is to contact the radiologist to inquire whether the bowel cleansing routine can be modified.

A clear liquid diet for 2 days instead of 1 day and the same cathartic regimen may be an acceptable alternative (Hageman & Goei, 1993). Another approach is to have the patient follow all the steps of bowel preparation but have the enema administered in the x-ray department 1 hour before the test.

If these measures are not possible, the patient will need some assistance at home. Perhaps a family member or close friend can perform the task. If not, suggest that the patient or a family member contact a community nursing agency, a home health care agency, or a nurse in private practice to obtain assistance. The elderly, arthritic patient could experience other problems related to the bowel preparation. Can you identify potential problems and suggest preventive measures?

### Critical Thinking 18–4

Safety considerations can focus on two areas of potential harm. One area of concern is the risk of fall or poor judgment by the patient because of the medications that provide conscious sedation. A second area is that of complication from either the conscious sedation or the procedure itself. The nursing role is to protect the patient from preventable injury and to monitor for complication so that medical treatment is initiated at a very early stage.

Once the narcotic-analgesics are administered, the patient will remain conscious but will become drowsy and relaxed. Judgment and motor skills are impaired. Protect the patient from a fall by use of bedrest and siderails and in transfer activities. After the test, many patients experience weakness and lightheadedness. They are often discharged after 2 hours, before all the effects of the medication have worn off. Preparation for discharge includes warning the patient about dizziness or weakness that can continue for a few hours and providing instruction on prevention of falls at home and not driving a car for the remainder of the day (Lugay et al., 1996).

The conscious sedation and the procedure can trigger cardiorespiratory events, particularly in the elderly patient (Phillips, 1995). During the procedure, monitor for changes in breathing patterns, such as depressed respirations, anoxia, apnea, and bronchospasm. The pulse oximeter should show an oxygen saturation greater than 90%, with oxygen administered by nasal cannula throughout the procedure. The electrocardiogram monitor is also observed for signs of arrhythmia during the procedure. The endoscopy room must be equipped with the emergency medications needed to correct the problem, as well as the equipment used for cardiopulmonary resuscitation.

### Chapter 19: Hepatic, Biliary, Pancreatic, and Splenic Function

### Critical Thinking 19–1

The serum bilirubin level is mildly elevated, and the infant requires monitoring. Because of the early discharge, the infant will be at home while the bilirubin level either rises to an abnormal level or falls to a normal range. The discharge plan should teach the parents how to observe for a problem and how to get help if the bilirubin level increases.

One focus of the discharge plan is assessment. Teach the parents to observe the infant daily for signs of jaundice of the sclera or skin (particularly the skin of the lower trunk and legs). Also teach them to assess for adequate hydration, as evidenced by urinary and fecal elimination and by moist mucous membranes (Schwoebel & Sakraida, 1997). Teach them to also assess for any signs of neurologic abnormality, such as convulsions, lethargy, or anorexia (Berrios & Jain, 1996). The parents should be taught to call the physician or health care professional about any abnormal findings.

A second focus of the discharge plan is to teach the mother how to feed the infant with formula or by breast-feeding. Adequate hydration and nutrition will promote urinary and fecal elimination. These elimination processes will lower the bilirubin level in cases of physiologic jaundice (Blackburn, 1995).

The third part of the plan relates to follow-up care. Some institutions schedule a phone call to the parents or a home visit to the parents and infant. In addition, instruct the parents to keep the follow-up pediatric appointment in 1 week. A repeat serum bilirubin test will be done at that time.

## Critical Thinking 19–2
The first step is to identify why the patient has refused. The negative response may be due to distaste, embarrassment, a lack of knowledge, or a strong sense of hygiene and cleanliness.

If the cause is emotional, a helpful response is to acknowledge the patient's feelings and to reassure that the feelings are shared and understandable.

The lack of knowledge can be met by explaining that the specimen will deteriorate and be useless unless it is kept chilled throughout the 72 hours of collection.

If the problem is a hygiene concern, alternative measures for chilling the specimen can be suggested. One option is to store the specimen and container in a sealable plastic bag. Place the bag and its contents in a plastic bucket filled with ice. Replace the ice as needed until the test is completed.

## Critical Thinking 19–3
One potential problem is a shift of the fluid from within the blood vessels to the extravascular tissues as edema or to an extravascular space as ascites. Assessment of the skin for pallor, cool temperature, and edema in dependent areas is done every 8 hours. Measurement of the circumference of each lower leg and checking for the presence of peripheral pulses may be done. Measurement of the abdominal girth may be done daily, to assess for a possible increase in size. The abdomen may be per-

cussed to detect tympany, the sound of the ascites fluid in the abdomen.

Hypovolemia will occur with a fluid shift. Vital signs are monitored every 1 to 8 hours, depending on the severity of the condition. Hypotension and a weak, rapid pulse may occur. The patient may become less responsive, with an altered level of consciousness. Monitoring of fluid intake and output is done because of the potential for dehydration and oliguria.

Observation for skin breakdown over bony areas is done each day. Edematous tissue is thin, poorly nourished, and poorly oxygenated. Tissue repair is slow when the serum protein level is low.

Observation of the nutritional intake and the patient's appetite is useful. Malnutrition and anorexia may contribute to the low serum protein level.

## Critical Thinking 19–4
In this example, the foreign language created a communication barrier. A lack of knowledge may also have interfered with following the instructions.

Explain the pretest preparation in Spanish; this can be done with the assistance of a translator. A bilingual family member or friend may be with the patient. Other employees or a visitor to the hospital may be available to translate. In regions with large populations of Spanish-speaking people, guidelines written in Spanish are helpful. After explanations are provided, ask the patient to repeat the instructions. Allow time for the patient to ask questions or clarify. It is frightening to be sick and unable to communicate. The tension or stress can interfere with comprehension.

## Chapter 20: Endocrine Function
### Critical Thinking 20–1
The administration of exogenous glucocorticoids (steroid therapy) will inhibit the release of adrenocorticotropic hormone (ACTH). ACTH and glucocorticoids are regulated by a negative feedback mechanism. As long as the glucocorticoid levels are maintained, the hypothalamus will not stimulate the pituitary gland to secrete ACTH.

### Critical Thinking 20–2
The best solution is prevention. The patient has the right to refuse, but two specimens are necessary. Before the first venipuncture was drawn, the patient should have been told about the need for two venipunctures. Now, however, the nurse needs to sit down with the patient and assess the patient's response. Does the patient "feel like a pin cushion"? Does the patient understand the need for the second venipuncture? Does the patient want control over what is happening? If the response is a result of feeling victimized and used, the nurse needs to give the patient emotional support and to include the patient more fully in the plan of care. If the response is a result of a lack of knowledge, teaching is indicated.

## Critical Thinking 20–3

Patients having serum aldosterone levels measured should maintain normal sodium levels for several weeks before the blood is drawn. You need to investigate with the patient whether he or she ate the pepperoni pizza, which is high in sodium, and if so, how many slices were eaten. Take a diet history. Evaluate sodium intake for the day and the previous 2 to 4 weeks. Report to the physician if the sodium intake was unusual. Although the physician probably asked the patient about his or her sodium intake, some patients do not consider "hidden salt," but only salt from the saltshaker.

## Critical Thinking 20–4

The patient is agitated and mistrustful. The nurse was correct in assessing the source of the patient's agitation. The nurse must continue the assessment step of the nursing process. Why is the patient distrustful of the physician? The nurse cannot plan or implement effective action until it is known what happened to the trust patients normally have for their doctors.

## Critical Thinking 20–5

Patients with Cushing's syndrome have high levels of glucocorticoids, which suppress the body's inflammatory response. Any infection, even a minor one, can be serious. When assigning roommates for patients with Cushing's syndrome, avoid any patient with local or generalized infection.

## Critical Thinking 20–6

Some patients with diabetes mellitus will develop a rebound effect in response to insulin-induced hypoglycemia. The hypoglycemia stimulates the secretion of various hormones, which cause a rise in serum glucose. This is called the *Somogyi effect*. Although the person experiences hyperglycemia, the real problem is hypoglycemia. Treatment is necessary to decrease the insulin level, which prevents hypoglycemia and the stimulation of the body's own hyperglycemic hormones.

## Critical Thinking 20–7

A teaching plan for diabetic patients usually includes supportive written material. If the patient has poor eyesight, determine if enlarging the written material will help. If not, record your instructions to the patient on audiocassette, so the patient can listen to them as often as needed. Patients who are visually impaired cannot assess color changes, so they need a glucometer with large digital numbers or one that gives an audible reading.

## Critical Thinking 20–8

Use positive reinforcement when teaching. Capillary glucose testing involves many steps. Point out to the patient the steps she is doing correctly. Explain the two points the patient can do better. Have the patient redemonstrate the corrected approach. Reinforce new

learning with praise. Reevaluate learning; it is difficult to change behaviors.

## Critical Thinking 20–9

Poorly controlled diabetics have serious complications. The adult patient must assume responsibility for his management, but do not assume the patient is noncompliant. Is the person a member of a group at risk for hemoglobin abnormality? You need to assess the patient's denial. Is it a lack of understanding, or is the anger a sign of nonacceptance of the diagnosis or of fear of the diagnosis or prognosis, or both? Start by building a trusting relationship. Do not allow the person's anger to develop antagonism between the patient and the other members of the health team. Emphasize your common goal: the health of the patient.

## Critical Thinking 20–10

Research has shown that American culture favors tall people. Parents become very aware of their child's height (especially that of sons) if it varies from that of other children. Height is usually inherited. Before referring the patient to an endocrinologist, observe the height of the parents. Ask about the grandparents' height. Also, question the parents about their growth patterns. Were they the shortest child in their elementary school graduation, but one of the taller graduates from their high school? These questions will help the parents clarify their concern and will give you insight into what needs to be done.

## Critical Thinking 20–11

Acromegaly causes significant changes in a person's appearance. It can make the person unrecognizable to friends and relatives. When the person looks into a mirror, he or she sees a stranger. Appearance can change rather quickly, over a period of months. The person frequently finds it difficult to integrate these changes into the self-image and may become isolated from others. A possible nursing diagnosis for the behavior described is body image disturbance.

## Critical Thinking 20–12

Age will influence not only the level of knowledge of the learner, the capacity to understand the relationship between cause and effect, and the ability to conceptualize and interpret information, but also the methodology used by the nurse as educator.

A child of 4 years is unable to integrate the essential information necessary for diabetic management. The nurse, therefore, teaches the parents or child care provider. The child should be included. The child can be given a syringe without a needle to become familiar with injections. Giving "shots" to a doll while the child observes helps assess the child's response to therapy. Parents need to be counseled to perceive the child as a child with diabetes, not as a diabetic, to prevent the child from assuming the self-image of a sick child.

As children grow, they begin to think logically, are able to identify cause and effect, and begin to generalize knowledge and experience. By early adolescence, the child is able to assume gradually increasing responsibility for diabetic management. The nurse should teach both the adolescent and the parents. Early adolescents are concerned about their self-image and fear of being different. Peer group instruction is effective at this age. Parents need to be warned not to let diabetic management become a factor in the adolescent struggle for independence.

Young adults hold a challenge for the nurse as educator. Young adults are fully responsible for their diabetic management. The nurse should assess young adults' ability to control their diabetes as it competes with the other demands on their life and time, such as building a career or caring for a growing family. Fears and concerns about their children inheriting diabetes must also be addressed.

## Critical Thinking 20–13

This is a challenge! First, assess the situation. When is the child most active? What activities does the child enjoy? Are the parents able to assist? *Upright* does not mean that the child has to stand still for 2 hours. Have distractions ready. Alternate caregivers. Control the environment to maintain an upright position.

## Critical Thinking 20–14

It is difficult for a mother to see a painful procedure done on her infant. Most find it distressing. This mother, however, is crying uncontrollably. The nurse needs to assess for several possible nursing diagnoses: (1) hopelessness, (2) powerlessness, (3) anxiety, (4) loss, and even (5) sleep pattern disturbance. The mother may feel her infant's illness is overwhelming and may not know what to expect or what is expected of her. She may not know how to care for or protect her child. The unfamiliar environment of the hospital, the limited knowledge of the disease process, and the loss of control may make the mother feel alone and alienated. The mother may feel guilty for wanting a healthy child or may feel responsible for the child's illness. Fatigue may be the problem. Has the mother been at the infant's bedside since admission or birth? The nurse needs to continue to assess and validate perceptions of the mother's behavior. The mother needs emotional support and comfort. The nurse should let the mother cry and reassure her that crying is normal. The nurse also should listen to her and identify her support systems.

## Critical Thinking 20–15

Patients with psychogenic polydipsia will compulsively drink. Even when a laboratory test requires that the patient refrain from drinking, the person with psycho-

genic polydipsia will seek out *any* source of water, such as an aquarium or watering cans. If psychogenic polydipsia is suspected, the patient must be kept under constant observation during the water deprivation test.

## Chapter 21: Renal and Urinary Tract Function

### Critical Thinking 21–1

Albumin is not the only protein that can be excreted in the urine. It is possible that the urine contains proteins (other than albumin) that are not measured by the reagent strip.

### Critical Thinking 21–2

With renal failure, both blood urea nitrogen (BUN) and serum creatinine levels will rise, so the urea-to-creatinine ratio remains close to normal. Discrepancies in the ratio usually indicate a nonrenal cause for the elevation.

### Critical Thinking 21–3

The dietary restrictions for a child with phenylketonuria (PKU) are significant. As the child matures, he or she needs to assume more responsibility for his or her care. Parents assume responsibility for the preschooler's diet, but once the child gains independence in school, he or she must assume partial responsibility. When the child has reached age 7 years, the nurse needs to sit down with the child and parents and investigate what happened to lead to a dietary indiscretion. Was it a lack of knowledge? Was it peer pressure or a desire to be like everyone else? Was it poor planning for snacks and lunch at school? Was it rebelling or denial? Actions will be based on the assessments made.

### Critical Thinking 21–4

Although it is recommended that the prostate-specific antigen (PSA) test *and* the digital rectal examination be done to screen for prostate cancer, the recommendation is controversial. The question arises when an elevated result occurs. Because aggressive therapy can cause impotence and incontinence, some physicians prefer a more conservative approach of monitoring and complementary therapy. This approach is supported by the fact that most patients with prostate cancer are older and die of other causes before the prostate cancer becomes clinically problematic.

### Critical Thinking 21–5

It is essential that all the urine be collected over a 24-hour period. If the time of initiation of the test is not documented, the patient or the nursing staff from the previous shift may know when the collection began. To avoid this problem, most institutions initiate a policy that all 24-hour urine specimens are collected during a specific time period, such as from 8 AM to 8 AM. It is also good practice to include the beginning time on the collection bottle.

If the time of the collection cannot be determined, discard the collected urine and begin the test again.

## Critical Thinking 21–6

The patient has been taught twice but still has not learned to discard the tissue into the collection container. The nurse needs to stay with the patient in the bathroom and guide the person through the procedure. A drape should be provided, if necessary, to ensure the patient's privacy.

## Chapter 22: Reproductive Function

### Critical Thinking 22–1

During a discussion, the patient may express feelings of uselessness or helplessness about the inability to conceive or about other aspects of her life. She may express guilt or shame because she has no children. She also may exhibit hesitancy or have an apparent inability to make decisions. If she previously had positive feelings about herself, her current feelings and beliefs are probably based on this situation.

### Critical Thinking 22–2

Because this laboratory value should progressively rise in a normal first trimester of pregnancy, the sudden decline of the human chorionic gonadotropin (hCG) level indicates that the viability of the fetus is in question. Follow-up serial testing of serum hCG and ultrasound will be used to provide additional diagnostic data.

Appropriate emotional support measures depend on the nursing assessment of the patient. When she has been informed of the situation, the mother is likely to be upset, sad, or anxious. She may cry, withdraw, or express fear, confusion, or even denial. Time is a factor in adjustment to loss or potential loss. It may be too soon for the patient to clearly express her thoughts, or she may have strong hope that other tests will show that the fetus is alive and well.

Nursing interventions encourage her to express her feelings and talk about the pregnancy and what it means to her. Listening with understanding helps support the mother in a caring way. Nonjudgmental acceptance of the patient's feelings helps promote communication. For example, the nurse should allow the patient to hope but should avoid statements that reinforce her denial. The nurse can also encourage the patient to communicate with the father of the child and other caring family members.

If the tests confirm that the fetus has died or that the patient has had a miscarriage, the mother is likely to experience depression, usually within the first month after the loss. The nurse should assess for signs of major depression. Referral for counseling or treatment with medication may be indicated.

### Critical Thinking 22–3

Our knowledge of genetics increases rapidly as the mapping of all human genetic material nears completion.

Diagnostic DNA tests are increasingly developed as a result of the knowledge of genetics. With amniocentesis, cordocentesis, or chorionic villus sampling used to obtain fetal cells, early DNA testing of the fetus is done to identify genetic abnormality. At this time and for the foreseeable future, no ability exists to correct a genetic defect in the fetus. The prospective parents are faced with the choices of abortion or delivery of an infant with an illness or disability that could last for a lifetime.

As knowledge of genetics and identification of genetic abnormalities continue to grow, that growth will have a profound effect on society, government, health care insurance providers, doctors and nurses, individuals, and fetuses. The direction of future change could easily affect our values and beliefs about life and health. It also raises many ethical questions.

Our government and society provide support for disabled individuals and families who have a severely ill or disabled child. Would that support continue when a genetic defect is known at an early stage of pregnancy and the woman or family decides to continue the pregnancy? Could the government pass laws to mandate screening for genetic defects in the fetus? Mandatory screening laws to detect genetic defects in newborns have been instituted already, as with phenylketonuria (PKU) and sickle cell anemia. If insurance companies refuse medical coverage for a genetic defect in the fetus, what impact would this have on the decision to abort or not?

Which genetic abnormalities are acceptable, and which would be considered unacceptable? Who decides that issue? How will society value the individual with a genetic disorder when early knowledge and an option to prevent the birth exist? Would the early knowledge of a genetic defect in the fetus affect the woman's decision to have an abortion? Will indigent and uninsured people have the same options for genetic screening as those who have greater financial resources? If not, would people with fewer financial resources be the only ones to bear children with genetic problems? In light of available genetic information, how does one define a "normal" fetus? What is a "perfect child"?

### Critical Thinking 22–4

Several possible reasons exist for why women avoid having a mammogram. Women may think that when no palpable lump exists or when no change in the appearance of the breast occurs, no need for the test exists. Additionally, most people fear cancer, and testing for this disease invokes some anxiety. If they know someone who died of breast cancer, they may have a sense of hopelessness about this disease or thoughts that death from breast cancer is inevitable. The cost of the examination may be a factor, although Medicaid, Medicare, and most insurance companies and health maintenance organizations (HMOs) pay for mammograms for women older than 50 years. Some women's physicians may not have recommended the mammogram. Other women may dislike the test because of the uncomfortable or painful breast compression. Older people sometimes believe that the mammogram cannot detect breast cancer very well.

Interventions could include discussion of the value of screening for and early detection of breast cancer. Early detection measures include breast self-examination, clinical examination of the breasts by the physician or nurse, and mammography. In a group discussion, ask why women do not have this test. Listen to their thoughts and answer the women's questions. Help dispel the myths associated with mammography.

Help women determine where they can obtain a mammogram in their community. Provide a list of addresses of the facilities and the phone numbers that can be used to make an appointment. Distribute printed educational materials from the local office of the American Cancer Society. Encourage the women to have the test.

## Chapter 23: Neurologic Function

### Critical Thinking 23–1

Fear and anxiety are common reactions to this procedure. You can ask what is bothering the patient. A specific part of the test may evoke fear, such as fear of pain. When the patient can verbalize the thought, the response can provide direct reassurance. The feelings may be more diffuse, so that the patient cannot identify any specific cause. In this case, general measures of comfort will help. Physically, you can reassure by being present next to the patient. Hold the patient's hand, and communicate in a calm voice. Explain that the procedure will be completed shortly. Most people can endure some discomfort when they know that it will not last very long.

### Critical Thinking 23–2

Unequal pupillary response to light is an abnormal neurologic finding. Additional neurologic testing should be done quickly. Include assessment for consciousness and the ability to respond correctly to verbal commands. Look at the patient's face as he or she speaks. Are the facial and mouth movements symmetrical? Test motor movements of the hands by testing the patient's ability to grasp and squeeze your hands. Is the strength of grip equal and strong? To test motor ability in the legs, ask the patient to move each leg. Does he or she move them equally, or does one remain still? Monitor the vital signs, assessing for bradycardia and an elevated pulse. Observe the breathing rate, effort, and pattern.

With the initial finding of unequal pupils, the follow-up assessments may add additional abnormal findings. Notify the physician of the pupillary change, and report other abnormal (or normal) findings. Record your assessments in the patient's chart. It is possible that the patient is having a complication of stroke.

## Chapter 24: Musculoskeletal Function

### Critical Thinking 24–1

Ask the patient how often he might go between floors during a normal day. Based on his responses, help him reorganize his activities so that he ambulates and uses the stairs infrequently. Demonstrate how to go up and down stairs with crutches or with a limited weight-bearing gait. Ask if other people live in the house or nearby who could provide assistance.

### Critical Thinking 24–2

The teaching plan can have several areas of focus. These include having a dual-energy x-ray absorptiometry (DEXA) scan and, if an abnormal result exists, discussing the need for medication to prevent or treat the problem of osteoporosis. Another focus is to modify the risk factors by cessation of smoking; increase in weight-bearing exercises, walking for exercise, and spending time in the sunshine; and reduction of caffeine consumption. Dietary modifications include increasing the intake of calcium in foods and with calcium supplement tablets. Additionally, teach the patients how to prevent falls that can result in a fracture. Measures include having a vision examination and correcting any vision impairment, working and living in a well-lit environment, and removing small objects and clutter from the floors and stairs of the home.

## Chapter 25: Sensory Function

### Critical Thinking 25–1

Because this procedure has no adverse effects afterward, the patient can do her activities as planned. A few precautionary suggestions should be made. Remind the patient that her pupils will remain dilated for a few hours. When in the sunlight, she should wear sunglasses to protect the retinas from glare. When indoors, however, the sunglasses should be removed because the lighting is subdued and she will not see well. Because her pupils are dilated, her vision will be blurry for a while. Ask her friend to assist her at curbs and stairs so that a fall does not occur. If they have a car, the friend must be the driver. Remind the patient to drink extra fluids during and after her outing.

### Critical Thinking 25–2

The teaching plan should address the following:

1. Use of sunscreen cream. Individuals who are very fair and white-skinned, often with red hair, are most vulnerable to sunburn. They burn easily and rarely tan from exposure to the sun. These people need maximum protection and should use a sunscreen product with a sun protection factor (SPF) of 15 or higher daily. Individuals who burn minimally to moderately and who tan slowly or easily are at risk to develop skin cancer, but it is not as high a risk. When exposure to

the sun is prolonged, this group should apply sun-screen cream with an SPF of 4 to 6. Individuals with darker pigment, such as darker-skinned Mediter-raneans, Indians, Mongolians, or those of African heritage, do not need to use sunscreen cream (Arndt, 1995).

2. Method of use. The sunscreen product should be applied 1 to 2 hours before exposure to the sun and reapplied at several intervals during the exposure. The cream tends to wash off during swimming and prolonged exercise and with sweating.

3. Use of lipstick sunscreen. This product can be applied to protect the lips. It also should be reapplied at inter-vals during sun exposure.

4. Protection of children. Parents and children should be taught that it is very important to protect children from sun exposure. Protection during childhood greatly reduces the risk of most skin cancers (non-melanoma) during one's lifetime.

# Therapeutic Drug Monitoring

Therapeutic drug monitoring provides exact information about the quantity of medication that is in the blood. This testing is performed for several reasons. In the patient with a normal metabolism, the standard dose and schedule of a particular medication usually results in a therapeutic blood level of the medication within a specific period. In other patients, such as elderly individuals, neonates, and obese persons, the standard dose may produce a diminished or excessive clinical result because of abnormal metabolism or diminished renal or hepatic function. Therapeutic drug monitoring is used to adjust the dose and schedule of medications as needed.

For a variety of reasons, many patients do not take their medication in the same amount as was prescribed. Therapeutic drug monitoring provides data to alert the physician or nurse about the need to investigate the cause of the problem.

Some medications have a narrow range of values for a therapeutic effect. A small increase beyond that range can have a toxic result. Therapeutic drug monitoring is carried out to protect the patient from the harm of excess medication.

In the case of overdose (accidental or deliberate), the laboratory tests can identify the medication and the amount that is in the blood. The patient may be comatose, psychotic, or agitated from the effect of the overdose and may be unable to describe what was ingested. The test results provide data for corrective action.

Table A–1 provides the range of blood values of selected medications to measure for therapeutic effect and for toxicity. For therapeutic drug monitoring, the tests are ordered at planned intervals to establish and maintain an effective medication level in the blood. To identify a problem of toxicity, the laboratory test may be ordered when the patient demonstrates side effects to the medication or when an unexplained change in behavior, such as loss of consciousness, occurs.

**Table A-1    Therapeutic Drug Monitoring**

| Drug | Collection Tube | Therapeutic Range | Toxic Value |
|------|-----------------|-------------------|-------------|
| Acetaminophen (Tylenol) | Red | 10–30 µg/mL<br>SI 66–199 µmol/L | >200 µ/mL<br>SI >1,324 µmol/L |
| Amikacin (Amikin) | Red | 25–35 µg/mL<br>SI 43–60 µmol/L | 35–40 µg/mL<br>SI 60–68 µmol/L |
| Amitriptyline (Elavil) | Red, green | 80–250 ng/mL<br>SI 289–903 nmol/L | >500 ng/mL<br>SI >1,805 nmol/L |
| Amiodarone (Cordarone) | Red | 1.0–2.5 µg/mL<br>SI 1.6–3.9 µmol/L | >2.5 µg/mL<br>SI >4 µmol/L |
| Amobarbital (Amytal) | Lavender, green, red | 5–15 µg/mL<br>SI 22–66 µmol/L | SI >20 µg/mL<br>SI >86 µmol/L |
| Carbamazepine (Tegretol) | Red | 4–12 µg/mL<br>SI 17–51 µmol/L | >15 µg/mL<br>SI >63 µmol/L |
| Chloramphenicol (Chloromycetin) | Red | 10–25 µg/mL<br>SI 31–77 µmol/L | >25 µg/mL<br>SI >77 µmol/L |
| Chlordiazepoxide (Librax, Librium) | Red | 0.7–1.0 µg/mL<br>SI 2.3–3.3 µmol/L | >5 µg/mL<br>SI >17 µmol/L |
| Chlorpromazine (Thorazine) | Red | 50–300 ng/mL<br>SI 157–942 nmol/L | >750 ng/mL<br>SI >2,355 nmol/L |
| Diazepam (Valium) | Red | 0.2–1.0 µg/mL<br>SI 0.7–3.5 µmol/L | >5 µg/mL<br>SI >18 µmol/L |
| Digoxin (Lanoxin) | Red | 0.8–2.0 ng/mL<br>SI 1.0–2.6 nmol/L | >2 ng/mL<br>SI >2.6 nmol/L |
| Disopyramide (Norpace) | Red, green, lavender | Atrial arrhythmias<br>2.8–3.2 µg/mL<br>SI 8.3–9.4 µmol/L<br>Ventricular arrhythmias<br>3.5–7.5 µg/mL<br>SI 9.7–22 µmol/L | >7 µg/mL<br>SI 20.6 µmol/L |
| Flucytosine (Ancobon) | Red | 25–100 µg/mL<br>SI 194–775 µmol/L | 100–125 µg/mL<br>SI 775–970 µmol/L |
| Fluoxetine (Prozac) | Red, green | 100–800 ng/mL<br>SI 289–1,735 nmol/L | >2,000 ng/mL<br>SI >5,784 nmol/L |
| Haloperidol (Haldol) | Red, green | 5–20 ng/mL<br>SI 10–43 nmol/L | >42 ng/mL<br>SI >84 nmol/L |
| Imipramine (Tofranil) | Red, green | 150–250 ng/mL<br>SI 530–890 nmol/L | >300 ng/mL<br>SI >1,070 nmol/L |
| Lidocaine (Xylocaine) | Red, green, lavender | 1.5–5.0 µg/mL<br>SI 6.4–21.4 µmol/L | >6 µg/mL<br>SI >25.6 µmol/L |
| Lithium (Eskalith) | Red | 0.6–1.2 mEq/L<br>SI 0.6–1.2 mmol/L | >1.5 mEq/L<br>SI >1.5 mmol/L |
| Methotrexate (Mexate) | Red, green, lavender | Variable (dosage dependent) | Low dose:<br>>9.1 ng/mL<br>SI >20 nmol/L<br>High dose: >454 ng/mL<br>SI >1,000 µmol/L |

## Table A–1    Therapeutic Drug Monitoring *(continued)*

| Drug | Collection Tube | Therapeutic Range | Toxic Value |
|---|---|---|---|
| Mexiletine (Mexitil) | Red | 0.75–2.0 µg/mL<br>SI 4–11 µmol/L | >2 µg/mL<br>SI >9 mmol/L |
| Phenobarbital (Luminal) | Red, green, lavender | 20–40 µg/mL<br>SI 86–172 µmol/L | >40 µg/mL<br>SI >172 µmol/L |
| Phenytoin (Dilantin) | Red, lavender | 10–20 µg/mL<br>SI 40–79 µmol/L | 25–50 µg/mL<br>SI 120–200 µmol/L |
| Procainamide (Pronestyl) | Red | 4–10 µg/mL<br>SI 17–42 µmol/L<br>*N*-Acetylprocainamide<br>(NAPA)<br><30 µg/mL<br>SI <127 µmol/L | >14 µg/mL<br>SI 59.5 µmol/L<br><br><br><br>>30 µg/mL<br>SI >127 µmol/L |
| Propoxyphene (Darvocet-N, Darvon) | Red | 0.1–0.4 µg/mL<br>SI 0.3–1.2 µmol/L | >0.5 µg/mL<br>SI >1.5 µmol/L |
| Propranolol (Inderal) | Red | 50–100 ng/mL<br>SI 190–390 nmol/L | >1,000 ng/mL<br>SI >3,860 nmol/L |
| Quinidine (Cardioquin) | Red | 2–5 µg/mL<br>SI 6.2–15.4 µmol/L | >8 µg/mL<br>SI >24.7 µmol/L |
| Salicylate (acetylsalicylic acid, aspirin) | Red, lavender | For analgesia:<br><10 mg/dL<br>SI <0.72 mmol/L<br>For anti-inflammatory effect:<br>15–20 mg/dL<br>SI 1.09–1.45 mmol/L | Mild: 30 mg/dL<br>SI 2.17 mmol/L<br>Severe: >80 mg/dL<br>SI >3.62 mmol/L |
| Theophylline (Aminophylline, Elixophyllin) | Red | 10–20 µg/mL<br>SI 56–111 mmol/L | Adult: >20 µg/mL<br>SI >111 µmol/L<br>Neonate: >10 µg/mL<br>SI >56 µmol/L |
| Thiocyanate (nitroprusside, Nipride) | Red, lavender | 1–4 µg/mL<br>SI 0.02–0.07 mmol/L | >35 µg/mL<br>SI >0.6 mmol/L |
| Tocainide (Tonocard) | Red, green | 4–10 µg/mL<br>21–52 µmol/L | >12 µg/mL<br>>52 µmol/L |
| Valproic acid | Red, green | 50–100 µg/mL<br>350–690 µmol/L | >200 µg/mL<br>>1,390 µmol/L |
| Vancomycin (Vancocin) | Red | 20–40 µg/mL<br>14–27 µmol/L | >80 µg/mL<br>>54 µmol/L |
| Verapamil (Isoptin, Calan) | Red, green | 100–400 ng/mL<br>SI 200–815 nmol/L | >400 ng/mL<br>SI >815 nmol/L |
| Warfarin (Coumadin) | Red, lavender | 2–5 µg/mL<br>SI 6.5–16.2 µmol/L | >10 µg/mL<br>SI 32.4 µmol/L |

# APPENDIX B

# Toxic Substances

Screening for toxic substances is performed to identify the agent responsible for an acute, chronic, or possibly life-threatening illness. Some of these toxic substances are drugs of abuse and have been taken in an unknown quantity. The clinical effect of the substance varies among individuals who are occasional or habitual users. It can also vary with the preparation or mixture that was inhaled, injected, or eaten.

Some toxic substances are ingested by small children. The poisons commonly ingested include rat poison, antifreeze, and insecticide. Other toxic substances that can be identified by laboratory testing are toxic chemicals and metals that poison the individual from an environ-

mental source, including inhalation of poisonous gases from a fire and exposure to hazardous industrial wastes. When the individual is acutely ill from any of these toxic substances, it is essential to identify the cause. Appropriate action can then be taken to reverse the effect and protect the organs from further damage. Some of the toxins pose a long-term threat because they cause mutation and eventual malignancy.

In Table B–1, the values for the normal range of a toxic substance vary from none to minute amounts. The values for toxicity levels are not always defined. The toxicity may vary among individuals, or its very presence may be considered toxic.

## Table B–1  Toxic Substances

| Substance | Specimen | Collection Tube | Normal Value | Toxic Level |
|-----------|----------|-----------------|--------------|-------------|
| Alcohol (ETOH, ethanol) | Blood | Red (clotted), blue, green, gray | Negative<br>Negative | >300 mg/dL<br>SI 65.1 mmol/L |
| Amphetamine | Urine (random) | Plastic cup | Negative<br>Negative | 25–250 µg/mL<br>180–1,850 µmol/L |
| Arsenic | Blood (20 mL) | Trace metal-free container | <23 µg/dL<br>SI <0.31 µmol/L | 600–9,300 µg/L<br>SI 8–124 µmol/L |
| | Urine (24-hr) | Plastic, acid-washed container | 0–50 µg/L<br>SI 0–0.065 µmol/L | >850 µg/L<br>SI >11.3 µmol/L |
| Cadmium | Urine (24-hr) | Plastic, acid-washed container | <1 µg/L<br>SI 8.9 µmol/L | >10 µg/L<br>SI 88.97 µmol/L |
| Cannabinoids (marijuana, hashish) | Urine (random) | Plastic cup | Negative | Not defined |
| Cocaine | Blood | Red, gray | Negative | >1,000 ng/mL<br>>3,300 nmol/L |
| | Urine (random) | Plastic cup | Negative<br>Negative | 1,000 ng/mL<br>3,300 nmol/L |
| Cyanide | Blood | Red, lavender | Smoker:<br>0.0006 mg/L<br>SI 0.23 µmol/L<br>Nonsmoker:<br>0.004 mg/L<br>SI 0.15 µmol/L | >1 µg/mL |
| Ethylene | Blood | Red, green | Negative | 0.3–4 g/L |
| Fluoride | Blood | Red (nonglass tube) | 0.1–20 µg/dL<br>SI 0.5–2.4 µmol/L | >28.5 µg/dL<br>SI >15 µmol/L |
| Lead | Blood | Lead-free tube with heparin | <10 µg/dL<br>SI 0.5 µmol/L | >80 µg/dL<br>SI >3.86 µmol/L |
| Mercury | Blood | Metal-free tube | <0.06 µ/mL<br>SI <0.3 nmol/L | 0.06–60 µg/mL<br>SI 3–300 nmol/L |
| | Urine | Plastic, acid-washed container | 10–50 µg/24 hr<br>SI 0.05–0.25 µmol/24 hr | >100 µg/24 hr<br>SI >0.50 µmol/24 hr |
| Opiates (codeine, morphine) | Urine (random) | Plastic cup | Negative | Not determined |

# APPENDIX C

# Abbreviations Associated with Laboratory and Diagnostic Testing

| | |
|---|---|
| A-a | Alveolar-arterial |
| ABI | Ankle-brachial index |
| ACE | Angiotensin-converting enzyme |
| ACT | Activated clotting time |
| ACTH | Adrenocorticotropic hormone |
| ADH | Antidiuretic hormone |
| AFAFP | Amniotic fluid alpha$_1$-fetoprotein |
| AFP$_1$ | Alpha$_1$-fetoprotein |
| AFP$_2$ | Alpha$_2$-fetoprotein |
| A/G | Albumin-globulin ratio |
| AGT | Antiglobulin test |
| ALB | Albumin |
| ALP | Alkaline phosphatase |
| ALT | Alanine aminotransferase |
| ANA | Antinuclear antibody |
| Anti-HAV | Hepatitis A antibody |
| Anti-HBc | Hepatitis B core antibody |
| Anti-HBe | Hepatitis B e antibody |
| Anti-HCV | Hepatitis C antibody |
| Anti-HDV | Hepatitis Delta antibody |
| Anti-HEV | Hepatitis E antibody |
| APTT | Activated partial thromboplastin time |
| ART | Automated reagin test |
| AST | Aspartate aminotransferase |
| BAO | Basal acid output |
| BE | Barium enema |
| BUN | Blood urea nitrogen |
| C&S | Culture and sensitivity |
| Ca$^{++}$ | Calcium ion |
| Ca$_i$ | Calcium, ionized |
| CA 19-9 | Carbohydrate antigen 19-9 |
| CA 125 | Cancer antigen 125 |
| CAT | Computed axial tomography |
| CBC | Complete blood count |
| CCr | Creatinine clearance |
| CEA | Carcinoembryonic antigen |
| CH$_{50}$ | Complement, total |
| CK | Creatine kinase |

| | |
|---|---|
| $Cl^-$ | Chloride ion |
| $CO_2$ | Carbon dioxide |
| CPK | Creatine phosphokinase |
| CRP | C-reactive protein |
| CSF | Cerebrospinal fluid |
| CST | Contraction stress test |
| CT | Calcitonin |
| CT | Computed tomography |
| cTnI | Cardiac troponin I |
| cTnT | Cardiac troponin T |
| DAT | Direct antiglobulin test |
| DOPAC | Dihydroxyphenyl acetic acid |
| DSA | Digital subtraction angiography |
| DVI | Digital vascular imaging |
| $E_2$ | Estradiol |
| $E_3$ | Estriol |
| EA | Early antigen |
| EBNA | Epstein-Barr nuclear antigen |
| ECG | Electrocardiogram |
| ECHO | Echocardiogram |
| ECT | Emissions computed tomography |
| ECT | Euglobulin clot test |
| EEG | Electroencephalography |
| EFM | Electronic fetal monitoring |
| EGD | Esophagogastroduodenoscopy |
| EIA | Enzyme immunoassay |
| EKG | Electrocardiogram |
| ELISA | Enzyme-linked immunosorbent assay |
| EMG | Electromyography |
| ENG | Electronystagmography |
| EP | Erythropoietin |
| EPS | Electrophysiologic studies |
| ERCP | Endoscopic retrograde cholangiopancreatography |
| ER/PGR | Estrogen–progesterone assay |
| ERV | Expiratory reserve volume |
| ESR | Erythrocyte sedimentation rate |
| EUG | Excretory urogram |
| EUS | Endoscopic ultrasound |
| FANA | Fluorescent antinuclear antibody |
| FBP | Fibrin breakdown products |
| FBS | Fasting blood sugar |
| FDP | Fibrin degradation products |
| FEF | Forced expiratory flow |
| FEV | Forced expiratory volume |
| FNA | Fine-needle aspiration |
| FNB | Fine-needle biopsy |
| FOB | Fecal occult blood |
| FRC | Functional residual capacity |
| FSH | Follicle-stimulating hormone |
| FSP | Fibrin split-products |
| $FT_3$ | Free triiodothyronine |

| | |
|---|---|
| $FT_4$ | Free thyroxine |
| FTA-ABS | Fluorescent treponemal antibody absorption test |
| FVC | Forced vital capacity |
| GB | Gallbladder |
| GED | Gastroesophageal duodenoscopy |
| GEST | Graded exercise testing |
| GEX | Graded exercise testing |
| GGT | Gamma-glutamyltransferase |
| GGTP | Gamma-glutamyltranspeptidase |
| GH | Growth hormone |
| GHb | Glycohemoglobin |
| GLU | Glucose |
| GPT | Glutamic pyruvic transaminase |
| G-6-PD | Glucose-6-phosphate dehydrogenase |
| GTP | Glutamyl transpeptidase |
| HAA | Hepatitis-associated antigen |
| HAP | Haptoglobin |
| HAV, Ab | Hepatitis A virus antibody |
| HAVAb | Hepatitis A virus antibody |
| Hb | Hemoglobin |
| $HbA_1$ | Glycosylated hemoglobin |
| HBcAb | Hepatitis B core antibody |
| HBeAb | Hepatitis B e antibody |
| HBeAg | Hepatitis B e antigen |
| HbF | Fetal hemoglobin |
| Hbg | Hemoglobin |
| HBsAb | Hepatitis B surface antibody |
| HBsAg | Hepatitis B surface antigen |
| HBsAgAb | Hepatitis B surface antigen antibody |
| hCG | Human chorionic gonadotropin |
| $HCO_3$ | Bicarbonate |
| Hct | Hematocrit |
| HDL | High-density lipoprotein |
| 5-HIAA | 5-Hydroxyindole acetic acid |
| HLA | Human leukocyte antigen |
| HSV | Herpes simplex virus |
| HVA | Homovanillic acid |
| IADSA | Intra-arterial digital subtraction angiography |
| I-ALP | Alkaline phosphatase isoenzymes |
| IAT | Indirect antiglobulin test |
| IC | Inspiratory capacity |
| IF | Intrinsic factor |
| IgG | Immunoglobulin G |
| IgM | Immunoglobulin M |
| IRV | Inspiratory reserve volume |
| ITT | Insulin tolerance test |
| IUG | Intravenous urography |
| IVC | Intravenous cholangiography |
| IVDSA | Intravenous digital subtraction angiography |
| IVFA | Intravenous fluorescent angiography |

| | |
|---|---|
| IVP | Intravenous pyelogram |
| IVU | Intravenous urography |
| IVUS | Intravascular ultrasound |
| $K^+$ | Potassium ion |
| 17-KGS | 17-Ketogenic steroid |
| 17-KS | 17-Ketosteroid |
| LAP | Leucine aminopeptidase |
| LATS | Long-acting thyroid stimulator |
| LDH | Lactate dehydrogenase |
| LDL | Low-density lipoprotein |
| LDM | Low-dose myelography |
| LH | Luteinizing hormone |
| LP | Lumbar puncture |
| L/S | Lecithin–sphingomyelin |
| MAO | Maximal acid output |
| Mb | Myoglobin |
| MBC | Maximum breathing capacity |
| MCH | Mean corpuscular hemoglobin |
| MCHC | Mean corpuscular hemoglobin concentration |
| MCV | Mean corpuscular volume |
| Mg, $Mg^{++}$ | Magnesium, magnesium ion |
| MHA-TP | Microhemoagglutination assay–*Treponema pallidum* |
| MMEF | Forced midexpiratory flow rate |
| MPV | Mean platelet volume |
| MRI | Magnetic resonance imaging |
| MUGA | Multiple gated acquisition angiography |
| MV | Minute volume |
| MVV | Maximum voluntary ventilation |
| 5'N | 5'-Nucleotidase |
| $Na^+$ | Sodium ion |
| NAP | Neutrophil alkaline phosphatase |
| NCS | Nerve conduction study |
| $NH_3$ | Ammonia |
| NPO | Nothing by mouth |
| NST | Nonstress testing |
| 5'NT | 5'-Nucleotidase |
| O&P | Ova and parasites |
| $O_2$sat | Oxygen saturation |
| OF | Osmotic fragility |
| OGTT | Oral glucose tolerance test |
| $P_4$ | Progesterone |
| PAO | Peak acid output |
| PAP | Papanicolaou smear |
| PAP | Prostatic acid phosphatase |
| PCA | Parietal cell antibody |
| $P_{CO_2}$ | Partial pressure of carbon dioxide |
| $P_{cr}$ | Plasma creatinine |
| PCR | Polymerase chain reaction |
| PCR | Pulse cuff recording |
| PCV | Packed cell volume |

| | |
|---|---|
| Pdi | Transdiaphragmatic pressure |
| PDW | Platelet distribution width |
| PET | Positron-emission tomography |
| $PET_{CO_2}$ | End-tidal partial pressure of carbon dioxide |
| pH | Partial pressure of hydrogen |
| Phe | Phenylalanine |
| $P_{I}max$ | Maximum intrathoracic pressure |
| PKU | Phenylketonuria |
| $P_{O_2}$ | Partial pressure of oxygen |
| $P_{O_4}{}^{3-}$ | Phosphate |
| PPD | Purified protein derivative |
| PRA | Plasma renin activity |
| PRL | Prolactin |
| PSA | Prostate-specific antigen |
| PT | Prothrombin time |
| PTC | Percutaneous transhepatic cholangiography |
| PTH | Parathyroid hormone |
| PTHC | Percutaneous transhepatic cholangiography |
| PTT | Partial thromboplastin time |
| PUBS | Percutaneous umbilical blood sampling |
| $P_{VO_2}$ | Partial pressure of oxygen in the venous system |
| RAIU | Radioactive iodine uptake |
| RBC | Red blood cell |
| RDW | Red cell distribution width |
| RF | Rheumatoid factor |
| RIA | Radioimmunoassay |
| RPR | Rapid plasma reagin |
| $RT_3U$ | Resin triiodothyronine uptake |
| RV | Residual volume |
| SACE | Serum angiotensin-converting enzyme |
| SAECG | Signal-averaged electrocardiogram |
| $Sa_{O_2}$ | Arterial oxygen saturation |
| SBGM | Self-blood glucose monitoring |
| SGOT | Glutamate oxaloacetate transaminase, serum |
| SGOT | Serum glutamic-oxaloacetic transaminase |
| SGPT | Serum glutamate pyruvate transaminase |
| SHBD | Serum hydroxybutyrate dehydrogenase |
| SMUG | Self-monitoring of urinary glucose |
| SPECT | Single photon emission computed tomography |
| SRT | Speech reception threshold |
| STH | Growth hormone; somatotropin |
| $Sv_{O_2}$ | Oxygen saturation in the venous system |
| T&C | Type and crossmatch |
| T-ALP | Total alkaline phosphatase |
| $T_3$ | Triiodothyronine |
| $T_4$ | Thyroxine |
| TBG | Thyroxine-binding globulin |
| $tCO_2$ | Total carbon dioxide |
| TEE | Transesophageal echocardiography |
| TIBC | Total iron-binding capacity |
| TLC | Total lung capacity |

| TP | Total protein |
|------|------|
| TRH | Thyroid-releasing hormone |
| TSH | Thyroid-stimulating hormone |
| TUS | Transluminal ultrasound |
| TV | Tidal volume |
| UA | Urinalysis |
| VA | Visual acuity |
| VC | Vital capacity |
| VCA | Viral capsid antigen |
| VCG | Vectorcardiogram |
| Vds | Dead space volume |
| VDRL | Venereal Disease Research Laboratory |
| VEST | Ventricular extrastimulus testing |
| VMA | Vanillylmandelic acid |
| V/Q | Ventilation–perfusion |
| WBC | White blood cell |
| WDS | Word discrimination score |

# Symbols and Units of Measurement

| | |
|---|---|
| α | alpha |
| AU | arbitrary unit |
| cm | centimeter |
| dL | deciliter |
| fL | femtoliter |
| γ | gamma |
| g | gram |
| IU | international unit |
| kg | kilogram |
| L | liter |
| μg | microgram |
| mEq | milliequivalent |
| mg | milligram |
| mIU | milli-international unit |
| mL | milliliter |
| mm | millimeter |
| mm Hg | millimeters of mercury |
| mmol | millimole |
| mOsm | milliosmole |
| ng | nanogram |
| % | percentage |
| pg | picogram |
| SI | Système International (International System of Units) |
| U | unit |
| μ | micro |

## Table E–1 Normal Values: Whole Blood, Serum, and Plasma Tests

| Name of Test | Conventional Values | SI Units | Chapter Number |
|---|---|---|---|
| Activated clotting time | 70–120 sec | Same | 6 |
| Activated partial thromboplastin time | 25–35 sec | Same | 6 |
| Newborn | <90 sec | Same | 6 |
| Premature infant | <120 sec | Same | 6 |
| Adrenocorticotropic hormone (adult) | | | |
| In AM | 25–100 pg/mL | 25–100 ng/L | 20 |
| In PM | 0–50 pg/mL | 0–50 ng/L | 20 |
| Adrenocorticotropic stimulation test: a rise of plasma cortisol in 30–60 min | 20 µg/dL | 276 nmol/L | 20 |
| Alanine aminotransferase | | | |
| Adult | 0–35 IU/L | Same | 19 |
| Male >60 yr | 13–40 IU/L | Same | 19 |
| Female >60 yr | 10–28 IU/L | Same | 19 |
| Male newborn–1 yr | 13–45 IU/L | Same | 19 |
| Female newborn–1 yr | 15–45 IU/L | Same | 19 |
| Albumin | | | |
| Adult >60 years | 3.4–4.8 g/dL | 34–48 g/L | 19 |
| Adult 18–60 years | 3.5–5 g/dL | 35–50 g/L | 19 |
| Child | 3.2–5.4 g/dL | 32–54 g/L | 19 |
| Newborn | 2.8–4.4 g/dL | 28–44 g/L | 19 |
| Albumin-to-globulin ratio | >1 | Same | 19 |
| Aldosterone | | | |
| Adult (average sodium diet) | | | |
| Supine | 3–10 ng/dL | 0.08–0.27 nmol/L | 20 |
| Upright | 5–30 ng/dL | 0.14–0.83 nmol/L | 20 |
| After fluorocortisone suppression or intravenous saline infusion | <4 ng/dL | <0.11 nmol/L | 20 |
| Adrenal vein | 200–800 ng/dL | 5.54–22.16 nmol/L | 20 |
| Child | | | |
| 11–15 yr | <5–50 ng/dL | <0.14–1.39 nmol/L | 20 |
| 3–11 yr | <5–80 ng/dL | <0.14–2.22 nmol/L | 20 |
| 1–3 yr | 5–60 ng/dL | 0.14–1.7 nmol/L | 20 |
| 1 wk–1 yr | 1–160 ng/dL | 0.03–4.43 nmol/L | 20 |
| Alkaline phosphatase | | | |
| Adult | 4.5–13 King-Armstrong units/dL | 32–92 U/L | 19 |
| Child | 15–30 King-Armstrong units/dL | 107–213 U/L | 19 |
| Infant | 10–30 King-Armstrong units/dL | 71–213 U/L | 19 |

(continued on the following page)

**Table E–1    Normal Values: Whole Blood, Serum, and Plasma Tests** (continued)

| Name of Test | Conventional Values | SI Units | Chapter Number |
|---|---|---|---|
| Alkaline phosphatase isoenzymes | Percent inactivation after 16 min at 55°C | Fractional inactivation after 16 min at 55°C | 19 |
| Liver | 50–70 | 0.50–0.70 | 19 |
| Bone | 90–100 | 0.90–1.00 | 19 |
| Intestine | 50–60 | 0.50–0.60 | 19 |
| Placenta | 0 | 0 | 19 |
| Regan | 0 | 0 | 19 |
| Alpha$_1$-fetoprotein | | | |
| Adult | <10 ng/mL | <10 µg/L | 19 |
| Third trimester of pregnancy | 550 ng/mL | 550 µg/L | 19, 22 |
| Ammonia | | | |
| Adult | 15–45 µg/dL | 11–32 µmol/L | 19 |
| Child | 29–70 µg/dL | 21–50 µmol/L | 19 |
| Neonate | 90–150 µg/dL | 64–107 µmol/L | 19 |
| Amylase | | | |
| Adult | 27–131 U/L | 0.46–2.23 µKat/L | 19 |
| Neonate | 5–65 U/L | 0.09–1.11 µKat/L | 19 |
| Androstenedione | | | |
| Adult | | | |
| Male | 75–205 ng/dL | 2.6–7.2 nmol/L | 22 |
| Female | 85–275 ng/dL | SI 3–9.6 nmol/L | 22 |
| Child | | | |
| 10–17 yr | 8–240 ng/dL | 0.3–8.4 nmol/L | 22 |
| 1–10 yr | 8–50 ng/dL | 0.3–1.7 nmol/L | 22 |
| 1–12 mo | 6–68 ng/dL | 0.2–2.4 nmol/L | 22 |
| Newborn | 20–290 ng/dL | 0.7–10.1 nmol/L | 22 |
| Angiotensin-converting enzyme | | | |
| Adult (≥20 yr) | | | |
| Male | 12–36 IU/L | Same | 14 |
| Female | 10–30 IU/L | Same | 14 |
| Anion gap | 3–11 mEq/L | 3–11 mmol/L | 14 |
| Anti-DNA | Negative | Same | 24 |
| | <70 IU/mL | Same | 24 |
| | Titer: <1:10 | Same | 24 |
| Antiglobulin test, direct | Negative | Same | 17 |
| Antiglobulin test, indirect | Negative | Same | 17 |
| Antinuclear antibody | Negative | Same | 24 |
| Antithrombin III | 21–30 mg/dL | 210–300 mg/L | 6 |
| | 85%–115% | 0.85–1.15 | 6 |
| Aspartate aminotransferase | | | |
| Average adult | 8–20 U/L | Same | 15, 19 |
| Male adult >60 yr | 11–26 U/L | Same | 15, 19 |
| Female adult >60 yr | 10–20 U/L | Same | 15, 19 |
| Child <5 yr | 19–28 U/L | Same | 15, 19 |
| Infant | 16–72 U/L | Same | 15, 19 |
| Newborn | 16–72 U/L | Same | 15, 19 |

## Table E–1    Normal Values: Whole Blood, Serum, and Plasma Tests *(continued)*

| Name of Test | Conventional Values | SI Units | Chapter Number |
|---|---|---|---|
| Bilirubin, direct | | | |
|   Adult | 0–0.2 mg/dL | <3.4 µmol/L | 19 |
| Bilirubin, indirect | | | |
|   Adult | <1.1 mg/dL | <19 µmol/L | 19 |
| Bilirubin, total | | | |
|   Child to adult | 0.3–1.2 mg/dL | 5–21 µmol/L | 19 |
|   Full-term neonate | 1.4–8.7 mg/dL | 24–149 µmol/L | 19 |
| Blood gases, arterial | | | 14 |
|   pH | 7.35–7.45 | 7.35–7.45 | 14 |
|   $Pco_2$ | 35–45 mm Hg | 4.7–5.3 kPa | 14 |
|   $HCO_3$ | 21–28 mEq/L | 21–28 mmol/L | 14 |
|   $Po_2$ | | | 14 |
|     Adult | 80–100 mm Hg | 10.6–13.3 kPa | 14 |
|     Newborn | 60–70 mm Hg | 8.0–10.33 kPa | 14 |
|   $Sao_2$ | | | |
|     Adult | >95% | Fraction saturated >0.95 | 14 |
|     Newborn | 40%–90% | Fraction saturated 0.40–0.90 | 14 |
|   Base excess | q 2 mEq/L | q 2 mmol/L | 14 |
| Blood gases, mixed venous | | | |
|   pH | 7.33–7.43 | 7.33–7.43 | 14 |
|   $Pco_2$ | 41–51 mm Hg | 5.3–6.0 kPa | 14 |
|   $HCO_3^-$ | 24–28 mm Hg | 24–28 mmol/L | 14 |
|   $Pvo_2$ | 35–49 mm Hg | Same | 14 |
|   $Svo_2$ | 60%–80% | Same | 14 |
| Calcitonin, serum | | | 20 |
|   Adult | <150 pg/mL | <150 ng/L | 20 |
|   Infant | | | |
|     Cord blood | 25–150 pg/mL | 30–240 ng/L | 20 |
|     7 days | 77–293 pg/mL | 77–293 ng/L | 20 |
| Calcitonin, plasma | | | |
|   Male | 19 pg/mL | 19 ng/L | 20 |
|   Female | 14 pg/mL | 14 ng/L | 20 |
| Calcium | | | |
|   Adult | 8.6–10.0 mg/L | 2.15–2.50 mmol/L | 5 |
|   Child | 8.8–10.8 mg/dL | 2.20–2.70 mmol/L | 5 |
|   Infant (0–10 days) | 7.6–10.4 mg/dL | 1.90–2.60 mmol/L | 5 |
| Calcium, ionized | | | |
|   Adult (whole blood) | 4.60–5.08 mg/dL | 1.15–1.27 mmol/L | 5 |
|   Adult (plasma) | 4.12–4.92 mg/dL | 1.03–1.23 mmol/L | 5 |
|   Infant (24–48 hr, whole blood) | 4.00–4.72 mg/dL | 1.00–1.18 mmol/L | 5 |
| Cancer antigen 125 | <35 U/mL | <35 kU/L | 22 |
| Carbohydrate antigen 19-9 | | | 19 |
|   Adult | <37 U/mL | <37 kU/L | 19 |

*(continued on the following page)*

## Table E–1    Normal Values: Whole Blood, Serum, and Plasma Tests (continued)

| Name of Test | Conventional Values | SI Units | Chapter Number |
|---|---|---|---|
| Carbon dioxide, total | | | |
| 2 yr–adult (venous) | 22–26 mEq/L | 22–26 mmol/L | 5 |
| 2 yr–adult (arterial) | 23–29 mEq/L | 23–29 mmol/L | 5 |
| Infant–2 yr | 18–28 mEq/L | 18–28 mmol/L | 5 |
| Carcinoembryonic antigen | | | |
| Adult nonsmoker | <2.5 ng/mL | 2.5 µg/L | 18 |
| Adult smoker | Up to 5 ng/mL | 5 µg/L | 18 |
| Catecholamines | | | 20 |
| Epinephrine | | | 20 |
| Supine | <50 pg/mL | <273 pmol/L | 20 |
| Standing | <900 pg/mL | <4,914 pmol/L | 20 |
| Norepinephrine | | | 20 |
| Supine | 110–410 pg/mL | 650–2,423 pmol/L | 20 |
| Standing | 125–700 pg/mL | 739–4,137 nmol/L | 20 |
| Dopamine | | | 20 |
| Supine | <87 pg/mL | <475 pmol/L | 20 |
| Standing | <87 pg/mL | <475 pmol/L | 20 |
| Ceruloplasmin | | | |
| Adult | 18–45 mg/dL | 180–450 mg/L | 19 |
| Newborn–3 mo | 5–18 mg/dL | 50–180 mg/L | 19 |
| Chloride | | | |
| Adult and child | 97–107 mEq/L | 97–107 mmol/L | 5 |
| Newborn | 96–106 mEq/L | 96–106 mmol/L | 5 |
| Premature | 95–110 mEq/L | 95–110 mmol/L | 5 |
| Cholesterol, total | 120–200 mg/dL | 3.11–5.18 mmol/L | 15 |
| Clot retraction time | 1–24 hr | Same | 6 |
| Coagulation factor assay | 0.50–1.50 µ/mL | 500–1,500 U/L | 6 |
| | 50%–150% | 50–150 AU | 6 |
| Complement, total | 75–160 $CH_{50}$ U/mL | 75–160 $CH_{50}$ kU/L | 17 |
| Complete blood count | | | |
| Hematocrit | | | |
| Male | 41.5%–50.4% | 0.415–0.504 (volume fraction) | 4 |
| Female | 35.9%–44.6% | 0.38–0.47 (volume fraction) | 4 |
| Hemoglobin | | | |
| Male | 14.0%–17.5 g/dL | 140–175 g/L | 4 |
| Female | 12.3%–15.3 g/dL | 123–153 g/L | 4 |
| Platelet count | | | |
| Adult | 150,000–450,000 cells/µL | $150–450 \times 10^9$/L | 4 |
| Newborn (1–3 days) | 150,000–400,000 | $150–400 \times 10^9$/L | 4 |
| Red cell count | | | |
| Male | $4.5–5.9 \times 10^6$/µL | $4.5–5.9 \times 10^{12}$/L | 4 |
| Female | $4.5–5.1 \times 10^6$/µL | $4.5–5.1 \times 10^{12}$/L | 4 |

## Table E–1    Normal Values: Whole Blood, Serum, and Plasma Tests *(continued)*

| Name of Test | Conventional Values | SI Units | Chapter Number |
|---|---|---|---|
| Red cell indices | | | |
|   Mean corpuscular volume | 80–96 µm³ | 80–96 fL | 4 |
|   Mean corpuscular hemoglobin | 27.5–33.2 pg | 27.5–33.2 pg | 4 |
|   Mean corpuscular hemoglobin concentration | 33.4%–35.5% | 0.334–0.355 (mean concentration fraction) | 4 |
|   Red cell distribution width | 13.1% (range: 11.6%–14.6%) | Same | 4 |
| Reticulocyte count | | | |
|   Adults | | | |
|     Percentage of cells | 0.5%–1.5% | 0.005–0.15 (number fraction) | 4 |
|     Cell count | 25,000–75,000 cells/µL | $25–75 \times 10^9$/L | 4 |
|   Newborn | | | |
|     Percentage of cells | 3.0%–7.0% | 0.03–0.07 (number fraction) | 4 |
|   White cell count | $4.5–11 \times 10^3$/µL | $4.5–11 \times 10^9$/L | 4 |
| Cortisol, total | | | 20 |
|   Adult | | | |
|     8 AM–10 AM | 5–23 µg/dL | 138–635 nmol/L | 20 |
|     4 PM–6 PM | 3–16 µg/dL | 83–441 nmol/L | 20 |
| Creatinine | | | 21 |
|   Adult male | 0.7–1.3 mg/dL | 62–115 µmol/L | 21 |
|   Adult female | 0.6–1.1 mg/dL | 53–97 µmol/L | 21 |
|   Adolescent | 0.5–1 mg/dL | 44–88 µmol/L | 21 |
|   Child | 0.3–0.7 mg/dL | 27–62 µmol/L | 21 |
|   Infant | 0.2–0.4 mg/mL | 18–35 µmol/L | 21 |
|   Newborn | 0.3–1 mg/dL | 27–88 µmol/L | 21 |
| Creatine kinase | | | |
|   Adult male | 38–174 U/L | 0.65–29.6 µKat/L | 15 |
|   Adult female | 26–140 U/L | 0.44–2.38 µKat/L | 15 |
|   Newborn | 50–525 U/L | 0.85–8.93 µKat/L | 15 |
| Creatine kinase isoenzymes | | | |
| CK-BB, CK-1 | Trace or 0% of total CK | Trace or 0.00 (fraction of total CK) | 15 |
| CK-MB, CK-2 | 0%–6% of total CK | 0.00%–0.06% (fraction of total CK) | 15 |
| CK-MM, CK-3 | 90%–97% of total CK | 0.90–0.97 (fraction of total CK) | 15 |
| C-Reactive protein | <1 mg/dL | <10 mg/L | 24 |
| Dexamethasone suppression test | | | |
|   serum cortisol | <5 µg/dL | <138 nmol/L | 20 |

*(continued on the following page)*

**Table E–1    Normal Values: Whole Blood, Serum, and Plasma Tests** (continued)

| Name of Test | Conventional Values | SI Units | Chapter Number |
|---|---|---|---|
| D-Dimer | <0.25 mg/mL | <250 µg/L | 6 |
| | Negative | Same | 6 |
| D-Xylose absorption | | | |
| Child (1 hr) | >30 mg/dL | >2.0 mmol/L | 18 |
| Adult (2 hr, 5-g dose) | >20 mg/dL | >1.33 mmol/L | 18 |
| Adult (2 hr, 25-g dose) | >25 mg/dL | >1.67 mmol/L | 18 |
| Epstein-Barr antibody titer | | | |
| IgM anti-VCA | <1:10 | Same | 7 |
| IgG anti-VCA | <1:10 | Same | 7 |
| Anti-EBNA | <1:5 | Same | 7 |
| Anti-EA | <1:10 | Same | 7 |
| Erythrocyte sedimentation rate | | | |
| Adult <50 yr | | | |
| Male | 0–15 mm/hr | Same | 24 |
| Female | 0–20 mm/hr | Same | 24 |
| Adult >50 yr | | | |
| Male | 0–20 mm/hr | Same | 24 |
| Female | 0–30 mm/hr | Same | 24 |
| Child | 0–10 mm/hr | Same | 24 |
| Erythropoietin | 5–36 µU/mL | 5–35 IU/L | 21 |
| Estradiol | | | 22 |
| Adult | | | 22 |
| Premenopausal female | 30–400 pg/mL | 110–1,468 pmol/L | 22 |
| Postmenopausal female | 0–30 pg/mL | 0–110 pmol/L | 22 |
| Male | 10–50 pg/mL | 37–184 pmol/L | 22 |
| Estriol, pregnancy | | | 22 |
| Weeks of gestation | | | |
| 28–30 wk | 38–140 ng/mL | 132–486 nmol/L | 22 |
| 32–34 wk | 35–260 ng/mL | 121–902 nmol/L | 22 |
| 36–38 wk | 48–570 ng/mL | 167–1,978 nmol/L | 22 |
| 40 wk | 95–460 ng/mL | 330–1,596 nmol/L | 22 |
| Euglobulin clot lysis | 2–4 hr | Same | 6 |
| Factor II | 0.6–1.5 U/mL | Same | 6 |
| | 60%–150% | 0.60–1.50 | 6 |
| Factor V | 0.5%–1.5 U/mL | Same | 6 |
| | 50%–150% | 0.50–1.50 | 6 |
| Factor VII | 0.65–1.35 U/mL | Same | 6 |
| | 65%–135% | 0.65–1.35 | 6 |
| Factor VIII | 0.5–1.5 U/mL | Same | 6 |
| | 50%–150% | 0.50–1.50 | 6 |
| Factor IX | 0.5–1.5 U/mL | Same | 6 |
| | 50%–150% | 0.50–1.50 | 6 |
| Factor X | 0.6–1.3 U/mL | Same | 6 |
| | 60%–130% | 0.60–1.30 | 6 |
| Factor XI | 0.65–1.35 U/mL | Same | 6 |
| | 65%–135% | 0.65–1.35 | 6 |

## Table E–1    Normal Values: Whole Blood, Serum, and Plasma Tests (continued)

| Name of Test | Conventional Values | SI Units | Chapter Number |
|---|---|---|---|
| Factor XII | 0.65–1.5 U/mL | Same | 6 |
| | 65%–150% | 0.65–1.50 | 6 |
| Factor XIII | Clot is stable for 24 hr | Same | 6 |
| Ferritin | | | |
| Adult male | 20–250 ng/mL | 20–250 µg/L | 17 |
| Adult female | 10–120 ng/mL | 10–120 µg/L | 17 |
| Child (6 mo–15 yr) | 7–140 ng/mL | 7–140 µg/L | 17 |
| Infant (2–5 mo) | 50–200 ng/mL | 50–200 µg/L | 17 |
| Newborn | 25–200 ng/mL | 25–200 µg/L | 17 |
| Fibrin breakdown products | <10 µg/mL | <10 mg/L | 6 |
| Fibrinogen | | | |
| Adult | 200–400 mg/dL | 2–4 g/L | 6 |
| Newborn | 125–300 mg/dL | 1.25–3 g/L | 6 |
| 5′-Nucleotidase (adult) | 2–17 IU/L | 0.03–0.29 µKat/L | 19 |
| Follicle-stimulating hormone | | | 22 |
| Adult | | | |
| Male | 1.42–15.4 mIU/mL | 1.42–15.4 IU/L | 22 |
| Female | | | |
| Follicular phase | 1.37–9.9 mIU/mL | 1.37–9.9 IU/L | 22 |
| Ovulatory peak | 6.17–17.2 mIU/mL | 6.17–17.2 IU/L | 22 |
| Luteal phase | 1.09–9.2 mIU/mL | 1.09–9.2 U/L | 22 |
| Postmenopausal phase | 19.3–100.6 mIU/mL | 19.3–100.6 IU/L | 22 |
| Child 1–10 yr | | | |
| Male | 0.3–4.6 mIU/mL | 0.3–4.6 IU/L | 22 |
| Female | 0.68–6.7 mIU/mL | 0.68–4.6 IU/L | 22 |
| Gamma-glutamyltransferase | | | 19 |
| Male adult | 22.1 ± 11.7 U/L | 0.38 ± 0.020 µKat/L | |
| Female adult | 15.4 ± 6.58 U/L | 0.26 ± 0.11 µKat/L | |
| Male child >6 mo | 2–30 U/L | 0.03–0.51 µKat/L | 19 |
| Female child >6 mo | 1–24 U/L | 0.02–0.41 µKat/L | 19 |
| Gastrin | | | |
| Adult (16–60 yr) | 25–90 pg/mL | 25–90 ng/L | 18 |
| Adult (>60 yr) | <100 pg/mL | <100 ng/L | 18 |
| Child | <10–125 pg/mL | <10–125 ng/L | 18 |
| Infant (0–4 days) | 120–183 pg/mL | 120–183 ng/L | 18 |
| Globulin | 2.8–4.4 g/dL | 28–44 g/L | 19 |
| Glucagon | | | |
| Adult | 20–100 pg/mL | 20–100 ng/L | 20 |
| Child | 0–148 pg/mL | 0–148 ng/L | 20 |
| Infant | 0–1,750 pg/mL | 0–1,750 ng/L | 20 |
| Glucose, capillary | 60–110 mg/dL | 3.3–6.1 mmol/L | 20 |
| Glucose, fasting | | | |
| Children 2 yr to adult | | | |
| Whole blood | 60–110 mg/dL | 3.3–6.1 mmol/L | 20 |
| Plasma or serum | 70–120 mg/dL | 3.9–6.7 mmol/L | 20 |

(continued on the following page)

## Table E–1    Normal Values: Whole Blood, Serum, and Plasma Tests (continued)

| Name of Test | Conventional Values | SI Units | Chapter Number |
|---|---|---|---|
| Glucose, fasting (continued) | | | |
|   Elderly individual | 80–150 mg/dL | 4.4–8.3 mmol/L | 20 |
|   Children <2 yr | 60–100 mg/dL | 3.3–5.6 mmol/L | 20 |
|   Infant | 40–90 mg/dL | 2.2–5.0 mmol/L | 20 |
|   Neonate | 30–60 mg/dL | 1.7–3.3 mmol/L | 20 |
| Glucose-6-phosphate dehydrogenase screen | Enzyme activity is present | Same | 17 |
| | | | 20 |
| Glucose tolerance test, oral | | | 20 |
|   Baseline fasting blood glucose | 70–105 mg/dL | 3.9–5.8 mmol/L | 20 |
|   30-min blood glucose | 110–170 mg/dL | 6.1–9.4 mmol/L | 20 |
|   60-min blood glucose | 120–170 mg/dL | 6.7–9.4 mmol/L | 20 |
|   90-min blood glucose | 100–140 mg/dL | 5.6–7.8 mmol/L | 20 |
|   120-min blood glucose | 70–120 mg/dL | 3.9–6.7 mmol/L | 20 |
| Glucose, 2-hr postprandial | <126 mg/dL | <6.993 mmol/L | 20 |
| Glycosylated hemoglobin assay | 5.5%–8.8% of total hemoglobin | 0.05–0.08 (fraction of total hemoglobin) | 20 |
| | | | 20 |
| Growth hormone | | | |
|   Adult | | | 20 |
|     Male | Undetectable–5 ng/mL | 0–5 µg/L | 20 |
|     Female | Undetectable–10 ng/mL | 0–10 µg/L | 20 |
|   Child | Undetectable–16 ng/mL | 0–16 µg/L | 20 |
| Growth hormone stimulation test | | | 20 |
|   With arginine | >7 ng/mL | >7 µg/L | 20 |
|   With insulin | >20 ng/mL | >20 µg/L | 20 |
|   With propranolol and glucagon | >10 ng/mL | >10 µg/L | 20 |
| Growth hormone suppression test | Undetectable to <3 ng/mL | Undetectable to <3 µg/L | 20 |
| Haptoglobin | | | |
|   Adult | 40–180 mg/dL | 0.4–1.8 g/L | 17 |
|   Newborn–4 mo | 5–48 mg/dL | 0.05–0.48 g/dL | 17 |
| *Helicobacter pylori* | | | |
|   Antibody, IgG | Negative | <15 AU | 18 |
| Hematocrit | | | |
|   Male | 41.5%–50.4% | 0.415–0.504 (volume fraction) | 4 |
|   Female | 35.9%–44.6% | 0.359–0.447 (volume fraction) | 4 |
| Hemoglobin | | | |
|   Male | 14.0–17.5 g/dL | 140–175 g/L | 4 |
|   Female | 12.3–15.3 g/dL | 123–153 g/L | 4 |
|   Child (5 yr) | 11.7–13.7 g/dL | 117–137 g/L | 4 |
|   Infant (5–7 mo) | 10.8–12.2 g/dL | 108–122 g/L | 4 |
|   Newborn (1 day) | 17.3–21.5 g/dL | 173–215 g/L | 4 |
| Hemoglobin electrophoresis | | | |
|   HbA | 95%–98% | 0.95–0.98 Hb fraction | 17 |

## Table E–1    Normal Values: Whole Blood, Serum, and Plasma Tests *(continued)*

| Name of Test | Conventional Values | SI Units | Chapter Number |
|---|---|---|---|
| Hemoglobin electrophoresis *(continued)* | | | |
| HbA$_2$ | 1.5%–3.5% | 0.015–0.035 Hb fraction | 17 |
| HbF | 0%–2% | 0–0.02 Hb fraction | 17 |
| HbC | Absent | Same | 17 |
| HbS | Absent | Same | 17 |
| Hemoglobin, fetal | | | |
| 6 mo–adult | <2% HbF | <0.02 mass fraction HbF | 17 |
| Infant (0–6 mo) | <75% HbF | <0.75 mass fraction HbF | 17 |
| Hepatitis A antibody | Negative | Same | 19 |
| Hepatitis B core antibody | Negative | Same | 19 |
| Hepatitis B e antibody | Negative | Same | 19 |
| Hepatitis B e antigen | Negative | Same | 19 |
| Hepatitis B surface antibody | Negative | Same | 19 |
| Hepatitis B surface antigen | Negative | Same | 19 |
| Hepatitis B viral DNA assay | Negative | Same | 19 |
| Hepatitis C antibody | Negative | Same | 19 |
| Hepatitis C-RNA assay | Negative | Same | 19 |
| Hepatitis D antibody | Negative | Same | 19 |
| Hepatitis E antibody | Negative | Same | 19 |
| High-density lipoprotein (HDL) | | | 15 |
| Male | 44–45 mg/dL | 1.24–1.27 mmol/L | 15 |
| Female | 55 mg/dL | 1.425 mmol/L | 15 |
| Histoplasmosis antibody titer | <1 : 4; negative | Same | 7 |
| Human chorionic gonadotropin | | | 22 |
| Male and nonpregnant female | Negative; <5 mIU/mL | Same; <5 IU/L | 22 |
| Pregnant female | Positive | Same | 22 |
| Human immunodeficiency virus tests | | | |
| Human immunodeficiency virus antibody | Negative | Same | 7 |
| p24 antigen | Negative | Same | 7 |
| DNA-PCR amplification | No HIV viral DNA detected | Same | 7 |
| CD4$^+$ (T4) lymphocytes | 800–1,100 cells/mm$^3$; 40% of total lymphocytes | Same | 7 |
| CD4$^+$ : CD8$^+$ (T4 : T8) ratio | 1.0–3.5 | Same | 7 |
| HIV-RNA concentration | No HIV viral RNA copies are detected | Same | 7 |
| Human leukocyte antigen | No destruction of lymphocytes | Same | 17 |
| Insulin | | | 20 |
| Adult | 5–25 µU/mL | 34–172 pmol/L | 20 |
| Newborn | 3–20 µU/mL | 21–138 pmol/L | 20 |

*(continued on the following page)*

**Table E–1   Normal Values: Whole Blood, Serum, and Plasma Tests** (continued)

| Name of Test | Conventional Values | SI Units | Chapter Number |
|---|---|---|---|
| Insulin (continued) | | | |
|   1 hr after eating | 50–130 µU/mL | 347.3–902.8 pmol/L | 20 |
|   2 hr after eating | <30 µU/mL | <208.4 pmol/L | 20 |
| Intrinsic factor antibodies | Negative | Same | 17 |
| Iron | | | |
|   Adult male | 65–175 µg/dL | 11.6–31.3 µmol/L | 17 |
|   Adult female | 50–170 µg/dL | 9–30.4 µmol/L | 17 |
|   Child | 50–120 µg/dL | 9–21.5 µmol/L | 17 |
|   Infant | 40–100 µg/dL | 7.2–17.9 µmol/L | 17 |
|   Newborn | 100–250 µg/dL | 17.9–44.8 µmol/L | 17 |
| Ketones | <2 mg/dL | <0.34 nmol/L | 20 |
| Lactic acid | 8.1–15.3 mEq/L | 0.9–1.7 mmol/L | 14 |
| | | | 15 |
| Lactic acid dehydrogenase | | | 15 |
|   Adult | 200–400 U/L | Same | 15 |
|   Neonate | 400–700 U/L | Same | 15 |
| LDH isoenzymes | | | 15 |
|   LDH$_1$ | 14%–26% | 0.14–0.26 (fraction of total LDH) | 15 |
|   LDH$_2$ | 29%–39% | 0.29–0.39 (fraction of total LDH) | 15 |
|   LDH$_3$ | 20%–26% | 0.20–0.26 (fraction of total LDH) | 15 |
|   LDH$_4$ | 8%–16% | 0.08–0.16 (fraction of total LDH) | 15 |
|   LDH$_5$ | 6%–16% | 0.06–0.16 (fraction of total LDH) | 15 |
| LDL : HDL Ratio | <3 | Same | 15 |
| LE test | Negative | Same | 24 |
| Leucine aminopeptidase | 55.2 ± 10.6 U/L | 0.94 ± 0.18 µKat/L | 19 |
| Lipase (adult) | <200 U/L | <3.4 µKat/L | 19 |
| Lipids, total | 400–800 mg/dL | 4.0–8.0 g/L | 15 |
| Long-acting thyroid stimulator | Negative | Same | 20 |
| Low-density lipoprotein (LDL) | <130 mg/dL | <3.37 mmol/L | 15 |
| Luteinizing hormone | | | 22 |
|   Adult male | 1–8 mU/mL | 1–8 U/L | 22 |
|   Adult female | | | |
|     Follicular phase | 1–12 mU/mL | 1–12 U/L | 22 |
|     Midcycle peak | 16–104 mU/mL | 16–104 U/L | 22 |
|     Luteal phase | 1–12 mU/mL | 1–12 U/L | 22 |
|     Postmenopausal | 16–66 mU/mL | 16–66 U/L | 22 |
|   Child (6 mo–10 yr) | 1–5 mU/mL | 1–5 U/L | 22 |
| Lyme disease antibody | Negative for *Borrelia burgdorferi* | Same | 7 |
| Magnesium | | | |
|   Adult | 1.6–2.6 mg/dL | 0.66–1.07 mmol/L | 5 |

**Table E–1    Normal Values: Whole Blood, Serum, and Plasma Tests** *(continued)*

| Name of Test | Conventional Values | SI Units | Chapter Number |
|---|---|---|---|
| Magnesium *(continued)* | | | |
| Child 12–20 yr | 1.7–2.2 mg/dL | 0.70–0.91 mmol/L | 5 |
| 6–12 yr | 1.7–2.1 mg/dL | 0.70–0.86 mmol/L | 5 |
| 5 mo–6 yr | 1.7–2.3 mg/dL | 0.70–0.95 mmol/L | 5 |
| Newborn | 1.5–2.2 mg/dL | 0.62–0.91 mmol/L | 5 |
| Malaria smear | No organisms identified | Same | 7 |
| Measles antibody | | | 7 |
| IgM | <1:10; negative | Same | 7 |
| IgG | <1:5; negative | Same | 7 |
| Metyrapone testing (11-deoxycortisol) | >7 µg/dL | 202 nmol/L | 20 |
| Microfilariae smear | No organisms identified | Same | 7 |
| Mononucleosis tests | | | 7 |
| Monotest | Negative, nonreactive | Same | 7 |
| Heterophil titer | <1:56 | Same | 7 |
| Mumps antibody | | | 7 |
| IgM | <1–10; negative | Same | 7 |
| IgG | <1–5; negative | Same | 7 |
| Myoglobin | 90 µg/L | Same | 15 |
| Neutrophil alkaline phosphatase | 40–130 | Same | 17 |
| Osmolarity | | | |
| Adult | 285–300 mOsm/kg H$_2$O | 280–300 mmol/kg | 20 |
| Child | 270–290 mOsm/kg H$_2$O | 270–290 mmol/kg | 20 |
| Osmotic fragility | | | 17 |
| Initial hemolysis | 0.45% NaCl | 4.5 g/L NaCl | 17 |
| Complete hemolysis | 0.35% NaCl | 3.5 g/L NaCl | 17 |
| Parathyroid hormone | | | |
| Intact parathyroid hormone | 210–310 pg/mL | 210–310 ng/L | 20 |
| N-terminal fraction | 230–630 pg/mL | 230–630 ng/L | 20 |
| C-terminal fraction | 410–1,760 pg/mL | 410–1,760 ng/L | 20 |
| Parietal cell antibody | Negative | Same | 17 |
| pH, adult, arterial | 7.35–7.45 | Same | 14 |
| Fetal scalp | 7.25–7.35 | Same | 22 |
| Adult, mixed venous | 7.33–7.43 | 7.33–7.43 | 14 |
| Phenylalanine | | | 21 |
| Guthrie test | <2 mg/day/L | 121 µmol/L | 21 |
| Fluorometry method | | | |
| Normal newborn | 1.2–3.4 mg/dL | 73–206 µmol/L | 21 |
| Premature newborn | 2–7.5 mg/dL | 121–454 µmol/L | 21 |
| Adult | 0.8–1.8 mg/dL | 48–109 µmol/L | 21 |
| Phosphorus | | | |
| Adult | | | |
| 12–60 yr | 2.7–4.5 mg/dL | 0.87–1.45 mmol/L | 5 |
| Male, >60 yr | 2.3–3.7 mg/dL | 0.74–1.2 mmol/L | 5 |
| Female, >60 yr | 2.8–4.1 mg/dL | 0.90–1.32 mmol/L | 5 |
| Child | | | |
| 2–12 yr | 4.5–5.5 mg/dL | 1.45–1.78 mmol/L | 5 |

*(continued on the following page)*

**Table E–1 Normal Values: Whole Blood, Serum, and Plasma Tests** *(continued)*

| Name of Test | Conventional Values | SI Units | Chapter Number |
|---|---|---|---|
| Phosphorus *(continued)* | | | 5 |
| 10 days–2 yr | 4.5–6.7 mg/dL | 1.45–2.16 mmol/L | 5 |
| 0–10 days | 4.5–9 mg/dL | 1.45–2.91 mmol/L | 5 |
| Plasma volume | 40–50 mL/kg | Same | 17 |
| Platelet aggregation | 3–5 min | Same | 6 |
| Platelet count | | | 4 |
| Adult | 150,000–450,000 cells/µL | 150–450 × 10⁹/L | 4 |
| Newborn (1–3 days) | 150,000–400,000 | 150–400 × 10⁹/L | 4 |
| Platelet indices | | | |
| Mean platelet volume | 7.4–10.4 fL | Same | 4 |
| Platelet distribution width | 2–4 microns in diameter | Same | 4 |
| Potassium | | | 5 |
| Adult | 3.5–5.1 mEq/L | 3.5–5.1 mmol/L | 5 |
| Child | 3.4–4.7 mEq/L | 3.4–4.7 mmol/L | 5 |
| Infant | 4.1–5.3 mEq/L | 4.1–5.3 mmol/L | 5 |
| Newborn | 3.7–5.9 mEq/L | 3.7–5.9 mmol/L | 5 |
| Premature (48 hr) | 3.0–6.0 mEq/L | 3.0–6.0 mmol/L | 5 |
| Progesterone | | | 22 |
| Adult male | 13–97 ng/dL | 0.4–3.1 nmol/L | 22 |
| Menstruating female | | | |
| Follicular phase | 15–70 ng/dL | 0.5–2.2 nmol/L | 22 |
| Luteal phase | 200–2,500 ng/dL | 6.4–79.5 nmol/L | 22 |
| Pregnant female | | | 22 |
| 1st trimester | 1,025–4,400 ng/dL | 32.6–139.9 nmol/L | 22 |
| 2nd trimester | 1,950–8,250 ng/dL | 62.0–262.4 nmol/L | 22 |
| 3rd trimester | 6,500–22,900 ng/dL | 206.7–728.2 nmol/L | 22 |
| Prolactin | | | 22 |
| Adult | 0–20 ng/mL | 0–20 µg/L | 22 |
| Pregnancy (third trimester) | 95–473 ng/mL | 95–473 µg/L | 22 |
| Newborn | <30–495 ng/mL | 30–495 µg/L | 22 |
| Prostate-specific antigen | | | 21 |
| 40–49 yr | <1.5 ng/mL | <1.5 µg/L | 21 |
| 50–59 yr | <2.5 ng/mL | <2.5 µg/L | 21 |
| 60–69 yr | <4.5 ng/mL | <4.5 µg/L | 21 |
| 70–80 yr | <7.5 ng/mL | <7.5 µg/L | 21 |
| Prostatic acid phosphatase | | | 21 |
| 4-Nitrophenyl phosphate method (male) | 0.13–0.63 U/L | 2.2–10.5 U/L | 21 |
| Tartrate resistance fraction (male) | 0.2–3.5 U/L | 2.2–10.5 U/L | 21 |
| Thymolphthalein monophosphate method | <1.9 U/L | Same | 21 |
| Protein C | 2.82–5.65 µg/mL | 2.82–5.65 mg/L | 6 |
| | 70%–140% | 0.70–1.40 | 6 |
| Protein electrophoresis | | | 19 |
| Adult | | | |
| Albumin | 3.5–5 g/dL | 35–50 g/L | 19 |
| Alpha₁-globulin | 0.1–0.3 g/dL | 1–3 g/L | 19 |

p.514

## Table E–1    Normal Values: Whole Blood, Serum, and Plasma Tests *(continued)*

| Name of Test | Conventional Values | SI Units | Chapter Number |
|---|---|---|---|
| Protein electrophoresis *(continued)* | | | |
| Adult | | | |
|   Alpha$_2$-globulin | 0.6–1 g/dL | 6–10 g/L | 19 |
|   Beta globulin | 0.7–1.1 g/dL | 7–11 g/L | 19 |
|   Gamma globulin | 0.8–1.6 g/dL | 8–16 g/L | 19 |
| Child | | | |
|   Albumin | 3.6–5.2 g/dL | 36–52 g/L | 19 |
|   Alpha$_1$-globulin | 0.1–0.4 g/dL | 1–4 g/L | 19 |
|   Alpha$_2$-globulin | 0.5–1.2 g/dL | 5–12 g/L | 19 |
|   Beta globulin | 0.5–1.1 g/dL | 5–11 g/L | 19 |
|   Gamma globulin | 0.5–1.7 g/dL | 5–17 g/L | 19 |
| Protein S | 21–42 µg/mL | 21–42 mg/L | 6 |
| | 67%–140% | 0.67–1.40 | |
| Protein, total | | | 19 |
|   Adult, ambulatory | 6.4–8.3 g/dL | 64–83 g/L | 19 |
|   Adult, recumbent | 6–7.8 g/dL | 60–78 g/L | 19 |
|   Child >3 yr | 6–8 g/dL | 60–80 g/L | 19 |
|   Newborn | 4–7 g/dL | 40–70 g/L | 19 |
| Prothrombin time | | | |
|   Average | 10–13 sec | Same | 6 |
|   Newborn to 6 mo | 13–18 sec | Same | 6 |
| Prothrombin time, INR | 1.00–1.30 | Same | 6 |
| Red cell count | | | |
|   Male | 4.5–5.9 × 10$^6$/µL | 4.5–5.9 × 10$^{12}$/L | 4 |
|   Female | 4.5–5.1 × 10$^6$/µL | 4.5–5.1 × 10$^{12}$/L | 4 |
| Red cell indices | | | |
|   Mean corpuscular volume | 80–96 µm$^3$ | 80–96 fL | 4 |
|   Mean corpuscular hemoglobin | 27.5–33.2 pg | 27.5–33.2 pg | 4 |
|   Mean corpuscular hemoglobin concentration | 33.4%–35.5% | 0.334–0.355 (mean concentration fraction) | 4 |
|   Red cell distribution width | 13.1% (range: 11.6%–14.6%) *p. 68* | | 4 |
| Red cell volume | | | 17 |
|   Male | 25–35 mL/kg | Same | 17 |
|   Female | 20–30 mL/kg | Same | 17 |
| Renin | | | 20 |
| Adult | | | |
|   Recumbent position | 0.2–1.6 ng/mL/hr | 0.2–1.6 µg/hr$^{-1}$ × L$^{-1}$ | 20 |
|   Upright position | 0.7–3.33 ng/mL/hr | 0.7–3.33 µg/hr$^{-1}$ × L$^{-1}$ | 20 |
|   Infant | 2.4–37.0 ng/mL/hr | 2.4–37 µg/hr$^{-1}$ × L$^-$ | 20 |
|   Young child | 1.0–11.2 ng/mL/hr | 1.0–11.2 µg/hr$^{-1}$ × L$^{-1}$ | 20 |
|   Child | 0.5–5.9 ng/mL/hr | 0.5–5.9 µg/hr$^{-1}$ × L$^{-1}$ | 20 |

*(continued on the following page)*

**Table E–1    Normal Values: Whole Blood, Serum, and Plasma Tests** (continued)

| Name of Test | Conventional Values | SI Units | Chapter Number |
|---|---|---|---|
| Resin triiodothyronine uptake | 25%–35% | 0.25–0.35 | 20 |
| Rheumatoid factor | Negative | Negative | 24 |
| Rubella antibody | | | |
|    IgM | Negative | Same | 7 |
|    IgG | <1:4; negative | Same | 7 |
| Serotonin | 50–200 ng/mL | 0.28–1.14 µmol/L | 18 |
| Sickle cell test | Negative | Same | 17 |
| Sodium | | | |
|    Adult | 136–145 mEq/L | 136–145 mmol/L | 5 |
|    Child | 138–145 mEq/L | 136–145 mmol/L | 5 |
|    Infant | 139–146 mEq/L | 139–146 mmol/L | 5 |
|    Newborn | 133–146 mEq/L | 133–146 mmol/L | 5 |
|    Premature (48 hr) | 128–148 mEq/L | 128–148 mmol/L | 5 |
| Syphilis tests | | | |
|    Venereal Disease Research Laboratory | Negative; nonreactive | Same | 7 |
|    Rapid plasma reagin | Negative; nonreactive | Same | 7 |
|    Fluorescent treponemal antibody absorption | Negative; nonreactive | Same | 7 |
|    Microhemagglutination assay–*Treponema pallidum* | Negative; nonreactive | Same | 7 |
| Testosterone, free | | | 22 |
|    Adult | | | 22 |
|       Male | 50–210 pg/mL | 174–729 pmol/L | 22 |
|       Female | 1.0–8.5 pg/mL | 3.5–29.5 pmol/L | 22 |
|    Child (6–9 yr) | | | 22 |
|       Male | 0.1–3.2 pg/mL | 0.3–11.1 pmol/L | 22 |
|       Female | 0.1–0.9 pg/mL | 0.3–3.1 pmol/L | 22 |
| Testosterone, total | | | 22 |
|    Adult | | | 22 |
|       Male | 280–1,100 ng/dL | 9.72–38.17 nmol/L | 22 |
|       Female | 15–70 ng/dL | 0.52–2.43 nmol/L | 22 |
|    Child (1–5 yr) | | | 22 |
|       Male | 0.3–30.0 ng/dL | 0.10–1.04 nmol/L | 22 |
|       Female | 2–20 ng/dL | 0.07–0.69 nmol/L | 22 |
| Thyroglobulin autoantibodies | Titer <1:100; negative | Same | 20 |
| Thyroid microsomal autoantibodies | Titer <1:100; negative | Same | 20 |
| Thyrotropin | | | 20 |
|    Adult | 0.4–8.9 U/mL | 0.4–8.9 mU/L | 20 |
|    Newborn | <20 U/mL | <20 mU/L | 20 |
| Thyrotropin-releasing hormone test | | | 20 |
|    Thyroid-stimulating hormone value | | | 20 |
|       Male | 14–24 µU/mL | 14–24 mU/L | 20 |
|       Female | 16–26 µU/mL | 16–26 mU/L | 20 |
| Thyroxine-binding hormone | | | 20 |
|    Adult | 1.2–3.0 mg/dL | 12–30 mg/L | 20 |
|    Child | 2.9–5.0 mg/dL | 29–50 mg/L | 20 |
|    Infant | 1.6–4.2 mg/dL | 16–42 mg/L | 20 |
| Thyroxine, free | 0.9–1.7 mg/dL | 11.5–21.8 nmol/L | 20 |

**Table E–1    Normal Values: Whole Blood, Serum, and Plasma Tests** (continued)

| Name of Test | Conventional Values | SI Units | Chapter Number |
|---|---|---|---|
| Thyroxine, total | | | 20 |
|   Adult | 5–12 µg/dL | 64.4–154.4 nmol/L | 20 |
|   Child | | | |
|     10–20 yr | 4.2–11.8 µg/dL | 54.11–151.9 nmol/L | 20 |
|     1–10 yr | 6.4–15 µg/dL | 82.41–93.1 nmol/L | 20 |
|     2–10 mo | 7.8–16.5 µg/dL | 100.4–212.4 nmol/L | 20 |
|     Newborn | 6.4–23.2 µg/dL | 82.4–298.6 nmol/L | 20 |
| Tolbutamide stimulation test | | | 20 |
|   Serum insulin level | <195 µU/mL | 1,354 pmol/L | 20 |
| Total blood volume | 60–80 mL/kg | Same | 17 |
| Total iron-binding capacity | 250–425 µg/dL | 44.8–76.1 µmol/L | 17 |
| Toxoplasmosis antibody | <1:16; negative | Same | 7 |
| Transferrin | | | |
|   Adult (>60 yr) | 190–375 mg/dL | 1.9–3.75 g/L | 17 |
|   Adult (16–60 yr) | | | |
|     Male | 215–365 mg/dL | 2.15–3.65 g/L | 17 |
|     Female | 250–380 mg/dL | 2.50–3.80 g/L | 17 |
|   Child (3 mo–16 yr) | 203–360 mg/dL | 2.03–3.6 g/L | 17 |
|   Newborn | 130–275 mg/dL | 1.3–2.75 g/L | 17 |
| Transferrin saturate | 20%–50% | 0.20–0.50 fraction saturation | 17 |
| Triglycerides | | | 15 |
|   Male (<40 yr) | 46–316 mg/dL | 0.52–3.57 mmol/L | 15 |
|   Male (>50 yr) | 75–313 mg/dL | 0.85–3.5 mmol/L | 15 |
|   Female (<40 yr) | 37–174 mg/dL | 0.42–1.97 mmol/L | 15 |
|   Female (>50 yr) | 52–200 mg/dL | 0.59–2.26 mmol/L | 15 |
| Triiodothyronine | | | 20 |
|   Adult | 40–204 ng/dL | 0.6–3.1 nmol/L | 20 |
|   Child | | | |
|     10–20 yr | 80–213 ng/dL | 1.2–3.3 nmol/L | 20 |
|     1–10 yr | 105–269 ng/dL | 1.6–4.1 nmol/L | 20 |
|     1–12 mo | 105–245 ng/dL | 1.6–3.7 nmol/L | 20 |
|     Newborn | 100–740 ng/dL | 1.5–11.4 nmol/L | 20 |
| Triiodothyronine, free | 260–480 pg/dL | 4.0–7.4 pmol/L | 20 |
| Troponin | | | |
|   Cardiac troponin T | <0.2 µg/L | Same | 15 |
|   Cardiac troponin I | <0.35 µg/L | Same | 15 |
| Trypsinogen | | | |
|   CIS method | <80 µg/L | Same | 19 |
|   ELISA method | | | |
|   Neonate 1–4 days | 55–109 µg/L | Same | 19 |
|   Infant 4–6 wk | 70–104 µg/L | Same | 19 |
| Urea nitrogen | | | 21 |
|   Adult (>60 yr) | 8–23 mg/dL | 2.9–8.2 mmol/L | 21 |
|   Child to adult (1–60 yr) | 5–20 mg/dL | 1.8–7.1 mmol/L | 21 |
|   Infant (birth–1 yr) | 4–19 mg/dL | 1.4–6.8 mmol/L | 21 |

(continued on the following page)

**Table E–1    Normal Values: Whole Blood, Serum, and Plasma Tests** (continued)

| Name of Test | Conventional Values | SI Units | Chapter Number |
|---|---|---|---|
| Uric acid | | | 24 |
|   Adult | | | |
|     Male | 4.4–7.6 mg/dL | 262–452 µmol/L | 24 |
|     Female | 2.3–6.6 mg/dL | 137–393 µmol/L | 24 |
|   Adult 60–90 yr | | | |
|     Male | 4.2–8 mg/dL | 250–476 µmol/L | 24 |
|     Female | 2.2–7.7 mg/dL | 208–434 µmol/L | 24 |
|   Child <12 yr | 2.0–5.5 mg/dL | 119–327 µmol/L | 24 |
| Varicella-zoster antibody | | | |
|   IgM | Negative | Same | 7 |
|   IgG | <1 : 4; negative | Same | 7 |
| Vasopressin | | | |
|   With serum osmolality >290 mOsm/kg | 2–12 pg/mL | 1.85–11.1 pmol/L | 20 |
|   With serum osmolality <290 mOsm/kg | <2 pg/mL | <1.85 pmol/L | 20 |
| Vitamin $B_{12}$ assay | | | |
|   Adult | 200–835 pg/mL | 148–616 pmol/L | 17 |
|   Adult (60–90 yr) | 100–770 pg/mL | 81–568 pmol/L | 17 |
|   Newborn | 160–1,300 pg/mL | 118–959 pmol/L | 17 |
| Vitamin D, activated | 25–45 pg/mL | 60–108 nmol/L | 20 |
| White cell count | | | |
|   Adult | 4.5–11 × $10^3$/µL | 4.5–11 × $10^9$/L | 4 |
|   Child (1 yr) | 6,000–17,500 cells/µL | 6–17.5 × $10^9$/L | 4 |
|   Newborn | 18,000–22,000 cells/µL | 18–22 × $10^9$/L | 4 |
| White cell differential | | | |
|   Segmented neurotrophils | 56% | 0.56 (mean number fraction) | 4 |
| | 1,800–7,800 cells/µL | 1.8–7.8 × $10^9$/L | 4 |
|   Bands | 3% | 0.03 (mean number fraction) | 4 |
| | 0–700 cells/µL | 0–0.07 × $10^9$/L | 4 |
|   Eosinophils | 2.7% | 0.027 (mean number fraction) | 4 |
| | 0–450 cells/µL | 0–0.45 × $10^9$/L | 4 |
|   Basophils | 0.3% | 0.003 (mean number fraction) | 4 |
| | 0–200 cells/µL | 0–0.2 × $10^9$/L | 4 |
|   Lymphocytes | 34% | 0.34 (mean number fraction) | 4 |
| | 1,000–4,800 cells/µL | 1–4.8 × $10^9$/L | 4 |
|   Monocytes | 4% | 0.04 (mean number fraction) | 4 |
| | 0–800 cells/µL | 0–0.8 × $10^9$/L | 4 |

## Table F–1  Normal Values: Urine Tests

| Name of Test | Conventional Values | SI Units | Chapter Number |
|---|---|---|---|
| Albumin | | | |
|   Microalbumin | <2 mg/dL | <0.02 g/L | 21 |
|   Reagent strip | Negative | Same | 21 |
| Aldosterone | 2–26 µg/24 hr | 6–72 nmol/24 hr | 20 |
| Amylase | | | 19 |
|   1-hr test | 2–19 U/1 hr | Same | 19 |
|   2-hr test | 4–37 U/2 hr | Same | 19 |
|   24-hr test | 170–2,000 U/24 hr | 2.89–34.0 µKat/L | 19 |
| Calcium | | | 21 |
|   Adult (normal calcium intake) | 100–300 mg/day | 2.5–7.5 mmol/day | 21 |
|   Adult (low calcium intake) | 50–100 mg/day | 1.25–3.75 mmol/day | 21 |
|   Adult (calcium-free diet) | 5–40 mg/day | 0.13–1 mmol/day | 21 |
|   Infant and child | <6 mg/kg/day | <0.15 mmol/kg/day | 21 |
| Catecholamines | | | 21 |
|   Norepinephrine | 15–56 µg/24 hr | 88.6–331 nmol/24 hr | 20 |
|   Epinephrine | <20 pg/mL | <109 nmol/24 hr | 20 |
|   Dopamine | 100–400 pg/mL | 625–2,750 nmol/24 hr | 20 |
|   Vanillymandelic acid | 2–7 mg/24 hr | 10–35 µmol/24 hr | 20 |
|   Metanephrine | 24–96 µg/24 hr | 131–524 nmol/24 hr | 20 |
|   Normetanephrine | 75–375 µg/24 hr | 409–2,047 nmol/24 hr | 20 |
|   Homovanillic acid | 2–12 mg/24 hr | 10.98–65.88 µmol/24 hr | 20 |
| Chloride | | | 21 |
|   Adult | 110–250 mEq/24 hr | 110–250 mmol/24 hr | 21 |
|   Adult (>60 yr) | 95–195 mEq/24 hr | 95–195 mmol/24 hr | 21 |
|   Child (<6 yr) | 15–40 mEq/24 hr | 15–40 mmol/24 hr | 21 |
|   Child (6–10 yr) | | | |
|     Male | 36–110 mEq/24 hr | 36–110 mmol/24 hr | 21 |
|     Female | 18–74 mEq/24 hr | 18–74 mmol/24 hr | 21 |
|   Child (10–14 yr) | | | |
|     Male | 64–176 mEq/24 hr | 64–176 mmol/24 hr | 21 |
|     Female | 36–173 mEq/24 hr | 36–173 mmol/24 hr | 21 |
|   Infant | 2–10 mEq/24 hr | 2–10 mmol/24 hr | 21 |
| Cortisol, free | 20–90 µg/24 hr | 55–248 nmol/24 hr | 21 |
| Creatinine clearance | | | 21 |
|   Adult male | 1–2 g/day | 8.8–17.7 mmol/day | 21 |
| | 90–139 mL/min/1.73 m² | 0.87–1.34 mL/sec/m² | 21 |
|   Adult female | 0.8–1.8 g/day | 7.1–15.9 mmol/day | 21 |
| | 80–125 mL/min/1.73m² | 0.77–1.2 mL/sec/m² | 21 |
|   Child | 70–140 mL/min/ 1.73 m² | 1.17–2.33 mL/sec/m² | 21 |

(continued on the following page)

## Table F–1    Normal Values: Urine Tests *(continued)*

| Name of Test | Conventional Values | SI Units | Chapter Number |
|---|---|---|---|
| Dexamethasone suppression | | | 20 |
|   17-hydroxycorticosteroid (17-OHCS) | <4 ng/24 hr | <138 nmol/L | 20 |
|   Free cortisol | <25 µg/24 hr | 691 nmol/L | 20 |
| D-Xylose absorption | | | 18 |
|   Child | 16%–33% of ingested dose/5 hr | 0.16–0.33 (fraction of ingested dose) | 18 |
|   Adult (5-g dose) | >1.2 g/5 hr | >8.00 mmol/L/5 hr | 18 |
|   Adult (25-g dose) | >4 g/5 hr | 126.64 mmol/L | 18 |
|   Adult (>65 yr) | 3.5 g/5 hr | 23.31 mmol/L | 18 |
| Estriol, pregnancy | | | 22 |
|   First trimester | 0–800 µg/24 hr | 0–2,776 nmol/24 hr | 22 |
|   Second trimester | 800–12,000 µg/24 hr | 2,776–41,640 nmol/24 hr | 22 |
|   Third trimester | 5,000–50,000 µg/24 hr | 17,350–173,500 nmol/24 hr | 22 |
| Estrogens, total | | | 22 |
|   Female | | | 22 |
|     Postmenopausal | <20 µg/24 hr | 69 µmol/24 hr | 22 |
|     Premenopausal | 15–80 µg/24 hr | 52–277 µmol/24 hr | 22 |
|   Male | 15–40 µg/24 hr | 52–139 µmol/24 hr | 22 |
|   Child | <10 µg/24 hr | <35 µmol/24 hr | 22 |
| Fibrin breakdown products | <0.25 µg/mL | <0.25 mg/L | 6 |
| Follicle-stimulating hormone | | | 22 |
|   Adult | | | |
|     Male | 3–11 U/24 hr | 3–11 IU/24 hr | 22 |
|     Female, non-midcycle | 2–15 U/24 hr | 2–15 IU/24 hr | 22 |
|     Child, prepuberty | <1.0–3.4 U/24 hr | <1.0–3.4 IU/24 hr | 22 |
| Hydroxyindoleacetic acid, quantitative, adult | 1–9 mg/24 hr | 5–48 µmol/24 hr | 18 |
| Glucose | Negative | Negative | 20 |
| Hemosiderin | Negative | Same | 17 |
| Human chorionic gonadotropin | | | 22 |
|   Male, nonpregnant female | Negative | Same | 22 |
|   Pregnant female | Positive | Same | 22 |
| Ketones | Negative | Same | 20 |
| Lactose (24 hr) | | | 20 |
|   Adult | 12–40 mg/dL | 0.7–2.2 mmol/L | 18 |
|   Child | <1.5 mg/100 dL | NA | 18 |
| Luteinizing hormone | | | 22 |
|   Adult | | | |
|     Male | 9–23 U/24 hr | Same | 22 |
|     Female | 4–30 U/24 hr | Same | 22 |
|   Child (1–10 yr) | | | |
|     Male | <1–5.6 U/24 hr | Same | 22 |
|     Female | 1.4–4.9 U/24 hr | Same | 22 |
| Magnesium | 7.3–12.2 mg/dl | 3–5 mmol/day | 21 |
| Myoglobin | Negative | Same | 24 |
| | <0.4 mg/dL | <4 mg/L | 24 |

## Table F–1   Normal Values: Urine Tests (continued)

| Name of Test | Conventional Values | SI Units | Chapter Number |
|---|---|---|---|
| Osmolarity | | | |
| 24-hr specimen | 500–800 mOsm/kg H$_2$O | 500–800 mmol/kg H$_2$O | 20 |
| Random specimen | 50–1,200 mOsm/kg H$_2$O | 50–1,200 mmol/kg H$_2$O | 20 |
| Ova and parasites | Negative | Same | 7 |
| Phenylalanine | Negative | Same | 21 |
| Potassium | | | |
| Adult | 25–125 mEq/24 hr | 25–125 mmol/24 hr | 21 |
| Child (6–10 yr) | | | |
| Male | 17–54 mEq/24 hr | 17–54 mmol/24 hr | 21 |
| Female | 8–37 mEq/24 hr | 8–37 mmol/24 hr | 21 |
| Child (10–14 yr) | | | |
| Male | 22–57 mEq/24 hr | 22–57 mmol/24 hr | 21 |
| Female | 18–58 mEq/24 hr | 18–58 mmol/24 hr | 21 |
| Infant | 4.1–5.3 mEq/24 hr | 4.1–5.3 mmol/24 hr | 21 |
| Pregnanetriol | | | 22 |
| Adult | | | |
| Male | 0.4–2.5 mg/day | 1.2–7.5 µmol/day | 22 |
| Female | | | 22 |
| Follicular phase | 0.1–1.8 mg/day | 0.3–5.3 µmol/day | |
| Luteal phase | 0.9–2.2 mg/day | 2.7–6.5 µmol/day | |
| Child | | | |
| 0–5 yr | <0.1 mg/day | <0.3 µmol/day | 22 |
| 6–9 yr | <0.3 mg/day | <0.9 µmol/day | 22 |
| Protein | 40–150 mg/24 hr | Same | 21 |
| Protein electrophoresis | 40–150 ng/24 hr | 40–150 mg/24 hr | 21 |
| Schilling test | | | 17 |
| Stage 1 | >10 cobalt 58, vitamin B$_{12}$ excretion/24 hr | >0.10 (fraction of dose excreted) | 17 |
| Stage 2 | 0%–42% cobalt 57, vitamin B$_{12}$ + intrinsic factor excretion/24-hr | 0.00–0.42 (fraction of dose excreted) | 17 |
| Cobalt 57 to cobalt 58 ratio | 0.7–1.3 | Same | 17 |
| 17-Hydroxycorticosteroids | | | 20 |
| Adult male | 4.5–12 mg/24 hr | 12.4–33.1 µmol/24 hr | 20 |
| Adult female | 2.5–10 mg/24 hr | 6.9–27.6 µmol/24 hr | 20 |
| Child | | | |
| 8–12 yr | <4.5 mg/24 hr | <12.4 µmol/24 hr | 20 |
| <8 yr | <1.5 mg/24 hr | <4.14 µmol/24 hr | 20 |
| 17-Ketogenic steroids | | | |
| Adult male | 4–14 mg/24 hr | 13–49 µmol/24 hr | 20 |
| Adult female | 2–12 mg/24 hr | 7–42 µmol/24 hr | 20 |
| Child | | | |
| 11–14 yr | 2–9 mg/24 hr | 7–31 µmol/24 hr | 20 |
| <11 yr | 0.1–4 mg/24 hr | 0.3–14 µmol/24 hr | 20 |

(continued on the following page)

**Table F–1   Normal Values: Urine Tests** (continued)

| Name of Test | Conventional Values | SI Units | Chapter Number |
|---|---|---|---|
| 17-Ketosteroids | | | |
|   Adult male | 10–25 mg/24 hr | 35–87 µmol/24 hr | 20 |
|   Adult female | 6–14 mg/24 hr | 21–49 µmol/24 hr | 20 |
|   Child | | | |
|     10–14 yr | 1–6 mg/24 hr | 2–21 µmol/24 hr | 20 |
|     <10 yr | <3 mg/24 hr | <10 µmol/24 hr | 20 |
| Sodium | | | |
|   Adult | 40–220 mEq/24 hr | 40–220 mmol/24 hr | 21 |
|   Child (6–10 yr) | | | |
|     Male | 41–115 mEq/24 hr | 41–115 mmol/24 hr | 21 |
|     Female | 20–69 mEq/24 hr | 20–69 mmol/24 hr | 21 |
|   Child (10–14 yr) | | | |
|     Male | 63–117 mEq/24 hr | 63–117 mmol/24 hr | 21 |
|     Female | 48–168 mEq/24 hr | 48–168 mmol/24 hr | 21 |
| Specific gravity | 1.003–1.029 | Same | 21 |
| Uric acid | | | 21 |
|   Average diet (adult) | 250–750 mg/24 hr | 1.48–4.43 mmol/24 hr | 21 |
|   Low purine diet (male) | <420 mg/24 hr | <2.83 mmol/24 hr | 21 |
|   Low purine diet (female) | <400 mg/24 hr | <2.36 mmol/24 hr | 21 |
|   High purine diet (adult) | <1,000 mg/24 hr | <5.9 mmol/24 hr | 21 |
| Urobilinogen | | | |
|   Male | 0.3–2.1 mg/2 hr | 0.5–3.6 µmol/2 hr | 19 |
|   Female | 0.1–1.1 mg/2 hr | 0.2–1.9 µmol/2 hr | 19 |
| Water deprivation test | | | 20 |
|   Specific gravity | 1.025–1.032 | Same | 20 |
|   Osmolality | >800 mOsm/kg | >800 mmol/kg | 20 |

## Table G-1    Normal Values: Body Fluids

| Body Fluid | Name of Test | Conventional Values | SI Units | Chapter Number |
|---|---|---|---|---|
| Amniotic fluid | Chromosome analysis | Normal karyotype | Same | 22 |
| | Alpha$_1$-fetoprotein | <2.5 MOM (multiple of median) | Same | 22 |
| | Acetylcholinesterase | Negative | Same | 22 |
| | Rh incompatibility | Negative to 1+ | Same | 22 |
| | Bilirubin | 0.01–0.03 mg/dL | 0.02–0.06 µmol/L | 22 |
| | Creatinine | | | |
| | 36 wk gestation | 1.6–1.8 mg/dL | 141–159 µmol/L | 22 |
| | 37–38 wk gestation | >2 mg/dL | >177 µmol/L | 22 |
| | Lecithin/sphingomyelin ratio | >2 | Same | 22 |
| | Phosphatidylglycerol | Present | Same | 22 |
| | Pulmonary surfactant | Present | Same | 22 |
| | | Foam stability index: >0.48 | N/A | 22 |
| | Meconium | Absent | Same | 22 |
| Cerebrospinal fluid | Pressure | 80–180 mm H$_2$O | Same | 23 |
| | Appearance | Clear, colorless | Same | 23 |
| | Leukocytes | | | |
| | Adult | 0–5 cells/µL | 0–5 × 10$^6$/L | 23 |
| | Child | 0–10 cells/µL | 0–10 × 10$^6$/L | 23 |
| | Infant | 0–30 cells/µL | 0–30 × 10$^6$/L | 23 |
| | Differential | | | 23 |
| | Adult | | | |
| | Lymphocytes | 40%–80% | 0.40–0.80 number fraction | 23 |
| | Monocytes | 15%–45% | 0.15–0.45 number fraction | 23 |
| | Neutrophils | 0%–6% | 0.00–0.06 number fraction | 23 |
| | Neonate | | | |
| | Lymphocytes | 5%–35% | 0.05–0.35 number fraction | 23 |
| | Monocytes | 50%–90% | 0.50–0.90 number fraction | 23 |
| | Neutrophils | 0%–8% | 0.00–0.08 number fraction | 23 |
| | Lactate | 10–22 mg/dL | 1.1–2.4 mmol/L | 23 |
| | Glucose | 50–80 mg/dL | 2.75–4.4 mmol/L | 23 |
| | Total protein | 15–45 mg/dL | 150–450 mg/L | 23 |
| | Albumin | 10–30 mg/dL | 100–300 mg/L | 23 |
| | IgG | 1–4 mg/dL | 10–40 mg/L | 23 |
| | Protein electrophoresis | | | 23 |
| | Prealbumin | 2%–7% | 0.02–0.07 number fraction | 23 |
| | Albumin | 56%–76% | 0.56–0.76 number fraction | 23 |

*(continued on the following page)*

**Table G–1** **Normal Values: Body Fluids** *(continued)*

| Body Fluid | Name of Test | Conventional Values | SI Units | Chapter Number |
|---|---|---|---|---|
| Cerebrospinal fluid *(continued)* | | | | |
| | Alpha$_1$ globulin | 2%–7% | 0.02–0.07 number fraction | 23 |
| | Alpha$_2$ globulin | 4%–12% | 0.04–0.12 number fraction | 23 |
| | Beta globulin | 8%–18% | 0.08–0.18 number fraction | 23 |
| | Gamma globulin | 3%–12% | 0.03–0.12 number fraction | 23 |
| | Myelin–basic protein | <2.5 ng/mL | <2.5 µg/L | 23 |
| | Lyme disease antibody | Negative for *Borrelia bergdorferi* | Same | 7 |
| | Measles antibody | | | 7 |
| |   IgM | <1:10; negative | Same | 7 |
| |   IgG | <1:5; negative | Same | |
| | VDRL | Negative; nonreactive | Same | 7 |
| Effusion fluid | Carcinoembryonic antigen | | | 22 |
| |   Adult (smoker) | Up to 5 ng/mL | Up to 5 g/L | 22 |
| |   Adult (nonsmoker) | <2.5 ng/mL | <2.5 g/L | 22 |
| Gastric secretions | Gastric stimulation | | | 18 |
| |   pH | 1.5–3.5 | Same | 18 |
| |   Basal acid output (BAO) | | | |
| |     Male | 0–10.5 mEq/hr | 0–10.5 mmol/hr | |
| |     Female | 0–5.6 mEq/hr | 0–5.6 mmol/hr | |
| |   Peak acid output | | | 18 |
| |     Male | 12–60 mEq/hr | 12–60 mmol/hr | |
| |     Female | 8–40 mEq/hr | 8–40 mmol/hr | |
| |   BAO to MAO ratio | <20% | <0.20 | 18 |
| Peritoneal fluid | Peritoneal fluid analysis | | | 18 |
| |   Appearance | Clear, odorless, pale yellow, scanty | | 18 |
| |   Ammonia | <50 µg/dL | <35.6 µmol/L | 18 |
| |   Amylase | 138–404 amylase units/L | Same | 18 |
| |   Bacteria-fungi | None present | Same | 18 |
| |   Cells | No malignant cells present | Same | 18 |
| |   Glucose | 70–90 mg/dL | 3.89–4.99 mmol/L | 18 |
| |   Protein | 0.3–4.1 g/dL | 3–41 g/L | 18 |
| |   Red blood cells | None | None | 18 |
| |   White blood cells | <300 cells per µL | Same | 18 |
| |   Cancer antigen 125 | <35 U/mL | <35 kU/L | 22 |
| Perspiration | Sweat chloride | 5–40 mEq/L | 5–40 mmol/L | 19 |
| Semen | Semen analysis | | | 22 |
| |   Appearance | Opalescent gray-white color | Same | 22 |
| |   Volume | 2–5 mL | 0.002–0.005 L | 22 |
| |   Liquefaction | 10–60 min | Same | 22 |
| |   pH | 7.2–7.8 | Same | 22 |
| |   Acid phosphatase | >200 U/ejaculate | Same | 22 |
| |   Citric acid | >52 µmol/ejaculate | Same | 22 |
| |   Fructose | >13 µmol/ejaculate | Same | 22 |

**Table G–1    Normal Values: Body Fluids** *(continued)*

| Body Fluid | Name of Test | Conventional Values | SI Units | Chapter Number |
|---|---|---|---|---|
| Semen *(continued)* | | | | |
| | Zinc | >2.4 µmol/ejaculate | Same | 22 |
| | Motility | >50% | >0.50 (number fraction) | 22 |
| | Concentration | $20-250 \times 10^6$/mL | $20-250 \times 10^9$/L | 22 |
| | Morphology | >50% normal sperm | >0.50 (number fraction) | 22 |
| | Viability | >50% live sperm | >0.50 (number fraction) | 22 |
| | Leukocytes | $<1 \times 10^6$/mL | $<1 \times 10^9$ | 22 |
| | Antisperm antibodies | Negative | Same | 22 |
| Synovial fluid | Synovial fluid analysis | | | 24 |
| | Appearance | Crystal clear, transparent, pale yellow | Same | 24 |
| | Viscosity | High | Same | 24 |
| | Volume | <3.5 mL | Same | 24 |
| | Red blood cells | Absent | Same | 24 |
| | White blood cells | $0-200$/mm$^3$ | $0-200 \times 10^6$/L | 24 |
| | Nucleated cell count | <200 cells/µL | $<200 \times 10^6$ cells/L | 24 |
| | Granulocytes | <25% of nucleated cells | <0.25 (number fraction) | 24 |
| | Protein | 3 g/dL | 30 g/L | 24 |
| | Uric acid | <8 mg/dL | 476 µmol/L | 24 |
| | Glucose | 70–110 mg/dL | 3.9–6.1 mmol/L | 24 |
| | Blood–synovial fluid glucose difference | <10 mg/dL | 0.56 mmol/L | 24 |
| | Fibrin clot | Negative; absent | Same | 24 |
| | Mucin clot | Positive; abundant | Same | 24 |
| | Mucin string test | Formation of a long string | Same | 24 |
| | Culture | No growth | Same | 24 |
| | Lyme disease antibody | Negative for *Borrelia bergdorferi* | Same | 7 |
| Vaginal secretions | Prostatic acid phosphatase | <2 U/L | Same | 21 |

# INDEX

Note: Page numbers in *italics* refer to illustrations; page numbers followed by t refer to tables.

# DIAGNOSTIC PROCEDURES